IAP Recent Advances in
PEDIATRICS

1

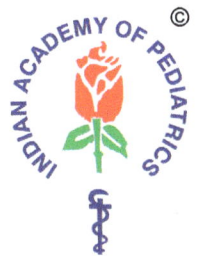

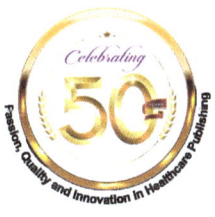

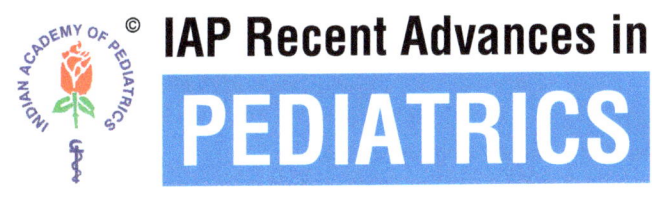 

IAP Recent Advances in PEDIATRICS — 1

Editor Emeritus
A Parthasarathy
MD (Ped) DCH DSc (Hon) FIAP
Senior Consultant Pediatrician, AP Child Care, Chennai
Former Distinguished Professor, Department of Pediatrics
The Tamil Nadu Dr MGR Medical University
Retired Senior Clinical Professor, Department of Pediatrics
Madras Medical College, Chennai
Deputy Superintendent
Institute of Child Health and Hospital for Children
Chennai, Tamil Nadu, India

Editor-in-Chief
PSN Menon
MD MNANS FIAP FIMSA
Consultant and Head
Department of Pediatrics
Jaber Al-Ahmed Armed Forces Hospital
Kuwait
Former Professor of Pediatrics
All India Institute of Medical Sciences
New Delhi, India

Executive Academic Editor
Alok Gupta
MD (Ped) FIAP
Pediatrician and Counselor
Pediatric Specialties Clinic, Jaipur
Formerly Assistant Professor in
Pediatric Medicine
Mahatma Gandhi Medical
College and Hospital
Jaipur, Rajasthan, India

Chief Academic Editors

MKC Nair
MD MMedSc PhD DSc MBA FIAP
Formerly Vice-Chancellor
Kerala University of Health Sciences, Thrissur
Founder Director
Child Development Center
Government Medical College
Thiruvananthapuram, Kerala, India

Piyush Gupta
MD FNNF FIAP FAMS
Professor
Department of Pediatrics
University College of
Medical Sciences and
Guru Teg Bahadur Hospital
New Delhi, India

Forewords
Digant D Shastri
Santosh T Soans
Bakul Parekh

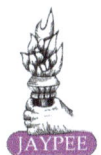

JAYPEE BROTHERS MEDICAL PUBLISHERS
The Health Sciences Publisher
New Delhi | London

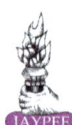 **Jaypee Brothers Medical Publishers (P) Ltd.**

Headquarters
Jaypee Brothers Medical Publishers (P) Ltd
4838/24, Ansari Road, Daryaganj
New Delhi 110 002, India
Phone: +91-11-43574357
Fax: +91-11-43574314
Email: jaypee@jaypeebrothers.com

Overseas Office
J.P. Medical Ltd
83 Victoria Street, London
SW1H 0HW (UK)
Phone: +44 20 3170 8910
Fax: +44 (0)20 3008 6180
Email: info@jpmedpub.com

Website: www.jaypeebrothers.com
Website: www.jaypeedigital.com

© 2020, Indian Academy of Pediatrics

The views and opinions expressed in this book are solely those of the original contributor(s)/author(s) and do not necessarily represent those of editor(s) of the book.

All rights reserved. No part of this publication may be reproduced, stored or transmitted in any form or by any means, electronic, mechanical, photocopying, recording or otherwise, without the prior permission in writing of the publishers.

All brand names and product names used in this book are trade names, service marks, trademarks or registered trademarks of their respective owners. The publisher is not associated with any product or vendor mentioned in this book.

Medical knowledge and practice change constantly. This book is designed to provide accurate, authoritative information about the subject matter in question. However, readers are advised to check the most current information available on procedures included and check information from the manufacturer of each product to be administered, to verify the recommended dose, formula, method and duration of administration, adverse effects and contraindications. It is the responsibility of the practitioner to take all appropriate safety precautions. Neither the publisher nor the author(s)/editor(s) assume any liability for any injury and/or damage to persons or property arising from or related to use of material in this book.

This book is sold on the understanding that the publisher is not engaged in providing professional medical services. If such advice or services are required, the services of a competent medical professional should be sought.

Every effort has been made where necessary to contact holders of copyright to obtain permission to reproduce copyright material. If any have been inadvertently overlooked, the publisher will be pleased to make the necessary arrangements at the first opportunity. The **CD/DVD-ROM** (if any) provided in the sealed envelope with this book is complimentary and free of cost. **Not meant for sale.**

Inquiries for bulk sales may be solicited at: jaypee@jaypeebrothers.com

IAP Recent Advances in Pediatrics

First Edition: 2020

ISBN: 978-93-89776-34-8

Dedicated to

The Academic-oriented Practitioners, Postgraduate Students in Pediatrics, its subspecialties and the Specialists in Neonatology, Pediatrics and Adolescent Medicine, who will be best benefited by selected topics in the subject to quench their thirst for recent advances in the field for their advanced learning and up-to-date knowledge and research. May they have the best of expertise to take care of the future generations in India and abroad.

Academic Editors

Dhanya Dharmapalan
MD PG Dip in PID (Oxford)
Consultant
Department of Pediatrics and
Pediatric Infectious Diseases
Apollo Hospitals
Navi Mumbai, Maharashtra, India

Jaydeep Choudhury
DNB (Ped) MNAMS FIAP
Professor
Department of Pediatrics
Institute of Child Health
Kolkata, West Bengal, India

P Ramachandran
MD (Pediatrics) DNB (Pediatrics)
Associate Dean (PG Studies) and
Professor of Pediatrics
Sri Ramachandra Medical College and
Research Institute (SRMC and RI), and
Sri Ramachandra Institute of Higher
Education and Research (SRIHER)
Chennai, Tamil Nadu, India

Remesh Kumar R
MD FIAP
Medical Superintendent and
Senior Consultant and Head
Department of Pediatrics
Apollo Adlux Hospital
Kochi, Kerala, India

Editorial Advisors

Digant D Shastri (President IAP 2019)

Bakul Parekh (President IAP 2020)

Piyush Gupta (President Elect 2020)

Remesh Kumar R (Hony Sec Gen IAP 2018-19)

Contributors

Anupam Sibal
MD FIMSA FIAP FRCP (Glasg) FRCP (Lon)
FRCPCH FAAP
Senior Consultant
Pediatric Gastroenterologist and
Hepatologist
Indraprastha Apollo Hospital
New Delhi, India
Group Medical Director
Apollo Hospitals Group
Clinical Professor
Faculty of Medicine and Health Sciences
Macquarie University
Sydney, Australia
anupamsibal@apollohospitals.com

Anupama Borker MD
Consultant and Head
Department of Medical Oncology
Goa Medical College
Bambolim, Goa, India
dranupamasb@gmail.com

Anuradha Sovani MPhil PhD
Professor and Head
Department of Psychology
Associate Dean Humanity
SNDT Women's University
Mumbai, Maharashtra, India
anuradhasovani@gmail.com

Ashish Pathak
DNB (Peds) FCPS Diploma in Global Health
(KI, Sweden) PhD (Sweden)
Professor
Department of Pediatrics
RD Gardi Medical College
Ujjain, Madhya Pradesh, India
drashish.jpathak@gmail.com

Ashok S Kapse MD
Professor and Head
Department of Pediatrics
Mahavir Superspecialty Hospital
Surat, Gujarat, India
ashok.kapse@gmail.com

Bakul Parekh MD DCH
Head
Bakul Parekh Children's Hospital (BPCH)
and Multispecialty Tertiary Care Centre
Mumbai, Maharashtra, India
bakulparekh55@gmail.com

Camilla Rodrigues MD
Consultant Microbiologist
PD Hinduja Hospital and Medical
Research Center
Mumbai, Maharashtra, India
dr_crodrigues@hindujahospital.com

Deepika Harit MD
Associate Professor
Department of Pediatrics
University College of
Medical Sciences and
Guru Teg Bahadur Hospital
New Delhi, India
deepikaharit@yahoo.com

Dhanya Dharmapalan
MD PG Dip in PID (Oxford)
Consultant
Department of Pediatrics and
Pediatric Infectious Diseases
Apollo Hospitals
Navi Mumbai, Maharashtra, India
drdhanyaroshan@gmail.com

Digant D Shastri
MD (Ped) PGDHHM FIAP
Senior Consultant Pediatrician and CEO
Killol Children Hospital
Surat, Gujarat, India
drdigantshastri@gmail.com

Ganesh Ramaswamy
DNB (Ped) MRCPCH MNAMS PhD
Senior Consultant (Pediatrics and
Metabolic Disorders)
Rainbow Children's Hospital
Chennai, Tamil Nadu, India
drganesh.r@rainbowhospitals.in

Ira Shah MD DCH FCPS DNB DPID (UK)
Professor and Head
Department of Pediatric Infectious
Diseases
Nodal Officer
Pediatric DR-TB Center and
Pediatric HIV/ART Center
BJ Wadia Hospital for Children
Mumbai, Maharashtra, India
irashah@pediatriconcall.com

Jaydeep Choudhury
DNB (Ped) MNAMS FIAP
Professor
Department of Pediatrics
Institute of Child Health
Kolkata, West Bengal, India
drjaydeep_choudhury@yahoo.co.in

K Siddhanth Shetty MD (Pediatrics)
Fellow Pediatric Intensive Care
Narayana Health City
Bengaluru, Karnataka, India
siddanth369@gmail.com

Krishna Mohan R
MBBS DNB Dip (Allergy & Asthma) MNAMS
Consultant Pediatrician
Government Taluk Hospital
Kozhikode, Kerala, India
meetkochu@yahoo.com

M Vijayakumar MD DCH DNB FIAP FRCP
Professor and Head
Department of Pediatrics
Government Medical College
Manjeri, Kerala, India
drmvijaycalicut@gmail.com

MR Lokeshwar MBBS MD DCH
Consulting Pediatrician and
Pediatric Hematologist/Oncologist
Lilavati Hospital and Research Centre,
Mumbai
Shushrusha Citizens Cooperative
Hospital Ltd
Mumbai, Maharashtra, India
mrlokeshwar@gmail.com

Malathi Sathiyasekaran
MD DCH MNAMS DM
Consultant Pediatric Gastroenterologist
Kanchi Kamakoti CHILDS Trust Hospital,
SMF
Rainbow Children's and
Apollo Children's Hospital
Chennai, Tamil Nadu, India
mal.bwcs@gmail.com

Moinak Sen Sarma MD DM
Assistant Professor
Department of Pediatric
Gastroenterology
Sanjay Gandhi Postgraduate Institute of
Medical Sciences
Lucknow, Uttar Pradesh, India
moinaksen@yahoo.com

Narendra Chaudhary
MD IAP Fellowship and FNB (Pediatric
Hematology Oncology)
Associate Professor
Department of Pediatrics
All India Institute of Medical Sciences
Bhopal, Madhya Pradesh, India
drnarendrapgi@rocketmail.com

Naveen Thacker MD
Director
Deep Children Hospital and
Research Centre
Gandhidham, Gujarat, India
drnaveenthacker@gmail.com

NC Gowrishankar MD DCH DNB FIAP
Pediatric Pulmonologist and
Bronchoscopist
Head
Pediatrics–Clinical
Operations and Quality
Mehta Multispecialty
Hospital India Pvt Ltd
Chennai, Tamil Nadu, India
cugowri@yahoo.com

Contributors

P Ramachandran
MD (Pediatrics) DNB (Pediatrics)
Associate Dean (PG Studies) and
Professor of Pediatrics
Sri Ramachandra Medical College and
Research Institute (SRMC and RI), and
Sri Ramachandra Institute of Higher
Education and Research (SRIHER)
Chennai, Tamil Nadu, India
ramachandran.paeds@gmail.com

PAM Kunju
MD DM (Neurology) WHO Fellowship Ped
Neuro (USA) FIAPN
Dean
Faculty of Medicine
University of Kerala
Professor and Head
Department of Pediatric Neurology
Government Medical College
Thiruvananthapuram, Kerala, India
drpamkunju@gmail.com

Pankaj Deshpande
MRCP (Ped) MD (Ped) FCPS (Child Health) DCH
Consultant Pediatric Nephrologist
Hinduja Hospital, Mumbai
Apollo Hospital, Belapur
Hinduja Surgical, Navi Mumbai
Maharashtra, India
drpankajdeshpande@gmail.com

Piyush Gupta MD FNNF FIAP FAMS
Professor
Department of Pediatrics
University College of
Medical Sciences and
Guru Teg Bahadur Hospital
New Delhi, India
prof.piyush.gupta@gmail.com

PSN Menon MD MNANS FIAP FIMSA
Consultant and Head
Department of Pediatrics
Jaber Al-Ahmed Armed Forces Hospital
Kuwait
Former Professor of Pediatrics
All India Institute of Medical Sciences
New Delhi, India
psnmenon@yahoo.com

Remesh Kumar R MD FIAP
Medical Superintendent and
Senior Consultant and Head
Department of Pediatrics
Apollo Adlux Hospital
Kochi, Kerala, India
drremesh2006@yahoo.com

Rhishikesh Thakre
DM (Neonatology) MD DNB DCH FCPS FIAP
Director
Neo Clinic and Hospital
Aurangabad, Maharashtra, India
rptdoc@gmail.com

Sanjay Khatri MD DNB FNB
Pediatric Cardiologist
Fortis Escorts Hospital
Jaipur, Rajasthan, India
drsanjaykhatri@yahoo.co.in

Santosh T Soans MD FIAP
Professor and Head, Chief
Neonatal and Pediatric Intensive Care
Division
AJ Institute of Medical Sciences and
Research Centre
Mangaluru, Karnataka, India
drsoans62@gmail.com

Senthil Ganesh Kamaraj
MS (Gen Surg) Mch (Paediatric Surgery) DNB
(Paediatric Surgery)
Consultant Pediatric Surgeon
Kanchi Kamakoti CHILDS Trust Hospital
Rainbow Children's Hospital
Apollo Children's Hospital
Chennai, Tamil Nadu, India
dr.senthilkamaraj@gmail.com

Sheikh Minhaj Ahmed
MD DNB MNAMS (Pediatric)
Fellowship Pediatric Critical Care
Pediatric Intensivist
Lilavati Hospital and Research Center
Mumbai, Maharashtra, India
minhaj1609@gmail.com

Shubha Phadke MD DM
Professor and Head
Department of Medical Genetics
Sanjay Gandhi Postgraduate Institute of
Medical Sciences
Lucknow, Uttar Pradesh, India
shubharaophadke@gmail.com

Smita Malhotra
DNB (Peds) MRCPCH (UK)
Consultant Pediatric Gastroenterology
and Hepatology
Indraprastha Apollo Hospitals
New Delhi, India
smitamalhotra172@gmail.com

Snehal Desai
DNB (Ped) IDPCC (Indian Diploma in Pediatric
Critical Care)
Fellowship in Neonatal Intensive Care
Amruta Hospital
Surat, Gujarat, India
snehalgdesai@gmail.com

Surender Kumar Yachha MD DM
Director
Pediatrics and Pediatric Superspecialty
Head
Department of Pediatric
Gastroenterology, Hepatology and Liver
Transplant
Sakra World Hospital
Bengaluru, Karnataka, India
skyachha@yahoo.co.in

Swati Kanakia MD DCH PhD
Pediatric Hematologist Oncologist
Lilavati Hospital and Research Centre and
Kanakia Healthcare
Mumbai, Maharashtra, India
drkanakia@gmail.com

Swati Bhave
MD DCH FCPS FIAP FAAP (HON)
Adjunct Professor (Adolescent Medicine)
Dr DY Patil Medical College, Pimpri and
Dr DY Patil Vidyapeeth, Pune
Senior Consultant (Adolescent Pediatrics)
Head and In-charge
Adolescent Wellness Clinic
Jehangir Hospital, Pune
Executive Director
Association of Adolescent and Child Care
in India (AACCI)
Mumbai, Maharashtra, India
sybhave@gmail.com

Tanu Singhal MD MSc (LSHTM, UK)
Consultant (Pediatrics and Infectious
Diseases)
Kokilaben Dhirubhai
Ambani Hospital and
Medical Research Institute
Mumbai, Maharashtra, India
tanusinghal@yahoo.com

Uday Bhaskar Post Graduate-DNB
(Paediatric Surgery)
Kanchi Kamakoti CHILDS Trust Hospital
Chennai, Tamil Nadu, India
kkcth@kkcth.org

Foreword

Indeed, it is proud privilege for me to write "Foreword" for *"IAP Recent Advances in Pediatrics".*

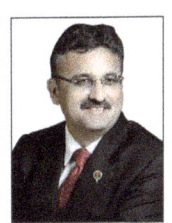

The medical science is ever expanding and in era of consumerism, Google learned patients and cut-throat competition, it is imperative for practitioners to get their knowledge updated regularly. The availability of literature is so vast that at times one gets confused which book to read and which guidelines to be put in practice. On one side, there is availability of too much material and on other side, the readers do not have enough time to read these available materials and it ends with failure. To address this problem, regular Annual Release of *IAP Recent Advances in Pediatrics* is the best possible solution. The idea was conceptualized when I visited Dr A Parthasarathy at his home in the month of June 2019 and on my humble request Professor A Parthasarathy agreed to take the lead and guide us. We feel blessed to have Dr PSN Menon, Dr MKC Nair, Dr Piyush Gupta, Dr Alok Gupta, Dr Remesh Kumar, Dr Jaydeep Choudhary, Dr P Ramachandran and Dr Dhanya Dharmapalan on board to give final shape to this concept.

For busy practitioners, reading this comprehensive book on recent updates will be big boon as they do not need to refer several books. For the postgraduate students, it will enhance their knowledge with recent developments which will ultimately help them to have better performance in the examination and also to appear as well updated doctor to the Google generation of parents.

This book has been brought out as a "Pediatric Digest" like Pediatric Clinics of North America and Best Clinical Practice Research Series, consisting of 568 pages incorporating 28 chapters. Each major subspecialty is covered in this book by at least one chapter on a selected topic. The write-up provides the most recent review on the topic with clinical practice points by a chosen Indian Pediatric Experts in the field. The first volume of the book is ready to be released during PEDICON-2020, Indore, Madhya Pradesh, India.

My heartiest congratulations to editorial team as well as contributors for coming out with this ready reckoner for the practitioners. I am sure that it will be popular amongst readers.

Digant D Shastri
President 2019
Indian Academy of Pediatrics

Foreword

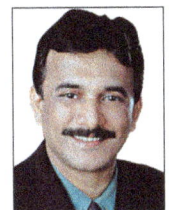

The first decade of the 21st century brought a number of discoveries, mistakes, and medical advances that have influenced medicine from the patient's bedside to medicine cabinet. Medical knowledge has been expanding exponentially. Whereas the doubling time was an estimated 50 years back in 1950, it accelerated to 7 years in 1980, 3.5 years in 2010, and a projected 73 days by 2020, medicine will advance more in the next 10 years than it did in the last 100 years according to a 2011 study in transactions of the American Clinical and Climatological Association.

In some cases, these advances changed deep-seated beliefs in medicine; in others, they opened up possibilities beyond what doctors thought was possible years ago. Medicine is built on progress. Looking back over the past few decades, we have come along in leaps and bounds. But what lies ahead for the future of medicine? Change does not happen overnight, but the future looks bright. The new technologies will also make the world truly globalized.....herald the age of *doctors without boundaries and patients without borders.* Focusing on exponential growth trends in medicine, I feel in future books we bring out there is a need to emphasize more on futuristic learning-like artificial intelligence deep learning, genomics, which is coming in a big way.

With membership touching 31,000, IAP has an unimaginably large talent pool of doctors which the organization should tap for furthering the cause of medicine through knowledge sharing. I am extremely proud and happy to learn this team is bringing out this book, *IAP Recent Advances in Pediatrics.* IAP is blessed to have academicians such as Drs PSN Menon, MKC Nair, Piyush Gupta, Alok Gupta, Remesh Kumar, Jaydeep Choudhary, P Ramachandran and Dhanya Dharmapalan, who have given their heart and soul to bring out this book. Compiling this book would have taken extraordinary effort and I congratulate the editorial board as well as the individual contributors for giving us a well-rounded work. I wish the reader a fruitful reading experience.

Santosh T Soans
President 2018
Indian Academy of Pediatrics

Foreword

Dear friends,

Season's Greetings!

It gives me great pleasure to write a foreword to a book which is edited by Professors A Parthasarathy, PSN Menon, MKC Nair, Piyush Gupta and Dr Alok Gupta.

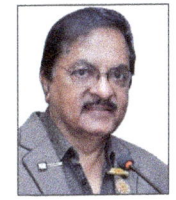

The world has seen a tremendous technology-driven change in the last couple of decades. Many things that were expensive and affordable only to the wealthiest people are now within reach of the common man. The Internet, Mobile Phones and Tablets have reduced the cost of communication nearly to zero. Ready access to knowledge is no longer the privilege of the few. Today, anybody has immediate ready access to the knowledge online which would have taken us hours to find a few decades back. Also, the knowledge from across the globe is accessible right from the first day to everyone, irrespective of the distance or amount of knowledge involved. Such is the impact of technology.

Technology is not without its own limitations though. One of the major ones being an explosion of knowledge which may be difficult to understand. In such a scenario, we must stick to the Gold standards of authors who keep on giving consistently great books year after year.

IAP Recent Advances in Pediatrics is another feather in the cap of IAP Publications. Chapters on Recent Advances in Pediatrics on selected topics by experts in the field covering all aspects of Neonatology, Pediatrics and Adolescence was much needed and the concept of having it every year with different topics and authors will be most welcomed by all practicing as well as research-oriented pediatricians and postgraduate students in India and abroad.

I can definitely say that there is absolutely no compromise made to the science or the simplicity with which any pediatrician can understand the book.

I am certain that this book will be a great asset to all the practicing pediatricians and would take this opportunity to congratulate them on the herculean task that the team have managed together so easily once again. I would like to offer my best wishes to them and urge the practicing pediatricians as well as postgraduate students to go through this digest completely from end to end so that you may derive maximum benefits from the hard work put in by the entire team.

Thank you once again Sirs, for giving me such an honor. May you and your efficient and passionate team continue enriching our lives with your wisdom.

Bakul Parekh
President 2020
Indian Academy of Pediatrics

Preface

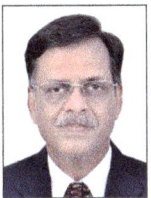

It gives us great pleasure to present to you, *IAP Recent Advances in Pediatrics*, a baby of the Indian Academy of Pediatrics (IAP). This treatise on pediatrics covering the perinatal age to adolescence, is designed to be a regular annual release during PEDICON every year from 2020. The idea conceptualized by our doyen of Pediatrics, Dr A Parthasarathy, solemnized by IAP President 2019, Dr Digant D Shastri and CIAP Team 2019, has taken form of Healthy Cuddly Newborn destined to grow into a perfect young adult. The process has been lovingly nurtured by all the esteemed authors and co-authors who have put in the best systems and organs in this creation.

This book has been brought out as a "Pediatric Digest" like Pediatric Clinics of North America and Best Clinical Practice Research Series, consisting of 568 pages incorporating 28 chapters. Each major subspecialty is covered in this book by at least one chapter on a selected topic. The write-up provides the most recent review on the topic with clinical practice points by chosen Indian Pediatric Experts in the field.

The first volume of the book is now in your hands, after being released during PEDICON-2020, Indore, Madhya Pradesh, India. The book is being published by M/s Jaypee Brothers Medical Publishers, New Delhi, India. I thank Shri Jitendar P Vij (Group Chairman), Mr Ankit Vij (Managing Director), Mr MS Mani (Group President), Ms Chetna Malhotra Vohra (Associate Director-Content Strategy), Ms Pooja Bhandari (Production Head), Ms Kritika Dua (Senior Development Editor) and team of M/s Jaypee Brothers Medical Publishers, for burning the midnight oil in bringing out this tome in a very timely manner. I request you to please give your feedback to enable us to plan future editions.

Alok Gupta MD
Executive Academic Editor
(On behalf of the Editorial Board, IAP-RAP)

Contents

1. Neonatology 1
- 1.1 Jaundice in the Newborn   *2*
  Rhishikesh Thakre
- 1.2 Respiratory Distress Syndrome in the Newborn   *16*
  Bakul Parekh, Snehal Desai

2. Nutrition 37
- 2.1 Current Status of Vitamin D Deficiency and Its Management   *38*
  Deepika Harit, Piyush Gupta

3. Immunity and Immunization 57
- 3.1 Ideal Vaccination Schedule 2020 for National Immunization Program and Indian Academy of Pediatrics   *58*
  Ashish Pathak, Naveen Thacker
- 3.2 Primary Immunodeficiency Disorders   *73*
  Jaydeep Choudhury

4. Infectious Diseases 89
- 4.1 Recent Advances in Diagnosis of Tuberculosis   *90*
  Tanu Singhal, Camilla Rodrigues
- 4.2 Diagnosis, Treatment and Management of Influenza (Indian Perspective)   *112*
  Digant D Shastri
- 4.3 Adenotonsillectomy: When it is Essential?   *125*
  Ashok S Kapse
- 4.4 HIV and AIDS: Diagnosis and Management   *143*
  Ira Shah
- 4.5 New Viral Infections   *155*
  Dhanya Dharmapalan

5. Neurology 169
- 5.1 Childhood Epilepsy Syndromes: Diagnosis and Management   *170*
  PAM Kunju
- 5.2 Acute Encephalopathy   *185*
  PAM Kunju

6. Cardiology 199

    6.1 **Managing Congestive Cardiac Failure in Children**   *200*
        Sanjay Khatri

7. Pulmonology 219

    7.1 **Diagnosis and Management of Bronchial Asthma**   *220*
        NC Gowrishankar

8. Allergy and Immunology 241

    8.1 **Recent Advances in Diagnostic Modalities of Pediatric-allergic Diseases**   *242*
        Remesh Kumar R, Krishna Mohan R

9. Gastroenterology 249

    9.1 **Inflammatory Bowel Disease**   *250*
        Surender Kumar Yachha, Moinak Sen Sarma

10. Hepatology 263

    10.1 **Spectrum of Hepatitis B in Children**   *264*
        Malathi Sathiyasekaran, Ganesh Ramaswamy

    10.2 **Pediatric Liver Transplantation**   *282*
        Smita Malhotra, Anupam Sibal

11. Nephrology 303

    11.1 **Urinary Tract Infections**   *304*
        Pankaj Deshpande

12. Urology 323

    12.1 **Vesicoureteric Reflux**   *324*
        Senthil Ganesh Kamaraj, Uday Bhaskar

13. Hematology 339

    13.1 **Thalassemia Syndromes**   *340*
        MR Lokeshwar, Swati Kanakia

    13.2 **Nutritional Iron Deficiency Anemia**   *371*
        MR Lokeshwar, Sheikh Minhaj Ahmed

14. Oncology 397

    14.1 **Acute Lymphoblastic Leukemia**   *398*
        Anupama Borker, Narendra Chaudhary

15. Endocrinology ... 415

15.1 Newborn Screening for Congenital Hypothyroidism *416*
M Vijayakumar, PSN Menon

16. Genetics ... 437

16.1 Down Syndrome: Rising Up *438*
Shubha R Phadke

17. Adolescent Medicine ... 457

17.1 Suicide in Adolescents: Causes and Prevention *458*
Swati Bhave, Anuradha Sovani

18. Intensive Care ... 479

18.1 Acute Respiratory Distress Syndrome *480*
Santosh T Soans, K Siddhanth Shetty

19. Emergencies and Poisoning ... 505

19.1 Rodenticide Poisoning *506*
P Ramachandran

Index ... 527

CHAPTER 1

NEONATOLOGY

1.1 Jaundice in the Newborn
Rhishikesh Thakre

1.2 Respiratory Distress Syndrome in the Newborn
Bakul Parekh, Snehal Desai

1.1 JAUNDICE IN THE NEWBORN

Rhishikesh Thakre

■ INTRODUCTION

Neonatal hyperbilirubinemia, "icterus neonatorum", is a "transitional" disorder which presents as jaundice characterized by yellowish discoloration of skin, sclera and mucous membrane. It manifests when bilirubin in circulation increases >5 mg/dL. The elevated unconjugated (indirect) bilirubin is most common, usually benign, but in few infants can lead to severe bilirubin-induced encephalopathy, kernicterus and impaired cognition. The rise in conjugated (direct) bilirubin is always pathological and warrants urgent evaluation and will not be detailed in the present chapter.

■ EPIDEMIOLOGY

Neonatal hyperbilirubinemia is a leading cause of hospitalization and ranked 7th globally among all causes of early neonatal deaths and ranked 9th among all causes of late neonatal deaths.[1] The burden is greatest in low-middle income countries. Up to 60% of term and 80% of preterm infants develop jaundice during the first week of life. In majority, the jaundice is benign but approximately 1 in 10 babies is likely to develop significant hyperbilirubinemia requiring treatment. The incidence of kernicterus ranges from about 0.2 to 2.7 cases per 100,000 live births. Disability-adjusted life year (DALY) represents 1 year of healthy life lost because of the condition at the population level. Globally, neonatal jaundice accounted for 113,401 DALYs [95% uncertainty interval (UI): 96,728–134,352] in 2016 and ranked 7th as a leading cause of DALYs in early neonatal period.[2]

■ RISK FACTORS

Knowledge of risk factors **(Table 1.1.1)** helps identify "at-risk" newborns and helps initiate appropriate measures for early detection and prompt management. Prematurity, hemolytic setting, perinatal infection and exclusive breastfeeding are leading risk factors predisposing to significant hyperbilirubinemia.[1]

■ BILIRUBIN METABOLISM

Nearly 75% of bilirubin is contributed by daily breakdown of red blood cells (RBCs) in reticuloendothelial system and 25% of bilirubin is contributed by nonheme sources and products of ineffective erythropoiesis. Alteration in one or more steps involved in bilirubin metabolism **(Flowchart 1.1.1)** leads to rise in bilirubin in blood circulation manifesting clinically as jaundice.

Neonatology

Table 1.1.1: Risk factors for hyperbilirubinemia.

Infant factors
- Prematurity
- Intrauterine growth restriction
- Inadequate breast milk intake
- Hypothermia
- Polycythemia
- Hypoglycemia
- Hypothyroidism
- Sepsis
- Bowel obstruction or ileus

Maternal factors
- Race or ethnicity
- Primigravida
- Exclusive breastfeeding
- Blood group incompatibility (e.g. ABO, Rh)
- Drugs (e.g. oxytocin, promethazine)
- Family history of jaundice
- Diabetes mellitus

Perinatal factors
- Assisted delivery
- Birth trauma (e.g. cephalhematoma, bruises)
- Asphyxia
- Delayed cord clamping
- Congenital infections (e.g. cytomegalovirus)

Genetic factors
- Glucose-6-phosphate dehydrogenase (G6PD) deficiency
- RBC defects (e.g. spherocytosis)
- β-thalassemia
- Galactosemia
- Gilbert syndrome
- Crigler-Najjar syndrome

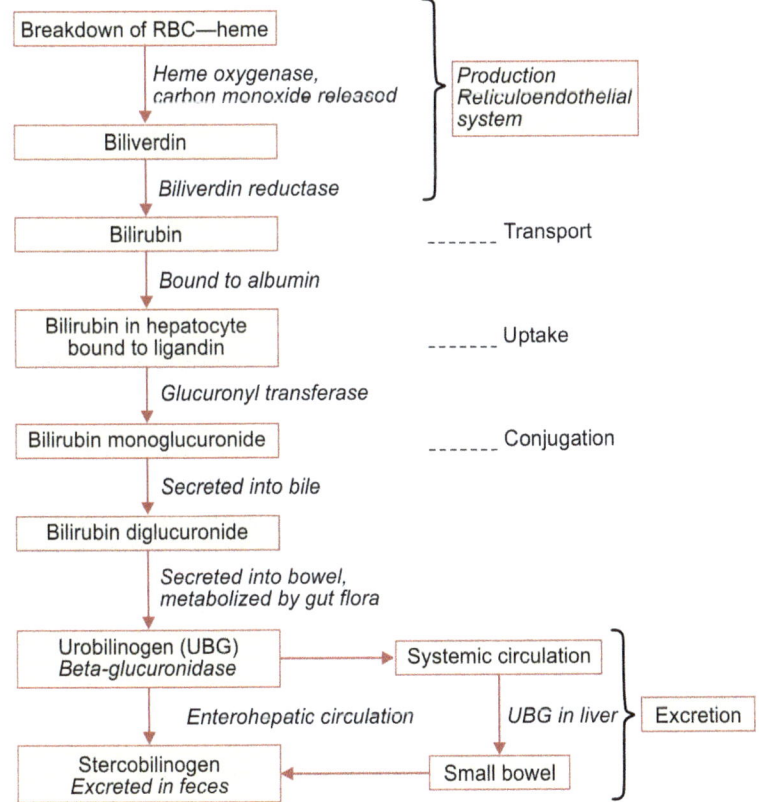

Flowchart 1.1.1: Bilirubin metabolism.

Bilirubin overproduction, reduced hepatic uptake or defective bilirubin conjugation leads to unconjugated (indirect) hyperbilirubinemia and bile canalicular transporter defects or impairment of bile flow through the intrahepatic and extrahepatic bile ducts results in conjugated (direct) hyperbilirubinemia.

The functional immaturity in bilirubin metabolism viz. increased fetal RBC breakdown, decreased liver uptake, immature conjugation, increased excretion and increased enterohepatic circulation predisposes to "physiologic hyperbilirubinemia" which is a self-limiting disorder requiring no treatment. It remains a "diagnosis of exclusion".

■ BILIRUBIN NEUROTOXICITY

Elevated indirect bilirubin has a potential to cause neurotoxicity which is a complex process not fully understood. Elucidation of structural-functional relationship between bilirubin and the brain, developmental and neurologic processes is needed. There is poor correlation between bilirubin values and neurotoxicity. Areas of the brain most susceptible to bilirubin damage are globus pallidus, hippocampus, lateral ventricular walls, cerebellum, and subthalamic nuclei of auditory and optic nerves. Studies show lipid peroxidation and protein oxidation at cellular level, impaired neuronal arborization, release of proinflammatory cytokines from microglia and astrocytes leading to loss of neurons, demyelination and gliosis.[3] The end result is characterized by tetrad of choreoathetoid cerebral palsy, high-frequency central hearing loss, vertical gaze palsy and dental enamel hypoplasia.

■ EARLY DETECTION OF JAUNDICE

Hyperbilirubinemia may develop both in the absence of risk factors and without clinically significant jaundice being present at the time of discharge. Hence one should *remain alert* for jaundice during first postnatal week **(Box 1.1.1)**.

Box 1.1.1: Predischarge assessment.

- Examine all the babies for jaundice at every opportunity especially in the first 72 hours
- Check whether there are risk factors associated with an increased likelihood of developing significant hyperbilirubinemia soon after birth
- Realize that visual inspection alone to estimate the bilirubin level in a baby with jaundice is error prone
- Measure and record the bilirubin level when in doubt
- Inform parents to report if the baby appears yellow or if there are any concerns
- Schedule a follow-up date based on "risk factors"

Table 1.1.2: Suggested follow-up schedule for all newborns.		
Scenario	Age at discharge	Follow-up
None of risk factors present	24–72 hours	48 hours after discharge
	>72 hours	Follow-up optional
Any risk factor present	24–48 hours	24 hours after discharge
	49–72 hours	48 hours after discharge
	73–120 hours	48 hours after discharge

All newborns should be assessed for one or more risk factors at time of discharge following birth. A suggested protocol is given in **Table 1.1.2**. The more the risk factors present, the greater is the risk of severe hyperbilirubinemia. The risk is extremely low if risk factors are absent.[4]

If facilities exist, all newborns at the time of discharge should undergo transcutaneous bilirubin (TcB) assessment. This serves as an objective screening tool. Babies with TcB >12 mg/dL should undergo serum total bilirubin estimation. The limitations of this approach include poor reliability in the first 24 hours, limited validity in preterm less than 34 weeks gestation and the high cost of the instrument.

If in doubt about the extent of jaundice or possibility of infant loss to follow-up, total serum bilirubin (TSB) should be done at discharge and hour-specific bilirubin nomogram used to predict "risk".

During the hospital stay and at every opportunity during first week of life, all newborns should be examined for jaundice (already detailed in **Box 1.1.1**). Jaundice is assessed by inspecting the baby's skin, sclera or mucous membranes preferably in natural light. The skin is blanched by digital pressure over bony parts to reveal underlying yellowing. The extent of jaundice can be estimated by Kramer's criteria. However, the clinical estimation is error prone, subjective, influenced by light, experience of the examiner and pigmentation of the infant.[5] Presence of bruising, cephalhematoma, lethargy, vomiting, excessive weight loss, pallor, plethora and hepatosplenomegaly points toward pathological jaundice. Abnormalities in tone, cry or sensorium must alert to the possibility of bilirubin neurotoxicity (**Fig. 1.1.1**). Certain features alert to the likelihood of pathological jaundice (**Box 1.1.2**).

Acute Bilirubin Encephalopathy

Acute bilirubin encephalopathy (ABE) describes the acute manifestations of neurologic dysfunction and can be reversible if corrected early enough. A bilirubin-induced neurologic dysfunction (BIND) score is used to assess the severity of jaundice (**Table 1.1.3**). A BIND score ≥4 is predictive of adverse outcome at 3–5 months of age with a specificity of 87.3% and sensitivity of 97.4%.[6]

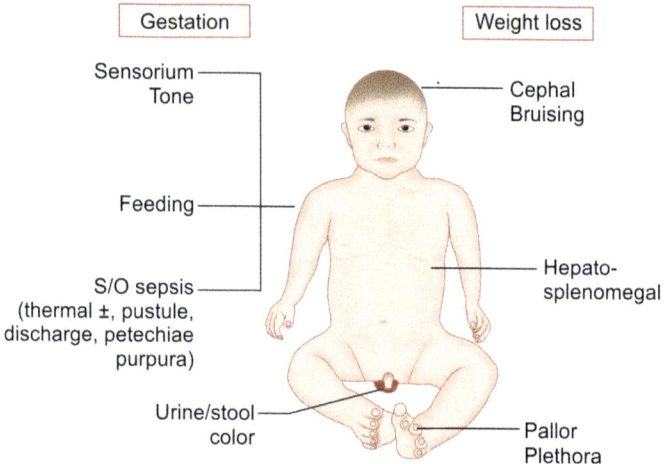

Fig. 1.1.1: Focused evaluation of newborn with jaundice.

> **Box 1.1.2:** Factors suggesting pathologic cause of jaundice.
>
> - Jaundice in the first 24 hours of life
> - Total serum bilirubin rising more than 5 mg/dL/24 hours
> - Direct reacting bilirubin >2 mg/dL
> - Pallor, hepatomegaly or splenomegaly
> - Failure of phototherapy to lower bilirubin

Table 1.1.3: Bilirubin-induced neurologic dysfunction (BIND) score.

Score	Mental status	Muscle tone	Cry
0	Normal	Normal	Normal
1	• Poor feeding • Sleepy-arousable	Mild hypotonia	High pitched
2	• Lethargy • Poor suck • Irritability	Moderate hypo- or hypertonia	Shrill
3	• Seizures • Apnea • Coma	• Retrocollis (**Fig. 1.1.2**) • Opisthotonus • Bicycling	• Inconsolable • Weak • Absent
BIND score	**Action**		**Outcome**
0–3	Intensive phototherapy		Good
4–6	Exchange transfusion		Fair, reversible
7–9	Exchange transfusion		Guarded, irreversible

■ INVESTIGATIONS

Not all jaundice infants need investigations (**Box 1.1.3**). In all neonates with jaundice that is severe, prolonged or nonphysiologic, investigations are done

Neonatology

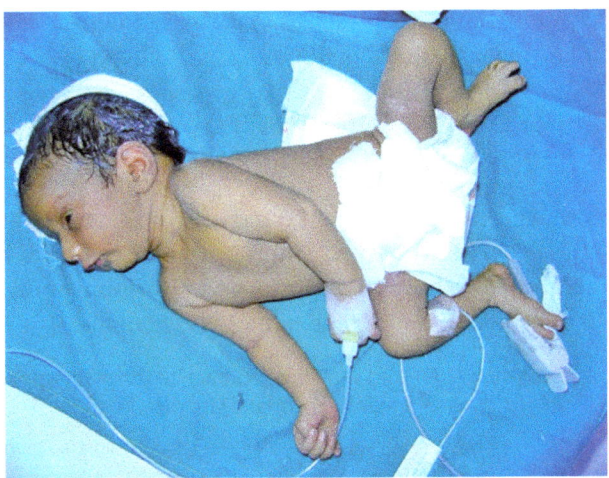

Fig. 1.1.2: Signs of bilirubin encephalopathy. Note the sun setting sign, retrocollis, and tightening of limbs in jaundiced newborn.

Box 1.1.3: Indications for measuring total serum bilirubin.

- Visible jaundice in the first 24 hours
- Jaundice in baby <38 weeks gestation
- Obstructive jaundice (dark urine or clay stools)
- Jaundice persisting beyond 3 weeks
- Jaundice requiring treatment
- Any baby, if there is clinical doubt about the extent of jaundice

---

Box 1.1.4: Investigations for significant hyperbilirubinemia.

- Total and direct bilirubin
- Mother and baby blood groups
- Hemoglobin or packed cell volume (PCV)
- Peripheral blood smear (for RBC shape, evidence of hemolysis)
- Reticulocyte count
- Direct Coombs' test (if mother is "O" or Rh negative)
- G6PD assay
- Urine examination and culture
- Evaluate for infection, as indicated
- Evaluate for cholestasis (if direct bilirubin is elevated)

---

to assess the severity of jaundice (for planning treatment) and etiology of the jaundice.

Box 1.1.4 summarizes the important investigations. The role of cord blood is limited for typing the baby blood group if mother's blood group is not known or is Rh negative or O Rh positive. The cord blood is collected for direct Coombs' test, TSB, reticulocyte count, peripheral smear and hemoglobin if there is setting of Rh incompatibility.[4] End-tidal carbon monoxide (ETCO) measurement in exhaled air may serve as indirect marker of ongoing hemolysis as equimolar concentrations of carbon monoxide and bilirubin are formed following breakdown of RBCs.

■ TREATMENT OF NONCONJUGATED HYPERBILIRUBINEMIA

The decision-making in jaundice management is based on gestation, weight, well-being and age in hours of baby. Supportive care is offered in addition to specific therapy. **Flowchart 1.1.2** provides an algorithm for diagnosis and management of neonatal jaundice including investigations.

Flowchart 1.1.2: Algorithm showing approach to the diagnosis and management of neonatal jaundice.

```
Jaundice ──▶ >2 weeks ──▶ Prolonged jaundice
                │
                ▼
           High colored urine ──▶ Conjugated hyperbilirubinemia
           Pale stools              (direct bilirubin
                                    >2 mg/dL or >20%
                                    of TSB).

Symptomatic
    │
    ▼
  • Sick, drowsy
    <34 weeks, <24-hour age
  • Pallor, hepatosplenomegaly ──▶ Hospitalize, investigate
  • Abnormal tone, cry or            and treat aggressively
    sensorium
  • Jaundice up to palms/soles

No ──▶ 

                                    Risk factors*
                                    • ABO or Rh setting
Well baby       Consider TSB or     • G6PD deficiency
at              transcutaneous      • Temperature instability
discharge  ──▶  bilirubin (TcB)     • Weight loss at discharge
+ risk          and interpret by      >3% per day or >7%
factors*        hour-specific       • Cumulative weight loss
                nomogram            • History of jaundice
                                      requiring treatment in
No                                    previous sibling/s
    ▼
            Re-evaluate after
              24 hours

Counsel
```

Investigations: for all	Rising bilirubin	Cholestasis	Prolonged jaundice
• Blood groups • Total serum bilirubin (TSB)	• PCV, peripheral blood smear • Reticulocyte count • Direct Coombs' test • G6PD assay • Sepsis evaluation (as indicated)	• Direct bilirubin • Urine examination and culture • Sepsis evaluation • Thyroid profile (T4, TSH) • USG liver • Expert referral	• Total and direct bilirubin • Evaluate for cholestasis/infection if indicated • Urine examination, reducing substances and culture

*Decision-making is based on TSB. Do not subtract direct bilirubin fraction.

(PCV: packed cell volume; G6PD: glucose-6-phosphate dehydrogenase; USG: ultrasonography; TSH: thyroid stimulating hormone)

Neonatology

Fluid Supplementation

Subclinical dehydration due to evaporative losses and poor intake of breast milk can lead to an increased incidence and severity of jaundice in newborns. Intravenous (IV) fluid administration has been reported to be a risk factor for development of nosocomial infection. There is no evidence that IV fluid supplementation affects important clinical outcomes such as bilirubin encephalopathy, kernicterus or cerebral palsy in healthy term newborn infants with unconjugated hyperbilirubinemia.[7]

Phototherapy

Phototherapy is an effective tool and must be considered as a key "drug" for jaundice management.[8] When bilirubin is exposed to blue light in the range of 420–480 nm, it undergoes change in structure to a product called lumirubin which can be excreted in urine without undergoing conjugation in the liver. The choice of device depends on the severity of jaundice. **Table 1.1.4** provides a comparison of various devices used in phototherapy and their advantages and disadvantages. The rule of thumb is to start phototherapy when TSB is 0.5% and 0.75% of the body weight in grams in sick and healthy infants respectively and to do an exchange transfusion when TSB is ≥1% of the body weight in grams.

Phototherapy is administered continuously and interrupted only for nursing and feeding purpose. The infant is placed naked with genitalia and eyes covered. Close attention is paid to the infant's temperature, daily

Table 1.1.4: Comparison of phototherapy (PT) devices.

Device	Advantages	Disadvantages
Blue-white PT	User friendly	• Variable dose • Blue hue • Intensity reduces with time • Risk of overheating
Fiberoptic PT	• No parental separation • No heat generated • No eye patches • Consistent intensity • Portable	Not recommended for terms due to size
Halogen PT	• Compact • Consistent intensity	• Generate heat • Area of focus and infant distance specifications • Fragile with heat
Light-emitting diode (LED) PT	• Long use up to 3,000 hours • Less heat • Consistent intensity	–

Table 1.1.5: Choosing phototherapy device.

Phototherapy	Conventional	Intensive
Wavelength (μW/cm²/nm)	Up to 10	>30
Devices	Blue white tubes, CFL, Halogen bulb, Fiberoptic, LED	Combination of PT LED
When?	Bili in PT range	• Rapidly rising bili • Bili in ET range

(LED: light-emitting diode; PT: phototherapy; CFL: compact fluorescent lamp; ET: exchange transfusion)

Table 1.1.6: Supportive care during phototherapy.

	Supportive care	
	Conventional PT	Intensive PT
Diaper	Use	Remove
IV fluids	Not routinely	Supplement
Duration	Intermittent	Continuous
Lactation support	Yes	Yes
Hydration check	Yes	Yes
Eye care	Yes	Yes
Thermal check	Yes	Yes
Adjuncts	No	White cloth, aluminum foil

(IV: intravenous; PT: phototherapy)

weight, intake and output. Breastfeeding is continued frequently. Hypoxia, hypothermia, hypoglycemia, acidosis and sepsis need to be prevented and if present and treated aggressively.

Table 1.1.5 details the choices of various phototherapy devices for conventional and intensive phototherapy. **Table 1.1.6** describes the differences in conventional and intensive phototherapy.

Compact Fluorescent Lamp

The response to phototherapy depends on cause, severity of hyperbilirubinemia and the light dose. A decrease in bilirubin levels of 6–20% of initial levels can be expected in the first 24 hours of standard phototherapy. Bilirubin levels decline most quickly in the first 4–6 hours of phototherapy. Intensive phototherapy can cause bilirubin drop by 30–40% within 24 hours and up to 10 mg/dL in first 6 hours when TSB levels are more than 30 mg/dL.

During phototherapy, depending on severity of hyperbilirubinemia, TSB should be monitored every 4–12 hours. Following discontinuation of phototherapy, a rebound increase in TSB levels of 1–2 mg/dL is most commonly seen in preterm, infants with hemolytic disease, or in infants treated with phototherapy in first 72 hours of age.

Neonatology

The treatment thresholds for phototherapy and exchange transfusion are in **Table 1.1.7**.[9]

Several factors affecting phototherapy are depicted in **Table 1.1.8**.

Table 1.1.7: Treatment thresholds for phototherapy and exchange transfusion of indirect hyperbilirubinemia.[9]

	Phototherapy		Exchange transfusion	
Age	Healthy newborns ≥35 weeks gestation	Newborns <35 weeks gestation	Healthy newborns ≥35 weeks gestation	Newborns <35 weeks gestation
Day 1	Any visible jaundice		15 mg/dL	10 mg/dL
Day 2	15 mg/dL	10 mg/dL	25 mg/dL	15 mg/dL
Day 3	18 mg/dL	15 mg/dL	25 mg/dL	20 mg/dL

Table 1.1.8: Evidence for issues in phototherapy (PT).[10]

Continuous or intermittent PT	No evidence to support the safe use of intermittent PT at moderate or high levels of serum bilirubin
Prophylactic PT for preterm/low birth weight (LBW)[11]	Helps to maintain a lower serum bilirubin concentration and may have an effect on the rate of exchange transfusion and the risk of neurodevelopmental impairment. Efficacy and safety on long-term outcomes including neurodevelopmental outcomes need to be determined
Light-emitting diode (LED) PT[12]	Efficacious in bringing down levels of serum total bilirubin at rates that are similar to PT with conventional [compact fluorescent lamp (CFL) or halogen] light sources
Reliability of transcutaneous devices with PT[13]	Moderate correlation between TcB and TSB during PT
Effect of positioning[14]	Unnecessary to alternate positions of the jaundiced neonates when conventional PT is delivered to lighten nurses' workload
Reflective materials around a PT[15]	Addition may be therapeutic for neonates with physiologic jaundice
Home- or hospital-based PT for term[16]	Inconclusive evidence
Blue light PT and melanocyte count[17]	No evidence
Fiberoptic PT[18]	Safe alternative to conventional PT in term infants with physiological jaundice
Chest shielding for preventing patent ductus arteriosus (PDA) under PT[19]	Very low-quality evidence

(TcB: transcutaneous bilirubin; TSB: total serum bilirubin)

Exchange Transfusion

Exchange transfusion is indicated for infants whose bilirubin levels cross the threshold indicated in **Table 1.1.6** or those who have clinical features of bilirubin encephalopathy. During exchange transfusion twice the infant's blood volume (160 mL/kg) is exchanged; this procedure can decrease the bilirubin level by approximately 50%. The procedure is invasive and carries a small risk of complications (1–5%)—fluid overload, infection, electrolyte imbalance, hypoglycemia, thrombocytopenia, thrombosis and death.

Intravenous Immunoglobulin

Routine use is not recommended. 500 mg/kg is used when serum bilirubin is rising despite intensive phototherapy or the value is within the exchange transfusion range in antibody-mediated hemolysis (Rh, ABO) settings.[20]

Phenobarbitone

Phenobarbitone by inducing the activity of uridine diphosphate-glucuronyl transferase enzyme can blunt the bilirubin rise seen in neonatal period. A meta-analysis of three studies has concluded that phenobarbitone reduces peak serum bilirubin, duration and need of phototherapy and need of exchange transfusion in preterm very low birth weight (VLBW) neonates. Although no major adverse events have been reported, reporting on neurodevelopmental outcome is lacking.[21]

Other Modalities

Several other interventions which have been studied for jaundice management are summarized in **Table 1.1.9**.

■ OUTCOME

Prognosis is excellent for uncomplicated newborn jaundice. Prognosis depends on gestation, age of onset, underlying cause, comorbid conditions and timing of intervention. Several other outcomes have been studied are summarized in **Table 1.1.10**.

■ SUMMARY

Jaundice is a sign and not a diagnosis. All newborns in first week of life and at every opportunity must be assessed for jaundice and risk factors. A structured follow-up and evaluation is mandatory to prevent significant jaundice. All efforts must be made to investigate the cause of jaundice. Phototherapy is the mainstay and should be used like a drug. All newborns with significant jaundice must have a long-term follow-up.

Table 1.1.9: Evidence for management of jaundice.

Use of bilirubin nomogram[22]	Transcutaneous bilirubin nomograms had the same predictive value as TSB nomograms. Result should be interpreted cautiously due to methodological limitation
Screening for bilirubin encephalopathy[23]	No robust evidence to suggest that screening is associated with favorable clinical outcomes
Preterm transcutaneous bilirubin reliability[24]	Reliable and could be used in clinical practice to reduce blood sampling
Prebiotics for prevention[25]	Not enough evidence
Prophylactic calcium during exchange transfusion (ET)[26]	Difficult to support or reject the continual use of prophylactic intravenous calcium
Clofibrate in combination with phototherapy6[27]	Insufficient data
Oral zinc for prevention[28]	Limited evidence with no effect on incidence or need of PT
Clofibrate[29]	Short-term benefits in term infants and infants without hemolytic diseases
Probiotics[30]	Routine use of probiotics to prevent or treat neonatal jaundice cannot be recommended
Yinzhihuang[31]	Yinzhihuang oral liquid combined with phototherapy seemed to be safe and superior to phototherapy alone for reducing serum bilirubin in neonatal jaundice
Meconium evacuation by per rectal laxative[32]	No significant clinical advantage for neonatal jaundice
Single- versus double-volume ET[33]	Insufficient evidence to recommend change from current use of double-volume ET
Metalloporphyrins[34]	Routine treatment cannot be recommended

(TSB: total serum bilirubin; PT: phototherapy)

Table 1.1.10: Evidence for association with hyperbilirubinemia.

Delayed cord clamping[35]	Increased risk of jaundice
Autism spectrum disorders (ASDs)[36]	Associated with ASD (OR, 1.43, 95% CI 1.22–1.67, random effect model). Not in preterm
Childhood allergic disorders[37]	Low quality evidence for significant increase in the odds of childhood allergic diseases after jaundice and/or PT
Urinary tract infection (UTI) with prolonged jaundice[38,39]	Overall prevalence of UTI was 11% in Iranian children. Screening is recommended. In the United Kingdom, the incidence was very low and hence urine screening is not recommended

REFERENCES

1. Olusanya BO, Kaplan M, Hansen TW. Neonatal hyperbilirubinaemia: a global perspective. Lancet Child Adolesc Health. 2018;2(8):610-20.

2. Olusanya BO, Teeple S, Kassebaum NJ. The contribution of neonatal jaundice to global child mortality: findings from the GBD 2016 study. Pediatrics. 2018;141(2). pii: e20171471.
3. Hansen TW. Core concepts: bilirubin metabolism. Neoreviews. 2010;11;e316-2.
4. Kumar P. Management of neonatal hyperbilirubinemia. In: Kumar P (Ed). Evidence-Based Clinical Practice Guidelines. New Delhi: National Neonatology Forum of India; 2011.
5. Perlman M. Clinical examination could not accurately predict neonatal jaundice. Evid Based Med. 2000;5:187.
6. El Houchi SZ, Iskander I, Gamaleldin R, et al. Prediction of 3- to 5-month outcomes from signs of acute bilirubin toxicity in newborn infants. J Pediatr. 2017;183:51-5.e1.
7. Lai NM, Ahmad Kamar A, Choo YM, et al. Fluid supplementation for neonatal unconjugated hyperbilirubinaemia. Cochrane Database Syst Rev. 2017;8:CD011891.
8. Lamola AA. A pharmacologic view of phototherapy. Clin Perinatol. 2016;43(2): 259-76.
9. World Health Organization (2017). WHO recommendations on newborn health: guidelines approved by the WHO Guidelines Review Committee. Geneva: World Health Organization; 2017. [online] Available from Https://Apps.Who.Int/Iris/Handle/10665/259269 [Last accessed December, 2019].
10. Jardine LA, Woodgate P. Neonatal jaundice: phototherapy. BMJ Clin Evid. 2015;2015. pii: 0319.
11. Okwundu CI, Okoromah CA, Shah PS. Prophylactic phototherapy for preventing jaundice in preterm or low birth weight infants. Evid Based Child Health. 2013;8(1):204-49.
12. Kumar P, Chawla D, Deorari A. Light-emitting diode phototherapy for unconjugated hyperbilirubinaemia in neonates. Cochrane Database Syst Rev. 2011;(12):CD007969.
13. Nagar G, Vandermeer B, Campbell S, et al. Reliability of transcutaneous bilirubin devices in preterm infants: a systematic review. Pediatrics. 2013;132(5):871-81.
14. Lee Wan Fei S, Abdullah KL. Effect of turning vs. supine position under phototherapy on neonates with hyperbilirubinemia: a systematic review. J Clin Nurs. 2015;24(5-6):672-82.
15. Lee Wan Fei S, Chew KS, Pawi S, et al. Systematic review of the effect of reflective materials around a phototherapy unit on bilirubin reduction among neonates with physiologic jaundice in developing countries. J Obstet Gynecol Neonatal Nurs. 2018;47(6):795-802.
16. Malwade US, Jardine LA. Home-versus hospital-based phototherapy for the treatment of non-haemolytic jaundice in infants at more than 37 weeks' gestation. Cochrane Database Syst Rev. 2014;(6):CD010212.
17. Lai YC, Yew YW. Neonatal blue light phototherapy and melanocytic nevus count in children: a systematic review and meta-analysis of observational studies. Pediatr Dermatol. 2016;33(1):62-8.
18. Mills JF, Tudehope D. Fibreoptic phototherapy for neonatal jaundice. Cochrane Database Syst Rev. 2001;(1):CD002060.
19. Bhola K, Foster JP, Osborn DA. Chest shielding for prevention of a haemodynamically significant patent ductus arteriosus in preterm infants receiving phototherapy. Cochrane Database Syst Rev. 2015;(11):CD009816.
20. Zwiers C, Scheffer-Rath ME, Lopriore E. Immunoglobulin for alloimmune hemolytic disease in neonates. Cochrane Database Syst Rev. 2018;3:CD003313.

21. Chawla D, Parmar V. Phenobarbitone for prevention and treatment of unconjugated hyperbilirubinemia in preterm neonates: a systematic review and meta-analysis. Indian Pediatr. 2010;47(5):401-7.
22. Yu ZB, Han SP, Chen C. Bilirubin nomograms for identification of neonatal hyperbilirubinemia in healthy term and late-preterm infants: a systematic review and meta-analysis. World J Pediatr. 2014;10(3):211-8.
23. Trikalinos TA, Chung M, Lau J, et al. Systematic review of screening for bilirubin encephalopathy in neonates. Pediatrics. 2009;124(4):1162-71.
24. Nagar G, Vandermeer B, Campbell S, et al. Effect of phototherapy on the reliability of transcutaneous bilirubin devices in term and near-term infants: a systematic review and meta-analysis. Neonatology. 2016;109(3):203-12.
25. Armanian AM, Jahanfar S, Feizi A, et al. Prebiotics for the prevention of hyperbilirubinaemia in neonates. Cochrane Database Syst Rev. 2019;8:CD012731.
26. Ogunlesi TA, Lesi FE, Oduwole O. Prophylactic intravenous calcium therapy for exchange blood transfusion in the newborn. Cochrane Database Syst Rev. 2017;2017(10):CD011048.
27. Xiong T, Chen D, Duan Z, et al. Clofibrate for unconjugated hyperbilirubinemia in neonates: a systematic review. Indian Pediatr. 2012;49(1):35-41.
28. Mishra S, Cheema A, Agarwal R. Oral zinc for the prevention of hyperbilirubinaemia in neonates. Cochrane Database Syst Rev. 2015;(7):CD008432.
29. Gholitabar M, McGuire H, Rennie J, et al. Clofibrate in combination with phototherapy for unconjugated neonatal hyperbilirubinaemia. Cochrane Database Syst Rev. 2012;12:CD009017.
30. Deshmukh J, Deshmukh M, Patole S. Probiotics for the management of neonatal hyperbilirubinemia: a systematic review of randomized controlled trials. J Matern Fetal Neonatal Med. 2019;32(1):154-63.
31. Wu RH, Feng S, Han M, et al. Yinzhihuang oral liquid combined with phototherapy for neonatal jaundice: a systematic review and meta-analysis of randomized clinical trials. BMC Complement Altern Med. 2018;18(1):228.
32. Srinivasjois R, Sharma A, Shah P, et al. Effect of induction of meconium evacuation using per rectal laxatives on neonatal hyperbilirubinemia in term infants: a systematic review of randomized controlled trials. Indian J Med Sci. 2011;65(7):278-85.
33. Thayyil S, Milligan DW. Single versus double volume exchange transfusion in jaundiced newborn infants. Cochrane Database Syst Rev. 2006;(4):CD004592.
34. Suresh GK, Martin CL, Soll RF. Metalloporphyrins for treatment of unconjugated hyperbilirubinemia in neonates. Cochrane Database Syst Rev. 2003;(2):CD004207.
35. McDonald SJ, Middleton P, Dowswell T, et al. Cochrane in context: effect of timing of umbilical cord clamping of term infants on maternal and neonatal outcomes. Evid Based Child Health. 2014;9(2):303-97.
36. Amin SB, Smith T, Wang H. Is neonatal jaundice associated with autism spectrum disorders: a systematic review. J Autism Dev Disord. 2011;41(11):1455-63.
37. Das RR, Naik SS. Neonatal hyperbilirubinemia and childhood allergic diseases: a systematic review. Pediatr Allergy Immunol. 2015;26(1):2-11.
38. Tola HH, Ranjbaran M, Omani-Samani R. Prevalence of UTI among Iranian infants with prolonged jaundice, and its main causes: a systematic review and meta-analysis study. J Pediatr Urol. 2018;14(2):108-15.
39. Steadman S, Ahmed I, McGarry K, et al. Is screening for urine infection in well infants with prolonged jaundice required? Local review and meta-analysis of existing data. Arch Dis Child. 2016;101(7):614-9.

1.2 RESPIRATORY DISTRESS SYNDROME IN THE NEWBORN

Bakul Parekh, Snehal Desai

■ INTRODUCTION

Prematurity is the leading cause of neonatal mortality worldwide. Respiratory distress syndrome (RDS) occurs almost exclusively in premature infants. The incidence and severity are inversely proportional to the gestational age. Modern neonatal pediatrics started in the 1970s with the introduction of assisted ventilation. Other advances that improved the survival of preterm infants included the use of antenatal corticosteroids widely used from the late-1970s onwards, and the exogenous surfactant, which became available from the early 1990s.

■ ANTENATAL CARE

A detailed discussion of antenatal management while delivering a preterm is beyond the scope of this discussion; however, a few salient points with reference to RDS are enumerated for awareness of the pediatrician.

It is ideal to transport the unborn preterm child in utero and deliver at a center where tertiary neonatal intensive care unit (NICU) facility is available. In a situation of preterm premature rupture of membranes (PPROM), antibiotics delay the preterm delivery and reduce neonatal morbidity. The use of co-amoxiclav should be avoided because it increases the risk of necrotizing enterocolitis (NEC).[1]

Magnesium Sulfate Therapy

The most common pathological lesion associated with cerebral palsy in preterm infants is periventricular white matter injury. It is observed that magnesium sulfate ($MgSO_4$) given to women with imminent preterm delivery reduces cerebral palsy at 2 years of age by about 30%.[2] Although the evidence is not new, there is no widespread use of $MgSO_4$ in preterm delivery as yet. The possible reasons include the lack of a statistically significant difference in primary outcome measures from the randomized controlled trials (RCTs); and the large number needed to treat for benefit as compared to the advantage of maternal administration of steroids. However, the use should be encouraged because the meta-analyses clearly show that magnesium reduces cerebral palsy and motor deficits.[3]

Second, unlike steroids that need to be administered up to 24 hours before preterm birth to have their optimal effect, magnesium has a much more rapid neuroprotective effect, making it more relevant. Finally, obstetricians are already familiar with giving a similar magnesium sulfate regime to women at risk of preeclampsia and know that major maternal adverse effects are uncommon. An intravenous 4 g loading dose over 20-30 minutes should be given followed by a 1 g/h maintenance regime to continue for 24 hours or until birth, whichever occurs sooner.[4]

Prenatal Corticosteroids

A single course of prenatal corticosteroids given to mothers with anticipated preterm delivery improves survival, reduces RDS, NEC and intraventricular hemorrhage and does not appear to be associated with any significant maternal or short-term fetal adverse effects.[5] Therefore prenatal corticosteroid therapy is recommended in all pregnancies with threatened preterm birth before 34 weeks of gestation where active care of the newborn is anticipated. Given the potential for long-term side-effects, steroids are not currently recommended for women in spontaneous preterm labor after 34 weeks.[6] The optimal treatment to delivery interval is more than 24 hours and less than 7 days after the start of steroid treatment; beyond 14 days, benefits are diminished. Beneficial effects of the first dose of antenatal steroid start within a few hours, so advanced dilatation should not be a reason to refrain from therapy.[7] WHO recommends that a single repeat course of steroids may be considered if preterm birth does not occur within 7 days after the initial course and there is a high risk of preterm birth in the next 7 days.[8] It is unlikely that repeat courses given after 32 weeks' gestation improve outcome.[9]

■ DELIVERY ROOM MANAGEMENT

Postnatal management of the preterm infant may be regarded simply as supportive care while the immature physiology and anatomy adapt to the postnatal environment independent of the placental circulation.

Umbilical Cord Clamping

Timing of *umbilical cord clamping* is an important first step. Clamping the cord immediately after delivery before initiation of respiration results in an acute transient reduction in left atrial filling leading to an abrupt drop in left ventricular output. Delayed "physiological" clamping after lung aeration results in much smoother transition and less bradycardia in animal models.[10] In premature infants, Cochrane review found that delayed (30-180 seconds) cord clamping versus early (within seconds) was associated with fewer infants requiring transfusions for anemia [relative risk (RR): 0.61], less intraventricular hemorrhage (RR: 0.59), lower risk for NEC compared with immediate clamping (RR: 0.62). For healthy women with term births, the National Institute for Health and Care Excellence (NICE) recommends that the cord is not clamped in the first 60 seconds, except where there are concerns about the baby's heart rate.[11]

In emergency situations where delayed cord clamping was not feasible, cord milking could be an alternative. There have been two RCTs suggesting that cord milking was equivalent to delayed clamping.[12] However, animal studies have shown that cord milking causes considerable hemodynamic disturbance leading to increased incidence of intraventricular hemorrhage raising concerns about the safety of this procedure.[13]

Continuous Positive Airway Pressure

Multiple animal studies and observational studies in humans have proved beyond doubt that positive pressure ventilation induces lung injury and triggers an inflammatory cascade immediately after delivery more so in a surfactant deficient lung.[14] Continuous positive airway pressure (CPAP) support is seen as a potentially "gentler" and less invasive modality to stabilize preterm neonates in the delivery room.[15] CPAP is to be used for infants born with a good heart rate but who are slow to establish a functional residual capacity (FRC) and effective spontaneous respiration. CPAP support with a pressure of at least 5–6 cm H_2O helps stabilize expanded or recruited alveoli and also works in synergy with endogenous surfactant by conserving the surfactant on the alveolar surface.[16]

Pragmatically, there is now increasing emphasis on minimizing ventilation-induced lung injury (VILI) and its consequence, chronic lung disease (CLD), starting in the delivery room.[15-17] Spontaneously breathing babies started on CPAP rather than intubation in the delivery room have a reduced risk of bronchopulmonary dysplasia (BPD).[18] The ideal level of CPAP is unknown, but most studies have used levels of at least 6 cm H_2O with some as high as 9 cm H_2O. Sustained inflation which is using pressures of 20–25 cm H_2O for 10 seconds at initiation of respiration to avoid intubation was considered, but subsequently abandoned because of excess death in infants.[19]

A T-piece resuscitator will be required to provide measurable CPAP in the delivery room from birth.[20] A self-inflating bag will not be able to give CPAP. In babies who are apneic or bradycardic, gentle, positive ventilation will need to be given which can also be delivered by a T-piece resuscitator.

Oxygen is a potentially toxic gas which can cause direct damage to respiratory epithelium. There is good evidence that 100% oxygen is harmful to most neonates and potentially more so in extremely preterm infants, in whom hyperoxia results in a 20% decrease in cerebral blood flow and a much worse alveolar-arterial oxygen gradient.[21]

During resuscitation, effort should be made to mimic normal transitional saturations, that is rising gradually from 60% to 90% over the first 10 minutes after birth. Therefore, blended air/oxygen should be available at the delivery room. For term babies requiring resuscitation, there is reduced mortality when using fraction of inspired oxygen (FiO_2) 0.21 rather than 1.0.[22] Observational studies have raised concerns about starting extremely preterm infants in air because of poorer recovery from bradycardia and increased mortality in the smallest babies.[23] Moreover, the combination of bradycardia (<100/min) and lower SpO_2 (<80%) in the first 5 minutes is associated with death or intracranial hemorrhage.[24]

Further trials are underway to resolve this issue. Presently, it is known that when titrating oxygen, most infants end up in about 30–40% oxygen by 10 minutes, so we believe it is reasonable to start preterm infants <28 weeks in about 30% oxygen until more evidence is available.[22] For those between 28 and 31 weeks' gestation, 21–30% oxygen is recommended.[25]

Practically, if self-filling resuscitation bag is used during resuscitation; ventilation can be initiated with room air. If oxygen is required, O_2 can be connected providing around 40% FiO_2 without and around 100% FiO_2 with the reservoir in place. However, PEEP cannot be given through this method. Majority of T-piece resuscitators use only oxygen to deliver the required CPAP and also positive pressure if required, thus delivering 100% FiO_2. A built-in air/oxygen blender in the T-piece resuscitator or an external blender in the delivery room is essential for optimum treatment but not very widely available as yet in India.

Preterm babies have immature skin, leading to rapid loss of heat from the body leading to early hypothermia. It is essential to immediately wrap the baby in a polythene bag under a radiant warmer and to increase the environmental temperature in the delivery room to around 26°C, especially for babies born below 28 weeks.

■ SURFACTANT

In 1959, surfactant deficiency was identified as the principle cause of RDS in preterm. The function of pulmonary surfactant is essentially to lower surface tension, thus preventing collapse of alveoli at the end of expiration. The surfactant is composed of a complex mixture of approximately 90% lipids and 10% proteins. The lipid is majorly a phospholipid, di-palmitoyl-phosphatidyl-choline (DPPC). The proteins are surface proteins (SP), composed of two hydrophobic proteins, SP-B and SP-C, and two hydrophilic proteins, SP-A and SP-D. SP-B and SP-C play significant roles in the adsorption and spread of DPPC to stabilize alveoli.

Surfactants used in clinical practice are either natural or synthetic. The natural surfactants are derived from bovine and porcine minced lungs or lung lavage extracts. The natural surfactants have limitations such as elevated cost and limited availability. They also contain animal proteins that may be potentially immunogenic and infectious. Therefore, to overcome these limitations, synthetic surfactants were developed which have evolved over the years. Animal-derived products have been proven superior to first-generation synthetic products demonstrating the significant role of surfactant proteins.

The first-generation synthetic surfactants were SP free, have been proven inferior to natural surfactants in terms of mortality, lower oxygen and ventilation requirements thus demonstrating the significant role of surfactant proteins.[26,27]

Currently, first-generation protein-free synthetic surfactants have been removed from most markets. Thereafter, second-generation surfactants were investigated, which are supplemented with peptides or proteins to mimic natural surfactant proteins. Lucinactant contains two phospholipids and a high concentration of sinapultide, a synthetic peptide designed to have similar activity to surfactant protein B. The available literature supports the fact that the newly approved second-generation synthetic surfactant lucinactant is equally effective as animal-derived surfactants.[28]

CHF5633, a third-generation synthetic surfactant containing SP-B and SP-C analog is also proven effective and safe in a multicenter cohort study for preterm infants.

Timing of Surfactant Administration

The initial clinical trials with surfactant were conducted in preterm intubated and ventilated for RDS. These studies demonstrated that early surfactant administration ($FiO_2 < 45\%$) was superior to late administration ($FiO_2 > 45\%$).[29,30] From this evolved the strategy of early intubation of very preterm infants in the delivery room and administration of prophylactic surfactant from 1990.

What is the Latest Consensus on Prophylactic Surfactant?

Over the years, there have been two major changes in the management of preterm babies. Antenatal corticosteroids have gained widespread acceptance thus reducing the severity of RDS and instead of intubation and ventilation, more and more babies are being managed on CPAP. Both these interventions have been associated with lower rates of BPD. Hence the dilemma is whether to intubate and prophylactically give surfactant or manage them on CPAP and administer surfactant to preterm failed on CPAP.

Several large clinical trials (COIN, SUPPORT, and VON-DRM) have addressed this question.[31-33] It was concluded that it was better to start with CPAP support in the delivery room if possible and intubate and administer surfactant only to infants with signs of RDS.

Studies have compared primary CPAP and surfactant to failed CPAP to prophylactic surfactant treatment with the "Intubate-Surfactant-Extubate (INSURE)" approach. During INSURE, infants are intubated, receive surfactant, and are supposed to be immediately extubated to minimize mechanical ventilation. These studies also did not find a benefit of prophylactic surfactant with INSURE over CPAP.[34] A possible explanation may be that even short periods of mechanical ventilation can damage the vulnerable lung. Many of the infants in whom INSURE was performed, were ventilated for a longer period thus causing more damage. Many, mainly extremely preterm infants, who were treated with INSURE failed to be extubated after surfactant administration, leading to a longer time on ventilation. Meta-analyses have demonstrated that prophylactic INSURE did not lead to a higher survival without BPD.[35,36]

Prophylactic surfactant has a role only in selected cases where antenatal steroids have not been possible and the preterm has needed intubation during resuscitation. If intubation is required as part of stabilization, then surfactant should be given immediately, as the main purpose of avoiding surfactant prophylaxis is to avoid intubation.

If not Prophylactic, at What Stage do we Administer Surfactant?

At present, severity of RDS can only be determined clinically using a combination of FiO_2 to maintain normal saturations, coupled with judgment of work of breathing and degree of aeration of the lungs on chest X-ray, all of which can be influenced by CPAP.

The 2013 Guideline suggested that surfactant should be administered when $FiO_2 > 0.30$ for very immature babies and > 0.40 for more mature infants based on thresholds used in the early clinical trials. Observational studies have confirmed that FiO_2 exceeding 0.30 in the first hours after birth in babies on CPAP is a reasonably good test for predicting subsequent CPAP failure.[37] Therefore, it is recommended that the threshold of $FiO_2 > 0.30$ is used for all babies with a clinical diagnosis of RDS, especially in the early phase of worsening disease.

Recent evidences still demonstrate that early rescue surfactant (<2 hours after birth) as compared to late rescue surfactant (>2 hours after birth) is associated with a reduction in BPD and/or death.[38] Therefore, the American Academy of Pediatrics (AAP) and the European guidelines on surfactant administration advise stabilization of preterm infants on CPAP and, if necessary, the administration of surfactant as early rescue therapy, preferably within 2–3 hours after birth if FiO_2 requirement is more than 30% at a pressure of at least 6 cm of H_2O.[39,40]

More than one dose of surfactant may be needed. Clinical trials comparing multiple doses to a single dose showed fewer air leaks, although these were conducted in an era when babies were maintained on mechanical ventilation. Today many infants are maintained on noninvasive ventilation even when surfactant is required. Need for redosing can be minimized by using the larger dose of 200 mg/kg of natural porcine lung surfactant (poractant alpha).[41]

A second and occasionally a third dose of surfactant should be given if there is ongoing evidence of RDS such as persistent high oxygen requirement and other problems have been excluded.

Newer Advances in the Pipeline

Lung ultrasound may be a useful adjunct to clinical decision making in experienced hands, with RDS lungs having a specific appearance that can be differentiated from other common neonatal respiratory disorders and it has potential to reduce X-ray exposure.[42,43]

Rapid bedside tests to accurately determine presence or absence of surfactant in gastric aspirate are currently being tested in clinical trials.[44]

Dose of Surfactant Administration

The only trial that has so far demonstrated differences between natural surfactant preparations compared two doses of poractant alpha (Curosurf), at either 100 or 200 mg/kg body weight, with beractant (Survanta) at 100 mg/kg body weight.[45] When the two surfactants were compared at 100 mg/kg body weight, the main outcome data showed no significant differences between the groups.

However, when poractant alpha was increased to 200 mg/kg body weight, it resulted in lower mortality rates at 36 weeks than beractant at 100 mg/kg body weight. At 100 mg/kg body weight, the three natural surfactant preparations mentioned earlier had comparable effects on gas exchange and survival without BPD.[45]

Table 1.2.1 provides the different preparations of surfactant and their source, dose, and formulations.

Method of Surfactant Administration

Surfactant administration requires an experienced practitioner with intubation skills and ability to provide mechanical ventilation if required. Most surfactant clinical trials to date have used tracheal intubation, bolus administration with distribution of surfactant using invasive positive pressure ventilation (IPPV), either manually or with a ventilator, followed by a period of weaning from mechanical ventilation as lung compliance improves.

Table 1.2.1: Different preparations of surfactant: Source, dose, and formulations.

Surfactant	Survanta	Curosurf	Neosurf
Source	Bovine lung extract	Porcine lung extract	Bovine lung lavage
Dose (Phospholipids)	4 mL/kg (100 mg/kg)	2.5 mL/kg (200 mg/kg)	5 mL/kg (135 mg/kg)
Formulations	4 mL and 8 mL	1.5 mL and 3 mL	3 mL and 5 mL

The disadvantages of mechanical ventilation in preterm, most importantly lung trauma and the importance of early CPAP are being widely recognized. Hence the administration of surfactant to preterm neonates during respiratory support on CPAP has been investigated.

The first was an interruption of CPAP for intubation for surfactant administration followed by a short interval of positive pressure ventilation administered through ventilator or resuscitator bag followed by rapid extubation. That is INSURE, intubation–surfactant–extubation. The INSURE technique allows surfactant to be given without ongoing MV and is endorsed as it reduces BPD.[30]

Another procedure is less invasive surfactant administration (LISA). In this method a thin small diameter catheter, such as feeding tube is placed in the trachea with the aid of Magill forceps under direct laryngoscopy. The surfactant is delivered intratracheally while the infant is spontaneously breathing supported by CPAP. This method does not require endotracheal intubation nor mechanical ventilation.[46] The LISA procedure reported a reduction in the need for mechanical ventilation and the rate of BPD compared with the classic procedure of intubation and mechanical ventilation.[47,48]

Since the distribution of surfactant is dependent on alveolar recruitment and the CPAP is continued during the surfactant administration, there is optimal distribution of surfactant and thus leads to an immediate increase in end-expiratory lung volume and oxygenation in preterm infants.[49,50]

Meta-analyses compared LISA and INSURE for the incidence of severe neonatal complications such as BPD and the rate was lower for neonates treated with the LISA method.[51] Another advantage of LISA is avoidance of large mechanical breaths, which are often required with intubation thus limiting lung trauma.

However, none of the included trials provided data regarding long-term neurodevelopmental outcomes. Recent cohort study using historical controls showed no difference in long-term outcomes at school age with LISA.

It is reasonable to recommend it as the optimal method of surfactant administration for spontaneously breathing babies who are stable on CPAP. Some units also employ strategies of prophylactic LISA for the smallest babies, although this has not yet been tested in RCTs. One of the advantages of LISA is that the temptation to continue MV following surfactant is removed.

Dargaville et al. from Australia described a novel method of administering surfactant to very preterm neonates between 25 and 28 weeks of gestation. They used small stiff vascular catheters, which did not need to be introduced with Magill forceps. They demonstrated that this stiff catheter technique, which they called minimally invasive surfactant therapy (MIST), was effective without increasing neonatal complications.[52]

Surfactant delivered by nebulization would be truly noninvasive. With development of vibrating membrane nebulizers, it is possible to atomize surfactant, although only one clinical trial has shown that nebulizing surfactant when on CPAP reduces need for MV compared to CPAP alone, and this finding was limited to a subgroup of more mature infants of 32–33 weeks.[53] Further trials of nebulization are ongoing.

Surfactant has also been administered by laryngeal mask airway, and one clinical trial shows that this reduces need for intubation and MV.[54] However, the size of currently available laryngeal masks limits the use of the method to relatively mature preterm infants, and routine use for smaller infants at greatest risk of BPD is not recommended.[55]

■ NONINVASIVE VENTILATION

Continuous Positive Airway Pressure

There is increasing awareness from animal studies and observational studies in human infants that positive pressure ventilation is capable of inducing lung injury and triggering an inflammatory cascade within minutes of birth, especially in a surfactant-deficient lung.[14] It is well-established that respiratory support should be noninvasive as far as possible. The best-known mode of noninvasive neonatal respiratory support is CPAP. CPAP is useful in infants with respiratory distress who are spontaneously breathing, and is widely used both in the early acute and late weaning/recovery phases of RDS. The continuous distending pressure of at least 5–6 cm of H_2O applied to the lung improves oxygenation by decreasing atelectasis, helping establish an FRC and eliminating fetal lung fluid, controlling pulmonary plethora in the presence of a patent ductus arteriosus (PDA) and improving ventilation–perfusion matching.[6,16,17] It may also reduce airway resistance by supporting the non-surfactant dependent upper airways.

CPAP is also useful in reducing apnea of prematurity which commonly coexists with RDS. This CPAP can be generated using mechanical ventilators, expiratory resistance valves, flow drivers, or underwater bubbling circuits.

Using an underwater seal to generate the pressure or "Bubble CPAP," generates small fluctuations around the set pressure which some believe offers additional advantage.[56] Using a flow driver to generate CPAP has the theoretical advantage of offloading expiratory work of breathing (the Coanda effect). There is no evidence that one is better than the other, but the simplicity of bubble CPAP systems allows their use in low-income settings.[57,58] The interface for delivering the continuous pressure through the nose could be nasal prongs, short pharyngeal tubes or nasal mask. Again evidence suggests all are equally effective for delivering the pressure.[59] Although for prolonged use, nasal masks are the best as they cause the least distortion of the face.[60] CPAP is now typically delivered via the nose; this can be via a nasal mask or short nasal prongs. Potential disadvantages of CPAP tend to be common to most methods of respiratory pressure support and include increased risk of pneumothorax and decreased pulmonary perfusion.

In the weaning/recovery phase of RDS, CPAP is invaluable after extubation from positive pressure ventilation by reducing the need for reintubation due to respiratory failure.[61]

Nasal Intermittent Positive Pressure Ventilation

Some infants need more support than CPAP. Nasal intermittent positive pressure ventilation (NIPPV) combines CPAP with intermittent pressure increases through the nasal prongs, generating peak pressures just slightly higher than baseline CPAP.[62]

In most of the studies comparing NIPPV with CPAP, no difference is found in tidal volumes; however, there is evidence that NIPPV reduces work of breathing.

NIPPV can be generated by ventilators and by the flow drivers used for CPAP. Synchronizing NIPPV with spontaneous breathing is possible but challenging because of air leaking around the prongs and from the mouth. Pneumatic abdominal capsules are most commonly used for synchronization but are only available with a few devices. Other potential synchronization methods include neurally adjusted ventilatory assist (NAVA) which is invasive and expensive and respiratory inductance plethysmography which is currently not readily available.

NIPPV improves extubation success and reduces the risk of BPD and it appears that synchronization improves its effectiveness. Nasal bilevel CPAP is a variant of NIPPV where two pressure levels alternate while the infant breathes independently; however, there is no clear benefit of bilevel CPAP compared with standard CPAP in preterm infants.

Nasal High-flow Therapy

Nasal high-flow therapy is a third noninvasive support mode to deliver heated, humidified gas via small binasal cannula designed not to occlude the nostrils at a rate of 2-8 L/min. Weaning of flow rate is done clinically when FiO_2 requirement reduces and the work of breathing decreases.[63]

The use of nasal high-flow therapy in neonatal respiratory care has spread rapidly, despite initial concerns that airway pressure is neither controlled nor measured. Nasal high flow (NHF) generates some distending pressure, which varies with leak, gas flow, and infant weight; it probably also improves nasopharyngeal gas washout.[64]

The perceived benefits of nasal high-flow therapy compared with CPAP, which include a simple interface, easy application, improved infant comfort and preference by parents and nurses, fuelled its early uptake in the NICUs despite limited evidence of safety or efficacy.[64]

However, the use of nasal high-flow therapy post-extubation in preterm infants has now been widely investigated; results of a recent Cochrane review of six RCTs showed that nasal high-flow therapy and CPAP were equally effective for post-extubation support in preterm infants and that infants randomly assigned to receive nasal high-flow therapy had less nasal trauma than infants who received CPAP.[65]

Heated humidified high-flow nasal cannula (HFNC) are increasingly used as an alternative to CPAP. Centers familiar with the use of HFNC argue that with experience it can be used for initial support even in some of the smallest babies.[66,67] In the HIPSTER trial, HFNC was compared with CPAP as a primary mode of support in the delivery room for infants >28 weeks, but the trial was stopped early because more infants started on HFNC needed rescue with CPAP.[68]

At present, CPAP remains the preferred initial method of noninvasive support. There are likely to be further refinements of noninvasive support over the next few years. Better synchronization of ventilator support with the baby's own breathing efforts can be achieved using NAVA, and large clinical trials of these newer modes of support are urgently needed.[69]

■ MECHANICAL VENTILATION

Despite our best efforts to maximize noninvasive support, many small infants will initially require mechanical ventilation (MV).

The aim of MV is to provide "acceptable" blood gases as our effort to reach normal values leads to higher pressures and higher volumes causing lung injury. Overinflation increases risk of air leaks such as pneumothorax and pulmonary interstitial emphysema and suboptimally low pressure leads to areas of atelectasis during expiration, which generates inflammation. Maintaining an "open lung" is achieved by optimizing PEEP, at which FiO_2 requirement is lowest with acceptable blood gases and hemodynamic stability.[70]

Volume-targeted Ventilation

Conventionally, the volume of gas delivered with each ventilator breath is clinician controlled by adjusting inspiratory pressure and time. The pressure is set to deliver an approximate tidal volume of 5 mL/kg. As the compliance of the lung improves with time or after surfactant administration, the same pressure will now deliver the much larger tidal volume. Much of the lung damage represented by BPD is thought to be mediated through excessive volume delivery—volutrauma. Similarly, if the lung pathology worsens the volume delivered will decrease leading to hypoventilation. Logically, it might be advantageous to allow the ventilator to deliver preset volumes rather than preset pressures. Volume-targeted ventilation (VTV) enables clinicians to ventilate with less variable tidal volumes and real-time weaning of pressure as lung compliance improves. VTV compared with time-cycled pressure ventilation results in less time on the ventilator, fewer air leaks and less BPD.[71]

This mode allows the ventilator to respond to rapid changes in lung compliance without clinician intervention. VTV mode enables automatic weaning of PIP in real-time as compliance improves facilitating faster weaning from mechanical ventilation.[72]

Pressure Support Mode

Pressure support mode is where the ventilator supports all the respiratory efforts of the infant and the rate of breathing is determined by the infant itself and the cycling (i.e. ending of inspiration and starting of expiration) is also determined by the patient itself. This is the purest form of patient-controlled ventilation, leading to best synchronization and patient comfort.[73] As there is no fixed setting of ventilator breaths, it is important to understand to use this mode only when there is no risk of apnea.

High Frequency Oscillatory Ventilation

High frequency oscillatory ventilation (HFOV) is an alternative strategy to conventional MV allowing gas exchange to be achieved using very small tidal volumes delivered at very fast rates with the lung held open at optimal inflation using a continuous distending pressure (CDP). Studies comparing HFOV to conventional MV show modest reductions in BPD favoring HFOV, although there is a paucity of trials where HFOV is compared with volume targeted ventilation.[74]

Neurally Adjusted Ventilator Assist

It is always beneficial to synchronize the ventilator-derived breath to the patient's effort to take a breath. This reduces work of breathing and fluctuations of pressures. Usually the flow or the negative pressure developed in the ventilator circuit acts as a trigger for the ventilator to deliver the breath. However, there is a lag period between the patient initiating a breath and the ventilator triggering the breath. Now, the act of taking a breath is controlled by the respiratory center of the brain, which decides the characteristics of each breath, timing, and size. The respiratory center sends a signal along the phrenic nerve, excites the diaphragm muscle cells, leading to muscle contraction. In this mode the electrical activity of the diaphragm is captured, fed to the ventilator, and used to assist the patients breathing in synchrony with and in proportion to the patient's own effort. As the work of the ventilator and of the lung is controlled by the same signal synchronization is achieved beautifully.[75]

Servo-controlled Oxygen Delivery

Modern ventilators now also have the option of servo-controlled oxygen delivery. This means the FiO_2 delivered by the ventilator keeps changing to achieve the set target saturation values. This increases time spent in the desired saturation range and reduces hyperoxia, but there are no trials to show this improves outcomes.[76]

Early extubation of even the smallest babies is encouraged provided it is judged clinically safe. Infant's size, absence of growth restriction, FiO_2 and blood gases are all determinants of extubation success. Extubation may be successful from 7 to 8 cm H_2O MAP on conventional modes and from 8 to 9 cm H_2O CDP on HFOV. Extubating to a relatively higher CPAP pressure of 7–9 cm H_2O or noninvasive positive pressure ventilation (NIPPV) will improve chance of success.[77]

Several other strategies have been used specifically to shorten duration of MV including permissive hypercarbia, caffeine therapy, postnatal steroid treatment, and avoiding overuse of sedation.

Permissive Hypercarbia

Targeting arterial CO_2 levels in the moderately hypercarbic range is an accepted strategy to reduce time on MV.[78] The PHELBI (Permissive Hypercapnia in Extremely Low Birthweight Infants) trial explored tolerating even higher $PaCO_2$ up to about 10 kPa (75 mm Hg) compared to 8 kPa (60 mm Hg) in preterm babies <29 weeks for the first 14 days. Follow-up of this cohort and others suggests no long-term adverse sequelae of permissive hypercarbia and it is therefore reasonable to allow moderate elevation of $PaCO_2$ during weaning provided the pH is acceptable.[79] This allows for more gentle ventilation at reduced pressures and volumes thus decreasing volutrauma and barotrauma.

■ OXYGEN TARGET AFTER STABILIZATION

The oxygen target after initial stabilization has undergone a sea change. Oxygen in the earlier times was considered the panacea in the management of respiratory distress but was soon realized as the culprit of an epidemic of retinopathy of prematurity and subsequent blindness. However, targeting lower levels of oxygen has increased death from hypoxia. Hence clinicians soon realized a middle way was needed and thus large multicentric trials were needed to determine the optimum range of oxygen target.

The Neonatal Oxygenation Prospective Meta-analysis (NeOProM) collaboration, was established in 2003 called NeOProM which coordinated a series of international RCTs to be included in a prospective meta-analysis.[80] These were the SUPPORT trial in the USA,[81,82] the BOOST-2 (Brain Oxygen Optimization in Severe Traumatic Brain Injury, Phase II) trials in the UK,[83] New Zealand[84] and Australia[85] and the Canadian COT trial.[86]

The results of a meta-analysis of the composite primary outcome of death or disability in all five trials revealed a higher risk in the low oxygen saturation target group (saturation target: 85-89%) than in the high oxygen saturation group (saturation target: 91-95%), an effect mainly attributable to the difference in mortality between groups.[87]

Hence the recommendation is to target saturations between 90% and 94% by setting alarm limits between 89% and 95% although it is acknowledged that ideal oxygen saturation targets are still unknown.[88,89]

At the ground level, while treating a patient, targeting any oxygen saturation range is difficult; compliance is low, alarm limits are often inappropriately set and it is human tendency to maintain oxygen saturations higher than the upper limit.[90]

Linking automated oxygen delivery systems with oxygen saturation monitoring might be an option. A paradigm shift could be to search alternatives to peripheral oxygen saturation measurement have been. One possibility is the use of near infrared spectroscopy (NIRS) to measure regional brain tissue oxygenation, for which some normal values for preterm infants have been established.[91]

NIRS has shown that not all desaturations detected peripherally correlate with cerebral hypoxia and common interventions such as handling and airway suctioning cause large fluctuations in cerebral oxygenation.[92]

■ SUPPORTIVE CARE

Always maintain body temperature at 36.5–37.5°C. Start parenteral nutrition immediately with amino acids and lipids in initial fluid volumes about 70-80 mL/kg/day for most babies and restrict sodium during the early transitional period. Enteral feeding with mothers' milk should also be started on day 1 if the baby is stable. Antibiotics should be used judiciously and stopped early when sepsis is ruled out. Blood pressure should be monitored regularly aiming to maintain normal tissue perfusion, if necessary, using inotropes. Hemoglobin should be maintained at acceptable levels. Protocols should be in place for monitoring pain and discomfort and consideration should be given for nonpharmacologic methods of minimizing procedural pain and judicious use of opiates for more invasive.[88]

■ REFERENCES

1. Kenyon S, Boulvain M, Neilson JP. Antibiotics for preterm rupture of membranes. Cochrane Database Syst Rev. 2013;(12):CD001058.
2. Magpie Trial Follow-Up Study Collaborative Group. The Magpie Trial: a randomised trial comparing magnesium sulphate with placebo for pre-eclampsia. Outcome for women at 2 years. Br J Obst Gynecol. 2007;114:300-9.

3. Conde-Agudelo A, Romero R. Antenatal magnesium sulfate for the prevention of cerebral palsy in preterm infants less than 34 weeks' gestation: a systematic review and meta-analysis. Am J Obstet Gynecol. 2009;200:595-609.
4. Australian Research Centre for Health of Women and Babies. Antenatal Magnesium Sulphate Prior to Preterm Birth for Neuroprotection of the Fetus, Infant and Child: National Clinical Practice Guidelines. Adelaide: ARCH; 2010.
5. Roberts D, Brown J, Medley N, et al. Antenatal corticosteroids for accelerating fetal lung maturation for women at risk of preterm birth. Cochrane Database Syst Rev. 2017;3:CD004454.
6. Kamath-Rayne BD, Rozance PJ, GoldenbergRL, et al. Antenatal corticosteroids beyond 34 weeks gestation: what do we do now? Am J Obstet Gynecol. 2016;215(4):423-30.
7. Norman M, Piedvache A, Borch K, et al. Effective Perinatal Intensive Care in Europe (EPICE) Research Group. Association of short antenatal corticosteroid administration-to-birth intervals with survival and morbidity among very preterm infants: results from the EPICE cohort. JAMA Pediatr. 2017;171(7): 678-86.
8. WHO recommendations on interventions to improve preterm birth outcomes. Geneva: WHO; 2015.
9. Asztalos, Murphy KE, Willan AR, et al. Multiple courses of antenatal corticosteroids for preterm birth study: outcomes in children at 5 years of age (MACS-5). JAMA Pediatr. 2013;167:1102-10.
10. Polglase GR, Dawson JA, Kluckow M, et al. Ventilation onset prior to umbilical cord clamping (physiological-based cord clamping) improves systemic and cerebral oxygenation in preterm lambs. PLoS One. 2015;10(2): e0117504.
11. Intrapartum care: care of healthy women and their babies during childbirth. NICE Clinical Guideline 190. Manchester: NICE; 2014.
12. Nagano N, Saito M, Sugiura T, et al. Benefits of umbilical cord milking versus delayed cord clamping on neonatal outcomes in preterm infants: A systematic review and meta-analysis. PLoS One. 2018;13(8):e0201528.
13. Katheria AC, Reister F, Hummler H, et al. Premature Infants Receiving Cord Milking or Delayed Cord Clamping: A Randomized Controlled Non-inferiority Trial (abstract LB 1). Am J Obstet Gynecol. 2019;220(Suppl):S682.
14. Ainsworth SB. Pathophysiology of neonatal respiratory distress syndrome. Treat Respir Med. 2005;4:423-37.
15. Halamek LP, Morley C. Continuous positive airway pressure during neonatal resuscitation. Clin Perinatol. 2006;33:83-98.
16. O'Donnell CP, Stenson BJ. Respiratory strategies for preterm infants at birth. Semin Fetal Neonatal Med. 2008;13:401-9.
17. Sweet D, Bevilacqua G, Carnielli V, et al. European consensus guidelines on management of neonatal respiratory distress syndrome. J Perinat Med. 2007;35:175-86.
18. Schmölzer GM, Kumar M, Pichler G, et al. Non-invasive versus invasive respiratory support in preterm infants at birth: systematic review and metaanalysis. BMJ. 2013;347:f5980.

19. Kirpalani H, Ratcliffe S, Keszler M, et al. The international "Sustained Aeration for Infant Lung" (SAIL) randomized trial. Presented at the Pediatric Academic Societies meeting, May 5-8, 2018, Toronto.
20. Szyld E, Aguilar A, Musante GA, et al. Delivery Room Ventilation Devices Trial Group. Comparison of devices for newborn ventilation in the delivery room. J Pediatr. 2014;165(2): 234-9.
21. Saugstad OD, Ramji S, Vento M. Resuscitation of depressed newborn infants in air or pure oxygen: a meta-analysis. Biol Neonate. 2005;87:27-34.
22. Welsford M, Nishiyama C, Shortt C, et al. International Liaison Committee on Resuscitation Neonatal Life Support Task Force. Room air for initiating term newborn resuscitation: a systematic review with meta-analysis. Pediatrics. 2019;143(1):e20181825.
23. Lamberska T, Luksova M, Smisek J, et al. Premature infants born at[{LT}]25 weeks of gestation may be compromised by currently recommended resuscitation techniques. Acta Paediatr. 2016;105(4):e142-50.
24. Oei JL, Finer NN, Saugstad OD, et al. Outcomes of oxygen saturation targeting during delivery room stabilisation of preterm infants. Arch Dis Child Fetal Neonatal Ed. 2018;103(5):F446-54.
25. Saugstad OD, Oei JL, Lakshminrusimha S, et al. Oxygen therapy of the newborn from molecular understanding to clinical practice. Pediatr Res. 2019;85(1): 20-9.
26. Engle WA, Committee on Fetus and Newborn. Surfactant-replacement therapy for respiratory distress in the preterm and term neonate. Pediatrics. 2008;121(2): 419-31.
27. Halliday HL. Surfactants: past, present, and future. J Perinatol. 2008;28(Suppl 1):S47-S56.
28. Garner SS, Cox TH. Lucinactant: New and Approved, But Is It an Improvement? J Pediatr Pharmacol Ther. 2012;17(3):206-10.
29. Bevilacqua G, Halliday H, Parmigiani S, et al. Randomized multicentre trial of treatment with porcine natural surfactant for moderately severe neonatal respiratory distress syndrome. The Collaborative European Multicentre Study Group. J Perinat Med. 1993;21:329-40.
30. Stevens TP, Harrington EW, Blennow M, et al. Early surfactant administration with brief ventilation vs. selective surfactant and continued mechanical ventilation for preterm infants with or at risk for respiratory distress syndrome. Cochrane Database Syst Rev. 2007;(4):CD003063.
31. SUPPORT Study Group of the Eunice Shriver NICHD Neonatal Research Network: Early CPAP versus surfactant in extremely preterm infants. N Engl J Med. 2010;362:1970-9.
32. Dunn MS, Kaempf J, de Klerk A, et al. Randomized trial comparing 3 approaches to the initial respiratory management of preterm neonates. Pediatrics. 2011;128:e1069-76.
33. Morley CJ, Davis PG, Doyle LW, et al. Nasal CPAP or intubation at birth for very preterm infants. N Engl J Med. 2008;358:700-8.
34. Finer NN, Carlo WA, Walsh MC, et al. SUPPORT Study Group of the Eunice Kennedy Shriver NICHD Neonatal Research Network. Early CPAP versus surfactant in extremely preterm infants. N Engl J Med. 2010;362(21):1970-9.

35. Rojas-Reyes MX, Morley CJ, Soll R. Prophylactic versus selective use of surfactant in preventing morbidity and mortality in preterm infants. Cochrane Database Syst Rev. 2012;(3):CD000510.
36. Isayama T, Chai-Adisaksopha C, McDonald SD. Noninvasive ventilation with vs without early surfactant to prevent chronic lung disease in preterm infants: a systematic review and meta-analysis. JAMA Pediatr. 2015;169:731-9.
37. Dargaville PA, Aiyappan A, De Paoli AG, et al. Continuous positive airway pressure failure in preterm infants: incidence, predictors, and consequences. Neonatology. 2013;104(1):8-14.
38. Bahadue FL, Soll R. Early versus delayed selective surfactant treatment for neonatal respiratory distress syndrome. Cochrane Database Syst Rev. 2012;11:CD001456.
39. Polin RA, Carlo WA. Surfactant replacement therapy for preterm and term neonates with respiratory distress. Pediatrics. 2014;133:156-63.
40. Sweet DG, Carnielli V, Greisen G, et al. European consensus guidelines on the management of respiratory distress syndrome: 2016 update. Neonatology. 2017;111:107-25.
41. Singh N, Halliday HL, Stevens TP, et al. Comparison of animal-derived surfactants for the prevention and treatment of respiratory distress syndrome in preterm infants. Cochrane Database Syst Rev. 2015;(12):CD010249.
42. De Martino L, Yousef N, Ben-Ammar R, et al. Lung ultrasound score predicts surfactant need in extremely preterm neonates. Pediatrics. 2018;142(3): e20180463.
43. Escourrou G, De Luca D. Lung ultrasound decreased radiation exposure in preterm infants in a neonatal intensive care unit. Acta Paediatr. 2016;105(5): e237-9.
44. Verder H, Heiring C, Clark H, Sweet D, et al. Rapid test for lung maturity, based on spectroscopy of gastric aspirate, predicted respiratory distress syndrome with high sensitivity Acta Paediatr. 2017;106(3):430-7.
45. Ramanathan R, Rasmussen MR, Gerstmann DR, et al. A randomized, multicentre masked comparison trial of poractant alfa (Curosurf) versus beractant (Survanta) in the treatment of respiratory distress syndrome in preterm infants. Am J Perinatol. 2004;21:109-19.
46. Herting E. Less invasive surfactant administration (LISA)–ways to deliver surfactant in spontaneously breathing infants. Early Hum Dev. 2013;89:875-8.
47. Kribs A, Hartel C, Kattner E, et al. Surfactant without intubation in preterm infants with respiratory distress: first multi-center data. Klin Padiatr. 2010;222(1):13-7.
48. Gopel W, Kribs A, Ziegler A, et al. Avoidance of mechanical ventilation by surfactant treatment of spontaneously breathing preterm infants (AMV): an open label, randomised, controlled trial. Lancet. 2011;378:1627-34.
49. Van der Burg PS, de Jongh FH, Miedema M, et al. Effect of minimally invasive surfactant therapy on lung volume and ventilation in preterm infants. J Pediatr. 2016;170:67-72.
50. Bohlin K, Bouhafs RK, Jarstrand C, et al. Spontaneous breathing or mechanical ventilation alters lung compliance and tissue association of exogenous surfactant in preterm newborn rabbits. Pediatr Res. 2005;57:624-30.
51. Aldana-Aguirre JC, Pinto M, Featherstone RM, et al. Less invasive surfactant administration versus intubation for surfactant delivery in preterm infants with

respiratory distress syndrome: a systematic review and meta-analysis. Arch Dis Child Fetal Neonatal Ed. 2017;102:F17-23.
52. Dargaville PA, Aiyappan A, De Paoli AG, et al. Minimally-invasive surfactant therapy in preterm infants on continuous positive airway pressure. Arch Dis Child Fetal Neonatal Ed. 2013;98:F122-6.
53. Minocchieri S, Berry CA, Pillow JJ et al. Nebulised surfactant to reduce severity of respiratory distress: a blinded, parallel, randomised controlled trial. Arch Dis Child Fetal Neonatal Ed. 2018:31;50-1.
54. Roberts KD, Brown R, Lampland AL, et al. Laryngeal mask airway for surfactant administration in neonates: a randomized, controlled trial. J Pediatr. 2018;193: 40-6.
55. Bansal SC, Caoci S, Dempsey E, et al. The laryngeal mask airway and its use in neonatal resuscitation: a critical review of where we are in 2017/2018. Neonatology. 2018;113(2):152-61.
56. Welty SE. Continuous positive airway pressure strategies with bubble nasal continuous positive airway pressure: not all bubbling is the same: the Seattle Positive Airway Pressure System. Clin Perinatol. 2016;43(4):661-71.
57. De Paoli AG, Davis PG, Faber B, et al. Devices and pressure sources for administration of nasal continuous positive airway pressure (NCPAP) in preterm neonates. Cochrane Database Syst Rev. 2008;1:CD002977.
58. Mazmanyan P, Mellor K, Doré CJ, et al. A randomised controlled trial of flow driver and bubble continuous positive airway pressure in preterm infants in a resourcelimited setting. Arch Dis Child Fetal Neonatal Ed. 2016;101(1):F16-20.
59. McCarthy LK, Twomey AR, Molloy EJ, et al. A randomized trial of nasal prong or face mask for respiratory support for preterm newborns. Pediatrics. 2013;132(2):e389-95.
60. Say B, Kanmaz Kutman HG, Oguz SS, et al. Binasal prong versus nasal mask for applying CPAP to preterm infants: a randomized controlled trial. Neonatology. 2016;109(4):258-64.
61. Davis PG, Henderson-Smart DJ. Nasal continuous positive airway pressure immediately after extubation for preventing morbidity in preterm infants. Cochrane Database Syst Rev. 2003;(2):CD000143.
62. Roberts CT, Davis PG, Owen LS. Neonatal non-invasive respiratory support: synchronised NIPPV, non-synchronised NIPPV or bi-level CPAP: what is the evidence in 2013? Neonatology. 2013;104:203-9.
63. Roehr CC, Yoder BA, Davis PG, et al. Evidence support and guidelines for using heated, humidified, high flow nasal cannulae in neonatology. Oxford Nasal High Flow Therapy Meeting, 2015. Clin Perinatol. 2016;43(4):693-705.
64. Manley BJ, Owen LS. High-flow nasal cannula: mechanisms, evidence and recommendations. Semin Fetal Neonatal Med. 2016;21:139-45.
65. Wilkinson D, Andersen C, O'Donnell CP, et al. High flow nasal cannula for respiratory support in preterm infants. Cochrane Database Syst Rev. 2016;2:CD006405.
66. Zivanovic S, Scrivens A, Panza R, et al. Nasal high-flow therapy as primary respiratory support for preterm infants without the need for rescue with nasal continuous positive airway pressure. Neonatology. 2019;115(2):175-81.
67. Reynolds P, Leontiadi S, Lawson T, et al. Stabilisation of premature infants in the delivery room with nasal high flow. Arch Dis Child Fetal Neonatal Ed. 2016;101(4):F284-7.

68. Roberts CT, Owen LS, Manley BJ, et al. Nasal high-flow therapy for primary respiratory support in preterm infants. N Engl J Med. 2016;375(12):1142-51.
69. Firestone KS, Beck J, Stein H. Neurally adjusted ventilatory assist for non-invasive support in neonates. Clin Perinatol. 2016;43(4):707-24.
70. Rimensberger PC, Cox PN, Frndova H, et al. The open lung during small tidal volume ventilation: concepts of recruitment and "optimal" positive end-expiratory pressure. Crit Care Med. 1999;27(9):1946-52.
71. Klingenberg C, Wheeler KI, McCallion N, et al. Volume-targeted versus pressure-limited ventilation in neonates. Cochrane Database Syst Rev. 2017;10:CD003666.
72. Keszler M, Abubakar KM. Volume guarantee ventilation. Clin Perinatol. 2007;34:107-16.
73. Unal S, Ergenekon E, Aktas S, et al. Effects of volume guaranteed ventilation combined with two different modes in preterm infants. Respir Care. 2017;62(12):1525-32.
74. Cools F, Offringa M, Askie LM. Elective high frequency oscillatory ventilation versus conventional ventilation for acute pulmonary dysfunction in preterm infants. Cochrane Database Syst Rev. 2015;3(3):CD000104.
75. Rossor TE, Hunt KA, Shetty S, et al. Neurally adjusted ventilatory assist compared to other forms of triggered ventilation for neonatal respiratory support. Cochrane Database Syst Rev. 2017;10:CD012251.
76. Mitra S, Singh B, El-Naggar W, et al. Automated versus manual control of inspired oxygen to target oxygen saturation in preterm infants: a systematic review and meta-analysis. J Perinatol. 2018;38(4):351-60.
77. Sever Buzzella B, Claure N, D'Ugard C, et al. A randomized controlled trial of two nasal continuous positive airway pressure levels after extubation in preterm infants. J Pediatr. 2014;164(1):46-51.
78. Woodgate PG, Davies MW. Permissive hypercapnia for the prevention of morbidity and mortality in mechanically ventilated newborn infants. Cochrane Database Syst Rev. 2001;2(2):CD002061.
79. Thome UH, Genzel-Boroviczeny O, Bohnhorst B, et al. Neurodevelopmental outcomes of extremely low birthweight infants randomised to different PCO_2 targets: the PHELBI follow-up study. Arch Dis Child Fetal Neonatal Ed. 2017;102(5):F376-82.
80. Askie LM, Brocklehurst P, Darlow BA, et al. NeOProM: Neonatal Oxygenation Prospective Meta-analysis Collaboration study protocol. BMC Pediatr. 2011;11:6.
81. Carlo WA, Finer NN, Walsh MC, et al. Target ranges of oxygen saturation in extremely preterm infants. N Engl J Med. 2010;362:1959-69.
82. Vaucher YE, Peralta-Carcelen M, Finer NN, et al. Neurodevelopmental outcomes in the early CPAP and pulse oximetry trial. N Engl J Med. 2012;367:2495-504.
83. Darlow BA, Marschner SL, Donoghoe M, et al. Randomized controlled trial of oxygen saturation targets in very preterm infants: two year outcomes. J Pediatr. 2014;165:30-5.
84. Stenson BJ, Tarnow-Mordi WO, Darlow BA, et al. Oxygen saturation and outcomes in preterm infants. N Engl J Med. 2013;368:2094-104.
85. Tarnow-Mordi W, Stenson B, Kirby A, et al. Outcomes of two trials of oxygen-saturation targets in preterm infants. N Engl J Med. 2016;374:749-60.

86. Schmidt B, Whyte RK, Asztalos EV, et al. Effects of targeting higher vs lower arterial oxygen saturations on death or disability in extremely preterm infants: a randomized clinical trial. JAMA. 2013;309:2111-20.
87. Stenson BJ. Oxygen saturation targets for extremely preterm infants after the NeOProM trials. Neonatology. 2016;109:352-8.
88. Sweet DG, Carnielli V, Greisen G, et al. European Consensus Guidelines on the Management of Respiratory Distress Syndrome: 2019 Update. Neonatology. 2019;115:432-51.
89. Saugstad OD. Oxygenation of the immature infant: a commentary and recommendations for oxygen saturation targets and alarm limits. Neonatology. 2018;114(1):69-75.
90. Zanten HA, Tan RN, van den Hoogen A, et al. Compliance in oxygen saturation targeting in preterm infants: a systematic review. Eur J Pediatr. 2015;174:1561-72.
91. Sood BG, McLaughlin K, Cortez J. Near-infrared spectroscopy: applications in neonates. Semin Fetal Neonatal Med. 2015;20:164-72.
92. Watkin SL, Spencer SA, Dimmock PW, et al. A comparison of pulse oximetry and near infrared spectroscopy (NIRS) in the detection of hypoxaemia occurring with pauses in nasal airflow in neonates. J Clin Monit Comput. 1999;15:441-7.

CHAPTER 2

NUTRITION

2.1 Current Status of Vitamin D Deficiency and Its Management
Deepika Harit, Piyush Gupta

2.1 CURRENT STATUS OF VITAMIN D DEFICIENCY AND ITS MANAGEMENT

Deepika Harit, Piyush Gupta

■ INTRODUCTION

Vitamin D is a prohormone which is essential for normal bone development in humans. Over the past two decades, substantial research has been published to ascertain its role in health and disease. Vitamin D serves a crucial role in maintaining the normal calcium metabolism and its deficiency causes altered chondrocyte differentiation. This results in poor mineralization of growth plate and abnormal osteoid mineralization. Since the discovery of vitamin D receptor (VDR) in various cells of our body (e.g. β cells of pancreas, mononuclear cells, osteoblasts and activated B and T lymphocytes), researchers have also explored the role of vitamin D in extraskeletal systemic disorders.

Deficiency of vitamin D and/or calcium causes nutritional rickets (NR), which remains the most common form of rickets in developing nations. Calcium deficiency is the main reason for development of rickets in Africa and some parts of tropical Asia. It is also being increasingly recognized in other parts of the world. Vitamin D deficiency rickets usually presents in the first 18 months of life, whereas calcium deficiency typically presents after weaning and often after the second year of life.[1] The overall incidence of nutritional rickets is high between 4 months and 18 months of age, though cases are not uncommon in older children. The incidence of rickets has decreased in developed nations due to fortification of dairy and other food products with vitamin D; however, the disease is highly prevalent in tropical countries.[2]

■ PROBLEM STATEMENT

Vitamin D deficiency is a global problem affecting all ages and ethnic groups. No country or ethnicity is devoid of vitamin D-deficient population. The prevalence of severe vitamin D deficiency is particularly high in women and girls in Middle East. Population representative data on vitamin D status is not available for many areas in Africa and Asia. Data on vitamin D levels in children and adolescents is also lacking from southern America and Africa. It is noteworthy that studies are not always directly comparable, since several different assays are used, and inter-laboratory variations can be considerable. More importantly, a vast difference occurs in the cut-off used to define vitamin D deficiency, based on serum levels of 25-hydroxyvitamin D [25(OH)D]. Areas with good sunlight throughout the year also have high prevalence of vitamin D deficiency.[2]

■ GLOBAL OVERVIEW OF VITAMIN D STATUS

A recent systematic review, involving 95 reports from across the globe, evaluated serum 25(OH)D concentrations in maternal and newborn populations. The review included studies from Europe, Eastern Mediterranean region, Western Pacific, South East Asia, Africa, and Americas. The prevalence of 25(OH)D levels <50 nmol/L and <25 nmol/L in pregnant women was as follows—Western Pacific (83%, 13%), Europe (57%, 23%), Eastern Mediterranean region (46%, 79%), South-East Asia (87%, not available), and Americas (64%, 9%). The prevalence in newborns with same two cut-offs was as follows—Western Pacific area (54%, 14%), Europe (73%, 39%), Eastern Mediterranean region (60%, not available), South-East Asia (96%, 45%), and Americas (30%, 14%). Maternal and newborn 25(OH)D concentrations had strong correlation.[2]

In another population-based health survey of national representative population of >25 years age (n = 5034) in Australia, about 43% participants were classified as insufficient (45% men; 42% women) and 20% (19% men; 21% women) were classified as vitamin D deficient. Vitamin D deficiency and insufficiency were defined as serum 25(OH)D concentrations <50 nmol/L and 50–75 nmol/L, respectively.[3]

In a large-scale study (n = 1,814) on vitamin D status in China, optimal (50–125 nmol/L) 25(OH)D level was observed in only 47.6%. Serum 25(OH)D levels were significantly higher among the age group of 40–49 years (50.7 ± 17.99 nmol/L) than among ≥ 70 years (48.45 ± 14.49 nmol/L) or 18–29 years (47.81 ± 13.08 nmol/L) age groups.[4]

In a recent cross-sectional study from Ethiopia, serum 25(OH)D levels were estimated in rural and urban school children aged 11–18 years. Vitamin D deficiency defined as 25(OH)D <50 nmol/L was observed in 42% participants. Students in urban settings had higher prevalence of deficiency as compared to rural areas (61.8% vs. 21.2%).[5] In the USA NHANES 2011–12 study, 1,981 out of 4,962 (39.9%) participants were vitamin D deficient (considering serum levels <150 nmol/L).[6]

Vitamin D Status in India

People living closer to equator are believed to receive abundant sunshine and therefore expected to have better vitamin D status. Contrary to this belief, residents of tropical countries, including India, have a very high prevalence of vitamin D deficiency or insufficiency **(Table 2.1.1)**.[7-13] In a recent study by Mandlik et al., 71% of children aged 6–12 years in semirural settings were vitamin D insufficient with serum 25(OH)D concentrations between 50 nmol/L and 74.9 nmol/L, despite >2 hours of sun exposure.[14] Sahu et al. reported that prevalence of vitamin D deficiency (25(OH)D <50 nmol/L) in adolescent girls was 88.6%. 74% of pregnant women had vitamin D deficiency.[15]

Table 2.1.1: Prevalence of vitamin D deficiency in Indian children.

Author	Site of study	Sample size	Age group	Prevalence of vitamin D deficiency
Bawaskar et al. 2017[7]	Maharashtra	640	No age preference	65.4%
Kapil et al. 2017[8]	Himachal Pradesh	626	6–18 years	93%
Chowdhary et al. 2017[9]	Delhi	960	6–30 months	34.5%
Basu et al. 2015[10]	Kolkata	310	1–16 years	52.9%
Angurana et al. 2014[11]	Chandigarh	338	3 months–12 years	40.2%
Khadagwat et al. 2012[12]	Delhi	62	6–17 years	99.8%
Marwaha et al. 2005[13]	Delhi	5137	10–18 years	84.9–92.6%

In a study by Jain et al., 66.7% of infants and 81.1% of mothers had vitamin D deficiency [25(OH)D <15 ng/mL]. An additional 19.8% infants and 11.6% mothers had vitamin D insufficiency [25(OH)D 15-20 ng/mL].[16] Aggarwal et al. observed vitamin D deficiency in 186 low birth weight (LBW) infants (87.3%) and 103 normal birth weight (NBW) infants (88.6%) at birth. The same newborns when reassessed at a median corrected age of 12 and 15 weeks (LBW and NBW, respectively) showed vitamin D deficiency in 77 (60.6%) of LBW and 55 (71.6%) of NBW infants. Vitamin D deficiency was near universal (93-97%) in all mothers.[17]

Comprehensive National Nutrition Survey (CNNS) is one of the largest nutrition surveys in the world, conducted from 2016-18, in 30 states of India with a multistage survey design, covering both urban and rural households.[18] The survey collected data from three target population groups; preschoolers (0-4 years), school-age children (5-9 years), and adolescents (10-19 years). Vitamin D was estimated by electrochemiluminescence assay and serum vitamin D level of <12 ng/mL (30 nmol/L) was considered as deficient in all three population groups. In this survey, overall prevalence of vitamin D deficiency was 14% in preschool children, 18% in school-age children, and 24% in adolescents. Vitamin D deficiency varied considerably over states. Highest prevalence was found in Punjab (52% in 1-4 year, 76% in 5-19 year, and 68% in 10-19 year age groups) and lowest prevalence was found in Assam (1.1% in 1-4 year, 4.0% in 5-19 year, and 7.1% in 10-19 year age groups). Other states with overall consistently high prevalence of vitamin D deficiency in all age groups were Uttarakhand, Delhi, Rajasthan, Haryana, Gujarat, Jammu & Kashmir, and Manipur. There were striking differences in vitamin D levels of the children according to the type of residence (rural/urban), type of diet (veg/veg with egg/non-veg), and wealth index (poorest/poor/middle/rich/richest) **(Table 2.1.2)**.

Table 2.1.2: Percentage of children with vitamin D deficiency in blood by selected background characteristics.[18]

	1–4 years	5–9 years	10–19 years
Residence			
Urban	19.1	27.8	33.2
Rural	12	15.2	20.6
Diet			
Vegetarian	17.4	24.9	27.8
Vegetarian with egg	16.6	22.9	28.1
Non-vegetarian	12.8	16.2	22.5
Wealth Index			
Poorest	14.1	13.3	18.9
Poor	13.1	13.2	18.8
Middle	9.6	14.8	19.8
Rich	4.4	20.4	28.7
Richest	13.8	30.2	32.9

■ PHYSIOLOGY OF VITAMIN D

Vitamin D is a secosteroid, which is produced in skin from 7-dehydrocholesterol by the action of ultraviolet B (UVB) rays (290–315 nm) from the sun. Most of the vitamin D (90%) in our body is synthesized in the skin. The diet contributes to only 10% of the vitamin D in the body. Vitamin D synthesis in the skin is affected by various factors, e.g. time of day, presence of clouds and/or smog, geographic latitude, time of year, melanin content in skin, and sunscreen application. The vitamin D formed in skin and the one ingested in diet, are then absorbed by the intestine, and carried to the liver via the bloodstream **(Fig. 2.1.1)**. In the liver, it is transformed into 25(OH)D (calcidiol), which is the primary circulating form of vitamin D. It is also the most commonly measured form of vitamin D in serum. It is later converted into 1,25 dihydroxyvitamin D (calcitriol) in the kidneys. The biologically active form of vitamin D is 1,25 dihydroxyvitamin D [1,25OH)2D]. When serum calcium falls below 8.8 mg/dL, it leads to a proportional increase in the secretion of parathyroid hormone (PTH). PTH increases the 25(OH)D-1α-hydroxylase production in the kidneys, which finally increases the production of 1,25(OH)2D. The increase in 1,25(OH)2D augments calcium absorption in the intestines to stimulate bone remodeling. Kidneys reduce the production of 1,25(OH)2D to a normal state after the phosphorus and bone genes levels signal a normal state of bone remodeling.

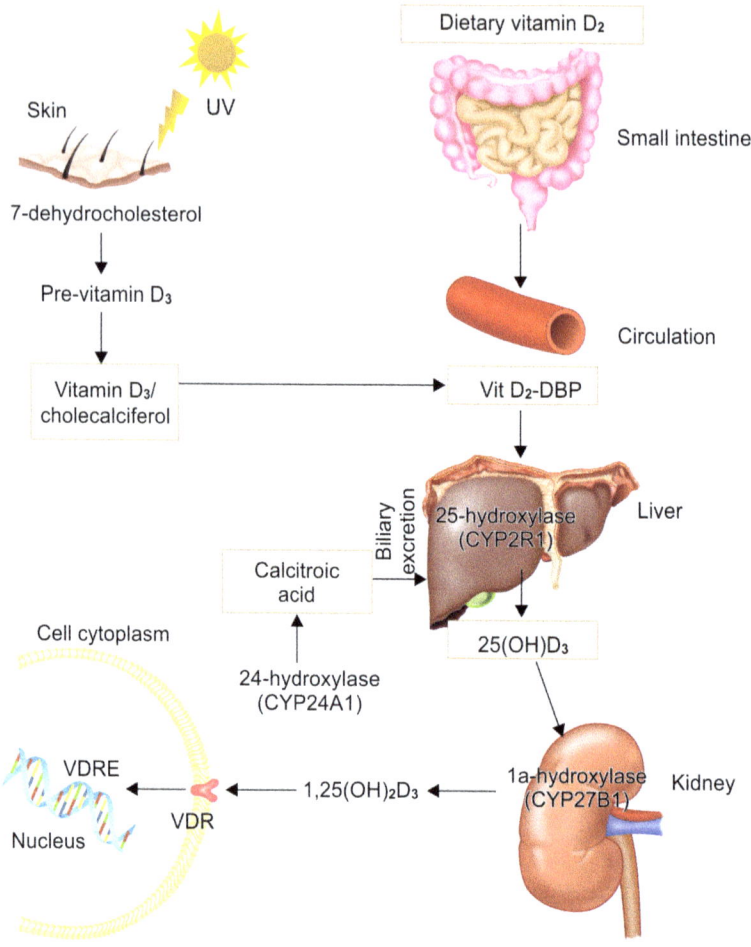

Fig. 2.1.1: Vitamin D metabolism.
(Vit D_2 DBP: vitamin D_2 binding protein; VDR: vitamin D receptor; VDRE: vitamin D response element)

Vitamin D has an established role in bone metabolism and calcium homeostasis. Pleiotropic effects of vitamin D are now being increasingly recognized and are currently a key research area. Vitamin D plays a role in immunomodulation by regulating both innate and adaptive immune system.

The physiological actions of vitamin D are exerted by its binding to and regulation of nuclear VDR. Essentially every organ and cell in the body has a VDR. Over 900 genes are expressed throughout the genome by VDR, which is a ligand-induced nuclear receptor. It affects gene transcription by forming vitamin 1,25(OH)2D–VDR complexes. This complex translocates from the cytosol to the nucleus on successful entry into the cells. There it combines with retinoid X receptor (RXR). This RXR-1,25(OH)2D-VDR complex binds to vitamin D response elements (VDRE), which are the promoter regions of target genes. VDR is commonly expressed in immune system cells, e.g. neutrophils, T lymphocytes, macrophages, and dendritic cells. VDRs are present abundantly in cells of colon, lungs, neurons, cardiomyocytes, and kidneys. VDR gene lies on chromosome 12 and >60 VDR polymorphisms have been identified. These polymorphisms can alter the transcription activity, which leads to modulation of cellular responsiveness to 1,25(OH)2D. These VDRs control the cellular proliferation, differentiation, apoptosis, and angiogenesis. 1,25(OH)2D is increasingly recognized as a potent inhibitor of cellular proliferation.

When an infective agent like *Mycobacterium tuberculosis* or its liposaccharides encounter a monocyte/macrophage through toll-like receptor (TLR), it stimulates VDR expression and increases the production of cathelicidin. Cathelicidin is a peptide, which promotes innate immunity and causes destruction of several infective agents. 1,25(OH)2D also induces autophagy in human monocytes via cathelicidin and causes localization of mycobacterial phagosomes with autophagosomes in human macrophages in a cathelicidin-dependent manner.[19]

■ RECOMMENDED DAILY ALLOWANCE AND SOURCES

Vitamin D, unlike other vitamins, is not abundantly available in foodstuffs. Dietary consumption usually accounts for only 5–10% of the total vitamin D. The amount in vegetable sources is negligible **(Table 2.1.3)**. This fat-soluble vitamin is found in fish (oily fish, e.g. salmon, mackerel, herring, sardine, trout, anchovy, and tuna), cod liver oil and other fish oils, egg yolk (20 IU/yolk), mushrooms, supplemented cereals, and fortified foods including formulas, milk, bread, and margarine. Human milk has a low vitamin D content, approximately 12–60 IU/L, and it is considered insufficient to prevent vitamin D deficiency in exclusively breastfed babies. Supplementation of 400 IU of

Table 2.1.3: Vitamin D content of food items.

Food items	Vitamin D content
Cow's milk	3–40 IU/L
Fortified infant formula	400 IU/L
Egg yolk	20–25 IU/yolk
Butter	35 IU/100 g
Cheese	12–44 IU/100 g
Cod liver oil	175 IU/g
Yogurt	89 IU/100 g
Fish	44–624 IU/100 g

Table 2.1.4: Recommended dietary allowance for calcium and vitamin D.[20-23]

	Calcium (mg)		Vitamin D (IU)	
	NIH (20)	ICMR (21)	NIH (20)	ICMR(21)
Infants: 0–6 months	200	500	400*	400
6–12 months	260	500	400*	400
Children (1–3 years)	700	600	600	400
(4–8 years)	1,000	600	600	400
(9–18 years)	1,300	800#	600	400
Adults (19–70 years)	1,000	600	600	400
71+ years	1,200	600	600	400
Pregnancy	1,000	1,200	600	400
Lactation	1,000	1,200	600	400

*Adequate intake
#10–17 years age
Source: National Institute of Health (NIH) USA 2010 and Indian Council of Medical Research (ICMR) Dietary guidelines for Indians–NIN 2011.

vitamin D helps in maintaining serum 25(OH)D concentrations at >50 nmol/L in breastfed infants. Though formula milk has vitamin D, infants needs to consume 1 liter of milk to get 400 IU/day vitamin D, which is not possible in neonates. *Thus, for all newborns, 400 IU of vitamin D supplementation is recommended till one year of age; it is also recommended that supplementation be started in the first few days of life.* Both Indian Academy of Pediatrics (IAP) and Global Consensus Recommendations advocate this endorsement.[22,23] Recommended daily allowance for calcium and vitamin D are given in **Table 2.1.4**.[20-23]

■ CLINICAL MANIFESTATIONS OF VITAMIN D DEFICIENCY

We will not discuss the details of clinical manifestations, as they are well-described elsewhere.[24] Rickets is identified as the well-known clinical presentation of vitamin D deficiency. The spectrum of extraskeletal manifestations of vitamin D deficiency varies from nonspecific complaints of irritability, body ache, bone pain, failure to thrive, and gross motor developmental delay to hypocalcemic seizures, tetany, life-threatening apneic spells, stridor, and cardiomyopathy. Hypocalcemic seizure and tetany due to vitamin D deficiency are more frequently seen in infancy and adolescence. There is rapid growth of the body during these phases of growth. This growing demand for calcium cannot be met with the body calcium stores and thus the patient may present with hypocalcemia even before the signs of rickets are observed.[25]

Directly or indirectly, vitamin D may affect every organ of the body either by the expression of VDR or by regulating other gene expressions. The extraskeletal effects of vitamin D have been a hot topic of debate and several studies (both observational and interventional) have been conducted with conflicting results. Data in children are limited. Most studies were designed to determine the beneficial effect of vitamin D supplementation on severity of various diseases, e.g. metabolic syndrome, diabetes mellitus, rheumatoid arthritis, psoriasis, systemic lupus erythematosus (SLE), inflammatory bowel disease (IBD), multiple sclerosis, asthma, food allergies, cancers, respiratory infections, and chronic hepatitis.[26]

Interventional studies in children with obesity, prediabetes, and type 2 diabetes show conflicting results. Obese adolescents have shown improved homeostatic model assessment of Insulin Resistance (HOMA-IR), quantitative insulin-sensitivity check index (QUICKI), and improved apo-B and low-density lipoprotein-C (LDL-C) following vitamin D administration.[25,26] Other studies have failed to demonstrate any beneficial effect.[27-30]

Meta-analyses to determine the effect of vitamin D supplementation on bronchial asthma have demonstrated improvement in exacerbation, but no effect on the severity of asthma.[31] A subsequent meta-analysis on 435 children (seven trials) and 658 adults (two trials) concluded that people receiving vitamin D supplementation had a reduction in asthma exacerbations requiring systemic corticosteroids. It also reduced the risk for exacerbation requiring an emergency department visit or hospitalization, but it had no effect on the measures of severity (percentage of predicted forced expiratory volume in one second or Asthma Control test Scores).[32] Another meta-analysis (2017) showed that asthmatic children had lower 25(OH)D levels as compared to nonasthmatic children, but the correlations between 25(OH)D and asthma incidence, asthma control, and lung functions were varied.[33]

Role of vitamin D in respiratory infections is also under scrutiny. A meta-analysis showed that vitamin D reduced the risk of overall acute respiratory infections in 0–95 years old. This benefit was maximum in people with low 25(OH)D levels (<10 ng/mL) and those receiving daily or weekly vitamin D supplementation as compared to bolus doses. In children aged 1–5 years, these effects were not so robust.[34,35] Cochrane systematic review on vitamin D supplementation (2016) for preventing infections in children under five years of age concluded that evidence from one large trial did not demonstrate benefit of vitamin D supplementation on the incidence of pneumonia or diarrhea in children under five years.[36] We conducted a randomized control trial (RCT) for evaluating the efficacy of single oral mega-dose of vitamin D3 for treatment and prevention of pneumonia in under-five children. There was no significant difference in the risk of recurrence of pneumonia over next 6 months in both the groups. Median (95% CI) time for resolution of severe pneumonia was 30 hours in the vitamin D group, as compared to 31 hours in the placebo group (p = 0.005). Serum immunoglobulin A (IgA), cathelicidin, and immunoglobulin G (IgG) concentrations were also comparable. We did not find any significant difference in the duration for complete recovery, hospital stay duration, and fever clearance time.[37]

Vitamin D supplementation exerts a protective effect against IBD. VDR genes (TaqI and ApaI) polymorphism affects the development of IBD. One recent meta-analysis found that patients of Crohn's disease and ulcerative colitis had lower levels of vitamin D than controls. They also reported an increased severity of Crohn's disease in those with vitamin D deficiency.[38] Another randomized controlled trial on vitamin D supplementation (400 vs 2,000 IU) in children and adolescents with IBD showed that a higher dose of vitamin D results in lower levels of proinflammatory markers.[39] More robust studies in children are required to determine the efficacy of vitamin D in reducing the severity of IBD.

A recent meta-analysis suggests that vitamin D levels in children with overt and latent tuberculosis (TB) infection are significantly lower than in controls. TB may contribute to vitamin D deficiency in children. Therefore, vitamin D deficiency may be associated with TB in children.[40]

In a cross sectional follow-up study on LBW term infants, 912 children aged 5 years who had participated in an earlier trial of vitamin D for term LBW infants in the first 6 months of life were assessed for gross motor development, using the Ages and Stages Questionnaire (ASQ), gross motor scale, and several measures of motor performance. Interestingly, children with poorer vitamin D status were able to perform more stands and squats. Greater handgrip strength was associated with lower tibia ultrasound Z score. The current height age Z score and arm muscle area showed the strongest associations with gross motor outcomes.[41] Authors concluded that this needs further research.

■ DIAGNOSIS

Diagnosis of nutritional rickets is based on the clinical features, biochemical findings, and characteristic radiological features. Since vitamin D and calcium deficiencies often coexist, performing only biochemical testing is not a good tool to diagnose and differentiate the primary cause of nutritional rickets as vitamin D and/or dietary calcium deficiency. The most readily available biochemical laboratory tests for nutritional rickets are serum calcium, phosphorus, and alkaline phosphatase (ALP). Serum calcium is usually normal but in severe cases it may be low. Serum phosphorus is usually low and a level <4 mg/dL is more specific than serum calcium values in making a diagnosis of rickets. ALP is generally raised (>500 IU/L in neonates and >1,000 IU/L in children up to 9 years).

The classical laboratory findings in nutritional rickets are decreased serum levels of 25(OH)D, phosphorus, calcium, and low urinary calcium. Alkaline

Table 2.1.5: Serum vitamin D status according to serum 25(OH)D levels.

Vitamin D Status	Serum Vitamin D (25 hydroxyvitamin D) levels	
	nmol/L	mg/dL
Sufficient	>50	>20
Insufficient	30–50	12–20
Deficient	<30	<12

Source: Global Consensus Recommendations on Prevention and Management of Nutritional Rickets.[23]

phosphatase, serum PTH, and urinary phosphorus levels are elevated. Normal levels and cut-offs for vitamin D status (as recommended by Global Consensus Recommendations on treating nutritional rickets) are depicted in **Table 2.1.5**.[23] The aim of all these guidelines is to achieve and maintain optimal vitamin D level with minimal risk for toxicity and adverse effects. These cut-off values have been based partly on the studies done in children for assessing relationship of PTH and vitamin D. Evidence suggest that decrease in 25(OH)D levels below 34 nmol/L cause an increase in PTH secretion. A level of 30–34 nmol/L of 25(OH)D may be a critical cut-off, below which there is a high likelihood of developing NR. These recommended cut-off values are aimed to prevent NR in population at large. However, it is noteworthy that NR has been reported in children with 25(OH)D concentrations >30 nmol/L and on the other hand, NR may not develop in people with very low 25(OH)D concentrations. NR is more likely to occur when there is prolonged deficiency over a long duration. Many patients with very low 25(OH)D may not have increased PTH production, and conversely, PTH suppression may not occur even if 25(OH)D levels are >30 ng/mL.[42] Most children with vitamin D deficiency or insufficiency according to these cut-offs are asymptomatic and have no evidence of any other marker of poor health or disease. Thus, the clinical relevance of these cut-offs can be ascertained only by global, population-based, and long-term prospective studies and correlating them with functional, rather than biochemical outcomes.

Vitamin D Assay

Commercially available vitamin D assays can measure 25(OH)D2, 25(OH)D3, and total 25(OH)D. Total 25(OH)D is recommended to evaluate vitamin D status, if both 25(OH)D2 and 25(OH)D3 are biologically equivalent. The accuracy of various tests varies widely between different tests and different laboratories. Various laboratory methods include enzyme-linked immunosorbent assays (ELISA), radioimmunoassay, chemiluminescent assays, high performance liquid chromatography (HPLC), and liquid chromatography-tandem mass spectrometry. Currently standard reference measurement procedure by

National Institute of Standards and Technology (NIST) and Ghent University is established for minimizing the inter-laboratory variations that recommend liquid chromatography tandem mass spectrometry method.

Radiological Changes

Apart from the biochemical and hormonal investigations, radiological findings readily help in confirming the diagnosis of rickets. The classical X-ray changes occur at open growth plate. The distal end of ulna is involved first, as the distal ulnar growth plate grows more rapidly than the distal radius. Thus, changes in ulna are a more sensitive indicator at wrist joint. Widening of the growth plate due to increase in the cartilaginous cell mass is the earliest finding. Disorganized spongy bone growth leads to irregular, indistinct metaphyseal margins (fraying). Later the protrusion of bulky mass of the cartilaginous cells in the poorly mineralized metaphysis leads to widening and cupping of metaphysis. The poor mineralization coupled with loss of mineral content manifests as rarefaction of the shaft bones and thinned cortex. As the child starts walking, radiological changes become appreciable in knee and ankle joints also. Some patients may develop greenstick fractures.

■ TREATMENT OF NUTRITIONAL RICKETS

Various regimens have been used for the treatment of vitamin D deficient rickets. Traditionally, Stoss therapy has been the standard mode of treating rickets, wherein mega doses of vitamin D (100,000–600,000 IU) are administered over 1–5 days or 60,000 IU weekly for 6–8 weeks. Stoss therapy is preferred for ensuring good compliance. A study in 56 Turkish children aged 3–36 months with NR, compared three single dose oral regimes (150,000 IU vs 300,000 IU vs 600,000 IU) and found them to be comparable.[43]

We compared a single mega-dose of 300,000 IU vs 600,000 IU and found them to be equally effective. The study also observed hypercalcemia in five children (2 in 300,000 and 3 in 600,000 group).[44] Mondal et al. found no difference in 25(OH)D, bone profile, and side effects in the two groups when single intramuscular (IM) dose of 600,000 IU vitamin D3 was compared to a weekly oral dose of 60,000 IU D3 for 10 weeks.[45]

Appropriate Route of Administration and Duration of Therapy

Rickets used to be treated with mega doses of intramuscular injection of vitamin D. For past two decades, treatment with oral doses has been in use. Currently, oral treatment is recommended over parenteral route, as it restores 25(OH)D levels much more rapidly than IM treatment.[23] Both vitamin D2 and D3 are equally effective for daily treatment. In single large dose therapy, D3 is preferable to D2 because the D3 has a longer half-life.

Minimum 12 weeks therapy is recommended. Some children may require treatment for more than 12 weeks. The current recommendations for treatment of nutritional rickets are summarized in **Table 2.1.6**.[22,23] Daily treatment is to be continued for minimum of 3 months and it should be followed by continued daily maintenance dose according to the age. The daily doses of vitamin D are similar in IAP and Global Consensus Recommendations guidelines but their schedules differ on single dose therapy.[22,23] While Global Consensus guidelines recommend single mega-dose in children above 3 months of age, IAP does not advocate injectable single mega-dose. IAP recommends 60,000 IU weekly doses for 6 weeks in children over 3 months of age. IAP recommends oral treatment with exceptions of patients with poor compliance and malabsorption. Injectable preparations are not recommended because in India, vitamin D is inadvertently used in very large doses for longer periods. Vitamin D can be consumed with meals or empty stomach.

According to Global Consensus Recommendations, all patients receiving vitamin D therapy for the treatment for nutritional rickets should also consume daily 500 mg oral calcium, either as dietary intake or supplement regardless of age or weight. Combined treatment with vitamin D and calcium is recommended because often the diet is deficient in both vitamin D and calcium.[46,47] Reassess the response after 3 months. Vitamin D refractory rickets should be suspected in patients showing no radiological or biochemical signs of healing after 12 weeks of therapy. Vitamin D refractory rickets is due to nonnutritional causes.

Table 2.1.6: Treatment doses of vitamin D for nutritional rickets.[22,23]

Age	Daily dose for 90 days, IU		Single dose, IU		Maintenance daily dose, IU	
	Global consensus	IAP	Global consensus	IAP	Global consensus	IAP
Premature neonates	2,000	1,000	-	-	400	400
Neonate	2,000	2,000	-	-	400	400
<3 months	2,000	2,000	-	-	400	400
3–12 months	2,000	2,000	50,000	60,000 weekly for 6 weeks	400	400
>12 months to 12 years	3,000–6,000	3,000–6,000	150,000	60,000 weekly for 6 weeks	600	600
>12 years	6,000		300,000		600	600

Source: Indian Academy of Pediatrics (IAP). Global Consensus Recommendations on Prevention and Management of Nutritional Rickets and Guideline for Vitamin D and Calcium in Children.

There is no strong evidence in support of any fixed duration of therapy for NR. Pediatric Endocrine Society recommends daily oral treatment for 8–12 weeks.[48] Reviews from United Kingdom also recommend 8 and 12 weeks of daily therapy.[49,50] Consensus statement from Australia and New Zealand also recommends 3 months treatment.[51]

Biochemical Vitamin D Deficiency: Should We Treat it?

Children of all ages are at risk for developing vitamin D deficiency but the optimal vitamin D levels for any functional outcome are not yet conclusive. All guidelines on vitamin D supplementation give a clear recommendation on the prevention of vitamin D deficiency and on treatment of nutritional rickets but there is lack of evidence on the dose, frequency, and duration of therapy for asymptomatic vitamin D deficiency. Global Consensus Recommendations, as well as IAP recommendations on rickets do not give any clear recommendation to treat asymptomatic vitamin D deficiency. Both Institute of Medicine and Endocrine Society recommend that in 0–18 years age group, treatment with 2,000 IU/day of vitamin D2 or D3 for at least 6 weeks or with 50,000 IU of vitamin D2 once a week for at least 6 weeks recommend to achieve a blood level above 30 ng/mL followed by a maintenance therapy of 400–1,000 IU/day in 0–1 year and 600–1000 IU/day in 1–18 years of age.[20,23]

■ PREVENTION OF NUTRITIONAL RICKETS

Global Consensus Recommendation on Prevention and Management of Nutritional Rickets 2015 advises that, to prevent rickets, all infants from birth to 12 months of age should be supplemented with 400 IU/day (10 µg) vitamin D, independent of their mode of feeding. Diet and/or supplementation are required in all children (>12 months of age) and adults to maintain an intake of at least 600 IU/day. High risk groups warranting regular vitamin D supplementation in the absence of food fortification include: (1) all children with a history of symptomatic vitamin D deficiency requiring treatment and (2) children and adults at high risk of vitamin D deficiency, with factors or conditions that reduce synthesis or intake of vitamin D.[23] IAP also recommends same dosages for prevention of rickets.[22] However, Indian Council of Medical Research (ICMR) recommends outdoor physical activity as a means of achieving adequate vitamin D status and daily supplementation should be done only under situations of minimal exposure to sunlight.[21]

Role of Sunlight Exposure

Ultraviolet B rays cause epidermal synthesis of previtamin D3. The risk of vitamin D deficiency and nutritional rickets is increased by decrease in sun exposure either due to covering body with clothes or by staying indoors purposefully. Environmental factors such as latitude, pollution, cloud cover, season, and time of day affect availability of UVB. This UVB dose–response and circulating 25(OH)D levels are also affected by personal factors, e.g. age, skin type, body composition, skin coverage, time spent outdoors, and genetic. It is seen that inhabitants of higher latitudes are more prone for vitamin D deficiency due to decrease in incident UVB radiation reaching their atmosphere. This reduction in UVB radiation at higher latitude is explained by the fact that at higher latitude, the sunrays form an oblique angle and thus traverse a longer path to reach earth surface. While passing through atmosphere and ozone layer, there is resultant more scattering and absorption of UVB rays in the atmosphere and only a minimal fraction reaches the surface.[52] Similar mechanisms operate in winter months, wherein the sun rays enter at a comparatively oblique path, leading to more UVB absorption by the atmosphere. During winter months in north, at above 37° latitude, the number of UVB photons reaching earth's atmosphere is decreased by 80-100% and thus little vitamin D is produced in the skin.[53] Vitamin D production requires a minimum amount of UVB, which may not be reached at a latitude of above 40 in winter even after prolonged sun exposure.[54] Specker et al. found that exposure to sunlight for 30 min/week for infants in diaper and 2 hr/week for fully clothed infants without that maintained vitamin D levels of >11 ng/dL.[55] Al-Daghri et al. studied 808 Saudi children and 526 adults. The study found that vitamin D status of children or adults was unaffected by sunlight exposure or skin color, except in boys with dark skin who had lower 25(OH)D concentrations associated with limited sun exposure.[56] Another study done was done on 3,127 apparently healthy schoolgirls (6-18 years age) in Delhi. Prevalence of biochemical hypovitaminosis D [serum 25(OH)D <50 nmol/L] was seen in 90.8% of girls. They also found a significant correlation between serum 25(OH)D levels and estimated sun exposure and percentage body surface area exposed.[57]

We studied the role of sunlight exposure on vitamin D status of predominantly breastfed urban poor infants from Delhi. We also tried to quantify the sunlight exposure required to achieve serum 25(OH)D level >20 ng/mL by 6 months of age. There was a significant positive correlation between infant's vitamin D levels and afternoon sunlight exposure, independent of maternal vitamin D status. Based on results of logistic regression, we recommended afternoon sun exposure of 30 min/week for 16-18 weeks (starting from 6 weeks) over 40% exposed body surface area to achieve sufficient vitamin D (20 ng/mL) in infants at 6 months of age.[58] However, there is no RCT comparing sunlight vs. oral vitamin D for prevention of rickets. Currently there is no determined safe threshold of UVB exposure for enough vitamin D synthesis across the population without increasing skin cancer risk.

THE WAY FORWARD

With growing evidence of the extraskeletal role of vitamin D, generation of more evidence is required on whether everyone needs to maintain a vitamin D level above a certain cut-off to reap the benefits of vitamin D or whether it is just a bubble waiting to burst. With so many studies all over the world showing a near universal presence of low vitamin D levels, it is a matter of concern whether low levels really cause so many problems. There is a need for multicentric global long-term prospective studies to find out if maintaining vitamin D levels in sufficient range makes a difference in long run by reducing the incidence of various disease processes and in improving the functional outcomes. Caution is needed to avoid overuse of vitamin D without clear indications. A strong political will can surely help in forming legislations regarding the food fortification of commonly consumed food, e.g. milk and *atta*/flour with vitamin D. People should be made aware of the need of vitamin D and how they can build optimal vitamin D levels by sun exposure and taking diet rich in vitamin D and calcium. On the other hand, we all need to understand that vitamin D is not a panacea for every illness. Routine supplementation as recommended by several agencies needs to be periodically reviewed and revised, based on its impact on functional outcomes and changing prevalence patterns of deficiency in the target population.

REFERENCES

1. Thacher TD, Fischer PR, Strand MA, et al. Nutritional rickets around the world: causes and future directions. Ann Trop Paediatr. 2006;26(1):1-16.
2. Saraf R, Morton SM, Camargo CA, et al. Global summary of maternal and newborn vitamin D status - a systematic review. Matern Child Nutr. 2016;12(4):647-68.
3. Malacova E, Cheang P, Dunlop E, et al. Prevalence and predictors of vitamin D deficiency in a nationally representative sample of adults participating in the 2011–2013 Australian Health Survey. Br J Nutr. 2019;121(8):894-904.
4. Fang F, Wei H, Wang K, et al. High prevalence of vitamin D deficiency and influencing factors among urban and rural residents in Tianjin, China. Arch Osteoporos. 2018;13(1):64.
5. Wakayo T, Belachew T, Vatanparast H, et al. Vitamin D deficiency and its predictors in a country with thirteen months of sunshine: the case of school children in central Ethiopia. PLoS One. 2015;10(3):e0120763.
6. Parva NR, Tadepalli S, Singh P, et al. Prevalence of Vitamin D deficiency and associated risk factors in the US population (2011-2012). Cureus. 2018;10(6):e2741.
7. Bawaskar PH, Bawaskar HS, Bawaskar PH, et al. Profile of Vitamin D in patients attending at general hospital Mahad India. Indian J Endocrinol Metab. 2017;21(1):125-30.
8. Kapil U, Pandey RM, Goswami R, et al. Prevalence of Vitamin D deficiency and associated risk factors among children residing at high altitude in Shimla district, Himachal Pradesh, India. Indian J Endocrinol Metab. 2017;21(1):178-83.

9. Chowdhury R, Taneja S, Bhandari N, et al. Vitamin-D deficiency predicts infections in young North Indian children: a secondary data analysis. PLoS One. 2017;12:e0170509.
10. Basu S, Gupta R, Mitra M, et al. Prevalence of Vitamin D deficiency in a pediatric hospital of Eastern India. Indian J Clin Biochem. 2015;30(2):167-73.
11. Angurana SK, Angurana RS, Mahajan G, et al. Prevalence of Vitamin D deficiency in apparently healthy children in North India. J Pediatr Endocrinol Metab. 2014;27(11-12):1151-6.
12. Khadgawat R, Thomas T, Gahlot M, et al. The effect of puberty on interaction between Vitamin D status and insulin resistance in obese Asian-Indian children. Int J Endocrinol. 2012;2012:173581.
13. Marwaha RK, Tandon N, Reddy DRH, et al. Vitamin D and bone mineral density status of healthy schoolchildren in Northern India. Am J Clin Nutr. 2005;82(2):477-82.
14. Mandlik R, Kajale N, Ekbote V, et al. Determinants of Vitamin D Status in Indian School-children. Indian J Endocrinol Metab. 2018;22(2):244-8.
15. Sahu M, Bhatia V, Aggarwal A, et al. Vitamin D deficiency in rural girls and pregnant women despite abundant sunshine in northern India. Clin Endocrinol (Oxf). 2009;70(5):680-4.
16. Jain V, Gupta N, Kalaivani M, et al. Vitamin D deficiency in healthy breastfed term infants at 3 months and their mothers in India: seasonal variation and determinants. Indian J Med Res. 2011;133:267-73.
17. Agarwal R, Virmani D, Jaipal ML, et al. Vitamin D status of low birth weight infants in Delhi: a comparative study. J Trop Pediatr. 2012;58(6):446-50.
18. Ministry of Health and Family Welfare (MoHFW), Government of India, UNICEF and Population Council. 2019. Comprehensive National Nutrition Survey (CNNS) National Report. New Delhi. [online] Available from https://nhm.gov.in › index1/ CNNS reports 2016-18 [Last accessed November, 2019].
19. Yuk JM, Shin DM, Lee HM, et al. Vitamin D3 induces autophagy in human monocytes/macrophages via cathelicidin. Cell Host Microbe. 2009;6(3):231-43.
20. Committee to Review Dietary Reference Intakes for Vitamin D and Calcium, Food and Nutrition Board, Institute of Medicine. Dietary Reference Intakes for Calcium and Vitamin D. Washington, DC: National Academy Press, 2010.
21. National Institute of Nutrition (ICMR). Dietary Guidelines for Indians –a manual. [online] Available from: http://ninindia.org/DietaryGuidelinesforNINwebsite.pdf [Last accessed November,2019] .
22. Khadilkar A, Khadilkar V, Chinnappa J, et al. Prevention and treatment of vitamin D and calcium deficiency in children and adolescents: Indian Academy of Pediatrics Guidelines. Indian Pediatr. 2017;54(7):567-73.
23. Munns CF, Shaw N, Kiely M, et al. Global Consensus Recommendations on Prevention and Management of Nutritional Rickets. J Clin Endocrinol Metab. 2016; 101(2):394-415.
24. Gupta P, Shah D. Nutritional disorders. In: Gupta P (Ed). Textbook of Pediatrics, 2nd edition. New Delhi: CBS Publishers; 2019. pp. 65-104.
25. Ladhani S, Srinivasan L, Buchanan C, et al. Presentation of vitamin D deficiency. Arch Dis Child. 2004;89(8):781-4.
26. Marino R, Misra M. Extra-skeletal effects of vitamin D. Nutrients. 2019;11:E1460.

27. Belenchia AM, Tosh AK, Hillman LS, et al. Correcting vitamin D insufficiency improves insulin sensitivity in obese adolescents: A randomized controlled trial. Am J Clin Nutr. 2013;97(4):774-81.
28. Kelishadi R, Salek S, Salek M, et al. Effects of vitamin D supplementation on insulin resistance and cardiometabolic risk factors in children with metabolic syndrome: A triple-masked controlled trial. J Pediatr. 2014;90(1):28-34.
29. Nader NS, Castaneda AR, Wallace J, et al. Effect of vitamin D3 supplementation on serum 25(OH) D, lipids and markers of insulin resistance in obese adolescents: a prospective, randomized, placebo-controlled pilot trial. Horm Res Paediatr. 2014;82(2):107-12.
30. Javed A, Vella A, Balagopal PB, et al. Cholecalciferol supplementation does not influence beta-cell function and insulin action in obese adolescents: a prospective double-blind randomized trial. J Nutr. 2015;145(2):284-90.
31. Jolliffe DA, Greenberg L, Hooper RL, et al. Vitamin D supplementation to prevent asthma exacerbations: A systematic review and meta-analysis of individual participant data. Lancet Respir Med. 2017;5(11):881-90.
32. Martineau AR, Cates CJ, Urashima M, et al. Vitamin D for the management of asthma. Cochrane Database Syst Rev. 2016;(9):CD011511.
33. Jat KR, Khairwa A. Vitamin D and asthma in children: a systematic review and meta-analysis of observational studies. Lung India. 2017;34(4):355-63.
34. Martineau AR, Jolliffe DA, Hooper RL, et al. Vitamin D supplementation to prevent acute respiratory tract infections: systematic review and meta-analysis of individual participant data. BMJ. 2017(15);356:i6583.
35. Martineau AR, Jolliffe DA, Greenberg L, et al. Vitamin D supplementation to prevent acute respiratory infections: individual participant data meta-analysis. Health Technol Assess. 2019;23(2):1-44.
36. Yakoob MY, Salam RA, Khan FR, et al. Vitamin D supplementation for preventing infections in children under five years of age. Cochrane Database Syst Rev. 2016;11:CD008824.
37. Gupta P, Dewan P, Shah D, et al. Vitamin D supplementation for treatment and prevention of pneumonia in under-five children: a randomized double-blind placebo controlled trial. Indian Pediatr. 2016;53(11):967-76.
38. Lu C, Yang J, Yu W, et al. Association between 25(OH) D level, ultraviolet exposure, geographical location, and inflammatory bowel disease activity: a systematic review and meta-analysis. PLoS One. 2015;10:e0132036.
39. Papa HM, Mitchell PD, Jiang H, et al. Maintenance of optimal vitamin D status in children and adolescents with inflammatory bowel disease: a randomized clinical trial comparing two regimens. J Clin Endocrinol Metab. 2014;99(9):3408-17.
40. Gou X, Pan L, Tang F, et al. The association between vitamin D status and tuberculosis in children: a meta-analysis. Medicine (Baltimore). 2018;97(35):e12179.
41. Filteau S, Rehman AM, Yousafzai A, et al. Associations of vitamin D status, bone health and anthropometry, with gross motor development and performance of school-aged Indian children who were born at term with low birth weight. BMJ Open. 2016;6:e009268.
42. Chapuy MC, Preziosi P, Maamer M, et al. Prevalence of vitamin D insufficiency in an adult normal population. Osteoporosis Int. 1997;7(5):439-43.

43. Cesur Y, Çaksen H, Gündem A, et al. Comparison of low and high dose of vitamin D treatment in nutritional vitamin D Deficiency Rickets. J Pediatr Endocrinol Metab. 2011;16(8):1105-10.
44. Mittal H, Rai S, Shah D, et al. 300,000 IU or 600,000 IU of oral vitamin D3 for treatment of nutritional rickets: a randomized controlled trial. Indian Pediatr. 2014;51(4):265-72.
45. Mondal K, Seth A, Marwaha R, et al. A randomized controlled trial on safety and efficacy of single intramuscular versus staggered oral dose of 600 000 IU Vitamin D in treatment of nutritional rickets. J Trop Pediatr. 2014;60(3):203-10.
46. Aggarwal V, Seth A, Aneja S, et al. Role of calcium deficiency in development of nutritional rickets in Indian children: a case control study. J Clin Endocrinol Metab. 2012;97(10):3461-6.
47. Balasubramanian K, Rajeswari J, Gulab, et al. Varying role of vitamin D deficiency in the etiology of rickets in young children vs. adolescents in northern India. J Trop Pediatr. 2003;49(4):201-6.
48. Misra M, Pacaud D, Petryk A, et al. Vitamin D deficiency in children and its management: review of current knowledge and recommendations. Pediatrics. 2008;122(2):398-417.
49. Pearce SH, Cheetham TD. Diagnosis and management of vitamin D deficiency. BMJ. 2010;340:b5664.
50. Shaw NJ, Mughal MZ. Vitamin D and child health: part 2 (extraskeletal and other aspects). Arch Dis Child. 2013;98(5):368-72.
51. Munns C, Zacharin MR, Rodda CP, et al. Prevention and treatment of infant and childhood vitamin D deficiency in Australia and New Zealand: a consensus statement. Med J Aust. 2006;185(5):268-72.
52. Diamond J. Evolutionary biology: geography and skin colour. Nature. 2005;435(7040):283-4.
53. Holick MF. Sunlight and vitamin D for bone health and prevention of autoimmune diseases, cancers, and cardiovascular disease. Am J Clin Nutr. 2004;80(6 Suppl):1678S-88S.
54. Matsuoka LY, Wortsman J, Haddad JG, et al. In vivo threshold for cutaneous synthesis of vitamin D3. J Lab Clin Med. 1989;114(3):301-5.
55. Specker BL, Valanis B, Hertzberg V, et al. Sunshine exposure and serum 25-hydroxy vitamin D concentrations in exclusively breastfed infants. J Pediatr. 1985;107(3);372-6.
56. Al-Daghri NM, Al-Saleh Y, Khan N, et al. Sun exposure, skin color and vitamin D status in Arab children and adults. J Steroid Biochem Mol Biol. 2016;164:235-8.
57. Puri S, Marwaha R, Agarwal N, et al. Vitamin D status of apparently healthy schoolgirls from two different socioeconomic strata in Delhi: Relation to nutrition and lifestyle. Br J Nutr. 2008;99(4):876-82.
58. Meena P, Dabas A, Shah D, et al. Sunlight exposure and vitamin D status in breastfed infants. Indian Pediatr. 2017;54(2):105-11.

CHAPTER 3

IMMUNITY AND IMMUNIZATION

3.1 Ideal Vaccination Schedule 2020 for National Immunization Program and Indian Academy of Pediatrics
Ashish Pathak, Naveen Thacker

3.2 Primary Immunodeficiency Disorders
Jaydeep Choudhury

3.1 IDEAL VACCINATION SCHEDULE 2020 FOR NATIONAL IMMUNIZATION PROGRAM AND INDIAN ACADEMY OF PEDIATRICS

Ashish Pathak, Naveen Thacker

■ INTRODUCTION

Vaccines are one of the greatest public health achievements of the modern era. It is estimated that vaccines help us to save 2–3 million lives each year. Vaccination successfully eradicated smallpox and has brought diseases such as polio and measles on the brink of eradication. Safe and effective licensed vaccines are now available to prevent more than 30 different infectious diseases, several of which can be combined into single vaccines or administered at a single visit. Given the number of vaccines available for use, it is imperative that pediatricians and those concerned with immunization are aware of the different vaccination schedules. In this chapter, we review the current vaccination schedule recommended by the Indian Academy of Pediatrics (IAP) and the immunization schedule **(Table 3.1.1)** in the National Immunization Program (NIP) schedule **(Table 3.1.2)** and also provide a guideline for an ideal immunization schedule for 2020 and beyond **(Table 3.1.3)**.

■ BRIEF OVERVIEW OF INDIVIDUAL VACCINE SCHEDULE

Bacillus Calmette–Guérin

The ideal time for bacillus Calmette-Guérin (BCG) vaccination is at birth. According to the NIP guidelines, BCG can be given till 1 years of age. The dose is 0.05 mL till the age of 1 month and 0.1 mL till the age of 1 year. There is no need to repeat BCG even if there is no visible scar at the BCG injection site, if the dose is documented. However, IAP guidelines of 2014 recommend a catch-up immunization till 5 years of age and a repeat dose in case BCG scar is not visible. These IAP recommendations need to be revisited in view of multiple studies in support of the Government of India (GOI) standpoint.

Bacillus Calmette-Guérin vaccination-related axillary lymphadenopathy is reasonably common because of wrong technique or high dose (more than 0.05 mL till 1 month of age). It needs to be given intradermally to avoid spread to lymph nodes, causing suppurative and nonsuppurative lymphadenitis. BCG reduces the risk of contracting tuberculosis (TB) by about 50% and appears to have maximum effect in preventing miliary and hematogenic spread of TB.

Immunity and Immunization

Table 3.1.1: Major recommendations for IAP immunization schedule, 2020.

Hepatitis B vaccine	• One dose of hepatitis B vaccine within 24 hours of birth • In case of use of a combination vaccine, a total of four doses of hepatitis B vaccine are justified
DTwP, DTaP, and combination vaccines	• DTwP or DTaP can be offered in primary series
Polio vaccines	• Ideally IPV should replace OPV as early as possible • Three doses of IM IPV in primary series are the best option • Two doses of IM IPV instead of three for primary series, if started at 8 weeks, with an interval of 8 weeks between two doses are an alternative • In case IPV is not available or feasible, the child should be offered three doses of bOPV. In such cases, the child should be referred for two fractional doses of IPV at a government facility at 6 and 14 weeks or at least one dose of IM IPV, either standalone or as a combination vaccine, at 14 weeks of age
Rotavirus vaccine	• RV1 can be used in 6, 10 weeks schedule
Influenza vaccine	• Inactivated influenza vaccine (either trivalent or quadrivalent) is recommended routinely to all children below 5 years of age starting from 6 months of age annually (2–4 weeks before influenza season)
Measles-containing vaccines	• Measles-containing vaccine (MMR/MR) should be administered after 9 months of age • MR vaccine as part of the national campaign is to be administered irrespective of previous vaccination
Typhoid vaccines	• Single dose of any of typhoid conjugate vaccine (TCV 25 mg) is recommended from 6 months onwards and can be administered with MMR also • Booster dose of typhoid conjugate vaccine is not recommended in subsequent years
Rabies vaccines	• ACVIP IAP endorses administration of a 4-dose schedule of rabies vaccine recommended by WHO 2018 for postexposure prophylaxis • ACVIP also endorses administration of rabies monoclonal antibody as an alternative to rabies immunoglobulin for category-III bites

(ACVIP IAP: Advisory Committee on Vaccines and Immunization Practices of Indian Academy of Pediatrics; bOPV: bivalent oral polio vaccine; MMR/MR: measles, mumps, and rubella; DTwP/DTaP: diphtheria, tetanus, and pertussis vaccines; IPV: injectable polio vaccine; RV1: monovalent rotavirus vaccine)

Hepatitis B Vaccine

The global coverage of the birth dose estimated as 39% is still low and thus burden of chronic hepatitis B virus infection is a potential threat. According

Table 3.1.2: National Immunization Schedule (NIS) for infants and children (vaccine-wise).[37]

Vaccine	When to give	Dose	Route	Site
For infants:				
Bacillus Calmette–Guerin (BCG)	At birth or as early as possible till 1 year of age	0.1 mL (0.05 mL until 1 month of age)	Intradermal	Left upper arm
Hepatitis B—birth dose	At birth or as early as possible within 24 hours	0.5 mL	Intramuscular	Anterolateral side of mid-thigh
Oral polio vaccine (OPV)—0	At birth or as early as possible within the first 15 days	2 drops	Oral	Oral
OPV 1, 2, and 3	At 6 weeks, 10 weeks, and 14 weeks (OPV can be given till 5 years of age)	2 drops	Oral	Oral
Pentavalent 1, 2, and 3	At 6 weeks, 10 weeks, and 14 weeks (can be given till 1 year of age)	0.5 mL	Intramuscular	Anterolateral side of mid-thigh
Pneumococcal conjugate vaccine (PCV)^	Two primary doses at 6 and 14 weeks followed by booster dose at 9–12 months	0.5 mL	Intramuscular	Anterolateral side of mid- thigh
Rotavirus (RV)^	At 6, 10, and 14 weeks (can be given till 1 year of age)	3	Oral	Oral
Inactivated polio vaccine (IPV)	Two fractional dose at 6 and 14 weeks of age	0.1 mL	Intradermal two fractional dose	Intradermal: right upper arm
Measles rubella^ (MR) 1st dose	9 completed months to 12 months. (Measles can be given till 5 years of age)	0.5 mL	Subcutaneous	Right upper arm
Japanese encephalitis (JE)-1*	9 completed months to 12 months	0.5 mL	Subcutaneous	Left upper arm
Vitamin A (1st dose)	At 9 completed months with measles-rubella	1 mL (1 lakh IU)	Oral	Oral

Contd...

Contd...

Vaccine	When to give	Dose	Route	Site
For children:				
Diphtheria, pertussis and tetanus (DPT) booster-1	16–24 months	0.5 mL	Intramuscular	Anterolateral side of mid-thigh
MR 2nd dose	16–24 months	0.5 mL	Subcutaneous	Right upper arm
OPV Booster	16–24 months	2 drops	Oral	Oral
JE-2	16–24 months	0.5 mL	Subcutaneous	Left upper arm
Vitamin A** (2nd to 9th dose)	16–18 months. Then one dose every 6 months up to the age of 5 years	2 mL (2 lakh IU)	Oral	Oral
DPT booster-2	5–6 years	0.5 mL	Intramuscular	Upper arm
TT/Td	10 years and 16 years	0.5 mL	Intramuscular	Upper arm

Note:
*JE vaccine is introduced in select endemic districts after the campaign.
**The 2nd to 9th doses of vitamin A can be administered to children 1–5 years old during biannual rounds, in collaboration with Integrated Child Development Scheme (ICDS).
^Rotavirus vaccine and PCV in selected states/districts as per details below:
- *Rotavirus:* It has been rolled out throughout the country from September, 2019.
- *PCV:* Bihar, Himachal Pradesh, Madhya Pradesh, Uttar Pradesh, Rajasthan (18 districts), and in Haryana using state funds.

Table 3.1.3: Indian Academy of Pediatrics (IAP) immunization timetable, 2018.[38]

Age (completed weeks/months/years)	Vaccines	Comments
Birth	BCG OPV-0 HB-1	Administer these vaccines to all newborns before hospital discharge
6 weeks	DTP-1 IPV-1 HB-2 HiB-1 Rotavirus-1 PCV-1	*DTP-1:* • The primary series should be completed with three doses of either wP or aP vaccines, irrespective of the number of components *Polio:* • All doses of IPV may be replaced with OPV, if administration of the former is unfeasible • Additional doses of OPV on all supplementary immunization activities (SIAs) • Two doses of IPV instead of 3 for primary series, if started at 8 week, and 8 week interval between the doses • No child should leave the facility without polio immunization (IPV or OPV), if indicated by the schedule • bOPV should be continued in place of IPV, only if IPV is not feasible, with a minimum of 3 doses at 6, 10, and 14 weeks of age *Rotavirus:* • *Minimum age:* 6 weeks for all available brands • Only two doses of RV1 are recommended at 6 and 10 weeks • If any dose in series was RV5 or RV-116E or vaccine product is unknown for any dose in the series, a total of three doses of RV vaccine should be administered
10 weeks	HB-3 DTP-2 IPV-2 HiB-2 Rotavirus-2 PCV-2	*Polio:* • bOPV should be continued in place of IPV, only if IPV is not feasible, with a minimum of 3 doses at 6, 10, and 14 weeks of age *Rotavirus:* • Only two doses of RV1 are recommended at 6 and 10 weeks • Recommendations on the age limit for the first dose and the last dose (16 and 32 weeks) should continue in spite of recommendation for increase in the age limit as per recent NIP guidelines

Contd...

Immunity and Immunization

Contd...

Age (completed weeks/months/years)	Vaccines	Comments
14 weeks	HB-4 DTP-3 IPV-3 HiB-3 Rotavirus-3 PCV-3	*Hepatitis B*: • Fourth dose of hepatitis B permissible for combination vaccine only *Polio*: • bOPV should be continued in place of IPV, only if IPV is not feasible, with a minimum of 3 doses at 6, 10, and 14 weeks of age *Rotavirus*: • Third dose not required for RV1. Catch-up up to 1 year of age in UIP schedule
6 months	Typhoid conjugate vaccine Influenza	*Typhoid conjugate vaccine*: • A single dose of TCV 25 µg is recommended from the age of 6 months onwards routinely • An interval of at least 4 weeks is not mandatory between TCV and measles-containing vaccine when it is offered at age of 9 months or beyond *Influenza*: • Begin influenza vaccination after 6 months of age, about 2–4 weeks before season; give 2 doses at the interval of 4 weeks during 1st year and then single dose yearly till 5 years of age
9 months	MCV-1 MMR-1	*MMR*: • MMR is administered instead of MR at 9 months, 15 months, and 4–6 years, or as two doses at 12–15 months of age with the second dose between 4 and 6 years of age. Additional dose of MR vaccine during MR campaign for children 9 months to 15 years, irrespective of previous vaccination status is to be administered, keeping in mind the need to support national programs *MCV*: • 9 months through 23 months; 2 doses at least 3 months apart; 2 years through 55 years; single dose
12 months	Hep-A1 MCV-2 JE-1	*JE*: • For individuals living in endemic areas and for travelers to JE-endemic areas provided there expected stay is for a minimum period of 4 weeks
13 months	JE-2	

Contd...

Contd...

Age (completed weeks/months/years)	Vaccines	Comments
15 months	MMR-2 Varicella-1 PCV booster-1	
16–18 months	DTP-B1 IPV-B1 HiB-B1	Polio: • bOPV, if IPV booster (standalone or combination) not feasible
2–3 years	MCV	
4–6 years	DTP-B2 MMR-3 Varicella-2	
9–14 years	PCV Tdap HPV-1 and -2	HPV: • 2 doses at 6 months interval 9–14 years of age; 3 doses (at 0, 1–2, and 6 months) 15 years or older and immunocompromised
15–18 years	Td HPV-1, 2, 3	

(BCG: Bacillus Calmette–Guérin; OPV: oral polio vaccine; HB: hepatitis B; HiB: *Haemophilus influenzae* type B vaccine; JE: Japanese encephalitis; PCV: pneumococcal conjugate vaccine; HPV: human papilloma virus; DTP: diphtheria, tetanus, and pertussis; MCV: meningococcal vaccine; MMR: measles, mumps, and rubella; TCV: typhoid conjugate vaccine; IPV: injectable polio vaccine; RV: rotavirus)

to World Health Organization (WHO) 2017 position paper, hepatitis B vaccine (HBV) should be administered at birth, preferably within the first 24 hours.[1] When the status of hepatitis-B surface antigen (HBsAg) in the mother is known to be negative at the time of delivery, then this dose can be delayed. However, this dose becomes crucially important when HBsAg report of mother is incorrect or unknown, or in case of infants born to HBsAg-positive mothers.[2] Therefore, the birth dose is critical for prevention of chronic complications associated with hepatitis B.

Recommendation on Hepatitis B Vaccine

The NIP schedule recommends one birth dose and three doses of hepatitis B in a combination vaccine. After considering the NIP recommendations, IAP has also recommended four doses of hepatitis B (e.g. three doses of hepatitis B from pentavalent combination vaccine and one dose from monovalent dose at birth).[1]

Diphtheria, Tetanus, and Pertussis Vaccines

Long-term efficacy of whole-cell pertussis vaccine (wP) is proven for more than 2 decades.[3] However, recent pertussis outbreaks in some developed countries have questioned the effectiveness of acellular pertussis (aP) vaccines. But countries facing the epidemics are not planning to revert to whole-cell pertussis vaccines primarily because in most countries, the cause of resurgence of pertussis was drop in coverage for the vaccine and not primarily the vaccine efficacy. The immunity after aP wanes more rapidly compared with wP 1 year after vaccination. The impact on transmission of pertussis in a given community is lower by aP vaccines compared to wP vaccines.[4-6] The WHO clearly states those countries currently using the wP vaccine for the primary series in their national programs should continue to do so.[7,8] WHO recommendation for countries using the aP vaccine is that they can continue aP vaccines but consider additional boosters and immunization of mothers in case of pertussis resurgence.[7] The duration of protection for both the aP and wP vaccines after the three primary doses and a booster dose at least after a year varies from 6 years to 12 years.[8] A study done among children in Germany reported 89% efficiency for aP vaccine.[9] Results from several studies suggest that multicomponent aP vaccines have greater efficacy than the single- or two-component aP vaccines.[10,11] However, there is insufficient data to conclude that the effectiveness of the aP vaccines is related to the number of components only.[7] NIP uses wP, whereas IAP has following recommendations related to aP: The primary series should be completed with three doses of either wP or aP vaccines, irrespective of the number of components. The wP vaccine is superior to aP vaccine in terms of efficacy and duration of protection but is more reactogenic. In view of parental anxiety and concerns for its reactogenicity, aP vaccine can also be administered even in the primary series.

Polio Vaccines

Efficacy of oral polio vaccine (OPV) is well established, which has resulted in the elimination of circulating wild poliovirus from our country and decline in number of cases worldwide. As a part of WHO's Endgame Plan, 126 countries decided to take initiative to withdraw type-2 poliovirus and initiate shifting from trivalent OPV (tOPV) to bivalent OPV (bOPV) in April, 2016.[12,13] However, introduction of injectable polio vaccine (IPV) in these countries has increased the demand globally, to over 200 million in 2016 from 80 million in 2013.[12,13] This increase in demand has not been met by increased production due to several technical challenges faced by two global IPV vaccine suppliers. Intradermal IPV administration with fractional doses of IPV (fIPV) (0.1 mL or one-fifth of a full dose) not only offers a potential cost reduction but also allows immunization of a larger number of children.[14] Higher immunogenicity can be obtained from two fractional doses administered via the intradermal route (ID) as compared to one full intramuscular (IM) dose of IPV.[15-18] WHO recommends a two-dose fIPV schedule to countries that are endemic and those with high import risk of wild poliovirus like India.[19]

The NIP schedule already has fIPV but scenario changes when it comes to private practitioners as they suffer irregular and inadequate access to standalone IPV and hence they are compelled to administer combination vaccines. Referring every patient to receive these vaccines is next to impossible for a pediatrician in a private setting.

Recommendations on Polio Vaccines

Regimen containing IPV as combination vaccine in the private settings is recommended. Birth dose of OPV should be set to mandatory. Supplementary immunization activities should continue to provide extra doses of OPV. All healthcare workers should ensure that no eligible child leaves the health facility without polio immunization either IPV or OPV. The bOPV should be continued in place of IPV, only if IPV is not feasible, with a minimum of three doses at 6, 10, and 14 weeks of age. Recommended minimum age of administration of IPV is 6 weeks with the best option being three doses of IM IPV 4 weeks apart in primary immunization schedule. In case of non-availability of standalone IM IPV, combination vaccines containing IPV can be used. If the primary series is started at 8 weeks with the minimum interval between them being 8 weeks then two doses of IM IPV, instead of three doses can be administered. If IPV is not available, the child should be given three doses of bOPV in a 6, 10, and 14 weeks schedule. In such cases, the child should be advised to receive two fractional doses of IPV at a government facility at 6 and 14 weeks of age or at least one dose of IM IPV either standalone or as a part of combination vaccine at 14 weeks.

Rotavirus Vaccines

Infants in developing countries are more susceptible for developing rotavirus gastroenteritis events (RVGE) than those in developed countries.[19] They are burdened with higher mortality and risk of lower vaccine coverage adds to the problem. A schedule of two doses at 10 and 14 weeks may result in incomplete course of vaccination, especially in developing countries because of restriction of upper age limit for rotavirus vaccine administration. Such children would remain immunologically susceptible to get rotavirus infection. The WHO recommends first dose of rotavirus vaccine at 6 weeks or as soon as possible thereafter.[19] No statistically significant difference in efficacy was found between the first dose of monovalent rotavirus vaccine (RV1) at age 6 weeks versus 10–11 weeks.[20] This lays the basis for recommending RV1 in a schedule of 6 and 10 weeks. The recommendations for the schedule of other vaccines remain the same.

Currently, the following live oral rotavirus vaccines are available in India: (1) human monovalent live vaccine (RV1); (2) human bovine pentavalent live vaccine (RV5); (3) Indian neonatal rotavirus live vaccine, 116 E; and (4) bovine rotavirus vaccine–pentavalent (BRV-PV). The most recent among them is BRV-PV, which is pentavalent rotavirus vaccine that contains serotypes G1, G2, G3, G4, and G9 obtained from bovine (UK) X human rotavirus reassortant strains. BRV-PV is a thermostable vaccine, is stable for 2 years at a temperature of 37°C and for 6 months at 40°C, and has a shelf life of 30 months.

Recommendation on Rotavirus Vaccines

The manufacturer's recommendations should be followed for routinely administering any of the available rotavirus vaccines. All the available vaccines have been verified to be safe and immunogenic. The recommended minimum age is 6 weeks for all available brands. Only two doses of RV1 are recommended at 6 and 10 weeks. In case the vaccine product is unknown for any dose in the series or any dose in series was RV5 or RV-116E, two more doses of the same RV vaccine or a total of three doses of RV vaccine should be administered. Age limit for the first dose and the last dose (16 and 32 weeks) should continue in spite of recommendation for increase in the age limit as per recent NIP guidelines.

Typhoid Vaccine

Global burden of typhoid, widespread prevalence of antibiotic-resistant strains of *Salmonella typhi*, and availability of favorable evidence on the efficacy, effectiveness, immunogenicity, safety, and cost-effectiveness of typhoid vaccines provide the bases for WHO's recommendation to use of typhoid vaccines in national programs for the control of typhoid fever.[21,22]

Typhoid conjugate vaccine (TCV) is preferred for all ages and can be safely used in younger children. It also has improved immunological properties and is expected to provide protection for longer duration. The WHO has also recommended TCV for infants and children from 6 months of age as a 0.5 mL single dose, and the same is our recommendation.[23] The need for revaccination with TCV needs more research.[23] Currently, three products of TCV are licensed in India. Two of them contain 25 μg of purified Vi-PS (Vi polysaccharide) of *S. typhi*, and one of them contains 5 μg purified Vi-PS of *S. typhi*. The WHO position paper in 2018 has remarked that the body of evidence for the 5 μg vaccine is very limited.

Recommendation on Typhoid Vaccines

Until more data is generated or available, we recommend only a single dose of TCV 25 μg from 6 months onward routinely. For a child who has received typhoid polysaccharide vaccine, a single dose of TCV is recommended. TCV should be given at an interval of at least 4 weeks after receiving the polysaccharide vaccine. Routine booster for TCV at 2 years is not recommended currently.

Measles, Mumps, and Rubella Vaccines

Measles-containing vaccine [measles, mumps, and rubella (MMR/MR)] should be administered after 9 completed months of age. There are many studies both from India and from other countries demonstrating efficacy and safety of MMR vaccine given at 9 months of age.[24-29] The MR (measles–rubella) vaccine is currently not available in the private sector.

Recommendation on MMR/MR Vaccines

To deal with prevailing mumps infection, we recommend continuing with the existing recommendation of administering MMR instead of MR at 9 months, 15 months, and 4–6 years,[24] or as two doses at 12–15 months of age with the second dose between 4 years and 6 years of age.[30] India successfully completed its MR campaign for children between age of 9 months and 15 years during which an additional dose of MR vaccine was administered, irrespective of previous vaccination status.

Influenza Vaccine

The burden of both mortality and morbidity associated with influenza is well known. Influenza circulation and influenza-associated hospitalization are major public health concerns worldwide and in India. It is estimated that between 1995 and 2010, children below 5 years of age got about 90 million new influenza episodes, out of which 20 million were cases of influenza-associated acute lower respiratory infections (ALRI), among which 1 million cases were of severe ALRI.[31] Total deaths associated with influenza ranged between 28,000 and 111,5000 and majority (99%) of these were from low-to-middle income countries.[31] About 0.16–0.45 million children below 5 years of age die in hospitals each year due to ALRI.[32] A systematic literature review of Indian studies identified that influenza accounted for 20–42% of monthly acute medical illness hospitalizations during the peak rainy season.[33]

As seen in past, the uptake of influenza vaccine is poor in India. Moreover, it was not feasible to recommend routine influenza vaccination to everyone in India and so IAP position paper on influenza in 2013 identified high-risk groups such as the elderly, children below 5 years, medical practitioners, and pregnant women and urged to consider them for this vaccine.[33]

Low-to-middle income countries are more prone for influenza infections and its incidence in children below 5 years of age is threefold higher than those from developed countries, with a 15 times higher mortality.[32] Thus, we can say that the magnitude of the problem is much higher in developing countries (including India) in relation to developed countries. According to geographical location of India, some parts of the country experience a distinct tropical environment because of its location close to the equator. Round the year circulation of influenza viruses peaking during monsoon is seen due to southern hemisphere seasonality. However, another peak season is seen in the northern part of India due to similar northern hemisphere pattern. Seasonal peaks during monsoon and winter increase influenza activity in India and influenza-associated morbidity and mortality are maximum during these peak seasons with high-risk groups being affected most, including children below 5 years. It is recommended to use influenza vaccine routinely in the high-risk group of children below age of 5 years.

Following combinations for the year 2020 (Southern Hemisphere) influenza vaccines are recommended:
- Trivalent vaccines to have—(1) A/Brisbane/02/2018 (H1N1) pdm09-like virus; (2) A/South Australia/34/2019 (H3N2)-like virus; and (3) B/Washington/02/2019-like (B/Victoria lineage) virus. Quadrivalent vaccines to contain the above three, and (4) A B/Phuket/3073/2013-like virus (B/Yamagata lineage).[34]

Recommendations on Influenza Vaccine

It is recommended to provide routine quadrivalent/trivalent inactivated influenza vaccine annually to all children between 6 months and 5 years of age. The latest available influenza vaccine can be administered after 6 months of age, 2–4 weeks prior to the influenza season: two doses at the interval of 1 month in the first year, and one dose annually before the influenza season up to 5 years of age.

Rabies Vaccine

Regarding rabies vaccine, it is suggested to continue with WHO's recommendation in 2018.[35] The WHO recommends to shorten the duration and number of doses for postexposure prophylaxis (PEP) as well as pre-exposure prophylaxis (PrEP). PrEP is recommended in two situations:
1. Children exposed to pets in home
2. Children identified to be vulnerable being bitten by dogs.

The WHO recommends a "1-site vaccine administration on days 0 and 7 for intramuscular administration".[35] For postexposure prophylaxis, recently the WHO35 has recommended a new 4-dose schedule of either of the following:[35]
- 1-site IM administration of vaccine on days 0, 3, 7 and between day 14 and 28, or
- 2-sites IM administration on days 0 and 1-site on days 7 and 21 (intramuscular).

Rabies Human Monoclonal Antibody

The new rabies human monoclonal antibody (RHMAB) is a monoclonal antibody, which has emerged as a safe and potent alternative to rabies immunoglobulin. RHMAB is a completely human IgG1 monoclonal antibody that binds to the ectodomain of the G glycoprotein produced by recombinant technology. It has been demonstrated to neutralize 25 different isolates of wild type or street isolates of rabies virus. RHMAB is not inferior to human rabies immunoglobulin (HRIG) in producing rabies virus-neutralizing antibody.[36] Because of its easy availability, standardized production quality, possibly greater effectiveness, no requirement of animals in its production, and less adverse events, WHO also recommends the use of RHMAB instead of HRIG.[35]

Recommendation on Rabies Vaccine

Rabies human monoclonal antibody is licensed in India (as Rabishield, Serum Institute of India; 40 IU/mL) since 2017. It is recommended to use RHMAB as an alternative to RIG—human or equine—along with rabies vaccines in all category-III bites. The recommended dose is 3.33 IU/kg body weight, preferably at the time of the first vaccine dose. It can be given up to the 7th day after the first dose of vaccine is given. It should be diluted in sterile normal saline to get a volume that is enough to be infiltrated around all the wounds.

■ REFERENCES

1. World Health Organization (2017). WHO position paper on hepatitis B vaccines – July 2017. [online] Available from https://www.who.int/wer/2017/wer9227/en/. [Last accessed December, 2019].
2. Barnett ED (2017). Give first dose of HepB vaccine within 24 hours of birth: AAP. Vol. 140. [online] Available from https://www.aappublications.org/news/2017/08/28/HepB082817. [Last accessed December, 2019].
3. Cherry JD (2014). Pertussis and Immunizations: Facts, Myths, and Misconceptions. Vol. 21. [online] Available from http://aap-ca.org/pertussis-and-immunizations-facts-myths-and-misconceptions/. [Last accessed December, 2019].
4. Winter K, Harriman K, Zipprich J, et al. California pertussis epidemic, 2010. J Pediatr. 2012;161(6):1091-6.
5. Centers for Disease Control and Prevention (CDC). Pertussis epidemic—Washington, 2012. MMWR Morb Mortal Wkly Rep. 2012;61(28):517-22.
6. World Health Organization. Pertussis vaccines: WHO position paper, August 2015—Recommendations. Vaccine. 2016;34(12):1423-5.
7. World Health Organization (2015). Pertussis Vaccine Evidence to Recommendations. [online] Available from https://www.who.int/immunization/position_papers/PertussisGradeTable3.pdf. [Last accessed December, 2019].
8. World Health Organization. Pertussis vaccines: WHO position paper. Wkly Epidemiol Rec. 2005;80(4):31-9.

9. Schmitt HJ, von König CH, Neiss A, et al. Efficacy of acellular pertussis vaccine in early childhood after household exposure. JAMA. 1996;275(1):37-41.
10. Jefferson T, Rudin M, DiPietrantonj C. Systematic review of the effects of pertussis vaccines in children. Vaccine. 2003;21(17-18):2003-14.
11. Carlsson RM, Trollfors B. Control of pertussis—Lessons learnt from a 10-year surveillance programme in Sweden. Vaccine. 2009;27(42):5709-18.
12. World Health Organization (2017). Use of fractional dose IPV in routine immunization programmes: Considerations for decision-making. [online] Available from: https://www.who.int/immunization/diseases/poliomyelitis/endgame_objective2/inactivated_polio_vaccine/fIPV_considerations_for_decision-making_March2017.pdf?ua=1. [Last accessed December, 2019].
13. Indian Academy of Pediatrics (IAP) Advisory Committee on Vaccines and Immunization Practices (ACVIP), Vashishtha VM, Choudhary J, et al. Introduction of Inactivated Poliovirus Vaccine in National Immunization Program and Polio Endgame Strategy. Indian Pediatr. 2016;53 (Suppl 1):S65-9.
14. Bahl S, Verma H, Bhatnagar P, et al. Fractional-Dose Inactivated Poliovirus Vaccine Immunization Campaign—Telangana State, India, June 2016. MMWR Morb Mortal Wkly Rep. 2016;65(33):859-63.
15. Resik S, Tejeda A, Mach O, et al. Immune responses after fractional doses of inactivated poliovirus vaccine using newly developed intradermal jet injectors: A randomized controlled trial in Cuba. Vaccine. 2015;33(2):307-13.
16. Clarke E, Saidu Y, Adetifa JU, et al. Safety and immunogenicity of inactivated poliovirus vaccine when given with measles–rubella combined vaccine and yellow fever vaccine and when given via different administration routes: a phase 4, randomised, non-inferiority trial in The Gambia. Lancet Glob Heal. 2016;4(8):e534-47.
17. Troy SB, Kouiavskaia D, Siik J, et al. Comparison of the immunogenicity of various booster doses of inactivated polio vaccine delivered intradermally versus intramuscularly to HIV-infected adults. J Infect Dis. 2015;211(12):1969-76.
18. Saleem AF, Mach O, Yousafzai MT, et al. Needle adapters for intradermal administration of fractional dose of inactivated poliovirus vaccine: evaluation of immunogenicity and programmatic feasibility in Pakistan. Vaccine. 2017;35(24):3209-14.
19. World Health Organization. Polio vaccines: WHO position paper, March 2016-recommendations. Vaccine. 2017;35(9):1197-9.
20. Weiser KS (2012). Rotavirus Vaccines Schedules: A systematic review of safety and efficacy from randomized controlled trials and observational studies of childhood schedules using RV1 and RV5 vaccines. [online] Available from https://www.who.int/immunization/sage/meetings/2012/april/Soares_K_et_al_SAGE_April_rotavirus.pdf. [Last accessed December, 2019].
21. World Health Organization (2018). Background Paper to SAGE on Typhoid Vaccine Policy Recommendations. [online] Available from: https://www.who.int/immunization/sage/meetings/2017/october/1_Typhoid_SAGE_background_paper_Final_v3B.pdf?ua=1. [Last accessed December, 2019].
22. World Health Organization (2013). Guidelines on the quality, safety and efficacy of typhoid conjugate vaccines. [online] Available from https://www.who.int/

biologicals/areas/vaccines/TRS_987_Annex3.pdf. [Last accessed December, 2019].
23. World Health Organization. Typhoid vaccines: WHO position paper, March 2018—Recommendations. Vaccine. 2019;37(2):214-7.
24. Vashishtha VM, Yewale VN, Bansal CP, et al. IAP perspectives on measles and rubella elimination strategies. Indian Pediatr. 2014;51(9):719-22.
25. Schoub BD, Path M, Johnson S, et al. Measles, mumps and rubella immunization at nine months in a developing country. Pediatr Infect Dis J. 1990;9(4):263-7.
26. Singh R, John TJ, Cherian T, et al. Immune response to measles, mumps & rubella vaccine at 9, 12 & 15 months of age. Indian J Med Res. 1994;100:155-9.
27. Forleo-Neto E, Carvalho ES, Fuentes IC, et al. Seroconversion of a trivalent measles, mumps, and rubella vaccine in children aged 9 and 15 months. Vaccine. 1997;15(17-18):1898-901.
28. Yadav S, Thukral R, Chakarvarti A. Comparative evaluation of measles, mumps & rubella vaccine at 9 & 15 months of age. Indian J Med Res. 2003;118:183-6.
29. Goh P, Lim FS, Han HH, et al. Safety and immunogenicity of early vaccination with two doses of tetravalent measles-mumps-rubella-varicella (MMRV) vaccine in healthy children from 9 months of age. Infection. 2007;35(5):326-33.
30. Centers for Disease Control and Prevention. Measles, Mumps, Rubella (MMR) Vaccination: What Everyone Should Know. [online] Available from https://www.cdc.gov/vaccines/vpd/mmr/public/index.html. [Last accessed December, 2019].
31. Nair H, Brooks WA, Katz M, et al. Global burden of respiratory infections due to seasonal influenza in young children: a systematic review and meta-analysis. Lancet. 2011;378(9807):1917-30.
32. Rudan I, Theodoratou E, Zgaga L, et al. Setting priorities for development of emerging interventions against childhood pneumonia, meningitis and influenza. J Glob Health. 2012;2(1):010304.
33. Venkatesh M, Doarn CR, Steinhoff M, et al. Assessment of burden of seasonal influenza in India and consideration of vaccination policy. Glob J Med Pub Health. 2016;5(5):1-10.
34. Grohskopf LA, Sokolow LZ, Broder KR, et al. Prevention and Control of Seasonal Influenza with Vaccines: Recommendations of the Advisory Committee on Immunization Practices—United States, 2018-19 Influenza Season. MMWR Recomm Reports. 2018;67(03):1-20.
35. World Health Organization. Rabies vaccines: WHO position paper, April 2018—Recommendations. Vaccine. 2018;36(37):5500-3.
36. Gogtay NJ, Munshi R, Ashwath Narayana DH, et al. Comparison of a Novel Human Rabies Monoclonal Antibody to Human Rabies Immunoglobulin for Postexposure Prophylaxis: A Phase 2/3, Randomized, Single-Blind, Noninferiority, Controlled Study. Clin Infect Dis. 2018;66(3):387-95.
37. National Health Mission I (2018). National Immunization Schedule. [online] Available from https://nhm.gov.in/New_Updates_2018/NHM_Components/Immunization/report/National_Immunization_Schedule.pdf. [Last accessed December, 2019].
38. Balasubramanian S, Shah A, Pemde HK, et al. Indian Academy of Pediatrics (IAP) Advisory Committee on Vaccines and Immunization Practices (ACVIP) Recommended Immunization Schedule (2018-19) and Update on Immunization for Children Aged 0 Through 18 Years. Indian Pediatr. 2018;55(12):1066-74.

3.2 PRIMARY IMMUNODEFICIENCY DISORDERS

Jaydeep Choudhury

■ INTRODUCTION

Primary immunodeficiencies (PIDs) are also known as inborn errors of immunity. These are genetic disorders that affect the immune cells either quantitatively or qualitatively leading to disruption of the performance of their functions.[1] It encompasses more than 350 inherited disorders. These disorders are usually due to single-gene mutations. The clinical presentation of PIDs is variable and includes severe or unusual infections, autoimmune diseases, and malignancies.

■ OVERVIEW OF IMMUNE SYSTEM

There are two broad systems of immunity—innate and adaptive.[2]

Innate Immunity

It is an immediate and nonspecific response to an infection. The main mediators are neutrophils, monocytes-macrophages, natural killer (NK) cells, and complement proteins.[2]

Adaptive Immunity

Adaptive immunity builds over time following antigenic challenge by an infection. But it is specific for that particular infection. It is mediated either by B cells or T cells or combined B and T cells. The process helps in generating immunologic memory.[2] As the particular organism has previously been encountered, the memory response to the same organism is quicker. T cell or B cell response by T-cell receptor (TCR) and B-cell receptor (BCR) recognizes different epitopes on the organism. "Immunologic memory" helps in generating quick and robust response.

The adaptive system can be either humoral (B cells) or cellular (T cells) or both. In reality, these T-cell and B-cell responses are functionally interdependent. B-cell response may be TD (T cell dependent) or TI (T cell independent).[1]

T-cells respond mainly to viral infections, intracellular organisms, opportunistic organisms, and tumors. B cells respond to *Staphylococcus aureus*, *Pneumococcus*, and *Haemophilus*. Complement helps B cells. Deficiency in complement function leads to *Neisseria* and *Meningococcus* infection. Macrophages engulf *Mycobacteria* and secrete cytokine IL-12/23. It goes to the T cells and NK cells and makes T-cells (Th-1 cells) and secretes their product interferon gamma (IFNγ). Interferon gamma is a cytokine. It activates macrophage and mononuclear cells to destroy *Mycobacteria*. Dendritic cells also participate in development of adaptive immunity. Dendritic cells and macrophages present antigens (bacteria, viruses, fungi, and parasites) to T and B cells. Thus, all the immune systems interact and coordinate to generate the most effective response.[1]

The summary of the major classification of primary immunodeficiency as per International Union of Immunological Societies is presented in **Table 3.2.1**.

CLASSIFICATION

Primary immunodeficiencies are divided into four groups based mainly on which immune cell is involved:[3]

1. *Phagocyte defects*:
   - *Neutrophils*:
     - *Increased numbers*: Leukocyte adhesion deficiency (LAD)
     - *Decreased numbers*: Severe congenital neutropenia (SCN)
     - *Functional defect*: Chronic granulomatous disease (CGD)
     - *Type of organism*: Abscess-forming pathogens (*Staphylococcus aureus*)
   - Monocyte/macrophage
   - Natural killer cells (NK cells).
2. *Serum complement*: Classical, lectin, and alternative pathways are rare causes.
3. *B-cell defects*: B cells mature into plasma cells, which produce immunoglobulins (antibodies) to contain an infection or prevent it. X-linked agammaglobulinemia (XLA), and common variable immune deficiency (CVID) are examples of B cell defects.
4. *T-cell defects*: T cells deal with viruses, tumors, intracellular pathogens, and opportunistic organisms, e.g. severe combined immune deficiency (SCID).

MANIFESTATIONS OF VARIOUS IMMUNODEFICIENCIES

Immunodeficiencies affecting Cellular and Humoral Immunity

It includes immunodeficiencies affecting both cellular and humoral immunity. There are three subcategories:[3]

1. T-cell-negative, B-cell-positive severe combined immunodeficiencies.
2. T-cell-negative, B-cell-negative severe combined immunodeficiencies.
3. Combined immunodeficiencies (CIDs). It is generally less profound than SCID.

T cells represent the major component of the cellular immune system. It is critical for defense against various viral and fungal infections. Children with

Table 3.2.1: Summary of International Union of Immunological Societies (IUIS) classification groups.

IUIS classification group	Primary immunodeficiency disease category	Characteristics	Examples
I	Cellular and humoral immunodeficiencies	• Recurrent viral, fungal, and bacterial infections • Autoimmunity	• SCID • DOCK8 deficiency • CD40L deficiency • MHC I/II deficiency
II	Syndromic combined immunodeficiencies	• Recurrent viral, fungal, and bacterial infections • Autoimmunity • Nonimmune features • Dysmorphology	• Hyper-IgE (STAT3) • Wiskott-Aldrich syndrome • Cartilage-hair hypoplasia • 22q11.2 deletion syndrome • NEMO deficiency
III	Antibody deficiencies	• Recurrent bacterial sinopulmonary infections	• X-linked (BTK) and autosomal-recessive agammaglobulinemia • Autosomal-recessive hyper-IgM • Selective IgA deficiency
IV	Immune dysregulatory diseases	• Lymphoproliferation • Autoimmunity • Hemophagocytic lymphohistiocytosis	• Chediak-Higashi syndrome • Perforin deficiency • ALPS • STAT3 gain of function • CTLA4 deficiency • LRBA deficiency • IL-10 deficiency
V	Phagocytic diseases	• Severe bacterial infections of the skin, lungs, and lymph nodes • Inflammatory bowel cisease	• Chronic granulomatous disease • Leukocyte adhesion deficiency • GATA2 deficiency • Congenital neutropenia

Contd...

Contd...

IUIS classification group	Primary immunodeficiency disease category	Characteristics	Examples
VI	Innate immunodeficiencies	• Invasive bacterial infections (sepsis, meningitis) often in the absence of fever • Recurrent fungal, mycobacterial, and viral infections	• IRAK4 and MyD88 deficiency • STAT1 gain of function • Interferon gamma receptor deficiency • IRF7 deficiency • TLR3 deficiency
VII	Autoinflammatory diseases	• Recurrent fever, rash, arthritis/arthralgia • Amyloidosis • Inflammatory bowel disease	• Familial Mediterranean fever • Mevalonate kinase deficiency • Muckle-Wells syndrome • NLRP1 deficiency
VIII	Complement deficiencies	• Disseminated neisserial infections • Recurrent pyogenic infections • SLE • Atypical hemolytic uremic syndrome	• Deficiency of complement components (C1 to C9) • Properdin deficiency • Factor D deficiency • Factor H deficiency
IX	Phenocopies of primary immunodeficiencies	• Various phenotypes	• ALPS-SFAS (somatic mutations in *TNFRSF6*) • Mucocutaneous candidiasis due to autoantibodies to IL-17 or IL-22 • Mycobacterial infections due to autoantibodies to IL-6 • Acquired angioedema due to autoantibodies to C1 inhibitor

(SCID: severe combined immunodeficiency; DOCK8: dedicator of cytokinesis 8; CD40L: CD40 ligand; MHC: major histocompatibility complex; IgE: immunoglobulin E; STAT3: signal transducer and activator of transcription 3; NEMO: nuclear factor-kappa-B essential modifier; BTK: Bruton tyrosine kinase; IgM: immunoglobulin M; IgA: immunoglobulin A; ALPS: autoimmune lymphoproliferative syndrome; CTLA4: cytotoxic T lymphocyte-associated antigen 4; LRBA: lipopolysaccharide-responsive beige-like anchor; IL: interleukin; GATA2: GATA-binding protein 2; IRAK4: IL-1 receptor-associated kinase 4; MyD88: myeloid differentiation primary response protein 88; STAT1: signal transducer and activator of transcription 1; IRF7: interferon regulatory factor 7; TLR3: toll-like receptor 3; NLRP1: NLR family pyrin domain-containing 1; SLE: systemic lupus erythematosus; ALPS-SFAS: autoimmune lymphoproliferative syndrome due to somatic FAS mutation; *TNFRSF6*: tumor necrosis factor receptor superfamily member 6)

Source: Adapted from Picard C, Bobby Gaspar H, Al-Herz W, et al. International Union of Immunological Societies: 2017 Primary Immunodeficiency Diseases Committee Report on Inborn Errors of Immunity. J Clin Immunol. 2018;38(1):96-128.

T-cell immunodeficiencies can have combined (T cell and B cell/antibody) defects due to impaired T cell "help" required for generation of antibodies from B cells (B cell positive) or due to defects in the B cells itself (B cell negative).

These children can present with viral, fungal, and bacterial infections, including infections from opportunistic infections like *Pneumocystis jirovecii* and also infections from live vaccines like measles, mumps, rubella, and varicella. The most severe form of T cell/CID is SCID. Children with this condition are born with almost no T cells. Although some patients with SCID have B cells but antibody production is deficient due to absence of T cell help. Children present within the first few months of life with various life-threatening infections. These patients typically die from overwhelming infection before 1 year of age. CIDs do not lead to death in the 1st year of life and typically have higher T cell numbers and T cell function compared with SCID. Initial screening of these children should include enumeration of T cell numbers by flow cytometry (CD3, CD4, and CD8) and assessment of T-cell function by testing proliferation to mitogens (proteins that stimulate T-cell division). Children with HIV infections (a secondary T-cell immunodeficiency) can present similarly to patients with primary T-cell immunodeficiency.

Combined Immunodeficiencies Associated with Syndromic Features

This category includes various subgroups of genetic syndromes with unique clinical features and typical underlying immune defects.[1,3]

CID with Congenital Thrombocytopenia

It is characterized by CID with reduced platelets. Wiskott-Aldrich syndrome (WAS) and WAS protein-interacting protein (WIP) deficiency are characterized by thrombocytopenia with small platelets, bloody diarrhea, and eczema.

CID due to DNA Repair Defects Other than Forms of SCID

Deoxyribonucleic acid (DNA) repair defects can result in both T and B cell abnormalities. Effective DNA repair is essential to generate T cell/B cell diversity. Other than a CID phenotype, many of these conditions are characterized by other clinical features such as intrauterine growth restriction (IUGR), facial dysmorphism, and radiosensitivity.

CID due to Thymic Defects with Congenital Anomalies

T cell precursors require thymus to complete development into functional T cells. Genetic disorders that result in impaired development of the thymus can result in CID. One of the common syndromes is DiGeorge syndrome. It is characterized by structural heart defects, hypoparathyroidism (leading to hypocalcemia), characteristic facial features, and T cell immunodeficiency due to impaired development of the thymus. CHARGE (coloboma of the eye, heart anomalies, choanal atresia, retardation, genital, and ear anomalies) syndrome due to mutations in the *CHD7* gene can present similarly, but they also suffer from eye colobomas, choanal atresia, and ear abnormalities.

CID with Immuno-osseous Dysplasias

These are characterized features of CID with skeletal abnormalities. Patients with cartilage-hair hypoplasia have short-limbed dwarfism with metaphyseal dysostosis. Patients with Schimke immuno-osseous dysplasia have short stature, spondyloepiphyseal dysplasia, and IUGR.

Hyper-IgE Syndromes

The characteristic feature is elevated immunoglobulin E (IgE). Autosomal dominant hyper-IgE syndrome (HIES) is characterized by eczema, hyperextensible joints, retained primary teeth, coarse facial features, and minimal trauma fractures. Children with Netherton syndrome have congenital ichthyosis and bamboo hair atopy. Patients with phosphoglucomutase 3 (PGM3) deficiency have severe atopy and autoimmunity.

Dyskeratosis Congenita, Myelodysplasia, Defective Telomere Maintenance

Telomeres are structures at the ends of linear chromosomes that prevent the loss of genetic material that normally occurs with every cell division. Without proper telomere maintenance, cell senescence and apoptosis can occur, especially in highly proliferative cell types such as lymphocytes. These children can develop nail dystrophy, sparse hair, abnormal skin pigmentation, lung fibrosis, and enteropathy.

CID due to Defects of Vitamin B_{12} and Folate Metabolism

Congenital defects in B_{12} and folate metabolism can result in a CID. These conditions are responsive to nutritional supplementation. Untreated patients suffer from features of intellectual disability.

Anhidrotic Ectodermal Dysplasia with Immunodeficiency

These disorders present with ectodermal dysplasia resulting in variable abnormal skin, conical teeth, and sparse hair.

CID due to Calcium Channel Defects

Lymphocyte activation following antigen stimulation is mediated by calcium entry into the cells. Patients also suffer from hypotonia and dental enamel abnormalities.

Other Defects

Apart from the above-mentioned conditions, there are few other CIDs with unique clinical phenotypes have also been described.

Predominantly Antibody Deficiencies

Predominantly antibody deficiencies are the most common type of immunodeficiency. B cells differentiate into plasma cells that produce antibodies or immunoglobulins such as IgG, IgA, and IgM. Antibodies can bind and opsonize pathogens to facilitate phagocytosis and activate complement proteins. Antibodies also contribute to the development of immune memory.

Children with antibody deficiency usually present with recurrent bacterial infections of the upper and lower respiratory tracts mainly from encapsulated bacteria such as *Streptococcus pneumoniae*. Invasive bacterial infections such as sepsis, meningitis, and osteomyelitis can also occur.

Followings are the subtypes in this category:[3]
- *Agammaglobulinemia with absent B cells*: It includes genetic defects that result in complete arrest of B cell development such as X-linked and autosomal recessive agammaglobulinemia.
- *Severe reduction in at least two serum immunoglobulins, common variable immunodeficiency (CVID) phenotype*: This includes patients with a CVID phenotype (severe reduction in at least two serum immunoglobulins or low numbers of B cells) with either no gene defect specified or a single gene defect.
- *Severe reduction in serum IgG and IgA with normal or elevated IgM, hyper-IgM*: Children in this category have severe reduction in serum IgG and IgA with normal to elevated IgM and normal numbers of B cells.
- *Functional deficiencies with generally normal numbers of B cells*: This includes specific deficiencies in immunoglobulin levels or impaired specific antibody response.

Initial screening for suspected antibody deficiency should include measurement of quantitative IgG, IgA, and IgM.

Diseases of Immune Dysregulation

These conditions result in autoimmune disease with or without recurrent infections:[1]
- *Inherited or familial hemophagocytic lymphohistiocytosis (FHL) syndromes*: These children develop recurrent life-threatening episodes of hemophagocytic lymphohistiocytosis (HLH) with fever and hepatosplenomegaly. They have reduced or absent natural killer (NK) and cytotoxic T lymphocyte (CTL) activity.
- *FHL syndromes with hypopigmentation*: Children in this condition develop recurrent life-threatening HLH and skin or hair hypopigmentation.

Chediak-Higashi syndrome, Griscelli syndrome type 2, and Hermansky-Pudlak syndrome type 2 are some examples.
- *Regulatory T cell (Treg) defects (e.g. IPEX)*: Impaired function of Treg results in systemic autoimmunity.
- *Autoimmunity with or without lymphoproliferation*: Autoimmune polyendocrinopathy with candidiasis and ectodermal dystrophy (APECED).
- *Autoimmune lymphoproliferative syndrome (ALPS)*.
- *Immune dysregulation with colitis*: Children suffer from severe, early-onset inflammatory bowel disease (Crohn's disease or ulcerative colitis) as early as infancy.
- *Susceptibility to Epstein-Barr virus (EBV) and lymphoproliferative conditions*: These children have a unique susceptibility to *EBV* infections that can lead to lymphoproliferation or HLH.

Congenital Defects of Phagocyte Number, Function, or Both

Phagocytes like neutrophils act as the first line of defense to protect the body from harmful bacteria and fungi by ingestion and destruction of these pathogens by activation of proteolytic enzymes. Children with impaired phagocyte immunity present with bacterial and fungal skin, lung and lymph node infections and abscesses:
- *Congenital neutropenia*: Children present with severe congenital neutropenia and infections but no other syndromic features. Some examples are elastase deficiency, X-linked neutropenia, and glycogen storage disease type 1b.
- *Defects of motility*: Along with severe congenital neutropenia and infections, they also have syndromic disease features such as dysmorphisms, developmental delay, and other nonimmune clinical features. Examples include leukocyte adhesion deficiency, Shwachman-Diamond syndrome, and cystic fibrosis.
- *Defects of respiratory burst*: Examples include chronic granulomatous disease and glucose-6-phosphate dehydrogenase (G6PD) deficiency class I.
- *Other nonlymphoid defects*: These children have defective phagocyte function but neutrophil oxidative burst testing (DHR assay) is normal. One example is pulmonary alveolar proteinosis.

Defects in Intrinsic and Innate Immunity

The adaptive immune system, which comprises B cells or antibodies and T cells, is designed to recognize and eliminate the specific pathogens. The limitation of the adaptive immune system is the lag period and slow response. It can take about 4 weeks to generate protective IgG antibodies following immunization. In contrast, the innate immune system is adept to counter the infection immediately by recognizing the unique features of pathogens that are not there in the host cells.

Defects in intrinsic and innate immunity are the following:
- *Mendelian susceptibility to mycobacterial disease (MSMD)*: MSMD is characterized by a narrow vulnerability to poorly virulent mycobacteria, such as bacillus Calmette-Guérin (BCG) vaccines and other environmental mycobacteria. The severe presentation is disseminated bacillus Calmette-Guérin (BCG) reaction.
- *Epidermodysplasia verruciformis (HPV)*: These patients suffer from recurrent cutaneous warts from human papillomavirus (HPV).
- *Predisposition to severe viral infection*: Severe recurrent viral infections such as influenza or herpes viral infections are the characteristic features.
- *Herpes simplex encephalitis (HSE)*: Children develop HSE during primary infection with herpes simplex virus type 1 (HSV1). Specific assays examining the toll-like receptor 3 (TLR3) pathway are required as routine immune screening tests are normal.
- *Predisposition to invasive fungal diseases*: These children have an unusual predilection to invasive fungal infections, particularly of the central nervous system (CNS).
- *Predisposition to mucocutaneous candidiasis*: Severe or persistent *Candida* infections can represent a defect in mucosal immunity.
- *TLR signaling pathway deficiencies with bacterial susceptibility*: Children with defects in TLR signaling suffer from various invasive bacterial infections like meningitis, sepsis, arthritis, osteomyelitis, and various abscesses, but fever is often not present in these patients. The usual pathogens include *S. pneumoniae*, *Staphylococcus aureus*, and *Pseudomonas aeruginosa*.
- *Other inborn errors of immunity related to nonhematopoietic tissues*: It includes isolated congenital asplenia, trypanosomiasis, acute necrotizing encephalopathy, osteopetrosis, and hidradenitis suppurativa that are due to genetic defects.

Autoinflammatory Disorders

These conditions are due to overactivation of innate inflammatory pathways that cause excessive release of proinflammatory cytokines, which causes recurrent fever and tissue damage. There is history of recurrent inflammation without evidence of other disorders like cyclic neutropenia or infections. Genetic testing can help to confirm the diagnosis:[3]
- *Type 1 interferonopathies*: These disorders usually have neurologic features.
- *Defects affecting the inflammasome*: This is characterized by secretion of proinflammatory cytokines such as tumor necrosis factor (TNF) and IL-1-

beta. Children suffer from recurrent episodes of fever, arthritis, arthralgia, and abdominal pain. Children are at risk for developing inflammatory bowel disease. Familial Mediterranean fever (FMF) is a typical example.
- *Noninflammasome-related conditions*: Children in this subgroup suffer from recurrent noninfectious inflammation of the skin, bone, and joints. Examples include pyogenic sterile arthritis, pyoderma gangrenosum, acne (PAPA) syndrome and deficiency of the IL-1 receptor antagonist (DIRA).

Complement Deficiencies

The complement arm of the immune system protects the body from bacterial pathogens by opsonizing bacteria and also forming a membrane attack complex to cause lysis of bacteria. Complement proteins also play a role in clearance of apoptotic cell debris, which can cause autoimmune inflammation. There are three main complement protein pathways—(1) classical complement, (2) alternative complement, and (3) lectin pathway.

Early classical complement component deficiencies (C1q, C1r, C1s, C2, C4, and C3) present with systemic lupus erythematosus (SLE) and susceptibility to infections from encapsulated bacteria. Terminal classical complement component deficiencies (C5, C6, C7, C8, and C9) present with a unique susceptibility to recurrent *Neisseria* meningitis.

Similar to terminal complement deficiency, alternative complement pathway defects due to properdin or factor D present with recurrent meningitis. A deficiency of factor H and factor I (both complement regulatory proteins) can cause a phenotype of recurrent atypical hemolytic uremic syndrome or neisserial susceptibility.

■ DIAGNOSIS OF IMMUNODEFICIENCY

History

Pre- and perinatal history are vital for information regarding congenital infection, prematurity, and intrauterine growth retardation.[4] These conditions may be associated with immune defects. Delayed separation of the umbilical cord, when local infection is not present, may suggest neutrophil defect.

Majority of the children with PID present with an infective problem.[5] The important considerations in such a condition are the age of onset of infections, site of infection, isolated or suspected organisms, and the time to recovery with standard treatments.

An immunodeficient child usually have more than usual infections, take longer to resolve, and may have an atypical course compared to other children.[5] The type of organism involved, particularly atypical infections, should direct further investigations.

It is generally believed that up to eight upper respiratory tract infections (URTI) per year are normal in the preschool years.[1] Hence, the occurrence of frequent URTI in a young child is not indicative of an underlying immune defect unless associated with frequent bacterial infections. Infections with common organisms may run an atypical course in a child with PID. They are unusually severe, or they fail to respond to standard treatments. Infections may be caused by atypical organisms also.

There may be various other clues from history. Failure to thrive is common in immunodeficiency. Diarrhea may be due to chronic or recurrent infection or autoimmune enteropathy. Features suggestive of bronchiectasis, such as productive cough, could also be present. Allergic or atopic features are common and may be severe. Autoimmune and malignant diseases, though not common, have an increased incidence.

A history of consanguinity may be present. Family history may reveal other children with unusual, sometimes fatal infectious complications in accordance with an autosomal recessive or X-linked inheritance. In some conditions, e.g. IgA deficiency, there may be a family history of collagen vascular or other immune-mediated disease. Older relatives who are carriers of or who are affected by milder variants of primary immune defects may have autoimmune manifestations like mouth ulcers and SLE variant in chronic granulomatous disease (CGD) or have a history of malignant disease or Wiskott-Aldrich syndrome.

Clinical Examination

Routine physical examination such as age and sex, vital signs, BCG scar, recurrent oral ulcers, absence of tonsils and adenoids, enlarged lymph nodes, hepatosplenomegaly, and dystrophic facial features in particular. Serial growth charts should be assessed to assess failure to thrive, poor weight gain, and loss of weight.

Physical examination should be focused toward potential sites of infection like throat, ears, and sinuses. Oral cavity and napkin area for candidiasis should be routinely examined. The presence or absence of lymphoid tissue should be noted. Cutaneous problems consistent with an immune defect should be looked into. In more severe antibody states such as X-linked agammaglobulinemia, there is a lack of tonsils and lymphoid tissues. Some diseases may have specific physical signs, such as oculocutaneous albinism in Chediak-Higashi syndrome, typical facies and/or cleft palate in DiGeorge syndrome, telangiectasia or neurological abnormalities in ataxia telangiectasia, and disproportionate short stature in some forms of combined immunodeficiency.[1,4]

The focus of systemic clinical examination is the three exposed mucocutaneous areas—skin, respiratory system, and gastrointestinal (GI) system.[2]

Followings are the signs and symptoms which should raise the suspicion of PID:
- *Skin*: Erythroderma, severe eczema, pustules, dystrophic nails, albinism, silvery hair, alopecia, and mucocutaneous candidiasis particularly around mouth and anus.
- *Respiratory system*: Sinusitis, otitis media, upper and lower respiratory tract infections including pneumonia after the age of 6 months in B-cell defects.
- *GI system*: Persistent diarrhea due to opportunistic organisms like *Cryptococcus*, Giardia, *Cryptosporidium*, *Clostridium difficile*.

Primary immunodeficiency should be suspected in:[1]
- Family history of immune deficiency
- Single infection with an unusual or opportunistic organism
- Single infection, which is severe, has an atypical course or occurs at an atypical age
- Recurrent minor bacterial infections or more than one episode of serious bacterial infection.

Presence of two or more of the following ten criteria proposed by Jeffrey Modell Foundation suggests the possibility of an underlying PID:
1. More than four ear infections in 1 year
2. More than two severe sinus infections in 1 year
3. More than 2 months treatment of antibiotics with little effect
4. More than two pneumonias per year
5. Insufficient weight gain or growth delay
6. Recurrent deep skin or organ abscesses (liver and lungs)
7. Persistent thrush in mouth or fungal infection on skin
8. Need for intravenous antibiotics to clear infections
9. More than two deep-seated infections (septicemia and meningitis)
10. Family history of a primary immunodeficiency.

Consequences of PID

- Repeated, persistent, or unusual infections and at unexpected ages
- Autoimmune phenomena like diabetes in infants or neutropenia
- *Malignancies*: Dysregulated immune cells are unable to check excessive growth of susceptible cells or cells susceptible to transformation.

Laboratory Investigations

Human immunodeficiency virus should be ruled out in all children with suspected immunodeficiency.

Hematology:
Complete blood count and peripheral smear examination often provides diagnostic clue:
- Absolute neutrophil count (ANC) for neutropenia
- Absolute lymphocyte count (ALC) at birth and later
- Platelet count including mean platelet volume (MPV)—helpful in diagnosing Wiskott-Aldrich syndrome (WAS)
- Peripheral blood smears for granules—Chediak-Higashi syndrome.

Tests of Innate Immunity

Complement: C3 and C4 can be measured. But normal levels of C3 and C4 do not exclude deficiencies of other complement components. Hence, it is better to assess the functional integrity of the complement pathway as deficiency in any one component will result in a failure of lysis.[1] However, the most common reason for failure of lysis is active infection, with consumption of complement components, or degradation of complement components.

Complement disorders are evaluated by checking the components of classic pathway by CH50 assay. The components of alternative pathway are checked by CH100 or AH50 assay.

Neutrophil function tests: The three main components of neutrophil function are chemotaxis, phagocytosis, and activation of the respiratory burst.

Chemiluminescence: This test evaluates the opsonizing capacity of patient serum.[1] Phagocytosis of organisms by neutrophils and monocytes results in the production of oxygen-free radicals. These react with unsaturated lipids, nucleic acids, and peptides of microbes to form unstable intermediates. When these intermediates return to their original state, light energy is emitted. This chemiluminescence is readily measured with a spectrophotometer or chemiluminometer.

Nitroblue tetrazolium reduction test (NBT): NBT is a yellow dye readily taken up by phagocytes. Upon stimulation, it is reduced to the purple dye formazan by the oxidative burst. In normal individuals, at least 95% of neutrophils should contain a purple deposit in stimulated cells.

Flow cytometric assays of neutrophil function:
- *Phagocytosis*: Fluorescently labeled organisms or inert agents can be used to assess the phagocytic ability of neutrophils.
- *Oxidative burst*: Neutrophils take up dihydrorhodamine and activation of the respiratory burst, which results in fluorescence within cells. It can be assessed using the flow cytometer. As with an NBT, carriers for CGD can also be detected.

Enzyme assays: Neutrophil-killing defects may occur in myeloperoxidase and glucose-6-phosphate dehydrogenase (G6PD deficiency). These can be assayed separately.

Tests for Adaptive Immunity

Immunoglobulins: IgG is the main circulating immunoglobulin.[2] IgA, IgM, IgD, and IgE are also found in serum but in lesser amount. IgG, IgA, and IgM are quantified by nephelometry. All five classes of immunoglobulin are low at birth and gradually mature over the first 5 years of life. A reduced or absent gamma IgG may be seen in hypogammaglobulinemia. Results should be evaluated with reference to age-specific normal ranges. Measurement of IgE is indicated, if hyper-IgE syndrome is suspected.

Specific antibody responses can be assessed to proteins in tetanus, diphtheria, and pneumococcal vaccines.

Cell-mediated immunity: Cell-mediated immunity can be assessed by measuring the number and function of cells. Lymphocytes can be enumerated using flow cytometry. The different light scatter properties of cells enable populations of neutrophils, monocytes, and lymphocytes to be differentiated.

Lack of a delayed hypersensitivity skin test response to candida, mumps, or tetanus in children older than 1 year indicates a T-cell disorder.

■ TREATMENT OF PRIMARY IMMUNODEFICIENCY DISORDERS

Supportive Care

Children with immunodeficiency require a holistic approach in supportive care. Particular focus should be on nutritional status and the management of dietary intolerances secondary to the gastrointestinal problems, which frequently occur. Prevention and treatment of infections is one of the most important aspects of supportive care.[2] Supporting the emotional needs of the family is also very important.

General Measures for Prevention of Infections

Newborns with severe immunodeficiency disorder should be in isolation, including limited numbers of persons involved with care. Breastfeeding should be encouraged. Strict handwashing procedures should be maintained. Proper immunization should be followed.

Specific Measures for Prevention of Infections

Cotrimoxazole prophylaxis against *Pneumocystis carinii* should be given for defects of cell-mediated immunity. Antifungal prophylaxis should be used in combined immunodeficiencies or phagocytic cell defects.

Treatment of Infections

Children with PID are prone to unusual infections. Broader spectrum antimicrobial cover may be needed. A policy of vigorous and early antimicrobial treatment of infections should be followed.

Replacement Immunoglobulin Therapy

This is the mainstay of treatment for the more severe antibody states and various combined immunodeficiencies. The need for immunoglobulin must be evaluated on an individual patient basis. Absolute indications include quantitative defects and qualitative defects.[4]

Hematopoietic Stem Cell Transplantation

All primary T lymphocyte and phagocyte immunodeficiency disorders are potentially correctable by hematopoietic stem cell transplantation (HSCT).[1]

Enzyme Replacement

Some reconstitution of immunological function can be achieved by administering replacement enzyme in ADA deficiency.

■ REFERENCES

1. Steihm RE, Ochs HD, Winkelstein JA. Immunological Disorders in Infants and Children, 5th edition. Philadelphia: WB Saunders; 2005.
2. Currimbhoy Z, Madkaikar D, Desai MM. Primary immunodeficiency diseases (PIDs). BJ Wadia Hospital for Children, Mumbai, India.
3. Bousfiha A, Jeddane L, Picard C, et al. The 2017 IUIS phenotypic classification for primary immunodeficiencies. J Clin Immunol. 2018;38(1):129-43.
4. Picard C, Bobby Gaspar H, Al-Herz W, et al. International Union of Immunological Societies: 2017 Primary Immunodeficiency Diseases Committee Report on Inborn Errors of Immunity. J Clin Immunol. 2018;38(1):96-128.
5. Yu JE, Orange JS, Demirdag YY. New primary immunodeficiency diseases: context and future. Curr Opin Pediatr. 2018;30(6):806-20.

CHAPTER 4

INFECTIOUS DISEASES

4.1 Recent Advances in Diagnosis of Tuberculosis
Tanu Singhal, Camilla Rodrigues

4.2 Diagnosis, Treatment and Management of Influenza (Indian Perspective)
Digant D Shastri

4.3 Adenotonsillectomy: When it is Essential?
Ashok S Kapse

4.4 HIV and AIDS: Diagnosis and Management
Ira Shah

4.5 New Viral Infections
Dhanya Dharmapalan

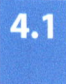

4.1 RECENT ADVANCES IN DIAGNOSIS OF TUBERCULOSIS

Tanu Singhal, Camilla Rodrigues

■ INTRODUCTION

Tuberculosis (TB) is one of the leading public health problems facing mankind today with an estimated 10 million new cases annually and approximately 1.45 million deaths in the year 2018. Human immunodeficiency virus (HIV) and TB together form a deadly intersection—around 8.6% of patients with TB are infected with HIV. Pediatric TB contributes to around 11% of the total burden of TB with an estimated 1 million cases annually. The annual incidence of rifampicin-resistant TB cases is estimated to be around 500,000 with 78% being multidrug-resistant (MDR) of which 10% are extensively drug-resistant (XDR). It is estimated that one-third of the world's population is latently infected with TB forming a pool of patients from which active cases arise.[1] India contributes to one-fourth of the incidence and mortality due to TB with 2.7 million annual cases.[1]

If we have to control the menace of TB, we need to diagnose it early and detect drug resistance at the outset. The diagnosis of pediatric TB is particularly challenging. Access to specimens whether pulmonary or extrapulmonary is difficult as compared to adults. Smear positivity is low as the disease is largely paucibacillary. We discuss herewith recent advances in diagnosis of TB in children along with what is currently practiced.

■ BASICS OF DIAGNOSIS OF TUBERCULOSIS

The diagnosis of TB is based on the following modalities:
- *Clinical diagnosis of pediatric TB* rests on symptoms, signs, and history of recent contact. The cardinal symptoms of pulmonary TB include history of fever, cough lasting for 2 weeks or more, and weight loss. A "recent contact" alludes to contact with a patient in the past 2 years who has "bacteriologically-positive pulmonary TB". The clinical manifestations of extrapulmonary TB (EPTB) depend on the site of involvement and include fever, weight loss, neck swellings, headache, vomiting, seizures, abdominal pain, back pain, and joint pains or swelling depending on the site of involvement.[2]
- *Radiology*: This includes X-rays, ultrasonography (USG), computerized tomography (CT) scan, magnetic resonance imaging (MRI), and the positron emission tomography (PET) scan.
- *Histopathology and cytology*: The classical histopathological feature of TB is necrotizing granulomatous inflammation with Langerhans giant cells

and acid-fast bacilli (AFB). Cytology and biochemistry of fluids [pleural, pericardial, ascitic, and cerebrospinal fluid (CSF)] show predominant lymphocytes with high protein.
- *Detection of latent infection* is done by skin tests and gamma interferon assays. However, these tests do not differentiate infection from disease; negative tests do not rule out disease either. These tests should not be used to diagnose active disease.
- *Microbiology*: This is the gold standard for diagnosis. It broadly includes smear microscopy, cultures, and molecular methods.

The diagnosis of TB disease is usually based on a combination of the above mentioned methods. While the aim is to establish a microbiologic diagnosis in each case for 100% specificity and knowledge of drug resistance, the same is always not possible and treatment may have to be initiated on an empiric basis.

Radiology

The diagnosis of TB has come a long way from the chest X-ray (CXR). CXR is undoubtedly the starting point for a suspected case of TB. Some features of CXR are pathognomonic for TB including miliary mottling, mediastinal adenopathy, and cavitatory consolidation. However, CXR is neither sensitive nor specific enough especially in early disease. CXR is, however, invaluable in follow-up of disease.

Ultrasonography

Ultrasonography is invaluable in picking up certain features of tuberculous cervical adenopathy such as matting and necrosis and also aids fine-needle aspiration cytology (FNAC) from the soft center of the node. It is invaluable in picking up small pleural effusions. Endobronchial ultrasound-guided transbronchial needle aspiration (EBUS-TBNA) is being increasingly done though more often in adults as against children.[3] USG is also able to pick up changes of abdominal TB including abdominal nodes, ileocecal thickening, ascites, and peritoneal thickening.

CT Scan

Contrast-enhanced CT has revolutionized the diagnosis of TB. Chest CT is more sensitive and specific for diagnosis of TB than CXR and is far superior in picking up necrotic mediastinal nodes, early miliary mottling, endobronchial nodules, and tree-in-bud appearance.[4] However, being very sensitive, it may pick up small necrotic nodes that are due to latent infection rather than active disease and hence the results should be interpreted carefully. Contrast-enhanced abdominal CT is also more sensitive than USG in picking up abdominal TB, especially granulomas in liver and spleen. CT plays an important role in guiding biopsy procedures. Cranial CT scan can pick up features of central nervous system (CNS) TB including leptomeningeal enhancement, granulomas, tuberculomas, and hydrocephalus.

MRI and Positron Emission Tomography Scan

MRI is superior to CT in the diagnosis of CNS and osteoarticular TB. Whole body PET-CT is emerging as an important investigation in pyrexia of unknown origin (PUO), but is expensive and does not differentiate TB from neoplastic etiology.[5] PET scans have been used to indicate extraneural sites of TB to upscale the diagnosis of TB meningitis (TBM) from possible TBM to probable TBM as per the TBM criteria.

ADVANCES IN SAMPLE COLLECTION

Pulmonary

Expectorated sputum is the simplest method in obtaining sample in patients with suspected pulmonary TB. This may not be always possible in young children and what is generally obtained is saliva. Alternate methods of sample collection have been developed.

Though *gastric aspirate* has been around for a long time, it has recently been evaluated in several trials and methods were standardized.[6] Obtaining a gastric aspirate sample after 4 hours of fasting in an ambulatory setup is more convenient than overnight fasting with only a slight reduction in yield.[7]

Induced sputum is another method of obtaining a respiratory sample. Here after premedication with a bronchodilator, hypertonic saline is administered to induce sputum that is either spontaneously expectorated or collected after nasopharyngeal suction. The sensitivity of gastric aspirate and induced sputum is almost similar. While gastric aspirate is more invasive and needs technical expertise as compared to induced sputum, it is less hazardous in transmission of infection to healthcare personnel and is more suited for infants and small children.

Bronchoscopy and bronchoalveolar lavage allow obtaining dedicated specimens from involved areas but is invasive, technically challenging, and not always available.[8] It is, therefore, indicated in cases of suspected drug-resistant TB or when the diagnosis is in doubt.

Extrapulmonary

Diagnosis of EPTB is more challenging since sample collection methods are more invasive. This may range from relatively simple methods such as pleural and peritoneal tap, lumbar puncture to tissue biopsies. Advances have been made in obtaining radiology-guided biopsies of involved sites for definitive diagnosis of TB. This is unlike the past where diagnosis of EPTB was largely based on clinical presentation and radiology, often leading to empiric therapy.

■ SMEAR MICROSCOPY

Ziehl-Neelsen Staining

Ziehl-Neelsen (ZN) staining of specimens is the conventional method for smear diagnosis of TB.[9] It is fast and cheap. It is, however, insensitive, as it needs at least 5,000–10,000 bacteria/mL for detection. The smear positivity in childhood pulmonary TB is only 10% in gastric aspirate or induced sputum specimens and even lower in extrapulmonary samples. Besides, differentiating tuberculous from nontuberculous mycobacteria (NTM) from smear examination is not reliable. Since microscopy cannot differentiate between dead and live bacilli, it cannot be used as a follow-up diagnostic test. The first smear examination detects 85% of the cases while the second smear detects another 12%. The third specimen adds only 2–3% to the diagnostic yield.[10] Therefore, the Revised National Tuberculosis Control Program (RNTCP) is now advocating only two specimens for diagnosis as against three earlier.

Advances in Smear Microscopy

Advances have been made in smear microscopy and these include *fluorescent stains* and *light-emitting diodes (LEDs) microscopy*. Fluorescent stains allow for rapid screening of slides unlike the ZN stain. Earlier fluorescent microscopes using the quartz-halogen lamps or high-pressure mercury vapor lamps were expensive, delicate, and required careful handling. LEDs are more robust, sustainable, and user-friendly, thus allowing advantages of fluorescence microscopy (FM) at peripheral healthcare systems. They require less power and thus reduce the cost incurred and the World Health Organization (WHO) has recommended replacement of conventional microscopy with LED microscopy.[11] There is a move in the RNTCP as well to replace conventional microscopy with LED microscopy at some centers. However, there have been problems reported with fluorescent stains including degradation in field conditions thus preventing a second examination.[12]

Sodium hypochlorite microscopy in which the sputum/sample is digested with household bleach is another method under evaluation. Preliminary data suggests that it increases the detection rate by 15%.[9]

Vital fluorescent staining is another development in the field of microscopy. As mentioned earlier, smears cannot differentiate between live and dead bacilli and hence cannot be used to monitor therapy. The definitive method for monitoring response to therapy is culture, which takes time to come in. A fluorescent dye called fluorescein diacetate (FDA), which only stains living cultivable cells, is being evaluated to monitor response to therapy.[13]

Automated Microscopy Techniques

Automated microscopy techniques by TBDx (Signature Mapping Medical Sciences, USA), which involve robotic loading of slides and analysis of high-resolution digital images, can analyze 200 slides in minutes. Preliminary studies show better sensitivity as compared to human reading but lower specificity and thus require manual review of positive slides. Further studies are planned. Another innovation is the *CellScope* that is a portable digital fluorescent microscope that provides digitally enlarged images for review.[14] *Automated smart microscopy* that scans for AFB using an artificial intelligence (AI)-based algorithm with machine learning and digital imaging is possibly the future of ZN microscopy. Automatic image capture and recognition tremendously reduce the workload of manual microscopy.

■ CULTURE TECHNIQUES AND PHENOTYPIC SUSCEPTIBILITY TESTING

Culture Techniques

Culture is the gold standard for diagnosis of TB and detects up to 10–100 bacteria/mL.[9] Cultures also allow for detection of drug resistance to first- and second-line drugs and assess response to therapy. Disadvantages of culture include need for technical expertise, long turnaround times (TATs), and false negativity if the patient has been on antitubercular drugs or antibiotics that also have antitubercular activity (e.g. quinolones, aminoglycosides, linezolid).

Conventional TB cultures entail the use of an egg-based culture media [Löwenstein–Jensen (LJ) media] or agar-based media (Middlebrook). The TAT is long ranging up to 6–8 weeks. Drug susceptibility takes another 2–3 weeks; thus, diagnosis of drug-resistant TB may take up to 70 days from the time of submission of sample.

Liquid cultures are a significant improvement over the conventional media. The mycobacterial growth indicator tube (MGIT) is based on the principle of nonradiometric detection of oxygen consumption by fluorescence. When bacteria grow, they utilize oxygen, allowing it to fluoresce when placed under ultraviolet (UV) light (either manual or automated). The MGIT 960 system allows for simultaneous processing of 960 cultures and is widely used in India.[15] Other liquid cultures in use and endorsed by the WHO include the MB/BacT, VersaTREK/ESP, microcolony detection [microscopic observation drug susceptibility (MODS)], and nitrate reduction or colorimetric assay. The TAT for liquid cultures for a smear-positive sample is around 9 days and that of a smear-negative sample is 16 days. A negative report is issued after 42 days of incubation. Drug susceptibility testing (DST) takes another 1–2 weeks. Liquid cultures are prone to contamination if care is not taken and require on-site maintenance by the manufacturer and strict quality control.

Identification of the mycobacterial culture as *Mycobacterium tuberculosis* (*M. tuberculosis*) complex (MTBC) is now done using the MPT64 test; the MTBC consists of *M. tuberculosis, M. bovis, M. microti, M. canetti,* and *M. africanum* among some other species. MPT64 is an antigen present only in MTBC and not in atypical mycobacteria. This test is a strip-based test with very high sensitivity and specificity and is much faster than the conventional para-aminobenzoic acid-based methods and is widely used in Indian laboratories for rapid identification of MTBC. Other methods for identification of *mycobacterium tuberculosis* (MTB) from a mycobacterial culture include matrix-assisted laser desorption and ionization time-of-flight (MALDI-TOF) analysis and molecular probes.

Phenotypic Susceptibility Testing

Phenotypic susceptibility testing is usually done by the 1% proportion method. Here the culture is inoculated into both drug-free and drug-replete media and the growth compared. Phenotypic susceptibility testing is faster with liquid cultures as compared to solid cultures. The breakpoints for defining resistance are based on epidemiologic cutoffs. Among the first-line drugs, susceptibility testing is very reliable for isoniazid (INH) and rifampicin, but less so for streptomycin and ethambutol (EMB). Susceptibility to pyrazinamide is tested by demonstrating the presence or absence of pyrazinamidase enzyme and is not very reliable. Phenotypic susceptibility testing for second-line drugs is even more complicated and only some laboratories are accredited for the same. Here again, susceptibility testing of quinolones and aminoglycosides is more accurate than that for ethionamide, para-aminosalicylic acid. Cycloserine and terizidone susceptibility testing is not available.[16] Laboratories are now testing susceptibility for other second-line drugs including clofazimine, linezolid, bedaquiline, and delamanid.[17]

Since mycobacterial cultures and susceptibility testing require expertise and logistics, in the public sector, these tests are reserved for suspected cases of drug resistance. However, the sensitivity of liquid cultures is more than the conventional molecular methods. Hence, in the private sector, one should always send samples for MGIT culture along with smear and molecular methods and request for phenotypic DST when indicated.

■ MOLECULAR DIAGNOSTICS

Molecular methods have been a game changer in the diagnosis of TB. Polymerase chain reaction (PCR)-based methods have been around for more than 2 decades, but these had limited sensitivity and specificity. Since most of these methods had separate systems for amplification and detection, contamination led to high rate of false positives. The current WHO guidelines recommend against the use of these older PCR methods for diagnosis of TB. The molecular methods available and the WHO endorsed for diagnosis of TB are discussed below.

Cartridge-based Nucleic Acid Amplification Methods

Cartridge-based nucleic acid amplification test (CBNAAT) has been the biggest game changer in the diagnosis of TB. *Xpert MTB/RIF* from the Foundation for Innovative New Diagnostics (FIND) was introduced exactly a decade ago.[18] It is a real-time semi-quantitative nested PCR system which can detect MTB and rifampicin resistance directly from clinical specimens as well as from cultures. The lower limit of detection is 131 cfu/mL. It uses three specific primers and five unique molecular probes to ensure high degree of specificity. The primers amplify a portion of the *rpoB* gene 81 bp RIF resistance determining region. The probes can differentiate between wild type (WT) and conserved sequence and mutations in the core region.

Though the test is approved only for sputum samples, it has been used in almost all types of pulmonary and extrapulmonary samples including stool and urine. The test cannot be carried out in blood or specimens with significant blood contamination (e.g. endometrial tissue). The sample is mixed with the sample reagent, which inactivates 99.9% of the TB bacilli and then is inserted in a cartridge, which is then inserted into the machine, which is small enough to be put on the desktop **(Fig. 4.1.1)**. Since the cartridge is self-contained, there is no risk of contamination. The TAT is 45 minutes and the result sheet mentions whether MTB complex is detected or not, the quantity of load (very low, low, medium, and high), and whether the isolate is rifampicin resistant. In some cases, if the load detected is very low, the rifampicin resistance results may be indeterminate or false positive (as the amplicon cannot bind the primer and the WT appears to absent).[19]

The sensitivity of Xpert MTB/RIF for smear-positive samples is more than 95% and specificity is more than 99%. For smear-negative but culture-positive sputum samples, the sensitivity is around 70%.[20] The sensitivity of Xpert for childhood pulmonary TB in gastric aspirate or induced sputum is lower and depends on the severity of disease. The sensitivity varies from 30% in primary complex to 70% in progressive primary disease or cavitatory disease.[21] The sensitivity of Xpert in extrapulmonary disease varies from 70% to 80% in pus, biopsies, and fine-needle aspirates, 50% to 70% in CSF, and only 20% to 30% in pleural, peritoneal, and pericardial fluid.[22,23] Xpert MTB/RIF in the stool has been found to be another novel sample for diagnosis of pulmonary TB in children, however with sensitivities lower than gastric aspirate.

The sensitivity and specificity of Xpert MTB/RIF for diagnosis of rifampicin resistance is around 99%. However, if the pretest probability of rifampicin resistance is low, the positive predictive value is low and needs to be confirmed

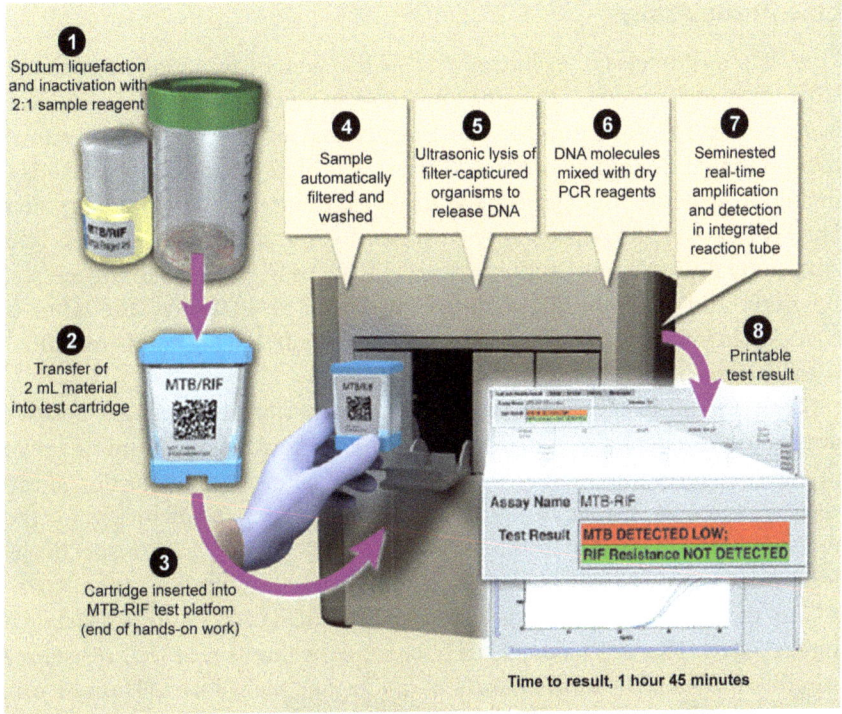

Fig. 4.1.1: Xpert MTB/RIF system.[18]
(DNA: deoxyribonucleic acid; MTB: *Mycobacterium tuberculosis*;
PCR: polymerase chain reaction; RIF: rifampicin)

by a second molecular test [Xpert/line probe assay (LPA)] in another sample.[24] Experience from the RNTCP, however, indicates that most samples which tested as rifampicin resistant on the Xpert even with low pretest probability of resistance tested as resistant in the second sample by a second method. Hence, there is a plan to modify the algorithm and eliminate the need for a second test for those samples, which tested rifampicin resistant even with low pretest probability of resistance (personal communication).

Xpert MTB/RIF has indeed revolutionized the diagnosis of TB and resistance. There are some limitations though. It does not give information about the INH susceptibility. About 10–15% of isolates that are rifampicin susceptible are INH resistant. Since it detects the deoxyribonucleic acid (DNA) of dead and living bacilli, it cannot be used as a follow-up test to monitor response to therapy. Besides, it does miss out on very paucibacillary disease. The Xpert is also not able to differentiate between different mycobacteria of the MTB complex, especially *M. tuberculosis* and *M. bovis*. Some of these limitations of the Xpert have been addressed in some other molecular methods that are discussed later.

Line Probe Assay

This strip test detects mycobacterial DNA and genetic mutations associated with drug resistance from smear-positive sputum specimens or culture isolates.[9] LPA identifies the species of the mycobacteria and detects resistance to both INH and rifampicin. Each strip consists of 27 reaction zones (bands), including six controls, eight *rpoB* WT and four mutants (MUT) probes, one *katG* WT and two MUT probes, and two *inhA* WT and four MUT probes. Two commercially available products are: (1) INNO-LiPA assay—Innogenetics, Belgium, and (2) Hain Lifescience GenoType® MTBDRplus (the latter is available in India). Theoretically, the TAT is 5–6 hours, but the entire procedure usually takes up to 72 hours.

It has a good sensitivity and specificity when performed on smear-positive and on culture isolates. Sensitivity, specificity, and positive and negative predictive values approximate between 98% and 99% for the detection of RIF resistance; while it is 94.2%, 99.7%, 99.1%, and 97.9%, respectively, for the detection of INH resistance and 98.8%, 100%, 100%, and 99.7%, respectively, for the detection of MDR compared to conventional results.

So, the advantage of LPA is that it gives information on INH resistance unlike Xpert. The LPA also tells us about the mechanism of INH resistance whether mediated by *inhA* or *katG*. In the former, high-dose INH may work, while in the latter, ethionamide is indicated. However, there may be phenotypic ethionamide resistance despite presence of *katG* mutation. Disadvantages of LPA include need for technical skill and false negativity in smear-negative samples. Hence, LPA is mainly for diagnosis of drug resistance and not so much for diagnosis of TB. The applicability in pediatric TB is, thus, limited since most disease is paucibacillary and hence smear negative.

We now have the second-generation LPA (MTBDRsl) version available for detection of resistance to second-line drugs.[25] These assays detect mutations in the *gyrA* gene [fluoroquinolone (FQ) resistance], *rrs* gene [kanamycin (KM), amikacin (AMK), and capreomycin (CM) resistance], and *embB* gene (EMB resistance). This test is recommended for smear-positive samples and culture samples that have tested rifampicin resistant. As against phenotypic susceptibility that takes 2–3 weeks for results to come back, the second-generation LPA detects quinolone and aminoglycoside resistance in a single day. This helps differentiation of pre-XDR and XDR-TB from MDR-TB. It, thus, helps in planning the treatment regimen, especially in sick patients.

The sensitivity for detecting quinolone, second-line injectable, and extensive drug resistance directly from clinical samples is 90.7%, 100%, and 92.3%, respectively, and the specificity for detection is 98.1%, 99.4%, and 99.6%, respectively. The type of *gyrA* mutations also help in predicting the degree of quinolone resistance. Some are associated with low-level resistance where high-dose moxifloxacin may be effective while other mutations are associated with high-level of moxifloxacin resistance. False-negative results are due to mutations not present in the test and false positive is due to silent mutations. This test is the first WHO-recommended rapid test for the detection of additional resistance in MDR-TB patients as well as XDR-TB. However, use of this test does not eliminate the need for phenotypic susceptibility testing for confirming the results and determining susceptibility to other second-line drugs.

Newer Molecular Methods

TrueNAT

TrueNAT is a chip-based polymerase reaction developed in India.[26,27] This is a battery-operated, low throughput device, but it requires two precision steps. The first step indicates whether MTB complex is present, and the second step tells about rifampicin resistance. Large-scale, multicenter evaluation is underway supported by the Indian Council of Medical Research (ICMR). Early data shows promise in terms of sensitivity and specificity. High concordance was observed between Xpert MTB/RIF and TrueNAT for case detection of TB.

Xpert Mycobacterium Tuberculosis/Rifampicin Ultra

This test was approved by the WHO in 2017 for diagnosis of TB and rifampicin resistance. The test is an improvement over the previous Xpert since it is more sensitive and can detect up to 16 bacilli/mL as against 131 bacilli/mL in the previous Xpert. It, thus, approaches the sensitivity of liquid mycobacterial cultures. This enhanced sensitivity is due to a larger cartridge chamber, which accommodates more sample and also presence of two new targets for detection of MTB complex. The test is particularly useful in diagnosing smear-negative disease, TB in HIV-infected patients, pediatric TB, and extrapulmonary disease.[28] The enhanced sensitivity comes at the cost of specificity. False-positive results are due to detection of dead bacteria in previously treated patients or scanty bacteria in the respiratory samples of latently infected people. The author in her own institution has seen high rates of false positivity in bronchoalveolar samples of patients who eventually were diagnosed to have illnesses other than TB. The specificity of the Xpert Ultra at detection of rifampicin resistance is also higher than the earlier Xpert, especially when the mycobacterial burden is low or very low. Whereas the previous Xpert would pronounce a sample to be rifampicin resistant when the load was very low (due to imperfect binding of the amplicon with the probes), the Xpert Ultra would either pronounce the rifampicin resistance as indeterminate or true positive.

The WHO has recommended replacement of the earlier Xpert with the new Ultra at all sites. The same machine can be used with new cartridges.

Xpert Extensively Drug-resistant

The Xpert XDR is a molecular assay to detect MTB as well as resistance to INH, quinolones, and aminoglycosides. In a way, it is like the second-generation LPA, but requiring less technical expertise. The test is in clinical trials currently.[29]

Pyrosequencing

It is a DNA sequencing technique that is based on the detection of the pyrophosphate released during DNA synthesis and is well suitable for large-scale screening for a short length DNA fragment.[30] Pyrosequencing (PSQ) can detect mutations associated with first- and second-line anti-TB drugs, with the additional advantage of being rapidly adaptable for the identification of new mutations.

Pyrosequencing data were compared to phenotypic MGIT 960 DST results for performance analysis. The PSQ assay illustrated good sensitivity for the detection of resistance to INH (94%), RIF (96%), FQ (93%), AMK (84%), CAP (88%), and KAN (68%). The specificities of the assay were 96% for INH, 100% for RIF, FQ, AMK, and KAN, and 97% for CAP.

The other advantages of PSQ are diagnosis of TB from smear-negative pulmonary and extrapulmonary samples and in resolving discordant results between phenotypic susceptibility and Xpert as well as confirm the status of rifampicin resistance when the Xpert is indeterminate or very low. The use of PSQ has found improved sensitivity in diagnosis of the XDR-TB in TBM.

Targeted Next Generation Sequencing

Targeted next generation sequencing (NGS) can be implemented through either an amplicon-based assay or a hybridization/capture-based assay to sequence large targets with a large depth of sequence coverage which offers high confidence for mutation detection and detection of mixed populations or heteroresistance within a sample.[31,32] Furthermore, this technology has been successfully implemented for the detection of TB drug resistance in clinical TB specimens.

Currently, targeted sequencing is being phased into the TB diagnostic pipeline for drug-resistant TB (DR-TB) detection direct from sputum samples is the Next Gen-RDST assay (Translational Genomics Research Institute, Phoenix, Arizona, USA) to detect mutations in *MTBC* gene regions associated with resistance to at least seven drugs. Likewise, the Deeplex®-MycTB assay (GenoScreen, Lille, France) is marketed for identification of mycobacterial species and prediction of MTBC drug resistance through targeted NGS of 18 resistance-associated gene targets in a 24-plexed amplicon mixture. These assays are undergoing evaluation.

Whole Genome Sequencing

Whole genome sequencing (WGS) of bacterial genomes allows simultaneous identification of all known resistance mutations as well as markers with which transmission can be monitored.[33] However, with the mean time to a positive MGIT culture being 14 days, most WGS results are not available for more than 2 weeks, which is too long a delay before starting therapy. Recently, a method has been developed to capture full *M. tuberculosis* genomes directly from infected sputum samples, allowing WGS without the requirement of culture. This has been developed to obtain the first *M. tuberculosis* genome sequences directly from both smear-positive and smear-negative sputum.[34]

■ SEROLOGIC DIAGNOSIS

The WHO has strongly recommended against the use of immunoglobulin G (IgG) and immunoglobulin M (IgM) serology for TB diagnosis because of poor sensitivity and specificity and has banned these tests.[35]

Lipoarabinomannan (LAM) is a glycolipid found in the outer cell wall of mycobacterial species. It is immunogenic and a major virulence factor promoting survival in human host and is excreted in the urine. The test is available as an enzyme-linked immunosorbent assay (ELISA) or dipstick method with a TAT of 4–6 hours or 20 minutes depending on the test kit used.[36] The WHO recommends that it should not be used for the diagnosis of TB, except for HIV positive in patients with signs and symptoms of TB (pulmonary and/or extrapulmonary) who have a CD4 cell count ≤100 cells/μL or HIV-positive patients who are seriously ill, regardless of the CD4 count.[9] For TB diagnosis among symptomatic patients, overall lateral flow-LAM pooled sensitivity was 44% and pooled specificity was 92%. The higher sensitivity of LAM in HIV-infected patients is due to higher bacillary burden and antigen load, greater likelihood of TB in the genitourinary tract, and greater glomerular permeability that allows increased antigen levels in urine. In a study evaluating 165 HIV-infected children below the age of 12 years with suspected TB of which 13 had confirmed TB (sputum/gastric aspirate culture positive), the sensitivity and specificity of urine LAM were 43% and 91% compared to 60% and 98% for sputum/gastric aspirate Xpert and 63% and 99% for stool Xpert.[37] The sensitivity increased with increasing immunosuppression. Hence, LAM may be used as a rapid method for diagnosis of TB in children with advanced HIV infection.

■ DETECTION OF LATENT INFECTION

Tuberculin Skin Test

The classic method for detection of latent infection is the *tuberculin skin test* (TST). The TST is the test, which has been the standard against which new methods have been evaluated and the basis of various clinical trials pertaining to latent infection and efficacy of chemoprophylaxis of latent infection.[38]

It can be administered through various methods—Mantoux, Heaf, and Tine being some of them. The antigen used for this purpose is purified protein derivative (PPD) Seibert and PPD RT23 with Tween 80. Five units of PPD-S are equivalent to 2 units of PPD RT23 with Tween 80. For the Indian population, an induration of 10 mm or more is considered positive for latent infection. This cutoff is downgraded to 5 mm for HIV-infected patients and upped to 15 mm in patients in low prevalence areas. The main issues with the TST are false positives in patients vaccinated with Bacillus Calmette-Guérin (BCG) and due to atypical mycobacteria and false negatives in patients with early infection, disseminated disease, and malnourished and immunocompromised hosts. Sensitivity and specificity are also affected by denatured product, faulty injection technique. Use of higher tuberculin unit (TU) is common in Indian clinical setting leads to false-positive results. Besides, use of the test needs the patient to return at 48–72 hours for measurement. Errors and interobserver variation in measurement of induration are not uncommon. An even greater problem facing us today is exhaustion of the seed stock of PPD RT23 with Tween 80[39] (personal communication).

Interferon-gamma Release Assays

It is owing to the disadvantages of the TST that other tests were evaluated for diagnosis of latent infection. Prominent were the *interferon-gamma release assays* (IGRAs).[9,40] These tests are based on the principle of stimulating the subject's lymphocytes *in vitro* with antigens including early secretory antigenic target-6 (ESAT-6), culture filtrate protein-10 (CFP-10), TB7.7, and then measuring the release of gamma interferon. Since these antigens are specific to MTB, false positivity due to previous BCG vaccination or NTM does not occur. A single visit is needed unlike the TST and results are available in 24 hours. Commercial IGRAs include QuantiFERON-TB Gold (QFT-G) and QuantiFERON-TB Gold in tube (QFT-GIT) (Cellestis, Australia) and T-SPOT.TB (Immunotec, UK).

These tests have been mostly evaluated in low-burden countries where they have been found fairly reliable in detecting latent infection. However, cost, need for laboratory infrastructure, and quick transport of the blood specimen are limitations. The older IGRAs need incubation within 16 hours of collection and for the newer IGRAs, this window is 8 hours. Hence, portable incubators may be needed if the reference laboratory is located distant from the site of collection.

The performance of these tests in high-burden settings has not been very promising. For this reason, the WHO in its 2011 statement does not recommend using these tests in high-burden settings for diagnosis of latent infection.[41] In its 2018 publication on diagnosis of latent TB infection, the

WHO has recommended using either IGRA or TST depending on the resources and logistics available even in high-burden countries.[39] Studies from India have reported poor agreement between TST and IGRA for diagnosis of latent infection with higher sensitivity of IGRA.[42,43]

In clinical practice, these tests for latent infection are widely used to diagnose active TB in adults and children.[44] The standards of TB care in India recommend against TST or IGRAs to diagnose active disease in adults and limit its use in diagnosis of pediatric TB.[24] There may, however, be some supporting role of the TST in diagnosis of TB in infants and young children.

C-Tb Test

The *C-Tb test* is a new skin test similar to TST, but uses the ESAT-6/CFP-10 proteins as the IGRAs.[45] Hence, it is not affected by prior infection with NTM or BCG. Due to the higher specificity, a cutoff of 5 mm is used to define a positive test in all individuals (children, adults, and HIV infected). Trials have shown sensitivity of C-Tb test to be same as TST and IGRAs in adults, children, and HIV-infected populations with active TB as well as those with presumed latent TB.[46] There is move by the RNTCP to evaluate the C-Tb test on a pilot basis.

Current Status

Tests for detection of latent infection have been extensively used in low-prevalence countries to diagnose and treat latent infection. In high-prevalence settings such as India, the focus is to diagnose and treat active TB. The emphasis on diagnosis and treatment of latent infection is less, especially when opportunities for reinfection abound. In patients with high risk of progression from latent infection to active disease such as childhood contacts of adults with pulmonary TB and people living with HIV (PLHIV), the WHO advocates chemoprophylaxis without doing any test for diagnosing latent infection.[39]

However, if the goal of ending TB by 2035 has to be met, then diagnosis and treatment of latent infection even in high-burden countries is important. Newer shorter regimens with 3 months of daily INH and rifampicin, 3–4 months of rifampicin alone, and weekly rifapentine with daily INH for 3 months have been found as effective as 6 months of daily INH with better adherence.[39] Hence, with the new WHO guidelines on diagnosis and treatment of latent infection, we are likely to witness an increased use of tests for detecting latent TB infection in the near future.

■ DIAGNOSTIC APPROACH FOR PEDIATRIC TUBERCULOSIS

The diagnostic algorithms for pediatric TB have evolved with time and current algorithms integrate symptoms, radiology, cytology or histopathology, molecular methods, and culture and susceptibility testing for diagnosing both pulmonary TB and EPTB.

Pulmonary Tuberculosis

In the earlier era, diagnosis of pulmonary TB was based on a tripod of clinical symptoms including history of contact, TST, and radiology. Microbiologic diagnosis was seldom possible due to inability to obtain a representative sample and low smear positivity rates. With better methods of sample collection and advent of CBNAAT, the scenario is different now. The current algorithm proposed by the Indian Academy of Pediatrics (IAP) and RNTCP integrates radiology, microbiologic diagnosis in a systematic manner **(Flowchart 4.1.1)**. The new algorithm does not include TST as a diagnostic

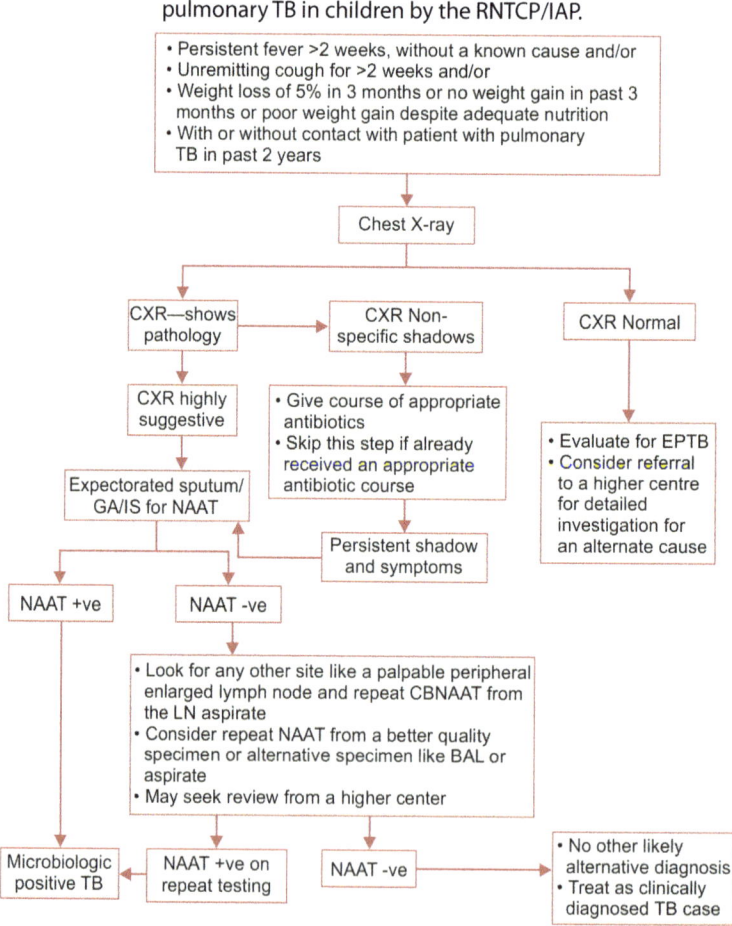

Flowchart 4.1.1: Proposed algorithm for diagnosis of pulmonary TB in children by the RNTCP/IAP.

(BAL: bronchoalveolar lavage; CBNAAT: cartridge-based nucleic acid amplification test; CXR: chest X-ray; EPTB: extrapulmonary tuberculosis; GA: gastric aspirate; IAP: Indian Academy of Pediatrics; IS: induced sputum; LN: lymph node; RNTCP: Revised National Tuberculosis Control Program)

criterion. Despite all efforts to make a microbiologic diagnosis, treatment of pediatric pulmonary TB is empiric in 30–50% of the cases.

Other novel samples that have also been evaluated for diagnosis of pulmonary TB include buccal swab, cough swabs from larynx, and stool samples.

Extrapulmonary Tuberculosis

Almost 50% of pediatric TB is extrapulmonary. The diagnosis is particularly challenging due to paucibacillary disease, need for obtaining samples by invasive methods, and presence of other TB mimics.

Lymph Node Tuberculosis

Lymph node TB is the most common form of EPTB in children. While earlier the diagnosis was usually based on radiology, TST, and FNAC, currently there is a focus on making a definitive diagnosis. The first step is to do FNAC of a necrotic node (USG-guided aspiration improves the pickup). The sample is subjected to cytology, CBNAAT, and liquid cultures. If cytology shows necrotizing granulomatous inflammation or AFB or a positive CBNAAT, treatment can be initiated. If the cytology shows ill-defined or absent granulomas and the CBNAAT is negative, excision biopsy is recommended for definitive diagnosis. This is to prevent mistaking TB from other differentials such as lymphoma, Kikuchi disease, and sarcoidosis. NTM should also be considered as a differential for TB lymphadenitis. Studies from India show that NTM contributes infrequently to mycobacterial lymphadenitis.[47] NTM should be suspected in children aged 1–5 years with rapidly enlarging nodes and abscess formation, absence of systemic symptoms, negative TST, and negative CBNAAT with presence of AFB on smear. Definitive diagnosis is by cultures, which sometimes must be incubated at low/high temperatures for better pick of NTM. NTM speciation can be done by molecular probes or MALDI-TOF.

Pleural Effusion

Pleural effusion is another common form of EPTB in children. Pleural tap is the initial investigation. It is an exudate with high protein and lymphocyte predominance on cytology. The smear positivity for AFB and the CBNAAT is 10–20%. Elevated adenosine deaminase level is not specific for childhood pleural TB. Culture positivity from pleural fluid is merely 20%. The CBNAAT and culture positivity from gastric aspirate are higher than the pleural fluid and are 20–30%. The highest sensitivity for diagnosis is from pleural biopsy histopathology, CBNAAT, and culture, but is often not possible. Hence, often empiric antitubercular therapy has to be resorted in children with lymphocytic pleural effusion when other causes such as malignancy are reasonably ruled out.

Central Nervous System Tuberculosis

Central nervous system TB is the most serious of all form of pediatric TB. For a suspect case of tuberculous meningitis (TBM), CSF analysis is the most crucial test. Unlike what was believed earlier, the cytology of CSF in TBM can range from lymphocyte predominance to polymorphonuclear predominance (only a polymorph percentage of greater than 90 is unlike TB). The protein is high, and sugar is low. CBNAAT positivity depends on the volume of CSF used for the test and 5 mL of CSF can yield a sensitivity of 50–70%. The sensitivity of the Xpert Ultra and PSQ for TBM is higher than the conventional CBNAAT methods. Smear positivity is less than 10% and culture positivity is around 70%. Contrast MRI imaging is helpful in supplementing diagnosis. Features suggestive of TBM include basal exudates, hydrocephalus, ring-enhancing lesions, and infarcts. Efforts should be made to look for extra CNS sites for diagnosis including cervical/mediastinal nodes. Despite the best of efforts, in 30–50% of cases, empiric therapy of TBM is necessary based on clinical presentation, radiology, and CSF cytology and biochemistry. The definitive diagnosis of tuberculomas is even more difficult than TBM. The CSF is negative if there is no meningeal involvement and biopsy of lesions is often not possible. Extra CNS sites should be looked for carefully.

Pericardial Tuberculosis

The definitive diagnosis of pericardial TB is also difficult. While echocardiographic features are suggestive, analysis of pericardial fluid is usually unrewarding with very poor culture and CBNAAT positivity. Contrast-enhanced computed tomography (CECT) may reveal associated mediastinal nodes, which can be biopsied.

Abdominal Tuberculosis

Abdominal TB includes peritoneal TB (presenting as ascites), ileocecal TB, abdominal lymphadenopathy or hepatosplenic TB, or a combination of these. Like other forms of serosal TB, ascitic fluid has very low rates of culture and CBNAAT positivity. The yield is higher from peritoneal, liver, lymph node, or ileocecal biopsies. USG, contrast CT scan, and CT enteroclysis are imaging modalities that help in diagnosis. Recent studies suggest that inflammatory bowel disease especially Crohn's disease is often misdiagnosed as TB in India.

Tuberculosis of Bone and Joints

A small percentage of pediatric TB involves bones and joints. The hip, knee, vertebrae, and small bones of hands and feet are the usual sites. MRI is a sensitive method to pick up early disease, especially of the spine. USG/CT-guided biopsies should be done and subjected to histopathology, CBNAAT, and culture. Yield from pus is higher than solid tissue.

Drug-resistant Tuberculosis

Children at risk of drug resistance include those that fail first-line therapy, those that default on treatment, those with recurrence of disease after previous therapy, and those who are in contact with an adult with DR-TB. Apart from this, children in contact with an adult who has died of TB and those with HIV are also at high risk of drug resistance.

In these children, obtaining an appropriate sample for evaluation is very crucial even if it has to be by invasive methods. The sample should be submitted for smear examination, CBNAAT, and liquid culture. Further workflow is depicted in **Flowchart 4.1.2**. Usually, the same sample is processed and subjected to all the three investigations. If the smear is positive, then LPA can be done directly from the specimen, which gives information about susceptibility to INH along with rifampicin. If rifampicin is resistant, then second-generation LPA can be done for detecting resistance to newer-generation quinolones, second-line aminoglycosides (KM, AMK, and CM), and EMB. This allows for rapid diagnosis of XDR and pre-XDR-TB and tailor therapy. Even for smear-positive samples, liquid cultures are important for phenotypic susceptibility and diagnosing susceptibility to second-line drugs.

If the smear is negative but CBNAAT is positive and confirms rifampicin resistance, second-line therapy should be initiated but liquid cultures inoculated. If available, one can subject the sample to new methods such as PSQ or WGS or Xpert XDR for differentiating MDR-TB from pre-XDR or XDR-TB. Once the culture is positive, first- and second-line LPA or PSQ can be done on the positive cultures for rapid diagnosis of resistance apart from phenotypic susceptibility testing.

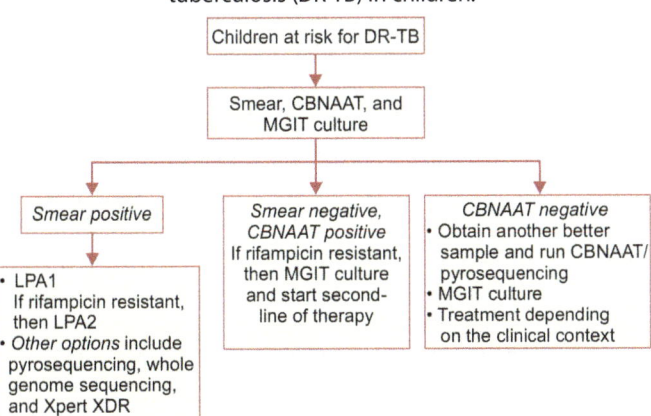

Flowchart 4.1.2: Flowchart showing workup for drug-resistant tuberculosis (DR-TB) in children.

(CBNAAT: cartridge-based nucleic acid amplification test; LPA: line probe assay; MGIT: mycobacterial growth indicator tube; XDR: extensively drug-resistant)

If the smear and CBNAAT is negative, a second sample from the same or alternative site should be obtained for repeat analysis. In case, the second sample is also CBNAAT negative, then one must wait for the liquid cultures to grow and then proceed. Alternatively, one can try performing PSQ or WGS for quick diagnosis of resistance.

There may sometimes be discordance between genotypic and phenotypic susceptibility. False-positive cases of rifampicin resistance may be due to detection of silent mutations or very low load. Similarly, false-negative results can be due to absence of the probe in the system for a particular mutation. These results have to be arbitrated on the basis of clinical presentation and alternative tests such as LPA, PSQ, and WGS.

■ CONCLUSION

Diagnosis of TB is one area of infectious disease where giant leaps have been made in technology. What is even more credible is that this technology has permeated from big fancy laboratories to the primary health level. The RNTCP has been ahead of the private sector in making these techniques available where they are needed most. The following points summarize the approach towards making a diagnosis of TB in children. The final aim is to make a definitive microbiologic diagnosis in all TB suspects.

- It all starts with selecting the correct candidate for diagnosis. A careful and detailed history and examination are needed to weed out patients who are not candidates for further testing to avoid unnecessary investigations. For example, a child with recurrent pulmonary symptoms may be suffering from reactive airway disease or bronchiectasis and not TB. A detailed contact history should be obtained.
- The next step is to conduct appropriate radiologic investigations, which may be a CXR for pulmonary TB, USG for lymph node TB, CT scan, and even MRI for CNS tuberculosis. Investigations such as complete blood count, erythrocyte sedimentation rate (ESR), and C-reactive protein (CRP) may be done, but these rarely support or exclude the diagnosis.
- The most crucial step is obtaining an appropriate sample for diagnosis. For pulmonary TB, it is sputum, gastric aspirate, or induced sputum and sometimes bronchoalveolar lavage. Novel samples such as stool can also be analyzed. For EPTB, the site-specific sample should be obtained even if it necessitates invasive methods. The specimen should be submitted for cytology and/or histopathology where applicable as well as AFB smear, CBNAAT, and liquid culture. The current preferred method for CBNAAT is Xpert MTB/RIF Ultra since it has a higher sensitivity than the earlier Xpert. The specificity, however, is lower than the earlier Xpert.
- For patients where the smear or CBNAAT is positive, treatment can be initiated, and the case is labeled as a microbiologic-confirmed case.

- If the sample is negative on smear or CBNAAT, attempt should be made to obtain a second better sample from the same or different site and repeat the test. If the same is not possible due to logistic issues or if the second sample is also negative, other diagnosis should be excluded and empiric first-line therapy initiated while waiting for the liquid cultures.
- If resources are available, then this negative sample can be subjected to PSQ for definitive microbiologic diagnosis. If the liquid cultures are positive, then susceptibility assessment should be done by CBNAAT, LPA, or phenotypic DST in all cases.
- If the sample was CBNAAT positive and rifampicin susceptible, an LPA or phenotypic INH DST should be done to look at INH susceptibility. INH-resistant isolates are better treated with a different regimen than the standard category 1 treatment.
- All patients with TB should be tested for HIV and notified to the RNTCP.
- Patients with suspected DR-TB should be referred to a higher center for evaluation. Here, microbiologic diagnosis is crucial even if it means getting the sample by invasive means. Determining rifampicin resistance alone is not enough; efforts should be made to determine susceptibility to INH and second-line drugs. The sample should be subjected to appropriate genotypic resistance determining methods including CBNAAT, Xpert XDR, first- and second-generation LPA, PSQ, or WGS. Positive liquid cultures should be processed for phenotypic susceptibility testing to first- and second-line drugs in accredited laboratories.

The task does not end with initiating anti-TB therapy. Follow-up microbiologic tests are indicated to demonstrate response to therapy and microbiologic cure. Here, it is only cultures that are indicated; molecular tests should not be used to follow-up response.

■ REFERENCES

1. World Health Organization (WHO). (2019). Global Tuberculosis Report: Executive Summary. [online] Available from: https://www.who.int/tb/publications/global_report/tb19_Exec_Sum_15October2019.pdf?ua=1. [Last accessed December, 2019].
2. Working Group on Tuberculosis, Indian Academy of Pediatrics (IAP). Consensus statement on childhood tuberculosis. Indian Pediatr. 2010;47(1):41-55.
3. Aljohaney AA. Utility and safety of endobronchial ultrasound-guided transbronchial needle aspiration in patients with mediastinal and hilar lymphadenopathy: Western region experience. Ann Thorac Med. 2018;13(2): 92-100.
4. Mukund A, Khurana R, Bhalla AS, et al. CT patterns of nodal disease in pediatric chest tuberculosis. World J Radiol. 2011;3(1):17-23.
5. Sánchez-Montalvá A, Barios M, Salvador F, et al. Usefulness of FDG PET/CT in the management of tuberculosis. PLoS One. 2019;14(8):e0221516.

6. Kumar P, Kumar A, Lodha R, et al. Childhood tuberculosis in general practice. Indian J Pediatr. 2015;82(4):368-74.
7. Lobato MN, Loeffler AM, Furst K, et al. Detection of *Mycobacterium tuberculosis* in gastric aspirates collected from children: hospitalization is not necessary. Pediatrics. 1998;102(4):E40.
8. Goussard P, Gie R. The role of bronchoscopy in the diagnosis and management of pediatric pulmonary tuberculosis. Expert Rev Respir Med. 2014;8(1):101-9.
9. Oommen S, Banaji N. Laboratory diagnosis of tuberculosis: advances in technology and drug susceptibility testing. Indian J Med Microbiol. 2017;35(3):323-31.
10. Mase SR, Ramsay A, Ng V, et al. Yield of serial sputum specimen examinations in the diagnosis of pulmonary tuberculosis: a systematic review. Int J Tuberc Lung Dis. 2007;11(5):485-95.
11. Fluorescent Light-Emitting Diode (LED) Microscopy for Diagnosis of Tuberculosis: Policy Statement. Geneva: World Health Organization; 2011.
12. Minion J, Shenai S, Vadwai V, et al. Fading of auramine-stained mycobacterial smears and implications for external quality assurance. J Clin Microbiol. 2011;49(5):2024-6.
13. Schramm B, Hewison C, Bonte L, et al. Field evaluation of a simple fluorescence method for detection of viable *Mycobacterium tuberculosis* in sputum specimens during treatment follow-up. J Clin Microbiol. 2012;50(8):2788-90.
14. Lewis JJ, Chihota VN, van der Meulen M, et al. "Proof-of-concept" evaluation of an automated sputum smear microscopy system for tuberculosis diagnosis. PLoS One. 2012;7(11):e50173.
15. Rodrigues C, Shenai S, Sadani M, et al. Evaluation of the bactec MGIT 960 TB system for recovery and identification of *Mycobacterium tuberculosis* complex in a high through put tertiary care centre. Indian J Med Microbiol. 2009;27(3):217-21.
16. Horne DJ, Pinto LM, Arentz M, et al. Diagnostic accuracy and reproducibility of WHO-endorsed phenotypic drug susceptibility testing methods for first-line and second-line antituberculosis drugs. J Clin Microbiol. 2013;51(2):393-401.
17. Ismail NA, Said HM, Rodrigues C, et al. Multicentre study to establish interpretive criteria for clofazimine drug susceptibility testing. Int J Tuberc Lung Dis. 2019;23(5):594-9.
18. Boehme CC, Nabeta P, Hillemann D, et al. Rapid molecular detection of tuberculosis and rifampin resistance. N Engl J Med. 2010;363(11):1005-15.
19. Ocheretina O, Byrt E, Mabou MM, et al. False-positive rifampin resistant results with Xpert MTB/RIF version 4 assay in clinical samples with a low bacterial load. Diagn Microbiol Infect Dis. 2016;85(1):53-7.
20. Steingart KR, Schiller I, Horne DJ, et al. Xpert® MTB/RIF assay for pulmonary tuberculosis and rifampicin resistance in adults. Cochrane Database Syst Rev. 2014;(1):CD009593.
21. Detjen AK, DiNardo AR, Leyden J, et al. Xpert MTB/RIF assay for the diagnosis of pulmonary tuberculosis in children: a systematic review and meta-analysis. Lancet Respir Med. 2015;3(6):451-61.
22. Denkinger CM, Schumacher SG, Boehme CC, et al. Xpert MTB/RIF assay for the diagnosis of extrapulmonary tuberculosis: systematic review and meta-analysis. Eur Respir J. 2014;44(2):435-46.

23. Kohli M, Schiller I, Dendukuri N, et al. Xpert® MTB/RIF assay for extrapulmonary tuberculosis and rifampicin resistance. Cochrane Database Syst Rev. 2018;8:CD012768.
24. World Health Organization (WHO). (2014). International Standards for Tuberculosis Care. [online] Available from: http://www.who.int/tb/publications/ISTC_3rdEd.pdf. [Last accessed December, 2019].
25. Barnard M, Warren R, Gey Van Pittius N, et al. Genotype MTBDRsI line probe assay shortens time to diagnosis of extensively drug-resistant tuberculosis in a high-throughput diagnostic laboratory. Am J Respir Crit Care Med. 2012;186(12): 1298-305.
26. Nikam C, Jagannath M, Narayanan MM, et al. Rapid diagnosis of *Mycobacterium tuberculosis* with Truenat MTB: a near-care approach. PLoS One. 2013;8(1):e51121.
27. Lee DJ, Kumarasamy N, Resch SC, et al. Rapid, point-of-care diagnosis of tuberculosis with novel Truenat assay: cost-effectiveness analysis for India's public sector. PLoS One. 2019;14(7):e0218890.
28. Zhang M, Xue M, He JQ. Diagnostic accuracy of the new Xpert MTB/RIF Ultra for tuberculosis disease: a preliminary systematic review and meta-analysis. Int J Infect Dis. 2019;90:35-45.
29. U.S. National Library of Medicine. (2019). Xpert MTB/XDR Clinical Evaluation Trial. [online] Available from: https://clinicaltrials.gov/ct2/show/NCT03728725. [Last accessed December, 2019].
30. Ajbani K, Lin SY, Rodrigues C, et al. Evaluation of pyrosequencing for detecting extensively drug-resistant *Mycobacterium tuberculosis* among clinical isolates from four high-burden countries. Antimicrob Agents Chemother. 2015;59(1): 414-20.
31. Daum LT, Konstantynovska OS, Solodiankin OS, et al. Next-Generation Sequencing for Characterizing Drug Resistance-Conferring *Mycobacterium tuberculosis* Genes from Clinical Isolates in the Ukraine. J Clin Microbiol. 2018;56(6):9-18.
32. Colman RE, Anderson J, Lemmer D, et al. Rapid Drug Susceptibility Testing of Drug Resistant *Mycobacterium tuberculosis* Isolates Directly from Clinical Samples by Use of Amplicon Sequencing: a Proof of-Concept Study. J Clin Microbiol. 2016;54(8):2058-67.
33. Cohen KA, Manson AL, Desjardins CA, et al. Deciphering drug resistance in *Mycobacterium tuberculosis* using whole-genome sequencing: progress, promise, and challenges. Genome Med. 2019;11(1):45.
34. Doyle RM, Burgess C, Williams R, et al. Direct Whole-Genome Sequencing of Sputum Accurately Identifies Drug-Resistant Mycobacterium tuberculosis Faster than MGIT Culture Sequencing. J Clin Microbiol. 2018;56(8):e00666-18.
35. World Health Organization (WHO). (2008). Laboratory-based evaluation of 19 commercially available rapid diagnostic tests for tuberculosis. [online] Available from: https://www.who.int/tdr/publications/documents/diagnostic-evaluation-2.pdf. [Last accessed December, 2019].
36. Kerkhoff AD, Lawn SD. A breakthrough urine-based diagnostic test for HIV-associated tuberculosis. Lancet. 2016;387(10024):1139-41.
37. LaCourse SM, Pavlinac PB, Cranmer LM, et al. Stool Xpert MTB/RIF and urine lipoarabinomannan for the diagnosis of tuberculosis in hospitalized HIV-infected children. AIDS. 2018;32(1):69-78.

38. Diagnostic Standards and Classification of Tuberculosis in Adults and Children. This official statement of the American Thoracic Society and the Centers for Disease Control and Prevention was adopted by the ATS Board of Directors, July 1999. This statement was endorsed by the Council of the Infectious Disease Society of America, September 1999. Am J Respir Crit Care Med. 2000;161(4 Pt 1):1376-95.
39. World Health Organization (WHO). (2018). Latent tuberculosis infection: Updated and consolidated guidelines for programmatic management. [online] Available from: https://apps.who.int/iris/bitstream/handle/10665/260233/9789241550239-eng.pdf;jsessionid=C223185408A728541271BB3EB8E11658?sequence=1. [Last accessed December, 2019].
40. Lu P, Chen X, Zhu LM, et al. Interferon-Gamma Release Assays for the Diagnosis of Tuberculosis: A Systematic Review and Meta-analysis. Lung. 2016;194(3):447-58.
41. World Health Organization (WHO). (2011). Tuberculosis IGRA TB Tests Policy Statement 2011. The use of TB Interferon-Gamma Release Assays (IGRAs) in Low- and Middle-income Countries. [online] Available from: http://www.who.int/tb/features_archive/igra_factsheet_oct2011.pdf. [Last accessed December, 2019].
42. Sharma SK, Vashishtha R, Chauhan LS, et al. Comparison of TST and IGRA in Diagnosis of Latent Tuberculosis Infection in a High TB-Burden Setting. PLoS One. 2017;12(1):e0169539.
43. Agarwal SK, Singh UB, Zaidi SH, et al. Comparison of interferon gamma release assay & tuberculin skin tests for diagnosis of latent tuberculosis in patients on maintenance haemodialysis. Indian J Med Res. 2015;141(4):463-8.
44. Bronner Murrison L, Ananthakrishnan R, Sukumar S, et al. How Do Urban Indian Private Practitioners Diagnose and Treat Tuberculosis? A Cross-Sectional Study in Chennai. PLoS One. 2016;11(2):e0149862.
45. Abubakar I, Jackson C, Rangaka MX. C-Tb: a latent tuberculosis skin test for the 21st century? Lancet Respir Med. 2017;5(4):236-7.
46. Aggerbeck H, Ruhwald M, Hoff ST, et al. C-Tb skin test to diagnose *Mycobacterium tuberculosis* infection in children and HIV-infected adults: A phase 3 trial. PLoS One. 2018;13(9):e0204554.
47. Reddy VC, Prasad CE, Aparna S, et al. A study of mycobacterial species causing lymphadenitis. Southeast Asian J Trop Med Public Health. 2008;39(1):130-5.

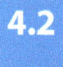

4.2 DIAGNOSIS, TREATMENT AND MANAGEMENT OF INFLUENZA (INDIAN PERSPECTIVE)

Digant D Shastri

■ INTRODUCTION

Influenza is acute viral infection of the respiratory tract caused by influenza viruses. There are three types of seasonal influenza viruses—A, B and C. Influenza A viruses are further categorized into subtypes. In 2009, A (H1N1) strain of influenza virus caused global influenza pandemic, but now it is a seasonal influenza virus, which cocirculates with other seasonal viruses.

Influenza viruses are genetically dynamic and evolve in unpredictable ways. Influenza viruses are further classified into strains based on antigenic properties. Humoral immunity to influenza viruses is generally thought to be strain-specific and acquired through infection or vaccination. Seasonal influenza epidemics can be caused by new virus strains that are antigenically distinct from previously circulating virus strains to which a population has immunity; this is known as antigenic drift. Uncommonly, a completely new strain of influenza will emerge to which there is little or no existing immunity, this is known as antigenic shift and such novel strains can give rise to influenza pandemics such as 2009 pandemic influenza.

Influenza virus spread from person-to-person. Inhalation of infectious droplets expelled through coughing or sneezing by infected individual is the predominant route of transmission, however contact with contaminate hands or other surfaces also can transmit the infection.

■ EPIDEMIOLOGY

Influenza virus infections cause substantial annual morbidity and mortality worldwide. Annual influenza epidemics result in an estimated three to five million cases of severe illness, and about 250,000-500,000 deaths globally. Influenza is an important cause of pneumonia or lower respiratory tract infection (LRTI) and approximately 8-10% of all patients with pneumonia test positive for influenza.[1-3]

■ CLINICAL FEATURES

Sudden, rapid onset of symptoms is the hallmark of influenza; the symptoms may include fever, chills, body aches, sore throat, nonproductive cough, runny nose and headache. Gastrointestinal symptoms and muscle inflammation occur more often in young children, and infants can present with a sepsis-like syndrome.

Physical Findings

There is rapid onset of fever spiking to 38-40°C (up to 41°C, especially in children), which typically lasts 4-8 days, which gradually diminishes. Face is flushed with hot and moist skin, congested eyes, watery discharge from eyes and nose, hyperemic mucous members and enlarged cervical lymph nodes (especially in children).

Clinical Course of Illness

Severity varies from afebrile symptoms mimicking common cold to severe prostration without major respiratory signs and symptoms, especially in the elderly. Fever and systemic symptoms typically last 3 days, occasionally 5–8 days, and gradually diminish. Cough and malaise may persist more than 2 weeks. Full recovery may take 1–2 weeks or longer, especially in the elderly.

Complications

In infants and children complications include sinus or ear infections, viral and bacterial pneumonia, bronchiolitis, croup, dehydration (with or without diarrhea) febrile seizures, and worsening underlying chronic conditions. Toxic shock syndrome and sudden death (may be due to cytokine dysregulation) have also been reported.

■ CATEGORIZATION

All individuals seeking consultations for flu-like symptoms should be screened at healthcare facilities, both government and private or examined by a doctor and categorized into A, B and C.[4] In order to prevent and contain outbreaks of Influenza, the following guidelines for screening, testing and isolation are to be followed:

Category A (Uncomplicated/Mild)

- *Symptomatology:* Patients with mild fever and cough or sore throat with or without body aches, headache, diarrhea and vomiting
- *Diagnostic test:* Not required

Category B (Uncomplicated but Severe Symptoms/High Risk Groups)

- *B1:* In addition to all the signs and symptoms mentioned under category A, if the patient has high grade fever (≥102°F) and severe sore throat
- *B2:* In addition to all the signs and symptoms mentioned under category A, individuals having one or more of the following high-risk conditions:
    - Age ≥ 65 years
    - Pregnancy (including up to two weeks postpartum)
    - Infants and children aged ≤ 5 years (especially < 2 years of age)
    - Chronic respiratory disease
    - Chronic heart, kidney, liver or neurological disease
    - Diabetes mellitus
    - Blood disorders (including hemoglobinopathies)
    - Persons with immunosuppression (including HIV/AIDS and use of long-term (≥ 2 weeks) corticosteroids, post-transplant patients)
    - Extreme obesity (BMI ≥ 40 kg/m^2)
    - Malignancy
- *Diagnostic test:* Testing of the category B patient for influenza is not required.

Category C (Complicated)

In addition to the above signs and symptoms of category A and category B, if the patient has one or more of the following signs as given in **Table 4.2.1**.

Table 4.2.1: Symptoms and signs of complicated influenza.

Symptoms	Signs
Breathlessness	Tachypnea
Hemoptysis	SpO_2 <90%
Altered mental status	Hypotension
Somnolence and poor feeding (in children)	Reduced urine output
Seizures	Cyanosis
Decreased urine output	
Persistence or worsening of initial symptoms beyond 72 hours	
Worsening of underlying chronic conditions like diabetes mellitus, chronic kidney disease, etc.	

■ LABORATORY DIAGNOSIS

In uncomplicated cases (patients who fit the ILI case definition) usually laboratory diagnosis is not recommended, as it provides no advantage in the management of patient. Testing can be considered for the following patients:
- Patients who meet the criteria for complicated or severe influenza, where a laboratory diagnosis will assist in patient management.
- Clusters of cases where a diagnosis of the cause of the outbreak is needed (e.g. within institutions such as healthcare facilities, nursing homes, hotels, day care centers). First 2–3 cases to be tested, thereafter testing not required.

Which Samples can be Tested?

A variety of respiratory specimens can be collected and include:[5]
- Throat swab (oropharyngeal swab)
- Nasal swab
- Nasopharyngeal swabs
- Bronchoalveolar lavage (BAL)
- Tracheal aspirates
- Nasopharyngeal or oropharyngeal aspirates as washes.

Bronchoalveolar lavage and tracheal aspirates are two preferred sample options in case of lower respiratory tract infection (pneumonia), and intubated patients. Swab specimens should be collected only on swabs with a synthetic tip (such as polyester/Dacron/rayon/flocked nylon swab) and mounted on aluminum or plastic shaft. Swabs with cotton and wooden shafts are not recommended. Specimens collected with swabs made of calcium alginate are not acceptable.

Bronchoalveolar lavage or tracheal aspirates should be collected in a sterile screw capped container in a sufficient quantity of 3–5 mL. Alternatively, the sample collected in mucus extractor can also be sent. Sputum is not a preferred sample for influenza testing.

Ideal Timing for Sample Collection

- As soon as possible preferably within 48 hours of onset of symptoms
- Preferably before antiviral medications are administered.

Biosafety Measures for Sample Collection

Before initiating collection of sample appropriate personal protective equipment (PPE) should be worn by the sample collector, e.g. N-95 mask, triple layered surgical masks, gloves, protective eyewear (goggles) (in case there is possibility of splash) and gown or apron.

Collection of Samples

Throat swab: Throat swab is the easiest sample to be collected. Ask the patient to open his/her mouth wide open. While the sample collection process is on, the patient should try to resist gagging and closing the mouth. Swabs from the posterior pharyngeal wall and tonsils are ideal.

Nasal swab: Insert swab into nostril along the lower floor of the nose till one reaches below the anterior turbinate. Leave the swab in place for a few seconds. Slowly remove swab while slightly rotating it. Use a different swab for the other nostril. Put tip of swab into vial containing VTM, breaking applicator's stick.

Nasopharyngeal swab: This can be collected through the nasal route or through oral route. For nasal route insert a thin flexible swab into nostril and right up to nasopharynx, leave the swab in place for a few seconds and then slowly remove swab while slightly rotating it. For oral route insert a thin flexible swab through mouth over the tongue and turn the swab upwards behind the soft palate to reach the nasopharynx, leave the swab in place for a few seconds and then slowly remove swab. Put the swab with tip downwards into vial containing VTM, breaking the extra portion of the swab stick.

Storage and Transport of the Sample

Sample should be sent to the laboratory as soon as possible at 4–8°C but not later than 48 hours. In case of delay beyond 48 hours, the specimens must be stored at –70°C. For intra-institution transfer sample should be transported to laboratory in a closed box (preferably vaccine carrier) with absorbent material (cotton/tissue paper) wrapped around the vial immediately after collection. For transportation of sample from the hospital or institution to the laboratory located elsewhere sample should be transpored after proper packaging using the standard triple packaging system.

■ LABORATORY TESTS FOR INFLUENZA DIAGNOSIS

In a person with an acute febrile respiratory illness laboratory confirmation of influenza virus infection is to be done by one or more of the following tests:[6,7]
- Molecular assays or nucleic acid amplification test (NAAT)
- Virus isolation—performed only for research/vaccine production purposes
- Other tests available (but not currently recommended) include:
  - Antigen detection tests
  - Antibody detection assays

Sensitivity and specificity of any test for influenza viruses in respiratory specimens might vary with the time from illness onset to specimen collection, respiratory source, the quality, handling and processing of the specimen and the time from specimen collection to testing.

Molecular Assays or Nucleic Acid Amplification Assays

Nucleic acid amplification assays have replaced culture techniques as the new gold standard in influenza diagnostics.
- Reverse transcriptase polymerase chain reaction (RT-PCR):
  - Real time reverse transcriptase PCR assay
  - Multiplex PCR systems
  - Conventional
- Other NAATs
- Rapid molecular assays

Reverse Transcriptase Polymerase Chain Reaction

Polymerase chain reaction detects viral RNA present in clinical specimens (also in virus cultures). Nasopharyngeal swabs, washes or aspirates are the best upper respiratory tract specimens; however other acceptable specimens include a nasal and/or throat swab. In patients with lower respiratory tract disease, lower respiratory tract specimens (endotracheal aspirate or BAL fluid) should be collected and tested if influenza is clinically suspected and testing of upper respiratory tract specimens is negative. The PCR provides increased sensitivity and possibility of quantitation of the viral target gene, can detect influenza viral RNA (positive results) for a longer duration than other influenza tests (e.g. antigen detection—immunofluorescence or rapid influenza diagnostic tests) and the interpretation of the result is less impacted by the level of influenza activity in the community. The PCRs has some limitations also—RT-PCR and other molecular assays may not be available in all outpatient or emergency room settings. For hospitalized patients, these assays are not always available on-site. Since respiratory specimens may need to be sent to a state public health laboratory for RT-PCR the actual time to receive results may be substantially longer. The test is more expensive than other influenza tests.[7]

The turnaround time varies from 45 minutes to several hours. In conventional RT-PCR assays it is 6–8 hours and in real time RT-PCR methods it is 3–4 hours.

Rapid Molecular Assays

These are mainly used as point-of-care use with sensitivity ranging 66–100%. They can produce results in a reasonable time period ranging from approximately 15–30 minutes to less than 1.5 hours. The Infectious Diseases Society of America (IDSA) recommends use of rapid influenza molecular assays over rapid influenza diagnostic tests (RIDTs) for detection of influenza viruses in respiratory specimens of outpatients.

Virus Isolation

Virus culture has been the gold standard for influenza diagnosis, however, is carried out only in reference laboratory. The virus can be isolated on cell lines or embryonated eggs. The advantages include:
- Viruses are available for further antigenic and genetic characterization essential for surveillance and antigenic characterization of new seasonal influenza A and B virus strains that may need to be included in the next year's influenza vaccine
- Culture in appropriate cell lines can also detect other clinically important respiratory viruses.

The disadvantages include:
- Important for public health purposes, but does not provide timely results to inform clinical management
- Positive influenza cultures may or may not exhibit cytopathic effects, thus a second step to specifically identify influenza viruses by immunofluorescence, hemagglutination-inhibition (HI) or RT-PCR is needed.

The turnaround time for shell vial culture is 1–3 days and for traditional tissue cell viral cultures is 3–10 days.

Antigen Detection Tests

Antigen detection tests (including rapid influenza diagnostic tests and immunofluorescence assays) are currently not preferred. Viral antigen detection may be carried out by enzyme immunoassay (EIA) methods or immunofluorescence assays.

Enzyme Immunoassay Methods

Most RIDTs are immunoassays that utilize antibodies against the nucleoproteins of influenza A and B viruses to detect viral antigens. It is simple and convenient to use and can detect influenza viral antigens in 10-15 minutes. The present tests are directed at conserved viral antigens (e.g. virus nucleoprotein, and matrix protein) The RIDTs are approved for specific kinds of respiratory specimens which vary by test, specific types of swabs and storage requirements and the specimen has to be collected with appropriate methods within 24-72 hours after illness onset.

Immunofluorescence Assays

They are not currently recommended for diagnosis. It requires the use of a fluorescent microscope and skilled technologists. The result is produced in approximately 2-4 hours (assays with an analyzer device produces results in approximately 15 minutes). It has moderate sensitivity and high specificity (superior to RIDTs).

Antibody-based Tests

They are not currently recommended for diagnosis. Serological tests available for the measurement of influenza A-specific antibody include:
- Hemagglutination inhibition test (HI)
- EIA
- Virus neutralization tests (VN)/microneutralization (MN) assay

They are impractical for routine diagnostic testing of clinical cases as timely results for clinical decision making is not possible as the antibodies take up to several weeks to develop and become detectable in serum and it requires paired acute and convalescent sera after 14 days. Wider nonavailability of standard panels of reagents for H5N1 and other novel strains, laboratory to laboratory variations in the test results and limited availability at number of public health or research laboratories are the other limitations of the antibody based tests.

■ TREATMENT

The guiding principles are:
- Early implementation of infection control precautions to minimize nosocomial/household spread of disease
- Prompt treatment to prevent severe illness and death
- Early identification and follow up of persons at risk.

Decision to start treatment with antiviral agents as well isolation policy depends on category of case.[4]

- *Category A (uncomplicated/mild):*
    - *Treatment:* They do not require oseltamivir and should be offered symptomatic treatment. The patients should be monitored for their progress and reassessed at 24–48 hours by the doctor
    - *Isolation:* Patients should confine themselves at home and avoid mixing up with public and high-risk members in the family.
- *Category B (uncomplicated but severe symptoms/high risk groups):*
    - *Treatment:* They should receive oseltamivir along with symptomatic treatment
    - *Isolation:* All patients of category B1 and B2 should confine themselves at home and avoid mixing up with public and high-risk members in the family.
- *Category C (Complicated):*
    - *Treatment:* Immediate hospitalization and treatment.
    - *Isolation:* For treating category C (Complicated) isolation facilities are preferred, however if dedicated isolation room is not available then patients can be grouped in a well-ventilated isolation ward with beds kept 1 m apart.

Supportive Therapy

To maintain hydration and nutrition start parenteral IV fluids. Those with hypoxia or respiratory distress will need oxygen therapy or ventilatory support depending on the severity of illness. Paracetamol or ibuprofen is prescribed for fever, myalgia and headache. Salicylate and aspirin are strictly contraindicated in any influenza patient due to its potential to cause Reye's syndrome.

Those patients who can take orally and retain the fluid per orally should be advised to drink plenty of fluids.

Indications of concurrent antibiotics in influenza include:
1. Patients presenting initially with severe disease (extensive pneumonia, respiratory failure, hypotension, and fever)
2. Investigate and empirically treat bacterial coinfection in patients who deteriorate after initial improvement
3. Patients who fail to improve after 3–5 days of antiviral treatment.

Suspected case should be constantly monitored for clinical and radiological evidence of lower respiratory tract infection and for hypoxia (respiratory rate, oxygen saturation, and level of consciousness).

Patients with signs of tachypnea, dyspnea, respiratory distress and oxygen saturation less than 90% should be supplemented with oxygen therapy. Patients with severe pneumonia and acute respiratory failure ($SpO_2 < 90\%$ and

PaO$_2$ <60 mm Hg with oxygen therapy) must be supported with mechanical ventilation. Invasive mechanical ventilation is preferred choice. To reduce spread of infectious aerosols, use of HEPA filters on expiratory ports of the ventilator circuit and high flow oxygen masks is recommended.[8]

Suspected cases not having pneumonia do not require antibiotic therapy. Antibacterial agents should be administered, if required, as per locally accepted clinical practice guidelines. Patient on mechanical ventilation should be administered antibiotics prophylactically to prevent hospital-associated infections.

Medications

Oseltamivir, peramivir, and zanamivir work by inhibiting influenza virus neuraminidase. Oseltamivir is the recommended drug for treatment. All patients in category B and C should receive oseltamivir. Empiric antiviral therapy is often necessary, and treatment should not be delayed while awaiting confirmatory test results. To be effective as treatment, these agents must be administered within 48 hours of symptom onset. For critically ill patients with H5N1 infection, evidence suggests that initiation of oseltamivir therapy up to 6–8 days from onset of symptoms may reduce mortality.[4,9-13] Studies also demonstrate the efficacy of these agents in preventing influenza A and B. For acute treatment, these agents are given twice daily for 5 days. For prevention, they are given once daily for 10 days.

Doses

In older children for treatment oseltamivir is to be prescribed in following dose (weight rage)
- *For weight <15 kg:* 30 mg BD for 5 days
- *15–23 kg:* 45 mg BD for 5 days
- *24–<40 kg:* 60 mg BD for 5 days
- *>40 kg:* 75 mg BD for 5 days

For young infants:
- < 3 months 12 mg BD for 5 days
- 3–5 months 20 mg BD for 5 days
- 6–11 months 25 mg BD for 5 days

The FDA approved baloxavir marboxil in October 2018 for use in adults and adolescents aged 12 years or older as a single weight-based oral dose for use within 48 hours of symptom onset. It is a prodrug that inhibits cap-dependent endonuclease, an enzyme specific to influenza, resulting in inhibition of viral replication. In clinical trials, single dose baloxavir was safe and effective in treating patients with uncomplicated influenza. It is active against influenza A and B, including strains resistant to neuraminidase inhibitors.[14]

PREVENTION

Prevention is the most effective management strategy for influenza. For prevention various general and specific measures are recommended.

General Measures

- Avoid going to overcrowded places
- Avoid close contact such as kissing or sharing drinks with patients with influenza
- Wash hands with soap and water or disinfect with an alcohol-based hand rub regularly
- Wipe down surfaces that are frequently touched or shared (door knobs, remote controls) with a standard household disinfectant.

Specific Measures

Vaccination

Influenza vaccination is the most effective method for prevention and control of influenza infection available currently. Because of the changing nature of influenza viruses, WHO monitors the epidemiology of influenza viruses throughout the world. Each year recommendations about strains to be included in the vaccine for the following influenza season are made. Separate recommendations are made for the Southern and Northern Hemisphere vaccines each year.

To prevent seasonal flu, the Advisory Committee on Immunization Practices (ACIP) of the US Centers for Disease Control and Prevention (CDC) and the American Academy of Pediatrics (AAP) recommend routine annual influenza vaccination for all persons aged 6 months or older, preferably before the onset of influenza activity in the community.[15]

Influenza vaccine provides reasonable protection against immunized strains. After the administration the vaccine takes 10–14 days' time to become effective. The influenza vaccine has had 50–60% efficacy against infection with influenza A viruses and 70% efficacy against influenza B viruses.[16]

IAP-ACVIP Recommendations

Indian Academy of Pediatrics Advisory Committee on Immunization Practices (IAP-ACVIP) recommends that quadrivalent/trivalent inactivated influenza vaccine (IIV) should be routinely offered annually to all children between 6 months and 5 years of age. The latest available influenza vaccine can be administered after 6 months of age, 2–4 weeks prior to the influenza season, two doses at the interval of 1 month in the first year and one dose annually before the influenza season up to 5 years of age **(Table 4.2.2)**.[17]

Table 4.2.2: Recommended dosage of influenza vaccine.		
Children 6 months through 36 months	0.25 mL (half the adult dose)	1 or 2 doses[†]
Children 36 months to 9 years	Adult dose (0.5 ml)	1 or 2 doses[†]
Children older than 9 years of age and adults	Adult dose (0.5 mL)	Single doe

[†]2 doses should be administered ≥ 1 month apart during 1st year of vaccination, thereafter one dose.

Vaccine strains:
The following combinations are recommended for 2018-19 influenza vaccines. Trivalent vaccines are recommended to have
1. A/Michigan/45/2015 (H1N1) pdm09-like virus,
2. A/Singapore/INFIMH-16-0019/2016 (H3N2)-like virus; and
3. B/Colorado/06/2017-like virus (Victoria lineage).

Quadrivalent vaccines are recommended to have above and B/Phuket/3073/2013-like virus (Yamagata lineage).

Chemoprophylaxis

Annual influenza vaccination is the best way to prevent influenza. WHO guidelines state that individuals at high risk of severe disease who have been exposed to a patient with influenza may benefit from chemoprophylaxis. Oseltamivir is the recommended drug. For prevention, it is to be given once daily for 10 days.

Doses

For chemoprophylaxis treatment oseltamivir is to be prescribed in following dose (weight rage):

Older children
- *For weight <15 kg:* 30 mg
- *15–23 kg:* 45 mg
- *24 to <40 kg:* 60 mg
- *>40 kg:* 75 mg

For young infants:
- *< 3 months:* 12 mg
- *3–5 months:* 20 mg
- *6–11 months:* 25 mg

Measures to Prevent Transmission of Influenza to Others

Patients should be advised to:
- Stay at home until symptoms have resolved (at least 24 hours after fever has defervescence)
- Avoid close contact with others especially those at high risk for severe influenza
- Avoid close contact such as kissing or sharing drinks
- Cover mouth and nose with tissue when sneezing or coughing
- Wash hands with soap and water or disinfect with an alcohol-based hand rub regularly
- Limit the number of visitors
- Wipe down surfaces that are frequently touched or shared (door knobs, remote controls) with a standard household disinfectant.

Measures to Prevent Transmission of Influenza to Healthcare Staff

- Use of universal personal protective equipment (PPE) by all health care staff in isolation wards/ICU
- Vaccination to be provided to health care workers as per national guidelines.
- Consider antiviral chemoprophylaxis for exposed health care staff for 10 days following the last exposure during epidemic/outbreak situation.

■ REFERENCES

1. Dawood FS, Iuliano AD, Reed C, et al. Estimated global mortality associated with the first 12 months of 2009 pandemic influenza A H1N1 virus circulation: a modelling study. Lancet Infect Dis. 2012,12:687-95.
2. Nair H, Brooks WA, Katz M, et al. Global burden of respiratory infections due to seasonal influenza in young children: a systematic review and meta-analysis. Lancet. 2011,378:1917-30.
3. World Health Organization. (2016). Seasonal influenza. [online] Available from http://www.who.int/mediacentre/factsheets/fs211/en/. [Last Accessed December, 2019].
4. Government of India. Guidelines on categorization of Seasonal Influenza cases during screening for home isolation, testing, treatment and hospitalization (25.02.2019). New Delhi: Ministry of Health and Family Welfare; 2019.
5. Heikkinen T, Marttila J, Salmi AA, et al. Nasal Swab versus Nasopharyngeal Aspirate for Isolation of Respiratory Viruses. J Clin Microbiol. 2002,40:4337-9.
6. Chartrand C, Leeflang MM, Minion J, et al. Accuracy of rapid influenza diagnostic tests: a meta-analysis. Ann Intern Med. 2012;156(7):500-11.
7. Centers for Disease Control and Prevention (2013). Seasonal Influenza (Flu): Guidance for Clinicians on the Use of RT-PCR and Other Molecular Assays for

Diagnosis of Influenza Virus Infection. [online] Available from http://www.cdc.gov/flu/professionals/diagnosis/molecular-assays.htm. [Last Accessed December, 2019].
8. World Health Organization Writing Group, Bell D, Nicoll A, et al. Non-pharmaceutical interventions for pandemic influenza, international measures. Emerg Infect Dis. 2006;(1):81-7
9. Gubareva LV, Kaiser L, Hayden FG. Influenza virus neuraminidase inhibitors. Lancet. 2000;355(9206):827-35.
10. Nicholson KG, Aoki FY, Osterhaus AD, et al. Efficacy and safety of oseltamivir in treatment of acute influenza: a randomised controlled trial. Neuraminidase Inhibitor Flu Treatment Investigator Group. Lancet. 2000,355:1845-50.
11. Muthuri SG, Venkatesan S, Myles PR, et al. Effectiveness of neuraminidase inhibitors in reducing mortality in patients admitted to hospital with influenza A H1N1pdm09 virus infection: a meta-analysis of individual participant data. Lancet Respir Med. 2014,2:395-440.
12. Heinonen S, Silvennoinen H, Lehtinen P, et al. Early oseltamivir treatment of influenza in children 1-3 years of age: a randomized controlled trial. Clin Infect Dis. 2010;51(8):887-94.
13. Centers for Disease Control and Prevention. Influenza Antiviral Medications: Summary for Clinicians. Georgia: Centers for Disease Control and Prevention; 2015.
14. Hayden FG, Sugaya N, Hirotsu N, et al. Baloxavir marboxil for uncomplicated influenza in adults and adolescents. N Engl J Med. 2018;379(10):913-23.
15. CDC. Prevention and Control of Seasonal Influenza with Vaccines: Recommendations of the Advisory Committee on Immunization Practices — United States, 2013–2014. Georgia: Centers for Disease Control and Prevention; 2013. pp. 1-43.
16. Osterholm M, Kelley N, Sommer A. Efficacy and effectiveness of influenza vaccines: a systematic review and meta-analysis. Lancet Infect Dis. 2012;12: 36-44.
17. Balasubramanian S, Shah A, Pemde HK, et al. Recommended Immunization Schedule (2018-19) and Update on Immunization for Children Aged 0 Through 18 Years. Indian Pediatr. 2018;55(12):1066-74.

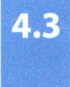

ADENOTONSILLECTOMY: WHEN IT IS ESSENTIAL?

Ashok S Kapse

■ INTRODUCTION

Across the world, tonsillectomy is one of the most common surgical procedures in children. The recent National Health Stat statement of USA, published in 2017, reported that 289,000 tonsillectomies were performed in children less than 15 years of age.[1] Tonsillectomy rates vary widely in different countries and within the country. Tonsillectomy rates in Spain, Italy, and Poland are much lower; in contrast, rates in Belgium, Finland, and Norway are high.[2] Childhood tonsillectomy rates in the US are three times higher than in England; rates within UK and New England vary sevenfold and fourfold.[3] This disparity is inexplicable in terms of need.

Last few decades have registered an additional indication for tonsil surgery. At the beginning of the 20th century, in the preantibiotic era, infection or recurrent tonsillitis was the main indication for tonsil surgery. Following the introduction of antibiotics in the 1950s and rationalization of indications, the number of tonsillectomies dramatically decreased over the subsequent decades. Data from the National Hospital Discharge Survey noted a decrease of more than 50% in inpatient tonsillectomy rates from 1977 to 1989. Then, in the 1970s, initial cases of pediatric obstructive sleep apnea (OSA) were identified and a shift in indication for adenotonsillectomy followed. Sleep-disordered breathing (SDB) became the primary indication for the adenotonsillectomy. A recent study reported significant increase in the incidence rates of tonsillectomy over the past 35 years. Today, SDB caused by upper airway obstruction is the most common indication for tonsil surgery in children and it has significantly exceeded other indication of recurrent tonsillar infection.

■ EVOLUTION: ROUTINE TO RATIONAL

In early 20's, British medical fraternity considered tonsillar disease as main culprit for almost all the ills of human body. An influential "focal theory" suggested that infected bodily sites acted as sources from which contamination spread through the body.[4] Certain elite surgeons considered tonsils as potent foci from which infected material could be swallowed and spread to nearby glands. The varied diseases including physical and mental under-development were attributed to infected tonsils. Tuberculosis, the greatest cause of death in adolescence at the start of the century, was thought to spread in this manner. George Ernest Waugh, one of the prominent ear, nose, and throat (ENT) surgeons, used this theory to present tonsillectomy as a technological solution to apparent social deterioration.[4]

Tonsillectomy was encouraged as routine surgery by general practitioners (GPs) and ENT surgeons; the operation had become a medical ritual that each 20th-century child had to pass through to access a "normal" childhood. It was elevated to a position of national political and moral importance.

Not everyone agreed; saner medical professional thought that tonsils were essential for human immunity; unfortunately, clinical proof was not forthcoming. In the 1940s and 1950s, poliomyelitis outbreaks became an increasing public health issue; a hypothesis relating tonsillectomy to serious bulbar poliomyelitis put tonsillectomy in trouble. A retrospective study of the 1947–48 South Australian poliomyelitis epidemic justified this theory. Many of the bulbar polio cases had undergone tonsillectomy and many of them much before bulbar poliomyelitis attack giving strong support to the concept that tonsillectomy leaves person vulnerable to polio much later than healed wounds.

Poliomyelitis outbreaks forced medical community to seriously analyze tonsillectomy indications; it compelled medical professionals to re-examine their concepts and actions. During the early 1960s, medical reformers made advisory panel to standardize and rationalize tonsillectomy.[4]

■ TONSILS: IMMUNOLOGICAL TRAINING CUM PRODUCTION UNITS

The tonsils consist of three masses of tissues: the lingual tonsil, the pharyngeal (adenoid) tonsil, and the palatine or faucial tonsil. Together they form Waldeyer's ring around the opening of the respiratory and digestive tract. Each tonsil includes lymphoid tissue covered by breathing epithelium that is invaginated into crypts. Tonsils are strategically positioned to serve as protective organs; they initiate immune responses against antigens entering the body through the mouth or nose. The greatest immunologic activity of the tonsils is found between the ages of 3 years and 10 years. As a result, the tonsils are usually enlarged and visible during this period of childhood.[5]

Current research suggests that tonsils and adenoids have a specialized role in immune system development and functioning. Helper T lymphocytes in the tonsils induce proliferation of B lymphocytes; these activated B lymphocytes develop into either antibody-expressing B memory cells capable of migration to the nasopharynx and other sites or into plasma cells that produce antibodies and release them into the lumen of the crypt.

Even though the tonsils generate all five immunoglobulin (Ig) isotypes, yet IgA is the most important creation of the tonsillar immune system. In its dimeric form, IgA combines with transmembrane secretory component and forms secretory IgA, which is one of the most vital components of the upper airway mucosal immune system.[6]

Shrinkage of tonsils particularly adenoids during adulthood is taken as evidence that they are redundant for adult health; however, recent research suggests that their activity in early life is of paramount importance for normal immune system development and early perturbations to their growth and development significantly enhance the risk of many diseases.

Diseased tonsils develop immunologic impairments and may become incapable of performing their normal immunological functions; it breeds the view that their removal may give therapeutic advantage; however, long-term implications of their abolition are uncertain.[7]

ADENOTONSILLAR HYPERTROPHY

Constant and/or recurrent stimulation could lead to adenotonsillar hypertrophy (ATH). Inflammatory stimuli secondary to microbial infection or allergy are the underlying root cause for ATH.

Inflammation and ATH

Increased expressions of various inflammatory cytokines in adenoid and tonsils suggest the role of inflammatory mediators in ATH. Presence of steroid receptors and messenger ribonucleic acid (mRNA) in hypertrophied adenoid tissue and an appropriate response to anti-inflammatory medicines such as corticosteroids further support the role of inflammatory factors in ATH.

Microbial Infection

Increased lymphocytic activity within the tonsils and adenoids suggested the microbial involvement in ATH; isolating pathogenic bacteria such as *Haemophilus influenzae* and other beta-lactamase–producing microorganisms from hypertrophied tonsils and adenoids further established their role.

Allergic Inflammation

Although ATH is multifactorial and its etiology has not been fully understood, it is generally agreed that chronic and recurrent inflammatory events occurring around the adenoid tissue are important factors; in this regard, allergic inflammation is among the most frequently occurring pathologic processes. In addition to viral and bacterial agents, adenoids are constantly exposed to allergens, which can initiate inflammatory processes that affect the adenoid tissue and can lead to the formation of an allergic adenoiditis.[8]

CLINICAL CONSEQUENCES OF ATH

Recurrent tonsillar infections and upper airway obstruction are two main health consequences of ATH.

Recurrent Tonsillitis

Children often get viral upper respiratory infections, which may be confused with recurrent tonsillitis. To clarify this issue, throat infection is defined as the episode of sore throat with more than one of the followings: temperature >101°F, cervical adenopathy, tonsillar exudates, or positive test for *group A beta-hemolytic streptococcus*.

Defining rate of recurrences was another dilemma. Paradise based on his elegantly conducted study in late 60s laid down criteria to define significant recurrences. As per paradise criteria, >7 episodes in the past year, >5 episodes per year in the past 2 years, or >3 episodes per year in the past 3 years should only be considered as severe enough for tonsillectomy.[9]

Natural History of Recurrent Tonsillopharyngitis

By and large tonsillopharyngitis has a favorable natural history. Recurrences tend to decrease with advancing age. Studies document that significant proportion of children waiting for surgery had decreased number of recurrences in the months preceding tonsillectomy and many of them no longer met criteria for surgery. Regardless of surgery, quality of life outcomes do improve with time.

Watchful Waiting

The favorable natural history of tonsillopharyngitis deserves at least a period of 12-month observation prior to tonsillectomy as an intervention for recurrent tonsillitis. During this period, patients should be closely monitored by regular clinic visits and episodes of pharyngotonsillitis should be accurately documented.

Watchful Waiting versus Surgery: Impact on Recurrent Throat Infections

A modest yet statistically significant reduction in frequency of throat infection among severely affected patients undergoing tonsillectomy has been documented by studies comparing surgery against watchful waiting; however, this benefit lasts only for first postoperative year and beyond first 12 months, there is no statistical difference between the tonsillectomy and watchful waiting groups. A Cochrane review also concluded that cases may resolve without surgery and, after the 1st year, there were minimal or no differences between groups. *Most significantly observations document that among less affected children, episodes of moderate-to-severe sore throat may increase after surgery as compared with controls.*

Panel Guidelines

A panel created to formulate guidelines commented that there was not a clear dominance of benefit over harm for tonsillectomy, even for children meeting the paradise criteria and it does not provide clinically significant improvements in children who do not meet the paradise criteria.[1,9]

Panel suggested that patients and caregivers should be informed about limited benefits of tonsillectomy particularly when performed in less severely affected children. *The option of surgery should be a shared decision between child's caregiver and primary care clinician.*

Indications beyond Paradise Criteria

Under certain clinical situations, paradise criteria could be exempted; severe infections requiring hospitalization; multiple antibiotic allergies, complications like peritonsillar abscesses or Lemierre syndrome (thrombophlebitis of the internal jugular vein); personal or family history of rheumatic heart disease; numerous repeat infections in a single household (ping pong spread); and periodic fever, aphthous stomatitis, pharyngitis, and cervical adenitis syndrome (PFAPA) are some of these circumstances.[1]

■ PARADIGM SHIFT

Off late, there has been a paradigm shift in the indication for tonsillectomy. With advent of potent antibiotics and strict rationalization of indications, there was a significant fall in the number of tonsillectomies in 1970s; however, ensuing decades saw new indication for tonsillar removal; upper airway obstruction causing obstructive sleep-disordered breathing (OSDB) has emerged as main indication for tonsillectomy. Swedish data scrutiny from 1987 to 2013 reported a doubling in the incidence rates of adenotonsillectomy. The increasing incidence of OSDB was the main reason for this transformation.[2,10]

Obstructive Sleep-disordered Breathing and OSA

Obstructive sleep-disordered breathing is a syndrome of partial or complete upper airway obstruction occurring during sleep; narrowed upper airway and pharyngeal collapsibility result into snoring and/or increased respiratory effort. OSDB may give rise to repeated, episodic reduction or cessation of airflow, a phenomenon known as obstructive sleep apneas/hypopneas (OSAS) that consequently disrupts normal oxygenation/ventilation and sleep patterns.

First described in the 1970s, obstructive sleep apnea syndrome in children is potentially harmful condition. Although this condition in children is multifactorial, still ATH and obesity are two significant risk factors. The most common age for OSAS is between 2 years and 10 years, which coincides with adenotonsillar lymphatic tissue growth. Snoring is hallmark finding for OSDB, any child who snores loudly for three or more nights per week needs thorough investigations.

Pediatric OSAS has been linked to metabolic changes, growth inhibition, and cardiovascular sequels; recent literature is increasingly showing the negative impact of OSAS on quality of life (QoL).[11]

Pathophysiology in OSAS

Intermittent upper airway obstruction during sleep causes patchy restless sleep, negative swings in intrathoracic pressure, and most importantly blood gas exchange abnormalities. These pathophysiological changes may have adverse impacts on the cardiovascular (CV) and central nervous (CNS) systems.

Cardiovascular system pathophysiology in OSAS: Exaggerated negative swings in intrathoracic pressure caused by upper airway obstruction culminate into increased systemic venous return, high preload to the right ventricle, and decreased ejection fraction. High-ventricular pre- and afterload result into increased cardiac strain, which is reflected as raised blood brain natriuretic peptide (BNP) levels. The high BNP levels may result into secondary enuresis. Fragmented sleep and hypoxemia resulting from OSAS cause sympathetic nervous system activation, peripheral vasoconstriction, and intermittent blood pressure elevation.

Central nervous system pathophysiology in OSAS: OSAS and ensuing blood gas disturbances like hypoxemia and hypercapnia may derange cerebral functions particularly in the prefrontal areas of the brain; these cortical dysfunctions may result into neurocognitive impairments (NCI). Growth hormone secretion decreases due to fragmented slow wave sleep; patchy sleep with increased calorie use in infants with OSAS may have a deleterious impact on child's growth.

The Spectrum of OSDB

From innocuous snoring to upper airway resistance syndrome to potentially damaging apnea/hypopnea, OSDB has a wide range of pathological spectrum.[12]

Primary snoring is a condition when child snores more than three nights per week; however, child has peaceful sleep without apneas, hypopneas, and gas exchange abnormalities. Prevalence of primary snoring is around 7.45%.

Upper airway resistance syndrome is defined as snoring associated with labored breathing, frequent arousals, but no recognizable obstructive events or gas exchange abnormalities.

Obstructive sleep apnea syndrome is the severest form of upper airway obstruction wherein recurring events of partial or complete upper airway obstruction (obstructive apneas and hypopneas) disrupt normal oxygenation, ventilation, and sleep pattern. Hypopneas are episodes of shallow breathing with airflow decreasing by at least 50%; while in obstructive apnea, no airflow occurs despite intense respiratory efforts.[12]

Clinical Implications of OSAS

Upper airway obstruction and resultant hypoxia result in wide spectrum of clinical morbidities. Pharyngeal obstruction may manifest as snoring, oral breathing, witnessed apneas, and patchy restless sleep (SOAP).[12-14] Sleep apnea/hypopnea may cause somnolence (excessive daytime sleepiness) academic regression, hypertension, secondary enuresis, behavioral disorders, and growth failure.

Abnormal breathing during sleep (snoring to apnea): Children snore loudly, which may get punctuated with audible intermittent gasps. Paradoxical chest and abdominal wall movements, labored breathing with retractions, cyanosis, sweating, and restlessness may occur in some cases.

Restless patchy sleep and frequent awakenings: Recurrent obstruction leads to restless and patchy sleep; children frequently wake up and may even fall out of bed; they may sleep in unusual positions, with extended head and neck and wide-open mouth. Children with obstructive sleep apnea may feel choking sensations during the night.

Oral (mouth) breathing: Adenotonsillar hypertrophy causes posterior nasal obstruction forcing child to breathe through mouth; daytime oral breathing is often closely linked with severity of obstruction.

Somnolence—excessive daytime sleepiness (EDS): Children with obstructive SDB tend to have excessive daytime sleepiness; children struggle to stay awake in classroom, while watching television, or reading, and may doze off at inappropriate times. They may show hyperactive and inattentive behavior and may develop academic regression.[15] Obese adolescents are extremely vulnerable to have EDS regardless of level of OSA severity. Young children may not have hypersomnia instead may perhaps demonstrate short attention spans, emotional lability, and behavioral problems.

Cognitive deficits and academic difficulties: Obstructive SDB is likely to cause cognitive deficits and academic difficulties in children; however, results of studies examining correlation between SDB and school performance in childhood are conflicting. A large community-based cohort of children revealed a relationship between SDB severity and impairments in cognitive function such as attention, executive functioning, language, memory, visual-spatial planning and analysis, and thought processing speed. In contrast, the Penn State Children's Cohort study failed to establish any relationship between mild OSAS and measures of IQ, verbal and non-verbal reasoning, executive functioning, memory, thought processing speed, and visual motor skill.

Hypertension: Many studies identified a significant association between OSAS and hypertension; a consensus statement on childhood hypertension even recommends exclusion of OSAS in children presenting with hypertension and snoring but a meta-analysis failed to find an association between OSAS and blood pressure.

Secondary enuresis: A number of studies showed that up to 50% of children with OSDB have secondary enuresis; hence, if a child who snores also develops secondary enuresis, it is mandatory to rule out obstructive sleep apnea. Many children and adults with obstructive apnea report increased nocturnal urinary frequency.

Behavioral problems: OSDB is believed to increase the risk for externalizing behaviors, e.g. aggression, hyperactivity, and internalizing behaviors, e.g. depression in some children.

Inattention/hyperactivity: Assessment of Sleep Apnea Study (TuCASA study) indicates a significant relationship between OSDB and hyperactivity/inattention. OSDB irrespective of its severity is associated with increased frequency of inattention/hyperactivity symptoms. However, studies using objective measures of sleep disturbance failed to identify any relationship between OSDB and attention deficit hyperactivity disorder (ADHD), except increased activity during the night.

Growth failure: Failure to thrive is common feature of OSDB; in a meta-analysis, growth failure was reported in significant proportion of participants with SDB, and therefore in any child being evaluated for growth failure, OSDB should always be an important consideration. Growth failure is especially pronounced among children of preschool age. Hormonal changes and excessive energy expenditures both contribute to growth failure. Adenotonsillectomy is generally successful in resolving physical parameters.

Comorbidities with ATH and OSDB

Recurrent Otitis Media

The link between OSAS and recurrent otitis media (ROM) or chronic otitis media with effusion (OME) is not very strong. In a large, retrospective population-based study, parents reported ROM in 44.8% of children with habitual snoring compared with 29.3% in the nonsnoring cohort. However, in another study, OSAS had no correlation with OME.

Recurrent Wheezing/Asthma

Obstructive sleep-disordered breathing and recurrent wheezing or asthma have important common risk factors namely allergic rhinitis and obesity. In a study, spanning over 1-year severity and frequency of asthma was found to have close link with OSDB. In a systematic review, Sanchez et al. concluded that when both conditions coexist, adenotonsillectomy for OSDB might significantly improve asthma control.

Metabolic Syndrome

Obstructive sleep apnea syndrome increases risk for metabolic syndrome; although obesity is a risk factor for both the metabolic syndrome and OSDB, yet growing evidence suggests that in children and adolescents, OSAS is an independent risk factor for the metabolic syndrome.[12,13,15]

Tonsillar Size and OSDB

Although ATH is usual cause of OSDB in children, the association between tonsillar size and OSAS severity as determined by polysomnography (PSG) is generally feeble. Grading systems for pharyngeal anatomy, such as the Friedman palate position or the Mallampati score **(Fig. 4.3.1)**, do not correlate with OSDB complications nonetheless combined volume of the tonsils and adenoids could have some bearing on OSDB severity. ATH has a familial tendency; overproduction of cysteinyl leukotrienes by genetic variants causing lymphoid proliferation explains familial predisposition.

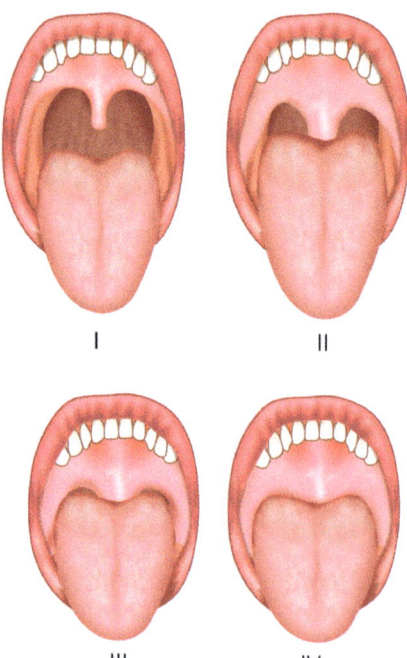

Fig. 4.3.1: Mallampati score for tonsillar hypertrophy.
(*Class I:* Soft palate, fauces, uvula, pillars visible; *Class II:* Soft palate, fauces, uvula visible; *Class III:* Soft palate, base of uvula visible; *Class IV:* Soft palate not visible at all)

■ TECHNIQUES FOR OBJECTIVE EVALUATION OF ATH

Lateral Neck X-ray

Assessment of tonsillar size usually does not require any type of imaging; however, determination of adenoid size needs lateral neck radiographs. Increased adenotonsillar tissue size as demonstrated by lateral neck radiography (adenoid/nasopharyngeal ratio or tonsillar/pharyngeal ratio >0.5) has high sensitivity but poor specificity for OSAS **(Fig. 4.3.2)**; studies suggest that increased adenotonsillar tissue size as detected by lateral neck radiography tends to overdiagnose OSAS in children. Neck radiography in a child presenting with SDB-associated comorbidities such as mouth breathing and enuresis can improve diagnostic specificity. Although MRI can provide very detailed images of soft tissues and bony structures underlying the nasopharynx, such images are generally not required, except in cases of suspected aberrant anatomy.[14]

Objective Evaluation of OSAS

A history of snoring alone is inadequate for making a diagnosis of obstructive sleep apnea or for determining its severity. The American Academy of Pediatrics Clinical Practice Guideline on childhood OSAS recommends objective testing for the diagnosis of OSAS; an overnight PSG performed in

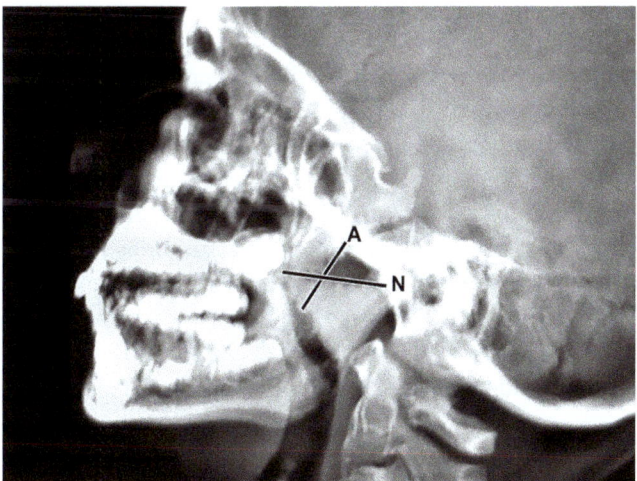

Fig. 4.3.2: Adenoid nasopharyngeal ratio (AN ratio).
Adenoid measurement (A) is the distance from the point of maximal convexity of the adenoid shadow to a line along the anterior margin of basiocciput. The nasopharyngeal (N) measurement is the distance between the posterior border of the hard palate and the anterior–inferior edge of the sphenobasioccipital synchondrosis.
Adenoid hypertrophy is classified as: AN ratio <0.5 minimal; AN ratio 0.5–<0.62 mild; 0.63–0.75 moderate; 0.76–0.88 severe.

properly attended sleep laboratory is gold standard test. The obstructive apnea–hypopnea index (the number of obstructive respiratory events per hour) determines the severity of disease.[14,16]

Apnea–Hypopnea Index

Apnea–hypopnea index (AHI) is a PSG-derived attribute, which is calculated by dividing total number of apneas and hypopneas that occur in a night sleep divided by the total duration of sleeping hours. AHI computes OSAS severity. An AHI of 1 or less is considered to be normal. An AHI of 1–5 is considered as very mildly increased, 5–10 is deemed as mildly increased, 10–20 is judged as moderately increased, and greater than 20 is regarded as severely abnormal.

An AHI of more than 5 events per hour is definite indication for treatment in children. An AHI of fewer than 3 events per hour does not require any intervention; the benefit of treatment in children with an AHI of more than 3 but fewer than 5 events per hour remains debatable.

Although PSG reliably measures the presence of OSA, it fails to correlate with the clinical implications of OSDB; child's general wellbeing, including emotional and behavioral health, does not always tally with PSG indices. Therefore, while evaluating treatment outcomes for pediatric OSA, it is essential to consider both PSG parameters and QoL assessments.

Is PSG Indicated for All Cases?

Being a pricey and laborious diagnostic modality, video PSG may not always be financially or practically feasible. Therefore, American Academy of Otolaryngology—Head and Neck Surgery Clinical Practice Guideline recommends that otherwise healthy, nonobese, and previously untreated children need not to undergo PSG prior to adenotonsillectomy.

Polysomnography prior to tonsillectomy is mandatory only for the children who are at risk for OSAS due to comorbidities like obesity, Down syndrome, craniofacial abnormalities, neuromuscular disorders, sickle cell disease, and mucopolysaccharidoses. PSG is also indicated in children who have discordance between the reported severity of SDB and the size of the adenoids and for whom the need for treatment is uncertain.[17]

Alternative Methods of OSDB Diagnosis

As PSG is not easily available everywhere particularly in low-resource settings, hence alternative methods are being evolved. Useful alternative methods are nocturnal pulse oximetry, the pediatric sleep questionnaire, the sleep clinical record, etc.; however, none of these methods are as reliable as PSG.

Nocturnal pulse oximetry is forthcoming as a cheaper alternative to PSG. In children with ATH, an abnormal oximetry according to the McGill criteria

(The McGill criteria: three or more clusters of desaturation events ≥4% and at least three desaturation to <90%) corresponds to OSAS of moderate severity but a negative result does not exclude OSAS with certainty.

The Pediatric Sleep Questionnaire and Sleep Clinical Record are useful for diagnosis; however, they are burdensome for routine clinical office practice.

■ CLINICAL CORRELATES OF OSAS SEVERITY

Secondary enuresis, daytime mouth breathing, elevated blood pressure, failure to thrive, academic regression and inattention, and hyperactivity are frequently present in children with OSDB. Among these morbidities, observed apnea, daytime oral breathing, secondary enuresis, and hypertension strongly correlate with OSA severity.[14,17]

Obesity the Worst Comorbidity

Obesity is a risk factor for OSAS; a prevalence of OSAS between 19% and 61% has been found in obese children and adolescents; this incidence is significantly higher than the prevalence of OSA in normal weight children.

Natural History of Mild OSAS

Studies document that up to two-thirds of children with mild OSAS (AHI 1-5 episodes/hr) are likely to recover completely as they grow older; others may persist with or deteriorate. OSAS is more likely to persist in male child, in an obese child, and in older age (>7 years) child. Childhood Adenotonsillectomy Trial (CHAT) study noted that the number of children with mild disease needed to treat with adenotonsillectomy to prevent persistence of OSAS was one in five children, *therefore in mild OSAS, medical management including montelukast and/or nasal steroids and reassessment after a period of observation is a valid therapeutic option.*

Natural History of Moderate-to-Severe OSAS

Moderate-to-severe OSAS (AHI >5 episodes/hr) is less likely to wane; only 26% patients would resolve spontaneously. The number of children with moderate-to-severe OSAS (AHI >4.7 episodes/hr) needed to treat to prevent persistence of disease in one in three.

■ OSDB DUE TO ADENOTONSILLAR HYPERTROPHY: GOALS OF THE TREATMENT

Treatment of ATH in children with OSDB has two main advantages: (1) it offers relief from the upper airway obstructive events occurring during sleep, and (2) it corrects sleep disordered breathing (SDB)-associated morbidities.

Quality of life, morbidity of the cardiovascular and central nervous systems, nocturnal enuresis, and somatic growth delay all show good improvements.

American Academy of Pediatrics suggests that any child who has OSAS of moderate severity (AHI >5) should receive treatment; however, if PSG or other investigations are unavailable, still treatment should be offered to every patient who has significant SDB-associated morbidity. In the presence of morbidity, treatment has been found to be beneficial even in mild OSAS cases.[17,18] *Therefore, irrespective of investigations results, SDB-associated clinical morbidity is the main determinant of treatment.*

Impact of Adenotonsillectomy on OSDB-related Morbidity

Adenotonsillectomy has favorable impacts on QoL and heals some of the SDB-associated morbidities; however, it may not cure all of them. Compared to moderate-to-severe OSAS, adenotonsillectomy is less efficacious regarding improvement in mild OSAS.

Morbidities originating out of CVS pathology like hypertension, pulmonary artery pressure, metabolic syndrome, and enuresis show better improvement after tonsillectomy. Physical growth and oral breathing improve in majority cases.

Results for disorders arising out of CNS pathology like cognitive impairments and behavioral changes are less satisfactory; resolution of SDB either spontaneously or following adenotonsillectomy or intranasally administered corticosteroids seemed to have little long-term effects on these abnormalities.

Quality of Life

Improvement in quality of life and symptom severity measures following adenotonsillectomy correlate poorly with PSG parameters and are feebly influenced by the baseline OSAS severity.

Adenotonsillectomy is not a panacea for all children with ATH; therefore, patients particularly without significant OSDB morbidities can be subjected to either watchful waiting or other medical treatment.

Watchful Waiting

Many studies sought to determine the prognosis for OSAS children kept under watchful waiting vis-a-vis adenotonsillectomy. Volsky et al.[19] studied children with mild OSA and compared 30 children who underwent tonsillectomy with 34 in the watchful waiting group. Baseline QoL measures which were worse in the tonsillectomy groups versus the observation group improved significantly immediately after surgery; however, the observation group also showed a significant improvement from baseline after 8 months.

Another study found that 42% of candidates for adenotonsillectomy had complete resolution of their OSAS and no longer met PSG criteria for surgery. In clinical practice, in patients without significant comorbidities, a normal waist circumference and a low AHI, adenotonsillectomy need not to be first line of treatment.[18]

■ MEDICAL MANAGEMENT OF OSDB

The medical management of ATH patients with OSDB is still under evolution. Anti-inflammatory medications have the potential to reduce mucosal inflammation and decrease ATH in children with OSA. Leukotriene inhibitors and/or inhaled nasal corticosteroids are the commonly utilized anti-inflammatory medications to treat pediatric OSA.

Role of Montelukast

Discovery of increased expression of leukotriene receptors in hypertrophied adenotonsillar tissue impelled montelukast, a leukotriene inhibitor, in the treatment of ATH-induced OSDB. A large retrospective review, involving 836 children with mild OSA (AHI between 1 and 5 on PSG), treated with 12 weeks of montelukast therapy, showed a significant (>50%) resolution rate for OSAS. Treatment incurred numerous benefits like decreased AHI, improved symptoms, and decreased radiographic adenoidal size.[20]

In addition to nonsevere primary OSA, montelukast is also utilized to treat post-adenotonsillectomy unresolved OSA. The duration of montelukast therapy required to treat pediatric OSA is still under investigation, yet the majority of studies use it for at least 3 months.

Montelukast Failure

Montelukast therapy may fail in about 20% of children; age greater than 7 years and obesity are predictors of a poor response to montelukast.

Intranasal Corticosteroids

The first successful use of intranasal steroid (INS) for adenoid hypertrophy was described by Demain and Goetz in 1995. They showed that properly administered aqueous nasal beclomethasone in standard doses can significantly reduce adenoidal hypertrophy and nasal airway obstructive symptoms in children. The authors hypothesize that by decreasing upper airway resistance and mucosal inflammation, intranasal corticosteroids reduce the disease burden of OSA, in addition, they also control allergic rhinitis, a common comorbid medical condition in children with OSA. Subsequently, several studies have demonstrated improvements in OSA severity in children treated with inhaled intranasal corticosteroids. Evidence suggests that by reducing adenoid size, intranasal steroids may significantly improve symptoms of nasal obstruction in children with ATH. Generally safe, INS can cause epistaxis in few cases. The safety and effectiveness of INS is yet to be established in children less than 2 years of age.[21,22]

INS of Choice

Mometasone furoate (MF) nasal spray is the INS of choice. Drug has three useful qualities: the potency of MF is similar to fluticasone propionate, the most potent steroid; the systemic absorption of the drug after topical administration is lowest of all steroids, hence it has no effect on growth and hypothalamic-pituitary-adrenal axis; lastly, drug does not cause any adverse effect on nasal mucosa on long-term use.[22]

Adenoidectomy versus INS + Montelukast

Study comparing surgical and medical treatment shows that adenotonsillectomy causes faster relief compared to MF nasal spray; however, nasal corticosteroids (MF nasal spray) and/or montelukast administered for 6–12 weeks were also associated with significant reduction in the adenoid size. Long-term topical intranasal mometasone nasal spray can be a good therapeutic option to decrease adenoid hypertrophy and nasal obstruction obviating the need for surgery. Thus, medical treatment is an effective alternative to surgery and deserves a fair trial in children; however, in patients of ATH with significant morbidities, steroid therapy should not delay surgical treatment.[23]

Persistent OSAS

In some cases, OSAS may persist despite adequate medical and surgical treatment. Older age >7 years and obesity are the main contributors to persistent OSA.[24]

■ IMPACT OF ADENOTONSILLECTOMY ON LONG-TERM RISK OF DISEASES

Long-term impacts of adenotonsillectomy were never thoroughly studied and by large have remained unknown. A recent Denmark study tried to analyze this issue.

In an arduous work spanning over three decades, 1,189,061 children were analyzed in this study (48% female), 17,460 underwent adenoidectomy, 11,830 tonsillectomy, and 31,377 adenotonsillectomy; 1,157,684 were in the control group. Analysis of 28 disease groups showed small but significant increases in relative risk for 78% of them.

Tonsillectomy was associated with a sizeable rise in absolute risk for the upper respiratory tract diseases, while increase in relative risk was almost three times; authors commented that tonsillectomy would substantially increase upper respiratory tract diseases in the later life.

Adenoidectomy was associated with twofold relative risk of upper respiratory tract diseases and 17% increased relative risk of infectious diseases; it was also associated with double relative risk for chronic obstructive pulmonary disorder.

Impacts on conditions that surgeries aimed to treat were found to be mixed. For 7 of 21 conditions, surgery was associated with significantly reduced long-term relative risk, 9 (43%) conditions there were no changes; however, 5 (24%) of the conditions registered significant raise. Tonsillectomy significantly reduced risk for tonsillitis and adenoidectomy markedly reduced relative risk for sleep disorders. Risk for otitis media and sinusitis increased significantly after adenotonsillectomy.[25]

These observations amply emphasize the significance of adenoids and tonsils for normal immune system development. Authors remarked that tonsils and adenoids are part of the lymphatic system and play a key role both in the pathogen screening and normal development of the immune system during childhood; therefore, removal of these immune organs during childhood is likely to impair pathogen detection and would increase risk of respiratory and infectious diseases in later life.

■ CONCLUSION

Adenotonsillectomy is performed for either recurrent tonsillar infections or obstructive sleep apnea. While performing surgery for recurrent infections, Paradise criteria should be strictly adhered to. OSA with only snoring should not constitute an indication for surgery; morbidities produced by OSDB should be the basis for procedure.

Tonsils and adenoids are important immunological organs and their removal in childhood can have far reaching impacts on human health. Moreover in majority of children, ATH has a favorable natural course. Therefore, a fair trial of 6 months to 1 year should always be offered and all long-term consequences should be thoroughly discussed with child's caregiver before the removal of tonsils.

■ REFERENCES

1. Mitchell RB, Archer SM, Ishman SL, et al. Clinical Practice Guideline: Tonsillectomy in Children (Update). Otolaryngol Head Neck Surg. 2019; 160(1_suppl):S1-S42.
2. Sumilo D, Nichols L, Ryan R, et al. Incidence of indications for tonsillectomy and frequency of evidence-based surgery: 12-year retrospective cohort study of primary care electronic records. Br J Gen Pract. 2018;69(678):e33-e41.

3. Wennberg J. Commentary: A debt of gratitude to J. Alison Glover. Int J Epidemiol. 2008;37(1):26-9.
4. Dwyer-Hemmings L. 'A Wicked Operation'? Tonsillectomy in Twentieth-Century Britain. Med Hist. 2018;62(2):217-41.
5. Scadding GK. Immunology of the tonsil: a review. JR Soc Med. 1990;83(2):104-7.
6. Brandtzaeg P. Immunology of tonsils and adenoids: everything the ENT surgeon needs to know. Int J Pediatr Otorhinolaryngol. 2003;67 Suppl 1:S69-76.
7. Casselbrant ML. What is wrong in chronic adenoiditis/tonsillitis anatomical considerations. Int J Pediatr Otorhinolaryngol. 1999;49 Suppl. 1:S133-5.
8. Bozkurt G, Dizdar SK, Korkut AY, et al. Adenoid Vegetation in Children with Allergic Rhinitis. Turk Arch Otorhinolaryngol. 2015;53(4):168-72.
9. Paradise JL, Bluestone CD, Bachman RZ, et al. History of recurrent sore throat as indication for tonsillectomy. Predictive limitations of histories that are undocumented. N Eng J Med. 1978;298(8):409-13.
10. Borgström A, Nerfeldt P, Friberg D, et al. Trends and changes in paediatric tonsil surgery in Sweden 1987–2013: a population-based cohort study. BMJ Open. 2017;7(1):e013346.
11. Katz ES, D'Ambrosio CM. Pathophysiology of pediatric obstructive sleep apnea. Proc Am Thorac Soc. 2008;5(2):253-62.
12. Kaditis AG, Alonso Alvarez ML, Boudewyns AN, et al. Obstructive sleep disordered breathing in 2–18 year-old children: diagnosis and management. Eur Respir J. 2016;47(1)69-94.
13. Rubinstein BJ, Baldassari CM. An Update on the Management of Pediatric Obstructive Sleep Apnea. Curr Treat Options Peds. 2015;1(3):211-23.
14. D Muzumdar H, Arens R. Diagnostic issues in pediatric obstructive sleep apnea. Proc Am Thorac Soc. 2008;5(2):263-73.
15. Redline S, Amin R, Beebe D, et al. The Childhood Adenotonsillectomy Trial (CHAT): rationale, design, and challenges of a randomized controlled trial evaluating a standard surgical procedure in a pediatric population. Sleep. 2011;34(11):1509-17.
16. Joosten KF, Larramona H, Miano S, et al. How do we recognize the child with OSAS? Pediatr Pulmonol. 2017;52(2):260-71.
17. Tan HL, Alonso Alvarez ML, Tsaoussoglou M, et al. When and why to treat the child who snores? Pediatr Pulmonol. 2017;52(3):399-412.
18. Alshammari SAG, Aljuhani AM, Alkhalaf AA, et al. Overview of Adenotonsillar Hypertrophy, Management Strategies. Int J Sci Eng Res. 2018;9(6):43-58.
19. Volsky PG, Woughter M, Beydoun H, et al. Adenotonsillectomy vs observation for management of mild obstructive sleep apnea in children. Otolaryngol Head Neck Surg. 2014;150:126-32.
20. Yang DZ, Liang J, Zhang F, et al. Clinical effect of montelukast sodium combined with inhaled corticosteroids in the treatment of OSAS children. Medicine (Baltimore). 2017;96(19):e6628.
21. Zhang L, Mendoza-Sassi RA, César JA, et al. Intranasal corticosteroids for nasal airway obstruction in children with moderate to severe adenoidal hypertrophy. Cochrane Database Syst Rev. 2008;(3):CD006286.
22. Berlucchil M, Barbieri D, Nassif N. Intranasal Steroid Treatment for Adenoids. In: Carmen Adkins (Ed). Corticosteroids and Steroid Therapy. New York: Nova Science Publishers, Inc.; 2015. pp. 41-61.

23. Pai VK, Shetty SS, Devan PP, et al. Adenoidectomy versus mometasone furoate nasal spray in treatment of nasal obstruction in children due to adenoid hypertrophy: a comparative study. Int J Otorhinolaryngol Head Neck Surg. 2019;5(2):310-3.
24. Jung YG, Kim HY, Min JY, et al. Role of Intranasal Topical Steroid in Pediatric Sleep Disordered Breathing and Influence of Allergy, Sinusitis, and Obesity on Treatment Outcome. Clin Exp Otorhinolaryngol. 2011;4(1):27-32.
25. Byars SG, Stearns SC, Boomsma JJ. Association of Long-term Risk of Respiratory, Allergic, and Infectious Diseases with Removal of Adenoids and Tonsils in Childhood. JAMA Otolaryngol Head Neck Surg. 2018;144(7):594-603.

4.4 HIV AND AIDS: DIAGNOSIS AND MANAGEMENT

Ira Shah

■ INTRODUCTION

HIV infection is a major cause of morbidity and mortality ever since this condition has been recognized. With the reporting of first cases in the early 1980s, the scenario is of a world-wide menace in a span of 40 years. India accounts for 13% of global HIV disease but it continuous to be among the low prevalence country because of its high population, the overall prevalence being <1%.[1]

When to Suspect HIV Infection in a Child?

Pediatric HIV primarily is a vertically transmitted infection with over 80% of the patients acquiring HIV through this route.[2] Children infected perinatally with HIV vary greatly in how rapidly they develop immune suppression and symptoms or signs of disease. Systemic and pulmonary infections including tuberculosis, chronic diarrhea, wasting, severe malnutrition, hepatosplenomegaly, lymphadenopathy, chronic dermatitis, pyrexia of unknown origin, recurrent otitis media are some of the common manifestations in children. In infancy, HIV encephalopathy, opportunistic infections especially with *Pneumocystis jirovecii* (PCP), cytomegalovirus (CMV), respiratory viruses and bacterial pneumonia are common. Systemic manifestations such as HIV cardiomyopathy, idiopathic thrombocytopenic purpura (ITP) are seen in older children and adolescents.[3]

■ DIAGNOSIS OF HIV

Diagnosis of HIV in Infants

All infants born to HIV-infected mothers carry maternal IgG antibodies which cross the placenta freely. These maternal antibodies may remain detectable in the infant's serum for up to 12–15 months after birth. As a result, serological diagnosis of HIV infection is only reliable after 15–18 months of age. Infants infected with HIV must be diagnosed as rapidly as possible to ensure the early institution of therapy to limit HIV-related morbidity and to prevent opportunistic infections. Tests that can be done for diagnosis of HIV infection in children below 18 months of age are HIV culture, detection of HIV-proviral DNA by polymerase chain reaction (PCR) or HIV antigen (p24). Detection of p24 antigen is cheaper, highly specific and easy to perform but it is less sensitive than other virological tests. Also false negativity is high in younger children as most of the p24 antigen is bound to maternal antibodies. HIV culture is done from peripheral blood mononuclear cells (PBMCs) but is technically difficult and time consuming. It is expensive and done in research institutes. Polymerase chain reaction is now the preferred tool for diagnosis of HIV in infants.[4-6]

Timing of PCR Test

As per the United States Agency for International Development (USAID), virologic testing at birth is considered for newborns born to HIV- infected women who did not receive antiretroviral (ARV) drugs adequately, or had an inadequate viral suppression. Testing HIV-exposed infants at the time of birth only identifies 20–58% of infants with HIV infection.[7] As per National AIDS Control Organization (NACO), early infant diagnosis (EID) by virological testing should be done at 6 weeks of age with a repeat testing at 6 months, 12 months and 6 weeks after cessation of breastfeeds. Confirmation of HIV status of all babies should be done at 18 months using all 3 antibody (Rapid) tests.[8]

Diagnosis of HIV in Children Above 18 Months of Age

Enzyme-linked immunosorbent assay (ELISA) is the time-tested reliable method for detection of anti-HIV antibodies with a sensitivity of >99.5% and specificity of 99%. As per NACO, confirmation of HIV status of should be done using three ELISA kits. For clinically symptomatic patients, the sample should be reactive with two different kits to confirm the HIV positivity state. For clinically asymptomatic persons, the sample should be reactive with all the three different kits to confirm the HIV positivity state.[4]

Diagnosis of HIV-2 Infection

The majority of commercially available HIV screening antibody tests can detect both HIV-1 and HIV-2 but do not distinguish between the two viruses. More than 60% of individuals with HIV-2 infection are misclassified as having HIV-1 by the HIV-1 Western blot. Confirmatory testing for HIV-2 infection uses an HIV-2 nucleic acid test. Infants born to HIV-2-infected mothers should be tested for HIV-2 infection with HIV-2-specific virologic assays (HIV-2 DNA PCR testing) at time points similar to those used for HIV-1 testing.[4]

■ MANAGEMENT OF HIV IN CHILDREN

Prior to starting antiretroviral therapy (ART), thorough assessment should be done to identify HIV-related illnesses and opportunistic infections. If opportunistic infection is suspected, then diagnosis and treatment of opportunistic infections (OIs) should take priority over ART initiation. After appropriate counseling, ART should be initiated.

Antiretroviral Drugs[9,10]

Antiretrovirals are a group of drugs that are used in the treatment of children living with HIV to decrease the viral burden. These drugs fall into three major classes—nucleoside and nucleotide analog reverse transcriptase inhibitors (NRTIs), non-nucleoside analog Reverse transcriptase inhibitors (NNRTIs) and protease inhibitors (PIs) along with pharmacokinetic enhancers. There are three new classes of drugs now approved for treatment of HIV in children. They are the entry/fusion inhibitors, integrase strand transfer inhibitors (INSTIs) and CCR5 (C-C chemokine receptor type 5) co-receptor antagonist.

Nucleoside Reverse Transcriptase Inhibitors[9,10]

The nucleoside reverse transcriptase inhibitors (NRTIs) were the first class of antiretroviral drugs that became available for treatment of HIV. They inhibit the reverse transcriptase enzyme. They have activity against both HIV-1 and HIV-2. Dual NRTI is the backbone of current combination of various antiretroviral therapies.

Drugs in this class include:
- Zidovudine (AZT/ZDV)
- Lamivudine (3TC)
- Abacavir (ABC)
- Emtricitabine (FTC)
- *Tenofovir disoproxil fumerate (TDF):* It is a nucleotide reverse transcriptase inhibitor (NtRTI). It also acts against Hepatitis B.
- *Tenofovir alafenamide (TAF):* It is a new NRTI similar to tenofovir disoproxil fumerate (TDF). TAF has lesser bone and renal toxicity than TDF, but equal antiviral efficacy as TDF.

Non-nucleoside Reverse Transcriptase Inhibitors[9,10]

Non-nucleoside reverse transcriptase inhibitors (NNRTIs) were the second class of anti-HIV agents to be developed. The parent compounds are the

active moieties, and are therefore immediately active on entering the cell. The NNRTI class of drugs rapidly reduces viral load; however drug resistance develops quickly after initiation of monotherapy and cross-resistance between drugs in this class is common. There are currently three NNRTIs used for treatment of HIV infection:
1. Nevirapine (NVP)
2. Efavirenz (EFV)
3. *Etravirine:* It is a second-line NNRTI used in children >6 years of age and is considered a 'second generation' NNRTI, in part because it retains activity against HIV-1 isolates which are resistant to other NNRTIs. The other second generation NNRTI is rilpivirine, which is only approved for use in adults.

Protease Inhibitors[9,10]

They are active against both HIV-1 and HIV-2. Low-dose ritonavir (RTV) is a potent protease inhibitor (PI) acts as a potent inhibitor of the cytochrome P450 3A4 (CYP3A4) isoenzyme, thereby inhibiting the metabolism of other PIs. It has been used in low doses combined with another PI as a "pharmacokinetic booster," increasing drug exposure by prolonging the second drug's half-life. Boosted PI-based regimens are commonly used in treatment of adults, but adequate pediatric data are only available for co-formulated lopinavir/ritonavir in children older than 2 weeks of age and for atazanavir, fosamprenavir, darunavir, and tipranavir with low-dose ritonavir in children age more than 6 years.

Entry Inhibitors[11]

These agents inhibit viral binding or fusion to host target cells. T-20 (Enfurvirtide) is currently used and is to be used only in children over 6 years of age. It is to be administered subcutaneously, twice daily. It prevents virus-cell fusion. It is used as part of salvage regime in patients who have multiple ART failures.

CCR5 Co-receptor Antagonist[12]

Maraviroc blocks the chemokine CCR5 co-receptor on the CD4 cell surface thereby preventing HIV from entering the cell. This was the first antiretroviral drug to be developed that does not actually target the virus itself. This drug is approved for use by children more than 2 years of age. Maraviroc is effective in combination with other ART in patients with multi-drug-resistant HIV-1. However, it is necessary to check for CCR5 or CXCR4 virus tropism before starting the drug. CCR5 antagonists will be inactive against CXCR4-tropic virus and mixed/dual tropic HIV virus. There are considerable interactions with both PI and NNRTI classes, requiring alteration in Maraviroc dosing depending on other drugs in the regimen.

Integrase Strand Transfer inhibitors[13]

They block the integrase enzyme thereby preventing incorporation of viral DNA into human genome. Raltegravir, dolutegravir, elvitegravir and bictegravir are integrase strand-transfer inhibitors (INSTIs). These drugs have been found to be useful in the treatment of patients with multidrug-resistant HIV-1. Raltegravir is FDA-approved for treatment of HIV-infected full-term neonates, infants and children. Raltegravir has a favorable safety profile and lacks significant drug interactions. FDA has recently approved dolutegravir for children >30 kg body weight. The drug has a very favorable safety profile and can be dosed once daily in treatment of INSTI-naive patients.

There appears to be increased risk of neural tube defects in infants born to women who were receiving dolutegravir (DTG) at the time of conception. Thus dolutegravir is not recommended for use in pregnant women during the first trimester and in non-pregnant women who are trying to conceive.

At present, highly active combination regimens including at least three drugs are recommended; and these regimens have shown increased survival, fall in the opportunistic infections, improved growth and neurocognition, and improved quality of life in children. The current guidelines for starting ART have been simplified. As per World Health Organization (WHO) July 2017 update on HIV treatment and care, ART should be initiated in everyone infected with HIV at any/all CD4 cell count, regardless of WHO clinical stage. NACO has adopted WHO guidelines to *treat all* people with HIV with ART regardless of CD4 count, clinical stage and age or population. Dual NRTIs backbone regimen includes, zidovudine with lamivudine or emtricitabine combination due to favorable safety profile and extensive experience and abacavir plus lamivudine or emtricitabine for children aged ≥3 months. Tenofovir alafenamide and emtricitabine as fixed dose combination tablet along with NNRTI (single tablet) is indicated in children ≥25 kg weight or ≥6 years with estimated CrCl ≥30 mL/min. Tenofovir disoproxil fumarate with lamivudine or emtricitabine combination is FDA approved for use in children ≥2 years. However, risk of decreased bone mineral density versus benefits should be considered. The preferred ART regimen in HIV-infected children is depicted in **Table 4.4.1**. ART should not be started in the presence of an active opportunistic infection (OI). In general, OIs should be treated or stabilized before commencing ART. *Mycobacterium Avium* Complex (MAC) and progressive multifocal leukoencephalopathy (PML) are exceptions in which commencing ART may be the preferred treatment, especially when specific MAC therapy is not available. In patients with TB co-infection, start TB treatment first and ART should be started after 2 weeks and before 2 months.[9,10]

Table 4.4.1: Preferred and alternative first-line regimens for children according to the World Health Organization (WHO), November 2015 consolidated guidelines.[13]

Age group	Preferred first-line regimens	Alternative first-line regimens (Children)
Children <3 years	ABC (or AZT)+ 3TC + LPV /r	ABC (or AZT) + 3TC + NVP
Children 3 years to <10 years	ABC + 3TC + EFV	ABC + 3TC + NVP AZT + 3TC + EFV (or NVP) TDF + 3TC (or FTC) + EFV (or NVP)
Adolescents	TDF + 3TC (or FTC) + EFV	AZT +3TC +EFV (or NVP) TDF or ABC + 3TC or FTC + DTG* or EFV$_{400}$* or NVP

*Safety profile and efficacy data on use of DTG and EFV$_{400}$ in people with HIV/TB coinfection and children <12 years are not yet available.
ABC: abacavir; AZT: zidovudine; 3TC: lamivudine; LPV/r: lopinavir-ritonavir; NVP: nevirapine; EFV: efavirenz; FTC: emtricitabine; TDF: tenofovir; DTG: dolutegravir; EFV$_{400}$: efavirenz at lower dose (400 mg/kg/day)

■ MONITORING RESPONSE TO ART[13-15]

By one month of starting an effective ART regimen in children, there is a substantial drop in the plasma HIV viral load and the CD4 count starts to rise. Infants, with an initial viral load of between 10^5 and 10^7 copies/mL, can take longer to become undetectable. As per World Health Organization (WHO) recommendations, routine viral load testing is encouraged at 6 followed by 12 months after initiating ART and if the patient is stable on ART (i.e. on ART for more than or at least 1 year, no present illness or pregnancy, good understanding of life-long adherence and evidence of treatment success which is two consecutive viral-load measures below 1000 copies/mL), then every year thereafter. WHO recommends measurement of the CD4 cell count 6 monthly until stable on ART, following which CD4 cell count monitoring can be withheld in patients who are virally suppressed and stable on ART.

Changing Antiretroviral Therapy

ART regimen may be changed in the following circumstances:
- Failure of current regimen
- Toxicity or intolerance to current regimen.

■ TREATMENT FAILURE[13]

Poor adherence, inadequate drug levels, prior existing drug resistance, drug-drug interaction or inadequate potency of the drugs chosen can all contribute to ARV treatment failure. Treatment failure is considered as either clinical failure, immunological failure or virological failure **(Table 4.4.2)**.

Table 4.4.2: WHO definition of clinical, immunological and virological failures for the decision to switch ART regimens.

Failure	Definition	Comment
Clinical failure	New or recurrent clinical event indicating severe immunodeficiency, WHO clinical stage 4 condition in adults and adolescents whereas WHO clinical stage 3 and 4 clinical condition with the exception of tuberculosis in children after 6 months of effective treatment.	The condition must be differentiated from immune reconstitution inflammatory syndrome (IRIS) occurring after initiating ART.
		For adults, certain WHO clinical stage 3 conditions (pulmonary TB and severe bacterial infections) may also indicate treatment failure.
Immunological failure	*Adults and adolescents:* CD4 count ≤250 cells/mm^3 following clinical failure[#] or persistent CD4 levels <100 cells/mm^3	Without concomitant or recent infection to cause a transient decline in the CD4 cell count.
	Children: • *<5 years:* Persistent CD4 levels below 200 cells/mm^3 • *>5 years:* Persistent CD4 levels below 100 cells/mm^3	Current WHO clinical and immunological criteria have low sensitivity and positive predictive value for identifying individuals with virological failure.
Virological failure	Viral load above 1000 copies/mL based on two consecutive viral-load measurements in 3 months, with adherence support following the first viral load test	An individual must be taking ART for at least 6 months before it can be determined that a regimen has failed.

[#]Previous guidelines defined immunological failure based on a fall from baseline, which is no longer applicable in the context of CD4-independent treatment initiation. The option of CD4 cell count at or below 250 cells/mm^3 following clinical failure is based on an analysis of data from Uganda and Zimbabwe.

When to Switch ARV Drugs for Treatment Failure[13]

Available drug regimens, viral resistance profiles, adherence issues and readiness of the family and child to switch; all need to be considered. Adding or substituting single drugs in a failing ART regimen without resistance testing risks giving the new drug as effective monotherapy which may result in rapid development of further resistance. It is therefore recommended that all changes in therapy with detectable viremia be preceded by a resistance test unless it is unequivocal that there is no cross-resistance with previous drugs received. Ideally resistance testing should be performed while the patient is still on the old regimen, or within a few weeks of stopping. Expert opinion should be sought in interpreting resistance genotypes. The general rule is to change all the drugs in the regimen after first-line ART failure with resistance. Regimen should include at least two, preferably three, fully active ARV drugs based on past treatment history and resistance pattern for durable and potent virologic suppression. The new WHO recommendations include use of DRV/r or RAL with LPV/r as alternative ART regimens for adults and adolescents. For children after failure of first-line LPV/r based regimen, RAL-based second line regimen is recommended. Failure of an NNRTI-based regimen is often as a result of viral drug resistance, and switching to a boosted PI or an INSTI based regimen is appropriate. Failure of a boosted PI-based regimen is more likely to be because of poor adherence than resistance. If resistance is detected, a switch to an NNRTI-based regimen or another PI without overlapping resistance may be appropriate. If resistance is not detected, continuing the PI with enhanced adherence support should be considered. Any change in regimen should be preceded by a thorough re-assessment of adherence, and a plan for adherence monitoring of the new regimen.

■ PREVENTION OF PARENT-TO-CHILD TRANSMISSION (PPTCT) OF HIV[16,17]

HIV can be transmitted from an HIV-positive woman to her child during pregnancy, childbirth and breastfeeding. Mother-to-child transmission (MTCT) which is also known as 'vertical transmission' accounts for most infections in children. Without treatment, the likelihood of the virus passing from mother-to-child is 15–45%. However, with antiretroviral treatment (ART) for the mother and a short course of antiretroviral drugs for the baby this risk is reduced to below 5%. Around 1.4 million HIV infections among children were prevented between 2010 and 2018 due to the implementation of PMTCT (Prevention of Mother-to-child transmission) services. In India, the PPTCT programme was launched in the year 2002 with an aim to prevent the perinatal transmission of HIV from an HIV infected pregnant mother to her newborn baby. The program entails counseling and testing of pregnant women in the ICTCs. In 2014, all pregnant women who are HIV positive are initiated on lifelong ART, irrespective of CD4 count and WHO clinical Staging. The recommended first-line regimen for HIV-infected pregnant women is Tenofovir (TDF) (300 mg) + Lamuvidine (3TC) (300 mg) + Efavirenz (EFV) (600 mg) (if there is no prior exposure to NNRTIs (NVP/EFV) at any gestational age. HIV-infected pregnant women who have had previous exposure to Sd-NVP (or EFV) for PPTCT prophylaxis in prior pregnancies, an NNRTI-based ART regimen such as may not be fully effective due to persistence of archived mutation to NNRTIs. Thus, these women will require a protease-inhibitor based ART regimen such as TDF + 3TC + LPV/r. The dose is TDF + 3TC (1 tablet daily) +LPV (200 mg)/r (50 mg) (2 tablets BD). However, the great majority of HIV infections in India are due to HIV-1, there are small foci of HIV-2 infection as well, primarily in western India. HIV-2 will also progress to AIDS, although progression is generally much slower. HIV-2 has the same modes of transmission as HIV-1 but has been shown to be much less transmissible from mother-to-child (transmission risk 0–4%). NNRTI drugs, such as NVP and EFV, are not effective against HIV-2 infection. Therefore, for women who are infected with HIV-2 alone should follow standard adult guidelines for HIV-2 treatment which consists of 2NRTIs + LPV/r. Prophylaxis NVP with AZT (instead of Syrup NVP) to be given to babies in mothers with HIV-2. If a pregnant woman is detected to have both HIV-1 and HIV-2 infections, she should receive standard first ART regimen (TDF+3TC + EFV) recommended for women with HIV-1 infection.

At the time of delivery, mother-to-child transmission risk is increased by the prolonged rupture of membranes, repeated per vaginal examinations, assisted instrumental delivery (vacuum or forceps), invasive fetal monitoring procedures (scalp/fetal blood monitoring), and episiotomy. Safe delivery techniques should be followed to reduce the transmission during delivery. Cesarean sections in HIV-positive pregnant women should be performed for obstetric indications only.

■ HIV-EXPOSED INFANT[16,17]

As per NACO prevention of parent-to-child transmission (PPTCT) guidelines, HIV-exposed infant (HEI) should be started on postpartum ARV prophylaxis for minimum of 6 weeks **(Table 4.4.3)**. They may be given exclusive breastfeeds for 6 months and continued breastfeeds along with complementary feeds from 6 months to 1 year. For babies who are HIV- infected and are on ART, breastfeed up to 2 years is recommended. Only when breastfeeding is contraindicated or cannot be done (maternal death, severe maternal illness) or is the individual mother's choice (at her own risk), exclusive replacement feeding may be considered. AFASS (A: Affordable, F: Feasible, A: Acceptable,

Table 4.4.3: Dose and duration of infant daily nevirapine (NVP) prophylaxis.[17]

Birth weight (kg)*	Daily NVP dose in mg	NVP dose in mL**	NVP dose in mL**
Less than 2 kg	2 mg/kg Once a day	0.2 mL/kg Once a day	Up to six weeks, irrespective of whether the baby is exclusively breastfed or exclusively replacement fed. The duration may be extended to 12 weeks if the mother had not received ART for at least 24 weeks, including women initiated on ART during labor and if she is breastfeeding the child.
2–2.5 kg	10 mg Once a day	1 mL Once a day	
More than 2.5 kg	15 mg Once a day	1.5 ml Once a day	

Formulation: 10 mg Nevirapine in 1 mL suspension
**Infant NVP:* Give first dose of NVP (within 6 to 12 hours of delivery and continue daily for 6 weeks.

S: Sustainable, S: Safe) criteria must be fulfilled to give exclusive replacement feeding. During the first six months, mixed feeding should not be done under any circumstance (Mixed feeding refers to breastfeeds and replacement feeds simultaneously in the first 6 months, and can lead to mucosal abrasions in the gut of the baby, which can facilitate HIV virus entry through these abrasions). Co-trimoxazole prophylaxis should be started from 6 weeks of age.

Co-trimoxazole Prophylaxis for HIV-exposed/ Infected Infants and Children[16,17]

Co-trimoxazole (CTX) prophylaxis is safe, inexpensive and highly effective in reducing morbidity and mortality among HIV-infected infants and children, as well as in adolescents and adults. Ideally, all infants exposed to HIV should be started on co-trimoxazole prophylaxis from six weeks of life. Providing co-trimoxazole prophylaxis protects against serious, often fatal, opportunistic infections (OIs). It has also been recognized that co-trimoxazole prophylaxis provides benefits beyond the prevention of *Pneumocystis jirovecii* pneumonia (PJP). Prophylaxis should be discontinued for children who are subsequently determined not to be infected with HIV. HIV-infected children and children whose infection status remains unknown should continue to receive prophylaxis for the 18 months of life.

In older children and adults (including pregnant women), co-trimoxazole prophylaxis is recommended for severe or advanced HIV clinical disease (WHO stage 3 or 4) and/or for a CD4 count ≤350 cells/mm^3. In settings where malaria and/or severe bacterial infections are highly prevalent, co-trimoxazole prophylaxis should be initiated regardless of CD4 cell count or WHO stage. Co-trimoxazole prophylaxis may be discontinued in adults (including pregnant women) with HIV infection who are clinically stable on antiretroviral therapy, with evidence of immune recovery and viral suppression.

Dose: 5 mg/kg/day of Trimethoprim once a day.

Isoniazid Prevention Therapy (IPT)

HIV-infected children without active tuberculosis should be offered isoniazid prevention therapy (IPT). HIV infection increases the susceptibility to new tuberculosis (TB) or activation of latent TB. There is a 30-fold greater risk of developing TB in HIV-infected patients as compared to those who are not infected with HIV. WHO recommends isoniazid preventative therapy (IPT) for six months in HIV-infected adults and children who are on anti-retroviral therapy (ART) and do not have active TB. The dose of Isoniazid (INH) to be used is 10 mg/kg/day for 6 months.

Immunization in HIV-infected Children

HIV-infected children should be protected from vaccine-preventable diseases. Most vaccines recommended for routine use can be administered safely to HIV-exposed or HIV-infected children. All inactivated vaccines can be administered safely. Varicella and measles-mumps-rubella vaccines can be considered for HIV-infected children who are not severely immunosuppressed (i.e. those with age-specific CD4 cell percentages of >15%). Oral polio, and intranasal influenza vaccine are contraindicated in HIV-infected patients. HIV-exposed infants should be given BCG at birth. However, it should not be given in HIV-infected children.

■ CONCLUSION

HIV has now evolved from a fatal condition to that of a chronic manageable disease. With newer advances both in antiretroviral drugs and diagnostics, HIV treatment has become simplified and available to all those who are infected. The recent protocol of PPTCT has simplified therapy as well as holds promise of <2% transmission of HIV, thus almost decreasing new cases of pediatric HIV.

■ REFERENCES

1. UNAIDS. HIV and AIDS Estimates. Available at URL: http://www.unaids.org/en/regionscountries/countries/india. Accessed on 15th March 2015.
2. Lyall H. Diagnosis, staging and clinical presentation of HIV in children: clinical and laboratory diagnosis. Available from Tr@inforPedHIV 2011.
3. Shah I. Age-related clinical manifestations of HIV infection in indian children. J Trop Pediatr. 2005;51(5):300-3.

4. CDC. MMWR. Revised Surveillance Case Definition for HIV Infection —United States, 2014. Available at URL: http://www.cdc.gov/mmwr/pdf/rr/rr6303.pdf. Accessed on 15th May 2015.
5. Shah Ira. Efficacy of HIV-PCR techniques to diagnose HIV in infants born to HIV-infected mothers: an Indian perspective. JAPI. 2006;54: 197-9.
6. Shah Ira. Diagnosis of perinatal transmission of HIV-1 infection by HIV DNA-PCR. JK Science. 2004;6:187-9.
7. UNAIDS. Antiretroviral Management of Newborns with Perinatal HIV Exposure or Perinatal HIV: Available at: https://aidsinfo.nih.gov/guidelines/html/3/perinatal/187/antiretroviral-management-of-newborns-with-perinatal-hiv-exposure-or-perinatal-hiv. (Accessed on 29th April 2019)
8. NACO. Prevention of Parent to Child Transmission. Available at URL: http://naco.gov.in/prevention-parent-child-transmissionpptct. (Accessed on 29th April 2019)
9. NACO. National Technical Guidelines on Antiretroviral Therapy. October 2018 Available at URL: http://naco.gov.in/sites/default/files/NACO%20-%20National%20Technical%20Guidelines%20on%20ART_October%202018%20%281%29.pdf. (Accessed on 29th June 2019)
10. WHO. Consolidated guidelines on the use of antiretroviral drugs for treating and preventing HIV infection: recommendations for a public health approach. Second edition. 2016. Available at URL: https://www.who.int/hiv/pub/arv/arv-2016/en. (Accessed on 29th April 2019)
11. Wiznia A, Church J, Emmanuel P, et al. Safety and efficacy of enfuvirtide for 48 weeks as part of an optimized antiretroviral regimen in pediatric human immunodeficiency virus 1-infected patients. Pediatr Infect Dis J. 2007;26(9): 799-805.
12. Maraviroc [package insert]. Food and Drug Administration. 2016. Available at https://www.accessdata.fda.gov/drugsatfda_docs/label/2016/208984_022128s017lbl.pdf. (Accessed on 29th April 2019)
13. WHO. Updated recommendations on first-line and second-line antiretroviral regimens and post-exposure prophylaxis and recommendations on early infant diagnosis of HIV. Available at URL: https://www.who.int/hiv/pub/guidelines/ARV2018update/en/. (Accessed on 29th April 2019)
14. NACO. National Guidelines for HIV-1 Viral Load Laboratory Testing. Available at URL: http://naco.gov.in/sites/default/files/NationalGuidelinesForHIV-1ViralLoadLaboratoryTestingApril2018%20%282%29.pdf. (Accessed on 29th April 2019)
15. WHO. What's new in treatment monitoring: viral load and CD4 testing. Available at URL: https://www.who.int/hiv/pub/arv/treatment-monitoring-info-2017/en/. (Accessed 31st March 2019)
16. World Health Organization (WHO). Mother-to-child transmission of HIV. Available at URL: https://www.who.int/hiv/topics/mtct/en/. (Accessed on 29th April 2019)
17. NACO. Prevention of Parent to Child Transmission. Available at URL: http://naco.gov.in/prevention-parent-child-transmissionpptct. (Accessed on 29th April 2019)

4.5 NEW VIRAL INFECTIONS

Dhanya Dharmapalan

■ INTRODUCTION

Noted Nobel Prize winner and American molecular biologist, Joshua Lederberg in his speech given before an audience of virologists in 1989 warned, "Our only real competitors remain the viruses; for it is by no means clear that antiviral antibiosis can generally be achieved in principle: the very essence of the virus is its fundamental entanglement with the genetic and metabolic machinery of the host".[1]

The emergence of new viral diseases results when a virus switches host from zoonotic species to humans and become recognized as new viral infections. Human immunodeficiency virus (HIV), Ebola, Nipah, severe acute respiratory syndrome coronaviruses (SARS-CoV), etc. are few such examples of viruses which have zoonotic origin. Once a virus is identified, it is classified as a member of a virus family based on the features of the virus, e.g. the genome [double-stranded deoxyribonucleic acid (dsDNA), single-stranded DNA (ssDNA), double-stranded ribonucleic acid (dsRNA), single-stranded RNA (ssRNA)(+), ssRNA(-)], structure of the viral capsid, whether enveloped or nonenveloped, host range, pathogenicity, and sequence similarity. This process of taxonomic classification of the virus is done by International Committee on Taxonomy of Viruses (ICTV). The committee then determines whether the newly discovered virus, based on its properties, belongs to an existing species or a new species.[2]

The epidemic potential of any virus can be explained by the concept of basic reproduction number R_0. R_0 is defined as the average number of secondary cases generated by a single primary case in a large, previously unexposed host population.[3] Factors that influence R_0 are pathogen traits and host traits which include demography, behavior, genetics, and adaptive immunity. Human activities like deforestation, urbanization, and agriculture have favored rodent and arthropod multiplication have led to increased incidence of zoonotic diseases in humans. Viruses are also capable of genetic reassortment. Spontaneous single point mutation in viruses, e.g. influenza A can lead to unpredictable pandemic in the immune naive human population.

The following are examples of application of this R_0 factor to the different stages of virus emergence due to cross-species switch in host **(Table 4.5.1)**.

■ SEVERE ACUTE RESPIRATORY SYNDROME CORONAVIRUS

Severe acute respiratory syndrome coronavirus was first reported from Guangdong province, China in 2003. It caused atypical pneumonia soon

Table 4.5.1: Understanding the emergence of viral pathogens based on stages of cross-species switch and the pathogen pyramid.[3,4]

Stages of cross-species host switch	Level as per the pathogen pyramid	Infection and transmission	R_0 factor	Comments
	1 (Exposure)	No infection in humans		
1	2 (Infection)	Infection in a new human host with no onward transmission (dead host)	$R_0 = 0$	Examples: Asfarviridae and Bornaviridae
2	3 (Transmission)	Continued onward transmission within the human population to cause local outbreaks with epidemic fade out	$0 < R_0 < 1$	37 species have been identified. Currently under high surveillance due to potential to evolve and cause a large epidemic. Examples: H5N1 influenza, Japanese encephalitis, Crimean–Congo hemorrhagic fever, West Nile virus, Middle East respiratory syndrome
3	4 (Epidemic)	Major epidemic or sustained endemic host-host transmission in the human population	$R_0 > 1$	More than 60 common human-pathogens identified including human influenza A virus ($R_0 < 2$), measles virus ($R_0 < 18$), and dengue virus ($R_0 < 22$)

complicating into and acute lung injury and acute respiratory distress syndrome (ARDS). The host switch of the virus occurred from zoonotic reservoirs like bats, Himalayan palm civets (*Paguma larvata*), and raccoon dogs *(Nyctereutes procyonoides)*. It affected mainly the elderly population with about 50% mortality during the epidemic.[5] However, the incidence in children was low, less than 10%. The transmission occurred mostly due to close contact with an infected adult in household or healthcare settings. The clinical outcome was favorable in SARS affected children and no death was reported.[6,7] SARS-CoV is not in circulation presently.

■ MIDDLE EAST RESPIRATORY SYNDROME CORONAVIRUS

Middle East respiratory syndrome coronavirus (MERS-CoV) caused fever and mild respiratory symptoms to severe respiratory distress. It was reported in clusters from the Middle East between 2012 and 2014. The virus mainly affected the adult population as there are few reports in pediatric population. Also, the mortality associated was less in children unless there was an underlying comorbidity.[8] Since human-to-human transmission occurred with droplets or by fomites, the Government of Kingdom of Saudi Arabia issued travel advisory in 2013. However, no sustained human-to-human transmission has been documented as the virus did not spread easily unless there was close contact. Majority of the cases occurred in Saudi Arabia where transmission was facilitated during Hajj, a mass annual religious gathering.[9] As a precautionary measure, it was advised to avoid contact with sick camels or consume unpasteurized camel milk or camel meat and wash hands before and after contact with camels.

■ OTHER NEW RESPIRATORY VIRUSES

Advances in molecular methods to detect virus in respiratory samples have led to the discovery of new respiratory pathogens like *human metapneumoviruses*, *Coronavirus NL63*, and *HKU1*. They clinically present with otitis media, bronchiolitis or pneumonia in children. However, the diagnostic methods of these new viruses are complex and limited by problems of amplification of nonviral related sequence artefacts.

■ NIPAH VIRUS

In May 2018, the southern state of Kerala witnessed an outbreak of Nipah virus encephalitis which killed 21 people. The previous outbreaks had occurred in eastern India in the West Bengal districts of Siliguri 2001 and Nadia 2007.

Evidence from Kerala outbreak suggested that fruit bats genus *Pteropus* were the natural hosts. Nipah is a paramyxovirus virus of *Henipavirus* genus. It was first isolated in March 1999 from the cerebrospinal fluid (CSF) of an encephalitis victim from Sungai Nipah village. Later it was named Nipah and classified into a new genus called *Henipavirus*.

Nosocomial transmission occurs by droplets or fomite. In Siliguri outbreak 75% cases occurred among visitors and healthcare workers who came in contact with the patient.[10] Hence in healthcare settings, in addition to standard precautions, droplet, contact, and airborne precautions should be strictly adhered to. In contrast, no human-to-human transmission was reported in 1998 Malaysian outbreak in which pigs were intermediate hosts.

The clinical presentation can be either or combined encephalitis with ARDS. The case fatality rate is 40–100%. Nipah should be therefore suspected in any outbreak of acute encephalitis with or without ARDS, high secondary attack, and case fatality, in a relevant geographical setting or contact with pigs/bats in a relevant epidemiological setting.

The diagnosis can be made by reverse transcription polymerase chain reaction (RT-PCR). Magnetic resonance imaging (MRI) brain shows multifocal discrete lesions in the subcortical and deep white matter of the cerebral hemisphere.[11]

The role of ribavirin has not been clearly evaluated and requires further studies. Other drugs being evaluated are m102.4 monoclonal antibody and Favipiravir.

■ HANTAVIRUS

Hantaviruses are RNA viruses belonging to family Bunyaviridae. *Hantaan virus, Seoul virus, Puumala virus, Sin Nombre virus,* and *Dobrava-Belgrade virus* are important species identified in this family. Rodents are the zoonotic reservoirs for hantaviruses which cause hemorrhagic fever with renal syndrome (HFRS) and hantavirus pulmonary syndrome (HPS).[12]

The transmission of the virus mostly occurs by inhalation of aerosolized viral particles from rodent excreta or saliva. Seroprevalence has been documented among health population. The clinical presentation has been described in five stages which may overlap: febrile, hypotensive, oliguric, diuretic, and convalescent.[12] In a week's time after onset, severe thrombocytopenia can occur mimicking dengue illness. Also, leptospirosis is an important differential in endemic settings because of renal involvement in some cases. There are reports from India among adults of ocular involvement in the form of low intraocular pressure, transient myopia, and conjunctival and retinal hemorrhages.[13]

Hantavirus has been infrequently reported in children. Serological diagnosis by anti-hantavirus immunoglobulin G (IgG) and immunoglobulin M (IgM) is the mainstay of diagnosis as molecular diagnosis can identify the virus in only 20% cases.[12]

■ CHIKUNGUNYA

Chikungunya re-emerged in India in 2005–06 with more than 1.38 cases in 14 states and union territories. The earlier outbreaks had been reported in 1963 in Kolkata, in 1964 in Southern India, and in 1973 in Maharashtra.

Chikungunya name has its origin from Makonde language which translates to "that bends up", based on the inability to stand or walk due to severe arthralgia. Chikungunya is a positive sense single-sided RNA virus which belongs to Togaviridae family, genus *Alphavirus*.

Human transmission takes place by the bite of Aedes mosquito, primarily by the *Aedes aegypti* and *Aedes albopictus* mosquito. The adaptation of the *Aedes albopictus* or the tiger mosquito to the South Asian climate, lack of vector control measures, urbanization are some factors postulated for the re-emergence of chikungunya in the Indian subcontinent.

The clinical features in children differ from adults.[14] Infants are more affected than older age groups. Vertical transmission from infected mother occurs mainly towards delivery. Both pediatric and adult age groups suffer from high grade fever. Maculopapular rash occurs earlier in children, mostly after 2-3 days of onset with a centrifugal spread. Brownish-black hyperpigmentation is seen in children over the centrofacial area and extremities. The characteristic pigmentation on the nose is called "brownie nose" or the "chik" sign. The pigmentation may also be scattered over body without any surrounding erythema. Intraepidermal retention of melanin by the chikungunya virus has been proposed as a possible mechanism for the hyperpigmentation. Symmetric, vesiculobullous lesions without any perilesional erythema occur mostly in young infants.[15]

Adults have more severe joint involvement than children. Arthralgia/arthritis is usually distal, symmetric, and affects multiple joints. Neurological complications like seizures, acute encephalopathy, and meningoencephalitis are seen in greater proportions among children than adults. Oral ulcers unlike adults are rare in children.

Reverse transcription polymerase chain reaction or serological evidence of IgG/IgM antibodies help in laboratory detection of this virus. It is advised to do both PCR and serological testing in the first week as PCR is positive in the first 5 days, while IgM becomes detectable between second and seventh day of onset and peaks around 1 month to decline after 2 months. IgG becomes detectable after a week and persists lifelong.

The treatment is supportive. It is better to avoid nonsteroidal anti-inflammatory drugs (NSAIDs) and use paracetamol so that there is no increased risk of bleeding.

■ ZIKA VIRUS

Zika virus was declared as a public health emergency by the World Health Organization (WHO) on 1st February 2016 after a massive outbreak in South America, predominantly in Brazil. The name of this *Flavivirus* can be traced to its discovery in rhesus monkeys in the Zika forest of Uganda in 1947 during yellow fever surveillance.

Zika is primarily transmitted by the *Aedes aegypti* mosquito but the secondary vector *Aedes albopictus* is predicted to become a major driver for urban transmission due to its wider global presence in both temperate and tropical regions.[16] The other modes of transmission are sexual, intrauterine, perinatal, laboratory exposure, and probably blood transfusion.[17]

Two lineages among the new stains detected are the Asian lineage and the African lineage. The first laboratory confirmation from India took place in Ahmedabad, Gujarat in 2016 from a patient who had no history of travel or contact with an international traveler. The detected virus was of Asian lineage. Earlier to this, there have been reports of seroprevalence in Indian population as early as 1954. In the 1954 study, the highest seropositivity was found to be in Bareja, Ahmedabad (Gujarat), the same site where the laboratory confirmation took place in 2016. This indicated that probably the virus was in circulation for over 60 years.[18,19] In 2018, Jaipur in Rajasthan State, India reported an outbreak and 159 Zika cases were confirmed. Viruses responsible for Gujarat and Rajasthan were identified as belonging to Asian lineage.

Infection in first trimester pregnancy is known to cause severe microcephaly and even fetal loss. The possible explanations for primary and secondary microcephaly are decrease in number of neurons during neurogenesis and in number of dendritic and synaptic connections, respectively. It is not yet clear if the strain identified in Gujarat and Rajasthan outbreaks can cause birth defects thereby needing extreme vigilance for any evolutionary changes.[20]

Zika is asymptomatic in majority. Incubation period is 4–10 days, 20–25% who become symptomatic present with low grade fever, maculopapular rash, nonpurulent conjunctivitis, and arthralgia. Most of these symptoms would subside as viremia settled but arthralgia can persist for months. Guillain–Barré syndrome has been strongly associated in the Zika outbreaks.[21]

In endemic settings, it becomes clinically challenging to differentiate Zika from dengue and chikungunya. There is relative higher association of nonpurulent conjunctivitis and milder joint involvement in Zika compared to chikungunya. In dengue fever, both conjunctivitis and joint involvement are uncommon.

Zika infection is diagnosed by RT-PCR and IgM-captured enzyme-linked immunosorbent assay (ELISA). However, there is significant cross-reactivity with other *Flavivirus* due to structural and genetic similarity, especially dengue virus.

The treatment of Zika infection is symptomatic as currently no antiviral is available.

■ CRIMEAN-CONGO HEMORRHAGIC FEVER VIRUS

In January 2011, Gujarat reported the first case of Crimean–Congo hemorrhagic fever (CCHF) cases, in India. Three people including an adult female, doctor, and nurse were killed due to multiorgan failure. It is caused by the CCHF virus, a RNA virus, which belongs to *Nairovirus* genus of Bunyaviridae family. The name of this disease is derived from the linkage between the first description in Crimea region in 1944 and the similar occurrence of disease in the Congo in 1956.

The disease is transmitted by bite of hard ticks. Farmers, workers who come in contact with cattle, and veterinarians are high risk for this zoonotic transmission. Human-to-human transmission occurs due to exposure to body fluids or infected tissues. Therefore, healthcare workers and laboratory workers are at high risk for getting nosocomial infection.

The virus mostly affected the adults. A study done in pediatric population suspected with CCHF in Iran between 2000 and 2006 confirmed 161 cases (17.7%) by CCHF IgM ELISA and RT-PCR. Of these 70.8% were male and more than 65.8% occurred in male children.[22] The disease manifests with sudden onset of high-grade fever with nonspecific symptoms like headache, myalgia, abdominal pain, and vomiting, which is followed suddenly by a hemorrhagic phase. In this phase, petechiae, ecchymoses develop. Bleeding can occur from other sites like hematemesis, melena, hemoptysis, and epistaxis or from venipuncture sites. Death can occur due to the hemorrhagic complications. The mortality rate is high, about 30–50%.[23]

Crimean–Congo hemorrhagic fever is managed by intensive care, hemodynamic support, and administration of blood products whenever necessary. WHO recommends ribavirin, oral or intravenous as a potential therapeutic drug for CCHF. The role of ribavirin is found to be controversial.[24]

Crimean–Congo hemorrhagic fever virus (CCHFV) is classified as WHO risk group IV which suggests maximum biocontainment facility on research on this virus. As infection with this virus carried a high mortality risk and can be transmitted via small particle aerosol, this virus is considered as a potential agent for biowarfare.

■ EBOLA VIRUS

The biggest outbreak of Ebola till date occurred in West Africa in 2014–15. Over 11,000 deaths were reported from Guinea, Liberia, and Sierra Leone. A retrospective cohort study of 8,448 children in Guinea recorded an overall case fatality rate of 62.9% with under-5 mortality of 82.9%. Bleeding signs were seen only in 24%.[25]

Ebola viruses belong to the genus *Ebolavirus* of the family Filoviridae. Zoonotic reservoirs for human transmission are infected nonhuman primates like chimpanzees, gorillas, fruit bats, and monkeys. The natural hosts are considered to be fruit bats belonging to the Pteropodidae family. The virus was named after Ebola River in Zaire now Democratic Republic of Congo, which documented the first outbreak in 1976. Human-to-human transmission occurs by direct contact with blood, and other body fluids of infected patients. Blood, vomitus, and semen are the most infectious. Sexual transmission is also reported. Since the virus can persist in seminal fluid for a long period, unless the seminal fluid is tested twice negative, unprotected sexual intercourse is to be avoided.

Ebola presents as fever with mild-to-severe gastrointestinal symptoms like vomiting and diarrhea which can cause severe dehydration. Hemorrhagic complications can occur in form of petechiae, hematemesis, and bleeding from venipuncture sites. Asymptomatic infections can also occur.

Ebola virus can be detected by RT-PCR from the body fluids of the infected person.

Treatment is mainly supportive in the form of fluid resuscitation and correction of electrolyte disorders. The leading candidate vaccines for Ebola include cAd3-ZEBOV and rVSV-ZEBO. Monoclonal antibodies ZMapp and TKM-Ebola are being researched for specific therapy.[26]

ENTEROVIRUSES

Enterovirus D68

Enterovirus D68 (EV-D68) has emerged as a new nonpolio enterovirus responsible for acute flaccid myelitis (AFM). This single-stranded positive-sense RNA virus belongs to Picornaviridae family. In 2014, US and Canada recorded the largest known EV-D68 outbreak. Another outbreak was reported from Netherlands in 2016.[27]

Enterovirus D68 caused severe respiratory illness. The weakness caused by AFM like polio was asymmetric, motor, and flaccid with reduced or absent deep tendon reflexes and mostly affected the upper limbs. The MRI of spine showed lesions in the anterior horn of the gray matter along the spinal cord. In some cases, brain stem was also affected. EV-D68 could be isolated from the respiratory specimens of these patients in only less than 50% cases; therefore the diagnosis of this condition is challenging.[27]

Other Enteroviruses

A recent surveillance during an outbreak of hand foot mouth disease (HFMD) among children in Navi Mumbai, India identified cocirculation of coxsackie A6 and coxsackie A16. Though classical HFMD is described to have vesicular lesions limited to the characteristic distribution over extremities and oral aphthous ulcers, this outbreak witnessed extensive lesions extending over the trunk and also reported recurrences. Though no neurological complications have been reported from India so far, enterovirus 71 causing HFMD have caused fatal neurological and cardiopulmonary complications in neighboring South Asian countries like China.[28] Though HFMD infection is presently considered as a benign self-limiting viral illness among children, extreme vigilance and surveillance is required for any change in the clinical presentation of this viral disease.

■ INFLUENZA VIRUS

Influenza will always continue to keep the humans on their toes due to the constant threat of a new pandemic. This is owing to its constantly evolving nature. India bore the maximum brunt during the 1918 Spanish flu epidemic which spread across the country after troops returned to Bombay from the First World War. It caused over 10-20 million deaths in India alone.[29] Since then over the past 100 years, the notable pandemics have been the Asian flu in 1957, Hong Kong flu in 1968, and Swine flu in 2009.

Influenza virus is a negative-stranded enveloped RNA belonging to Orthomyxoviridae family. The glycoproteins—hemagglutinin (HA) and neuraminidase (N) are responsible for the pathogenesis of the virus. HA helps in the binding of the virus to the receptors present in the epithelial lining of the respiratory tract while N is responsible for the release of virion from host cell and propagation of the virus along the tract.

New pandemics occur due to a sudden genetic reassortment with creation of a novel HA/NA and its entry into human population. This phenomenon, which is only seen in influenza A, is called as antigenic shift. Whereas minor antigenic changes which occur in influenza A, B, and C viruses causing a different antigenic strain, this is known as antigenic drift.

Influenza pandemics are named as per the nomenclature defined by the WHO in 1980.[30] It is described as antigenic type (A, B or C); host of origin (if not humans); geographical region of origin; number of lineage; year of isolation and; and, for influenza A viruses only, HA and NA subtype, described by letter and number, H1 to H16 known to date, and N1 to N9. For example A/California/04/2009 (H1N1).

It usually runs a benign course with fever, coryza, headache, and malaise. Over 50% may be asymptomatic. Influenza can cause severe complications in extremes of age, immunocompromised, and those with a chronic illness. Viral pneumonia, ARDS, secondary bacterial infections, myocarditis, and acute myositis are some of the complications associated. The diagnosis is mainly by RT-PCR.

Oseltamivir and zanamivir are the current therapeutic options.

The best preventive measure is by use of annual influenza vaccine, which is currently available as trivalent or quadrivalent formulation. These vaccines contain an H1N1 strain, an H3N2 strain and one or two influenza B strains—B/Victoria or B/Yamagata. These vaccines are produced with a lead time of 6 months after annual matching with the circulating strains in the peak season of October-May in the Northern hemisphere and May-October in the Southern hemisphere. Therefore, for this process of matching the WHO conducts meetings twice a year to review data of the circulating strains from its Global Influenza Surveillance and Response System (GISRS) to make formal recommendations of vaccine composition for next Northern or

Southern hemispheres flu seasons. Any case of human infection due to a new influenza A virus subtype is notified to the GISRS of WHO, within 24 hours of its detection. This network thus helps in robust global surveillance for a timely alert of any new influenza viruses.

■ COMBATING THE CHALLENGE OF NEW VIRAL INFECTIONS

Surveillance

Effective surveillance is the only way to combat the challenges faced by the continued emerging viruses. Biological details of the new virus, its mode of transmission, and pathogenesis are crucial to identify the best management and preventive strategies. Timely review could help to contain the outbreak of these viruses in human population.

In 2018, the WHO listed the viruses which have the potential to cause public health emergency due to lack of vaccines or antiviral drugs against them.[31] These are CCHF, Ebola viral disease, Marburg viral disease, Lassa fever, MERS-CoV and SARS, Nipah and Henipaviral diseases, Rift Valley fever (RVF), Zika disease, and Disease X.[31] Majority of these belonged to the level 3 of pathogen pyramid. A close monitoring was also suggested for chikungunya; highly pathogenic coronaviral diseases other than MERS and SARS; emergent nonpolio enteroviruses (including EV71 and D68); and severe fever with thrombocytopenia syndrome (SFTS) and arenaviral hemorrhagic fevers other than Lassa fever.

Some viruses which have high mortality rate and have the potential to cause rapid aerosol transmission, have been limited for research in biosafety level 4 (BSL-4) laboratories. Examples of such viruses are Ebola, CCHF, Nipah, Marburg, Lassa virus, etc. Indian Council of Medical Research (ICMR) established its first BSL-4 laboratory in December 2012.

Novel viral pathogens have been identified by newer molecular methods like random-primed PCR amplification and DNA microarrays. In India, a network of more than 160 viral research laboratories has been set up to deal with at least 30–35 viruses of public health importance.

In 2014, the Global Health Security Agenda (GHSA) was launched for capacity building across the world to detect infectious diseases of public health importance and activate coordinated emergency response.[32] In India, it partners with 17 institutions, including National Centre for Disease Control (NCDC), Manipal Centre for Virus Research (MCVR), National Institute of Virology (NIV), and the ICMR.

In the past Nipah outbreaks in India in 2001 and 2007, specimens were required to be transported out of the country for confirmation to US Centers for Disease Control and Prevention (CDC) at Atlanta. But in Kerala outbreak in 2018, the research scientists at MCVR, a Grade I Virus Research and Diagnostic Laboratory of the ICMR were able to identify Nipah virus as the pathogen responsible by using next-generation sequencing (NGS) analysis, in a turnaround time of only 12 hours. This early detection helped to manage the cases effectively and contain the spread of infection.

Cheaper and rapid methods need to be developed for early detection in case of a large outbreak, especially in setting of a developing country where the public health system is overburdened.

Vaccines

Challenges for production of a vaccine for a new viral infection include conducting efficacy trials for uncommon diseases, or manufacturing with shorter lead-time and lesser cost for diseases with potential for becoming pandemic. Except for influenza, vaccines are not available presently for the new viruses of public health importance. In case of influenza, there are lots of efforts ongoing for development of universal vaccine which can avoid the need for biannual matching with the circulating influenza strains in the Northern and Southern hemispheres.

Antiviral Medicines

There are very few antivirals developed that have proved their efficacy for treating the newly emerging viruses. Though oseltamivir and zanamivir are being used as the best therapeutic options for influenza, there are challenges of developing parenteral formulations and reduce the growing resistance to these drugs. Ribavirin has been recommended in treatment of Nipah and CCHF. Other antiviral agents including antibodies m102.4 monoclonal antibody and Favipiravir are being researched for Nipah. Monoclonal antibodies are also being evaluated for Ebola.

Public Health Interventions

On identification of new viruses, timely dissemination of information to medical professionals and health care is important for early detection of illnesses caused by new viruses. The public health system should be geared up to combat any emergence with effective health interventions in the community. For example, mosquito control measures during suspected Zika/chikungunya epidemics or rodent control measures for hantaviruses. Similarly cough/sneeze etiquettes and hand hygiene need to be reinforced during any outbreak of an airborne viral infection like for example influenza and SARS-CoA. Travel advisories for outsiders can help in containing local outbreaks.

Nosocomial infections need to be prevented by proper isolation and use of personal protective equipment while caring for such victims. WHO has released guidelines for safe and dignified burial for those who died from suspected or confirmed Ebola or Marburg to prevent secondary infections due to contact with body fluids.[33]

There is a need for screening high-risk populations and protecting them during an outbreak. For example, the public health authorities need to frame evidence-based guidelines to protect pregnant women from acquiring Zika infection.[34]

On a larger level, the deforestation activities need to be controlled to protect the wildlife habitats. Urgent measures should be adopted by global leaders to minimize the detrimental effect of human activities of the environment and thereby prevent radical climatic changes.

■ CONCLUSION

New viruses will continue to evolve with increased contact of humans with animal/bird species. Rapid urbanization and deforestation activities have only helped in multiplication of vectors like mosquitoes and rodents which help in viral transmission. Easy and fast means to travel have fueled dissemination of infections across the globe. There is a need to keep a constant vigilance of the viruses, especially of those with the potential to cause large or fatal outbreaks in humans. Despite the availability of molecular tests to detect viruses, a lot of research is needed to produce cheaper and reliable tests, effective antiviral drugs and vaccines for protection against these viruses. The public health system needs to be strengthened to control an outbreak of new viral infection in the community with an emergency response and prevent its further spread.

■ REFERENCES

1. Lederburg J. Viruses and humankind: Intracellular symbiosis and evolutionary Competition. In: Morse SS (Ed). Emerging Viruses. Oxford: Oxford University Press; 1993. pp. 3-9.
2. Lefkowitz EJ, Dempsey DM, Hendrickson RC, et al. Virus taxonomy: the database of the International Committee on Taxonomy of Viruses (ICTV). Nucleic Acids Res. 2018;46(D1):D708-17.
3. Woolhouse ME, Brierley L, McCaffery C, et al. Assessing the Epidemic Potential of RNA and DNA Viruses. Emerg Infect Dis. 2016;22(12):2037-44.
4. Parrish CR, Holmes EC, Morens DM, et al. Cross-species virus transmission and the emergence of new epidemic diseases. Microbiol Mol Biol Rev. 2008;72(3):457-70.
5. Graham RL, Donaldson EF, Baric RS. A decade after SARS: strategies for controlling emerging coronaviruses. Nat Rev Microbiol. 2013;11(12):836-48.
6. Stockman LJ, Massoudi MS, Helfand R, et al. Severe acute respiratory syndrome in children. Pediatr Infect Dis J. 2007;26(1):68-74.
7. Li AM, Ng PC. Severe acute respiratory syndrome (SARS) in neonates and children. Arch Dis Child Fetal Neonatal Ed. 2005;90:F461-5.

8. Thabet F, Chehab M, Bafaqih H, et al. Middle East respiratory syndrome coronavirus in children. Saudi Med J. 2015;36(4):484-6
9. Gautret P, Gray GC, Charrel RN, et al. Emerging viral respiratory tract infections—environmental risk factors and transmission. Lancet Infect Dis. 2014;14(11): 1113-22.
10. WHO. Nipah virus—FAQs. [online] Available from: http://www.searo.who.int/entity/emerging_diseases/links/nipah_virus_faq/en/. [Last accessed December, 2019].
11. Banerjee B, Gupta N, Kodan P, et al. Nipah virus disease: a rare and intractable disease. Intractable Rare Dis Res. 2019;8(1):1-8.
12. Chandy S, Boorugu H, Chrispal A, et al. Hantavirus infection: a case report from India. Indian J Med Microbiol. 2009;27(3):267-70.
13. Mehta S, Jiandani P. Ocular features of hantavirus infection. Indian J Ophthalmol. 2007;55(5):378-80.
14. Ritz N, Hufnagel M, Gérardin P. Chikungunya in Children. Pediatr Infect Dis J. 2015;34(7):789-91.
15. Seetharam KA, Sridevi K, Vidyasagar P. Cutaneous manifestations of chikungunya fever. Indian Pediatr. 2012;49(1):51-3.
16. Song BH, Yun SI, Woolley M, et al. Zika virus: history, epidemiology, transmission, and clinical presentation. J Neuroimmunol. 2017;308:50-64.
17. Hills SL, Fischer M, Petersen LR. Epidemiology of Zika Virus Infection. J Infect Dis. 2017;216(suppl_10):S868-74.
18. Khaiboullina S, Uppal T, Martynova E, et al. History of ZIKV Infections in India and Management of Disease Outbreaks. Front Microbiol. 2018;9:2126.
19. Sapkal GN, Yadav PD, Vegad MM, et al. First laboratory confirmation on the existence of Zika virus disease in India. J Infect. 2018;76(3):314-7.
20. Yadav PD, Malhotra B, Sapkal G, et al. Zika virus outbreak in Rajasthan, India in 2018 was caused by a virus endemic to Asia. Infect Genet Evol. 2019;69:199-202.
21. Rather IA, Lone JB, Bajpai VK, et al. Zika Virus: An Emerging Worldwide Threat. Front Microbiol. 2017;8:1417.
22. Aslani D, Salehi-Vaziri M, Baniasadi V, et al. Crimean-Congo hemorrhagic fever among children in Iran. Arch Virol. 2017;162(3):721-5.
23. Lahariya C, Goel MK, Kumar A, et al. Emergence of viral hemorrhagic fevers: is recent outbreak of Crimean Congo Hemorrhagic Fever in India an indication? J Postgrad Med. 2012;58(1):39-46.
24. Tezer H, Ozkaya-Parlakay A, Gulhan B, et al. Ribavirin use in pediatric patients with Crimean Congo Hemorrhagic Fever: is it really necessary? Braz J Infect Dis. 2016;20(2):222-3.
25. Chérif MS, Koonrungsesomboon N, Kassé D, et al. Ebola virus disease in children during the 2014-2015 epidemic in Guinea: a nationwide cohort study. Eur J Pediatr. 2017;176(6):791-6.
26. Khalafallah MT, Aboshady OA, Moawed SA, et al. Ebola virus disease: essential clinical knowledge. Avicenna J Med. 2017;7(3):96-102.
27. Cassidy H, Poelman R, Knoester M, et al. Enterovirus D68—The New Polio? Front Microbiol. 2018;9:2677.
28. Koh WM, Bogich T, Siegel K, et al. The Epidemiology of Hand, Foot and Mouth Disease in Asia: A Systematic Review and Analysis. Pediatr Infect Dis J. 2016;35(10):e285-300.

29. Chandra S, Kassens-Noor E. The evolution of pandemic influenza: evidence from India, 1918-19. BMC Infect Dis. 2014;14:510.
30. A revision of the system of nomenclature for influenza viruses: a WHO Memorandum. Bull World Health Organ. 1980;58(4):585-91.
31. World Health Organization. (2018). Blueprint for R&D preparedness and response to public health emergencies due to highly infectious pathogens. [online] Available from: https://www.who.int/emergencies/diseases/2018prioritization-report.pdf. [Last accessed December, 2019].
32. Sadanadan R, Arunkumar G, Laserson KF, et al. Towards global health security: response to the May 2018 Nipah virus outbreak linked to Pteropus bats in Kerala, India. BMJ Global Healt. 2018;3:e001086.
33. WHO. (2017). How to conduct safe and dignified burial of a patient who has died from suspected or confirmed Ebola or Marburg virus disease. [online] Available from: https://www.who.int/csr/resources/publications/ebola/safe-burial-protocol/en/. [Last accessed December, 2019].
34. John TJ. Neonatal Chikungunya: Spotlight on Gaps in Public Health. Indian Pediatr. 2018;55(8):659-60.

CHAPTER 5

NEUROLOGY

5.1 Childhood Epilepsy Syndromes: Diagnosis and Management
PAM Kunju

5.2 Acute Encephalopathy
PAM Kunju

5.1 CHILDHOOD EPILEPSY SYNDROMES: DIAGNOSIS AND MANAGEMENT

PAM Kunju

■ INTRODUCTION

The International League against Epilepsy (ILAE) released a new classification of seizure and epilepsy in 2017, which envisages a three-level of diagnosis. After excluding seizure mimics, first step is to identify the *seizure type*. Once the *seizure type* is determined, the next step is to diagnose the *epilepsy type*. Third level of diagnosis is *epilepsy syndrome*. Identifying the *etiology* is emphasized at each step as it provides significant treatment options.[1-3]

Seizures types are divided into four types: (1) *focal* onset, (2) *generalized* onset, (3) *unknown* onset, and (4) *unclassified*. Both focal and generalized can be of motor or nonmotor onset seizures.[1] Focal seizures were also divided into seizures with awareness and with impaired awareness. Instead of the term "secondary generalization", *focal to bilateral tonic-clonic* terminology is proposed.[1] Similarly, "simple, partial, and complex partial seizure" terminologies have been replaced by *focal seizures with awareness and with impaired awareness,* respectively **(Fig. 5.1.1)**.

ILAE 2017 classification of seizure types expanded version[1]

Focal onset	Generalized onset	Unknown onset
Aware / Impaired awareness	**Motor** Tonic-clonic Clonic Tonic Myoclonic Myoclonic-tonic-clonic Myoclonic-atonic Atonic Epileptic spasms[2]	**Motor** Tonic-clonic Epileptic spasms **Nonmotor** Behavior arrest
Motor onset Automatisms Atonic[2] Clonic Epileptic spasms[2] Hyperkinetic Myoclonic Tonic **Nonmotor onset** Autonomic Behavior arrest Cognitive Emotional Sensory	**Nonmotor (absence)** Typical Atypical Myoclonic Eyelid myoclonia	**Unclassified**[3]
Focal to bilateral tonic-clonic		

[1] Definitions, other seizure types and descriptors are listed in the accompanying paper and glossary of terms.
[2] These could be focal or generalized, with or without alteration of awareness.
[3] Due to inadequate information or inability to place in other categories.

Fig. 5.1.1: The International League against Epilepsy (ILAE) seizure types: 2017 Classification.
Source: Fisher RS, Cross JH, D'Souza C, et al. Instruction manual for the ILAE 2017 operational classification of seizure types. Epilepsia. 2017;58(4):531-42.

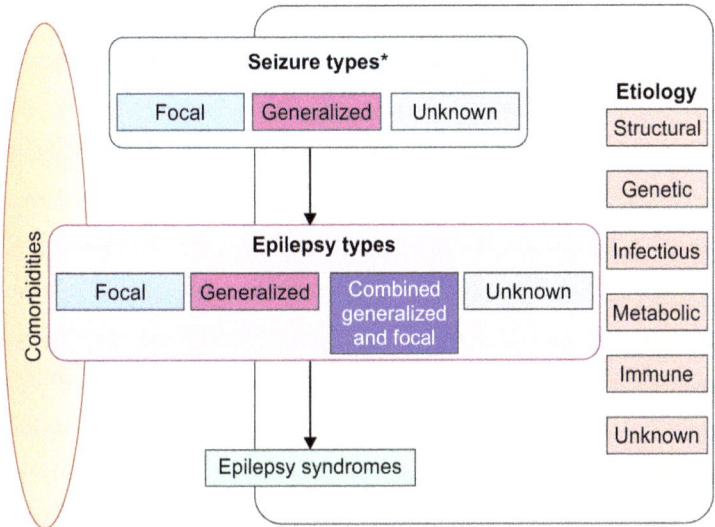

Fig. 5.1.2: The International League against Epilepsy framework of epilepsy classification.
*Denotes onset of seizure

Epilepsy types include the following:
- Focal epilepsy
- Generalized epilepsy
- Combined generalized and focal epilepsy
- An unknown epilepsy group.

Etiology is broken into six subgroups. These include structural, genetic, infectious, metabolic, immune, and unknown **(Fig. 5.1.2)**.

■ APPROACH TO EPILEPSY SYNDROME

The syndromic classification helps in giving some importance to the heterogeneity of seizures and the epilepsies as well as gives a common platform for evaluation, treatment, and research. A syndrome is defined by seizure behavior, electroencephalogram (EEG) manifestations, imaging findings, age of onset, remission, triggers, diurnal variation, intellectual and psychiatric dysfunction, and family history.

Though ILAE does not give a formal syndrome classification, it can be grouped according to the age. Idiopathic generalized epilepsies, self-limited focal epilepsies, and developmental and epileptic encephalopathies are some of the terms used for different syndromic categories.

■ SELF-LIMITED FOCAL EPILEPSIES IN CHILDHOOD[4,5]

Benign Epilepsy with Centrotemporal Spikes (Benign Rolandic Epilepsy)

Benign partial epilepsy of childhood with centrotemporal spikes (BECTS) is a common pediatric epilepsy syndrome, and accounts for around 25%

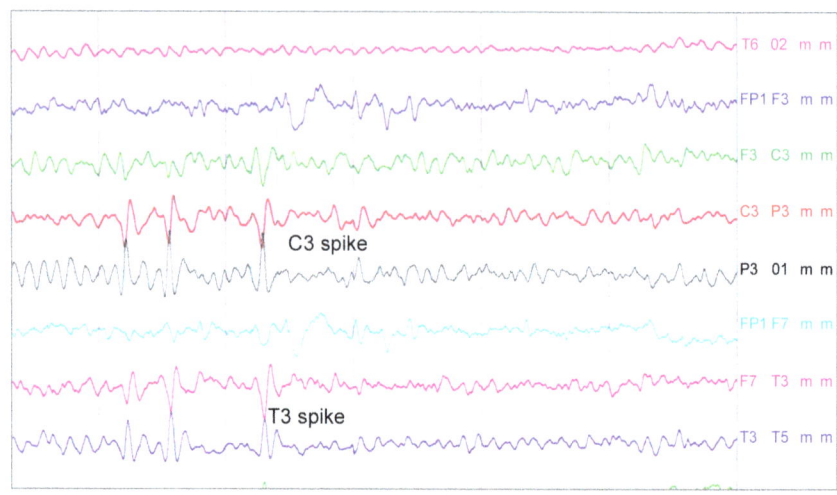

Fig. 5.1.3: Left centrotemporal spike. Observe the phase reversal of spike at C3 and T3.

of childhood epilepsies. The usual age of onset is 4–11 years with male predominance. The timing of seizures is usually shortly after sleep onset or just before awakening. The seizure is usually preceded by paresthesia on one side of tongue or mouth, followed by dysarthria or gagging type noises, jerking of ipsilateral face, and excessive drooling. Duration is brief, in the range of seconds to minutes but status epilepticus as well as postictal Todd paresis may occur. EEG shows typical broad-based centrotemporal spikes that are markedly increased in frequency during drowsiness and non-REM (non-rapid eye movement) sleep **(Fig. 5.1.3)**.

Benign partial epilepsy of childhood with centrotemporal spikes has usually very good prognosis either self-limiting or it responds to drugs like carbamazepine. However, one-fifth may have frequent seizures (early onset) with cognitive, behavioral, or oromotor deficits sometimes, linked to spike frequency or location. They may evolve into Landau Kleffner syndrome in a few situations. Remission is seen finally in all by changing to sodium valproate or adding clobazam.

Panayiotopoulos Syndrome (Early-onset Childhood Epilepsy with Occipital Paroxysms)

Childhood epilepsy with occipital paroxysms (CEOP) should be considered when a normal preschool (3–5 years) child presents with severe nocturnal vomiting followed by eye deviation and status epilepticus, usually hemiclonic. The most prominent feature is an autonomic component.

A later age *Gastaut variant of CEOP* is characterized by diurnal focal seizures with visual hallucinations or amaurosis and migraine-like headaches. Post-ictal headache is a common and prominent symptom. Neuroimaging is considered in cases with an abnormal perinatal history or examination, atypical EEG, or poorly controlled seizures. The EEG has a classic appearance of bilateral occipital spike and wave discharges precipitated by eye closure and attenuated by eye opening. The latter is sometimes called *"fixation off phenomenon"* because visual fixation will abort the spike wave discharges.

■ GENETIC GENERALIZED EPILEPSIES

These are detailed in **Table 5.1.1**.

Table 5.1.1: Genetic generalized epilepsies – characteristics and treatment.

Epilepsy syndrome	Age of occurrence	Seizure types	Electroencephalogram	Treatment
Childhood absence	3–10 years	Absence (several to many per day)	Normal background (BG) 3–3.5 per sec, bilateral, synchronous and symmetrical spike and wave activity	Monotherapy with ethosuximide, sodium valproate. If this fails add small doses of lamotrigine to valproate
Juvenile absence	Adolescence	Absence, generalized tonic-clonic (80%)	Normal BG, 3–3.5/sec, generalized spike and wave activity, polyspikes	Sodium valproate is efficacious. Phenytoin, carbamazepine, gabapentin, vigabatrin and pregabalin to be avoided
Epilepsy with myoclonic absences	First months of life to the early teens (peak 7 years)	Myoclonic absences	BG normal at onset; may deteriorate	High doses of valproate often combined with ethosuximide or small doses of lamotrigine
Juvenile myoclonic epilepsy	Range 10–20 year (Absences 5–16 years; myoclonus follows 1–9 years later; generalized tonic-clonic seizures (GTCTs) appear a few months later	Myoclonic, generalized tonic-clonic, absence (rare)	Normal BG, 3–4/sec generalized spike-wave discharges, polyspike-wave discharges with myoclonic seizures, photoparoxysmal response	Valproate, levetiracetam, lamotrigine. May require lifelong

Contd...

Contd...

Epilepsy syndrome	Age of occurrence	Seizure types	Electroen-cephalogram	Treatment
Epilepsy with GTCS on awakening	6–47 years with a peak at 16 years	GTCS	Normal BG generalized spike/polyspike-wave discharges	Valproate, levetiracetam, lamotrigine Avoid sleep deprivation with early awaking and alcohol consumption

Childhood Absence Epilepsy (Petit Mal)

This syndrome comprises approximately 15% of the childhood onset epilepsies and has a typical age of onset between 4 years and 10 years. Earlier onset (before age 4 years) raises concern regarding underlying glucose transporter type 1 deficiency. Typical absence seizure refers to abrupt impairment of consciousness, often associated with behavioral arrest, staring, eye fluttering, or automatisms. Atypical absence seizures are prolonged, seen in syndromes like Lennox–Gastaut. An EEG characterized by frontally predominant generalized 3 Hz spike wave complexes (precipitated by hyperventilation) with abrupt onset is diagnostic.

Genetic Generalized Epilepsies of Adolescence

When a patient presents with absence, myoclonic or generalized tonic-clonic seizures (GTCS) for the first time after 10 years, a diagnosis of genetic generalized epilepsies of adolescent onset is considered. EEG shows generalized paroxysms of spike or polyspike wave discharges. Photosensitivity is common. *Juvenile myoclonic epilepsy (JME), juvenile absence epilepsy (JAE), and epilepsies with only GTC seizures* should be considered in diagnosis. JME presents in adolescent girls with early morning myoclonic jerks (dropping of objects). It occurs often in sleep-deprived individuals, especially if suddenly awakened. They have additionally absences and GTCS **(Fig. 5.1.4)**. The most constant clinical feature is myoclonic seizures predominantly involving the upper extremities, especially upon awakening.

Juvenile absence epilepsy is similar to CAE, though the number of absences is much less and the onset is usually later. GTCS typically occur on awakening or in the evening. EEG background is preserved but features of abrupt paroxysmal generalized 4-6 Hz spike or polyspike and slow wave activity, sometimes described as having W configuration.

Sodium valproate is the most effective drug, but it may cause weight gain, hair loss, and menstrual irregularities and has a higher incidence of

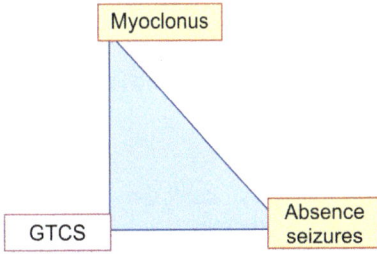

Fig. 5.1.4: Triad of juvenile myoclonic epilepsy seizures. (GTCS: generalized tonic-clonic seizures)

teratogenicity. Therefore, lamotrigine/levetiracetam may be preferable in adolescent girls.

■ SEVERE EPILEPSY SYNDROMES OF EARLY CHILDHOOD/ EPILEPTIC ENCEPHALOPATHIES

These are detailed in **Table 5.1.2**.[6-8]

Early myoclonic encephalopathy (Aicardi) is seen in neonatal period with fragmentary erratic myoclonus, multiple other seizure types, and encephalopathy with delay in developmental milestones. EEG shows burst suppression pattern **(Fig. 5.1.5)**. It is usually associated with metabolic disorders like nonketotic hyperglycinemia.

Early infantile epileptic encephalopathy (Ohtahara) presents with tonic spasms in neonatal period associated with structural malformations of cerebral cortex or genetic mutations in *ARX* or *STXBP1* genes.

Both syndromes have refractory seizures, require multiple antiepileptic drugs (AEDs), have poor prognosis, and evolve into West syndrome.

West Syndrome

This occurs in the first year of life with triad of epileptic spasms, developmental deterioration, and hypsarrhythmia in EEG **(Fig. 5.1.6)**. Neurometabolic and chromosomal disorders like Down syndrome and genetic disorders related to *ARX, CDKL5, SPTAN1, FOXG1, GRIN1, GRIN 2A, MAGI2, MEF2C,* and *SLC25A22* should be considered in the etiology.

For treatment, adrenocorticotropic hormone (ACTH) is preferred over oral steroids. Oral prednisolone is given 2-4 mg/kg or ACTH 30-40 units/day (3-6 U/kg) for 2 weeks with rapid taper over the next 2-4 weeks. Vigabatrin (VGB) is the first choice in tuberous sclerosis. It should be used for a period of 3-6 months only, due to the fear of visual field defects. A recent multicentric

Table 5.1.2: Severe epilepsy syndromes of early childhood according to age.

- *Neonatal period:*
  - Ohtahara syndrome
  - Early myoclonic encephalopathy
- *Infancy:*
  - Epilepsy of infancy with migrating focal seizures
  - West syndrome
  - Dravet syndrome
- *Childhood:*
  - Epilepsy with myoclonic atonic (previously astatic) seizures (Doose syndrome)
  - Lennox–Gastaut syndrome
  - Epileptic encephalopathy with continuous spike-and-wave during sleep (CSWS)/Encephalopathy with status epilepticus in sleep (ESES)
  - Landau Kleffner syndrome (LKS)

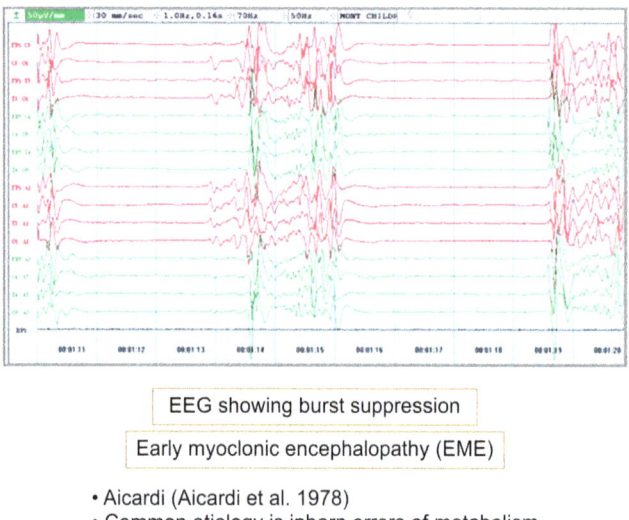

EEG showing burst suppression

Early myoclonic encephalopathy (EME)

- Aicardi (Aicardi et al. 1978)
- Common etiology is inborn errors of metabolism

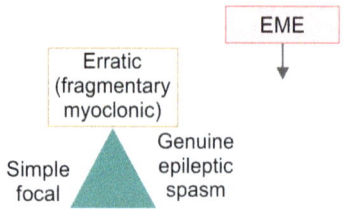

Fig. 5.1.5: EEG showing burst suppression and triad of seizure types in early myoclonic epileptic encephalopathy.

study [International Collaborative Infantile Spasms Study (ICISS)] done in 102 hospitals in five countries showed that a combination of hormonal

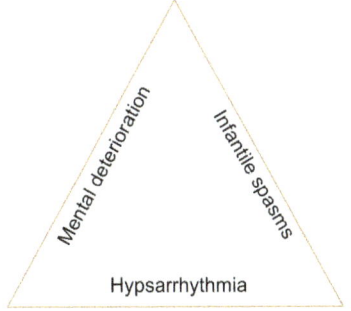

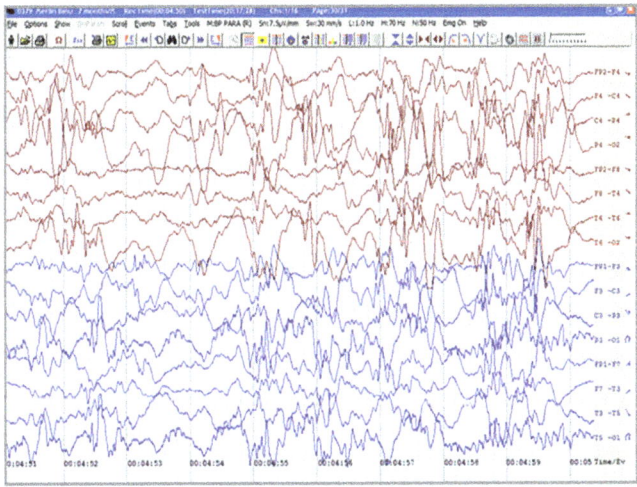

Fig. 5.1.6: Triad of West syndrome and EEG showing hypsarrhythmia.

(tetracosactide or high-dose prednisolone) and VGB therapy is significantly more effective at stopping spasms between days 14 and 42 than hormonal therapy alone [spasms stopped in 133 (72%) of 186 on hormonal therapy with VGB vs. 108 (57%) of 191 patients on hormonal therapy alone].

Lennox–Gastaut Syndrome

Lennox–Gastaut syndrome (LGS) is a severe epileptic encephalopathy with *atypical absences, tonic and atonic* (drop attacks) seizures, and slow spike wave activity in the EEG **(Fig. 5.1.7)**. Any toddler, who has epileptic drop attacks and is delayed or has arrest in development, should be considered to have LGS **(Fig. 5.1.8)**. LGS has a male predominance. Tonic seizures are more common. EEG background of slow (less than 3 Hz) spike and wave discharges plus paroxysmal fast activity during sleep and cognitive impairment are characteristic.

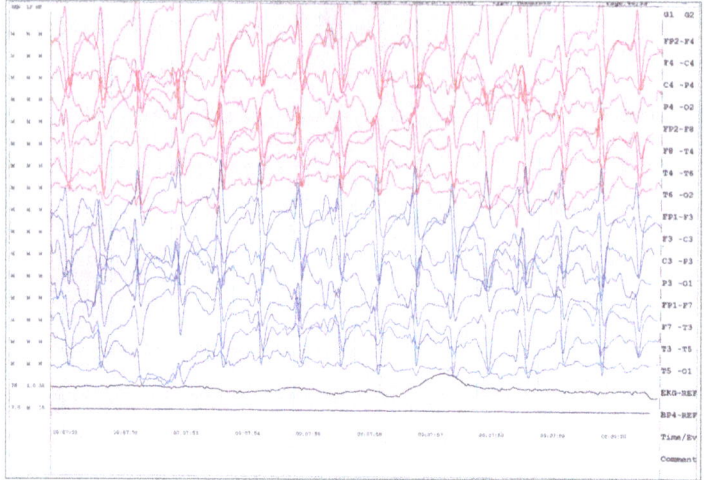

Fig. 5.1.7: Lennox–Gastaut syndrome: EEG 1–2/sec spike wave.

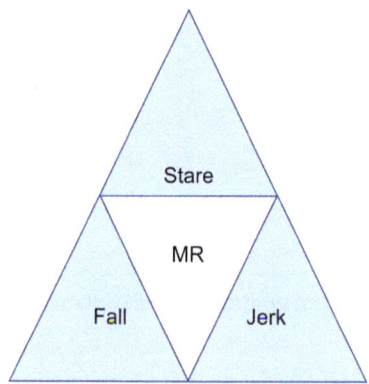

Fig. 5.1.8: Lennox–Gastaut syndrome: Triad of seizure + MR.
[Stare (Atypical absence); Fall (Atonic seizure); Jerk (Tonic seizure)]

Dravet Syndrome (Severe Myoclonic Epilepsy of Infancy)

Dravet syndrome begins between 2 months and 10 months with febrile hemiclonic convulsions. The tendency of fever as trigger factor decreases progressively and seizures occur without any fever. Myoclonic and absence seizures, often photosensitive, become prominent after the first year. *SCN1A* mutation is found in >75% cases. Valproate, clobazam, and topiramate (TPM) are likely to help in the management.

A recognized association exists with status epilepticus as well as sudden unexpected death in epilepsy. Treatment options include sodium valproate, clobazam, and stiripentol as well as ketogenic diet (KD). A role may exist for cannabidiol. Lamotrigine and carbamazepine may worsen seizures and should be avoided.

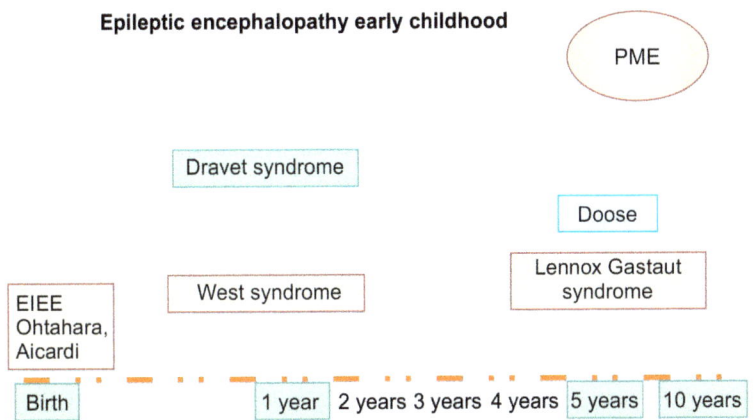

Fig. 5.1.9: Age wise epileptic syndromes. (EIEE: early infantile epileptic encephalopathy; PME: progressive myoclonic epilepsy)

Doose Syndrome

Doose syndrome is characterized by myoclonic atonic seizures, with onset between 18 months and 36 months. The myoclonus manifests as large amplitude symmetric jerks of the arms, legs, neck, and shoulders that may result in a head drop and upper limb flexion or abduction. This is followed by loss of muscle tone and a fall.

Standard antiseizure drug administered is valproic acid, ethosuximide or benzodiazepines. TPM, lamotrigine, rufinamide, and levetiracetam may show a benefit. KD and its variants have been found to be useful in some.

A calendar of epileptic encephalopathy of childhood is depicted in **Figure 5.1.9** and their characteristics and treatment are given in **Table 5.1.3**.

■ REFRACTORY EPILEPSIES IN OLDER CHILDREN AND ADOLESCENTS[8-11]

Mesial Temporal Lobe Epilepsy

Focal seizures with and without impaired consciousness are the most common seizure types in mesial temporal lobe epilepsy (MTLE). History of febrile seizures is common (up to two-thirds), though other causes including head trauma, perinatal injury, congenital brain malformation, central nervous system (CNS) infection, and brain tumors may be evident. Prolonged, febrile seizures may induce hippocampal edema that progresses to hippocampal sclerosis. The onset of MTLE characteristically occurs at the end of the first or second decade. Hippocampal sclerosis is a pathologic finding of atrophy and gliosis of the hippocampus as well as the amygdala, para-hippocampal gyrus, and entorhinal cortex.

Table 5.1.3: Severe epilepsy syndromes of early childhood/epileptic encephalopathies.

Epilepsy syndrome	Age of occurrence	Seizure types	EEG	Association/etiology	Treatment
Neonatal epileptic syndromes					
Benign familial neonatal convulsions	First week – 2nd or 3rd day	(Tonic-clonic) Start as tonic posturing with apnea, followed by vocalizations, ocular and autonomic features	Theta pointu alternant pattern (Runs of theta of 4–7 Hz mixed with sharp waves alternating sides)	Otherwise normal neonates *KCNQ2* mutation	• Remit spontaneously • Benzodiazepines and phenytoin for prolonged seizures
Benign neonatal seizures (non-familial)	5th day	Clonic	Focal or multifocal, or discontinuous pattern	Zinc deficiency?	Discontinue AED soon after the seizures subside
Early infantile epileptic encephalopathy (Ohtahara)	First 10 days of life, within the uterus or up to 3 months	Tonic seizures	Suppression-burst (occur in the sleeping and waking states)	Malformations of brain like hemimegal-encephaly	Severe outcome ACTH therapy and any type of AEDs
Early myoclonic encephalopathy (Aicardi)	Before 10 days of age	Triad of fragmentary myoclonus, simple focal seizures and epileptic spasms	Suppression-burst (more apparent during deep sleep)	• Psychomotor development abnormal • Inborn errors of metabolism	• Severe outcome • ACTH and AEDs • Sodium benzoate 120 mg/kg daily
West syndrome	3–12 months (peak age)	Epileptic spasms	Hypsarrhythmia	• Multiple and diverse develop-mental delay/Deterioration • Common with tuberous sclerosis complex and Down syndrome	• ACTH • Vigabatrin
Dravet syndrome	First year	Partial and generalized seizures, myoclonias	Normal EEG at onset; later: generalized spike-waves and multifocal spikes		Severe outcome valproate, clobazam, and stiripentol

Contd...

Contd...

Epilepsy syndrome	Age of occurrence	Seizure types	EEG	Association/etiology	Treatment
Lennox–Gastaut syndrome	1–7 years with a peak at 3–5 years	Polymorphic intractable seizures—tonic, atonic and atypical absences	EEG with paroxysms of fast activity and slow (<2.5 Hz) GSWD	Severe cognitive and behavioral abnormalities	• Intractable • *Multiple drugs:* Topiramate, Felbamate, Hormonal, and nonpharmacological treatments
Myoclonic astatic epilepsy	First year	Generalized myoclonic and astatic seizures	Interictal parietal theta activity and bilateral spike-waves		Variable outcome
Malignant migrating partial seizures of infancy *(Epilepsy of infancy with migrating focal seizures)*	First year	• Continuous electrographic seizures, multiple areas of onset • Both sides are alternately affected	Discharges involve multiple independent sites randomly, moving from one cortical area to another in consecutive seizures	*KCNT1* mutations	Severe outcome, variety of AEDs, ketogenic diet, vagal nerve stimulation
Genetic epilepsy with febrile seizures plus (GEFS+)	First months of life to childhood, (FS beyond 6 year)	Variable seizure and developmental phenotype in addition to febrile seizures (FS) and afebrile generalized and focal	EEG diverse and depend on the clinical phenotype. *Brief generalized polyspike–wave discharges* (GPSWD)	*SCN1A, SCN1B GABRG2*, mutations	Sodium channel blockers phenytoin, carbamazepine, oxcarbazepine, and lamotrigine may be deleterious
Hemiconvulsion-hemiplegia-epilepsy (HHE) syndrome	Before 4 years	Prolonged unilateral febrile seizures; (super-refractory status epilepticus [longer than 24 hours])	• EEG—*acutely* bilateral, ictal and interictal • Chronic, ictal EEGs poorly localizing but lateralize to the involved side	Subsequent hemiparesis and partial epilepsy	Epilepsy surgery, including lobar or multilobar resection and hemispherectomy
Benign myoclonic epilepsy	First 3 years	Myoclonic seizures	Normal interictal EEG	Normal development	Valproate with photosensitivity. Response to AED treatment is usually excellent
Benign familial/nonfamilial seizures	First year	Partial seizures		Normal development	

(ACTH: adrenocorticotropic hormone; AEDs: antiepileptic drugs; EEG: electroencephalogram; GSWD: generalized spike-wave discharges)

Mesial temporal seizures are often preceded by autonomic or abdominal auras such as déjà vu, jamais vu, fear, rising epigastric sensations or experiencing bad odors or tastes. It is found to be relatively refractory to antiseizure medications and seizure freedom is achievable in up to 90% of selected patients undergoing temporal lobectomy.

Epilepsia Partialis Continua

Epilepsia partialis continua (EPC) is a rare form of focal status epilepticus. It may have vascular, immune-mediated, neoplastic or metabolic-toxic causes. EPC should be suspected when focal, fairly constant myoclonic/clonic jerks involve one or more parts of the body (face/limb/tongue) only unilaterally.

In Rasmussen's encephalitis, a progressive hemiplegia with deterioration in cognition and behavior is usual, as the epilepsy is resistant to all AEDs. After a trial of intravenous immunoglobulin (IVIG), hemispheric resection/disconnection is the procedure that seems to benefit a large number.

Granuloma in Children

New-onset partial or generalized convulsive seizures occurring in clusters in an otherwise normal child are the most common presentation of single small contrast enhancing CT lesion. The most common etiology is neurocysticercosis (outside Kerala) followed by tuberculomas. Parenchymal neurocysticercosis cysts should be classified as an active vesicular form (cystic, without enhancement or edema, with occasional eccentric hyperdense nodule signifying scolex), a transitional colloidal/granular-nodular form (ring/disk enhancement with edema) or an inactive form (nonenhancing calcified lesions without edema).

Management of seizures in children is given in **Box 5.1.1**.[11]

■ DRUG-RESISTANT EPILEPSY

Drug-resistant epilepsy is defined by ILAE as failure of adequate trials of two tolerated, appropriately chosen, and used AED schedules (whether as monotherapies or in combination) to achieve sustained seizure freedom. In such children, reconfirm the diagnosis, exclude pseudoseizures, and ensure compliance. Then the following can be tried.

Nonpharmacological Treatment

Ketogenic Diet and Modified Atkins Diet

Ketogenic diet: It is a medically supervised high fat, low carbohydrate, and protein diet that maintains ketosis. Composition of KD is 80% fat, 15% protein, and 10% carbohydrate, making it a 4:1 diet ratio of fat: nonfat. Ratio of fat:

> **Box 5.1.1:** Choice of conventional antiepileptic drug (AEDs) and newer AEDs.
>
> - *Focal seizures (motor, nonmotor- with and without awareness and focal evolving to GTCS)*
>   - *First line:* Carbamazepine or lamotrigine (NICE guideline)
>   - *Second line:* Primidone; offer levetiracetam, oxcarbazepine or sodium valproate
>   - *Others:* Clobazam, gabapentin, topiramate, or zonisamide
> - *Refractory focal seizures:* Eslicarbazepine acetate, lacosamide, phenobarbital, phenytoin, pregabalin, tiagabine, vigabatrin and zonisamide
> - *Generalized seizures*
>   - Tonic-clonic seizures
>   - *First line:* Valproate, or lamotrigine
>   - *Adjunctive treatment:* Clobazam, lamotrigine, levetiracetam, sodium valproate or topiramate.
>   - *Absence seizures:* Theta pointu alternant pattern
>   - *First line:* Ethosuximide, valproate
>   - *Second line:* Lamotrigine, clonazepam
>   - *Adjunctive treatment:* Consider a combination ethosuximide, lamotrigine or sodium valproate
>   - Myoclonic seizures:
>   - *First line:* Valproate.
>   - Levetiracetam or topiramate if sodium valproate is not tolerated
>   - *Adjunctive treatment:* Levetiracetam, sodium valproate or topiramate
>   - *Infantile spasm* (West syndrome)
>   - *First line:* ACTH followed by prednisolone in infantile spasm
>   - *Second line:* Valproate, nitrazepam
>   - *Newer AED:* Vigabatrin, topiramate, levetiracetam
>   - Tonic, clonic, atonic seizures:
>   - Any of the above except ethosuximide
>
> (ACTH: adrenocorticotropic hormone; AEDs; antiepileptic drugs; GTCS: generalized tonic-clonic seizures; NICE: National Institute for Health and Care Excellence)

protein ranges from 2.5:1 to 4:1. The traditional KD, with 4:1 ratio of fat: carbohydrate + protein, has its drawbacks. It restricts calories and fluids, and requires a weighing of foods. Protein is generally restricted to 1 g/kg/day, with the majority of the remaining calories in the form of fat.

Modified Atkins diet (MAD): MAD encourages intake of fat and restriction of carbohydrates but does not restrict protein intake or daily calories or fluid. It allows a meal with 60% fat, 30% protein, and 10% carbohydrate. A number of uncontrolled studies in the last five years have shown a similar efficacy to the ketogenic diet. Approximately, half of the patients show more than 50% improvement in seizures with this diet.[11] Other dietary treatment includes low glycemic index treatment (LGIT) diet, which is more liberal than KD with carbohydrate content of glycemic index of 50 or lower and total daily carbohydrate intake restricted to 40–60 g/day.

Surgical Treatment

All infants and children with refractory focal or generalized epilepsy should be referred as early as possible to a comprehensive epilepsy center for possible surgical evaluation. Ideal surgically remediable syndromes include:
- Hemispheric epilepsies with pre-existing contralateral hemiplegias/visual field defects caused by large unilateral gliotic lesions/atrophy, Rasmussen's encephalitis, hemispheric dysplasias, etc. where hemispherectomy/ *hemispherotomies* could offer possible surgical cure.
- Discrete lesions without involvement of functional motor, visual and language cortex, where a *lesionectomy* will often result in a complete cure. Common lesions would include developmental tumors, cortical dysplasias, arteriovenous malformations (AVMs), etc. Sometimes lesions like large dysplasias/infarcts may need *lobectomies/multilobar resections*.
- Mesial temporal lobe epilepsy caused often by hippocampal sclerosis is not uncommon in teenagers and is amenable to an *anterior temporal lobectomy*.
- Drop attacks with injuries respond well to *corpus callosotomy* and should be offered as a palliative procedure.

■ REFERENCES

1. Scheffer IE, Berkovic S, Capovilla G, et al. ILAE classification of the epilepsies position paper of the ILAE Commission for Classification and Terminology. Epilepsia. 2017;58(4):512-21.
2. Co JP, Elia M, Engel J Jr, et al. Proposal of an algorithm for diagnosis and treatment of neonatal seizures in developing countries. Epilepsia. 2007;48(6):1158-64.
3. Pack AM. Epilepsy Overview and Revised Classification of Seizures and Epilepsies. Continuum (Minneap Minn). 2019;25(2):306-21.
4. Camfield C, Camfield P. Management guidelines for children with idiopathic generalized epilepsy. Epilepsia. 2005;46(Suppl 9):112-6.
5. Nabbout R, Dulac O. Epileptic encephalopathies: a brief overview. J Clin Neurophysiol. 2003;20(6):393-7.
6. Pearl PL. Epilepsy Syndromes in Childhood. Continuum (Minneap Minn). 2018;24(1):186-209.
7. Hussain SA. Epileptic Encephalopathies. Continuum (Minneap Minn). 2018;24(1):171-85.
8. Grill MF, Ng YT. "Simple febrile seizures plus (SFS+)": more than one febrile seizure within 24 hours is usually okay. Epilepsy Behav. 2013;27(3):472-6.
9. American Clinical Neurophysiology Society. Guideline 1: Minimum technical requirements for performing clinical electroencephalography. J Clin Neurophysiol. 2006;23(2):86-91.
10. NICE Clinical guideline. The Epilepsies: The diagnosis and management. [online] Available from: https://www.nice.org.uk/guidance/cg137/chapter/update-information#update-information. [Last accessed December, 2019].
11. Panayiotopoulos CP. A Clinical Guide to Epileptic Syndromes and their Treatment, Revised Second Edition, Based on the ILAE classifications and practice parameter guidelines. New York: Springer Healthcare Ltd; 2010.

5.2 ACUTE ENCEPHALOPATHY

PAM Kunju

■ INTRODUCTION

Acute encephalopathy in children is mainly caused by viruses. However, encephalopathy may be produced by various acquired and inherited metabolic disorders, which may be associated with fever. Recently a wide occurrence of viral epidemics had threatened the public health system and led to huge mortality and morbidity. H1N1, Nipah, Ebola, Zika, etc. were some of the viruses that had created global threats. WHO in its list of "Blueprint priority diseases" for research and development includes these and "Disease X" represents the knowledge that a serious international epidemic could be caused by a pathogen currently unknown to cause human disease.[1]

Initial clinical management of such meningoencephalitis is aimed at empirical treatment of both bacterial meningitis and herpes encephalitis.[2] Though this is a good practice in the early clinical setting, distinguishing between bacterial and viral infection of the brain versus meninges, and searching for the specific pathogen is highly essential as outcomes can be vastly different and it may be the first case of an epidemic.

■ DEFINITION OF TERMS

- *Encephalitis:* It is inflammation of the brain parenchyma, manifest by neurologic dysfunction (e.g. altered mental status, behavior or personality; motor or sensory deficits; speech or movement disorders; seizure)
- *Encephalopathy:* It is a disruption of brain function in the absence of a direct inflammatory process in the brain parenchyma (e.g. caused by metabolic disturbance, hypoxia, ischemia, drugs, intoxications, organ dysfunction, or systemic infection)
- *Acute febrile encephalopathy (AFE):* It is characterized by altered mental state that accompanies a short febrile illness.[3]

In febrile illnesses, encephalopathy can occur as a result of direct pathologic involvement of the nervous system. It can also be due to systemic complications like sepsis associated toxicity, hypotension, hypoxia, hypoglycemia, electrolyte imbalance or hyperpyrexia.

Common causes in India are bacterial meningitis, viral encephalitis like Japanese encephalitis (JE), cerebral malaria (CM), and typhoid/shigella encephalopathy. Tuberculous meningoencephalitis (TBM) usually has a subacute or chronic presentation but can also have an acute presentation. Most of these cases may have a complete recovery if the underlying cause is identified and treated promptly.

Central nervous system (CNS) infections are one of the commonest neurological emergencies in children. They can be broadly classified into meningitis (inflammation of the meninges) or encephalitis (inflammation of the brain parenchyma) even though both may coexist (meningoencephalitis).

The acute meningitis may have two presentations. The less common one is of dramatic onset with rapidly progressive shock, purpura and disseminated intravascular coagulation (DIC). The more common presentation is many days of respiratory or gastrointestinal symptoms followed by increasing lethargy and irritability. Death or serious sequelae may occur due to delay in diagnosis and treatment. A high index of suspicion is essential for early diagnosis and emergency management.[4]

Different etiological agents like pyogenic bacteria, *Mycobacterium tuberculosis,* viruses, fungi or parasites can cause meningitis. Bacterial infections produce acute fulminant meningitis. The tubercle bacilli and fungi cause subacute to chronic meningitis. Viral meningitis is relatively milder and subsides on its own.

The mode of transmission is person-to-person contact through respiratory tract or droplet infection. Immunosuppression due to immunoglobulin subclass deficiency, HIV infection and the like increases the risk of meningeal infection.

The term encephalopathy refers to any cause of brain dysfunction without actual inflammation of brain. The etiology includes metabolic, toxic, endocrine or electrolyte disturbance **(Table 5.2.1)**.

ACUTE ENCEPHALITIS SYNDROME

Clinically, a case of acute encephalitis syndrome (AES) is defined as a person of any age, at any time of year with the acute onset of fever and at least one of:
- Change in mental status (symptoms such as confusion, disorientation, coma or inability to talk)
- New onset of seizures (excluding simple febrile seizures). A simple febrile seizure is defined as a seizure that occurs in a child aged 6 months to less than 6 years, whose only finding is fever and a single generalized convulsion lasting less than 15 minutes.

Evolution of AES is characterized by a prodromal phase (1–3 days) of fever, malaise and headache followed by an encephalitic phase with persistent fever, decreasing level of consciousness, seizures, abnormal movements and or weakness.

CLINICAL CLUES

The symptoms of fever, headache, photophobia, anorexia, irritability, vomiting with features of meningeal irritation point towards the diagnosis of pyogenic meningitis. Meningeal irritation is manifested as nuchal rigidity, back pain, Kernig sign (flexion of the neck to *90°* with subsequent pain on

Table 5.2.1: Causes of acute encephalopathy[11] (Remember AEIOU).

A. Anoxic encephalopathy

E. Epilepsy related
- Nonconvulsive status
- Postictal
- Epileptic encephalopathy

I. Infection and postinfectious demyelination/autoimmune
- Meningitis
- Encephalitis
- Intracerebral abscess
- Systemic infection leading to altered mental state (SAE - sepsis-associated encephalopathy)
- Acute disseminated encephalomyelitis

Autoimmune encephalitis
- N-methyl-D-aspartate receptor antibody encephalitis
- Hashimoto's encephalopathy

O. Outside poisoning (toxins, drugs)

U. (Uremia/other metabolic)
- Uremia
- Hyperammonemia
- Hyper/hypoglycemia
- Lactic acidosis
- Liver failure
- Mitochondrial disorders, organic acidopathies
- Hypertensive encephalopathy

Infectious causes:
- Viral encephalitis
  - Herpes simplex
  - Varicella zoster
  - Japanese encephalitis
  - Rabies virus
  - HIV
- Bacterial
  - Bacterial meningitis (*S. pneumoniae, H influenzae, N meningitides*)
  - Leptospirosis
  - Mycoplasma
  - Tuberculosis
  - Rickettsial—scrub typhus
- Parasitic
  - Cerebral malaria
  - Toxoplasma
- Fungal

(HIV: human immunodeficiency virus)
Source: Solomon T, Thao TT, Lewthwaite P, et al. A cohort study to assess the new WHO Japanese encephalitis surveillance standards. Bull world health organ. 2008; 86(3):178-86.

extension), and Brudzinski sign (passive flexion of neck in supine position causes involuntary flexion of knees). But in newborns and young infants, the meningeal signs may be minimal. The only presentation may be with nonspecific symptoms like fever, irritability, poor activity, lethargy or refusal to feed. Seizures are a common presenting symptom of meningitis. A bulging fontanel is an important diagnostic clue.

The clinical findings like petechiae, ecchymoses and skin rashes and evidence of shock point towards meningococcemia. Cerebrospinal fluid (CSF) rhinorrhea, chronic otitis media, cochlear implants and postsplenectomy state predispose to pneumococcal meningitis. Complement deficiency predisposes to meningococcal meningitis.

Tuberculous meningitis often presents subacutely with irregular fever, altered sensorium, focal neurologic signs or signs of increased intracranial pressure. Malnutrition, history of contact with tuberculosis or immunodeficiency may give clues to diagnosis.

Encephalitis or inflammation of brain parenchyma is mainly caused by viruses. It can cause greater alteration of sensorium than bacterial meningitis. Encephalitis is usually associated with fever, altered sensorium and asymmetric focal neurological deficits. Bacterial meningitis is characterized by fever, headache, and stiffness without profound alteration of sensorium. When both coexist it is called meningoencephalitis.

Clinical Diagnostic Criteria of Encephalitis

The clinical diagnostic criteria include the following:
- Altered mental status (i.e., decreased or altered level of consciousness, lethargy, or personality change) lasting ≥24 hours with no alternative cause identified, plus
- ≥2 of the following for a "possible" diagnosis or ≥3 of the following for a "probable" diagnosis:
  - Documented fever ≥38°C (100.4°F) within 72 hours (before or after) presentation
  - Generalized or partial seizures not fully attributable to pre-existing seizure disorder
  - New onset focal neurologic findings
  - CSF WBC count ≥5 cells/mm^3
  - Abnormality of brain parenchyma on neuroimaging suggestive of encephalitis that is new or appears to have acute onset
  - Abnormality on EEG that is consistent with encephalitis and not attributable to another illness.

In encephalopathy fever is not marked, and neurological deficits will be symmetrical.

Though clinical presentation will be similar in most, regardless of the etiology, careful history and physical examination give clues to the etiology of meningitis and encephalitis. Investigations like imaging, electroencephalogram (EEG) and lumbar puncture (LP) with specialized studies help to clinch a specific etiology in many.[5-8]

Historical Clues

Some clues in history are very helpful in arriving at a diagnosis:
- *Epidemics:* Arboviral encephalitis like Japanese encephalitis (JE)
- Contact with pigs, monkeys, living near paddy field—arboviral encephalitis
- *Sporadic:* Herpes simplex virus (HSV) encephalitis
- *History of animal bite:* Rabies

- *History of working or playing in waterlogged fields/contact with rat urine/rainy season*: Leptospirosis
- *Contact with tuberculosis*: Tuberculosis meningitis (TBM)
- *History of diarrhea*: Enteroviral; Dysentery: Shigella encephalopathy
- Behavioral changes/psychiatric manifestation—autoimmune encephalitis.

General and Systemic Examination Clues

A few important clues seen during general and systemic examination are listed below.
- *Fever with rash:*
  - Maculopapular rash in measles, dengue, chikungunya, meningococcemia, scrub typhus, West Nile virus (WNV) disease[9]
  - *Vesicular rash in neonates with CNS HSV infection*: Varicella—Varicella encephalopathy; Zoster—vasculitis
  - Hand, foot and mouth disease (coxsackieviruses A and B)
  - *Herpetic lesions around lips*: Herpes labialis, HSV
- *Parotitis*: Mumps, Epstein-Barr virus
- *Fever, throat pain, respiratory symptoms*: H1N1 virus
- *Hypotension and shock:* Meningococcemia, dengue, leptospirosis
- ARDS, cardiac involvement– Nipah virus.

Specific Neurological Signs

Specific neurological signs that help in diagnosis are listed below.
- *Choreo-athetotic movements*: JE, West Nile virus, autoimmune encephalitis
- *Minimal alteration of sensorium, prominent headache, vomiting, meningeal signs*: Bacterial meningitis
- *Ataxia*: Varicella zoster, acute disseminated encephalomyelitis (ADEM)
- *Cranial nerve signs*: JE, West Nile virus, brainstem encephalitis
- *Papilledema*: Tuberculous meningitis, tumors
- *Visual loss*: ADEM with optic neuritis, hypertensive encephalopathy
- *Anterior horn cell involvement*: Polio, enterovirus, JE.

As the child comes to the emergency with decreased level of consciousness, the first priority is to stabilize the patient. Special attention should be given for airway, breathing and circulation. Check blood sugar and manage hypoglycemia. Check for features of shock, monitor BP and manage hypo/hypertension.

■ INVESTIGATIONS

The usual investigations for establishing a diagnosis include the following:[9,10]
- Complete blood count, differential count, and platelet count
- Peripheral smear for malarial parasites

- C-reactive protein (CRP)
- Liver function and renal function tests
- Blood culture, urine culture
- Throat swab for H1NI in epidemics.

When meningitis is clinically suspected, LP and CSF study are mandatory within 30 minutes and before starting antibiotics.

Contraindications for LP includes severe thrombocytopenia, a Glasgow coma scale (GCS) level of less than 9, papilledema and other features of raised intracranial pressure (ICP) and local infections at the LP site. In these cases, first dose of empirical antibiotics should be started after taking blood for culture and sensitivity.

When there is raised intracranial pressure suspected on the basis of papilledema, hypertension, bradycardia, and asymmetric pupils, an emergency computed tomography (CT) scan should be performed before LP to rule out any space occupying lesion like tumor, abscess, etc. If a delay of more than a few hours is expected before imaging or stabilization of patient, empirical treatment with a broad-spectrum antibiotic plus acyclovir is advised. If the CT scan does not show any mass lesion or severe brain edema LP can be done provided there is no contra-indication.

Cerebrospinal Fluid (Table 5.2.2)

Note the opening pressure, cells, protein, sugar, Gram stain and culture, latex agglutination test for pneumococci, *H. influenzae* and meningococci, virological assay, acid fast bacillus (AFB) stain and culture, tuberculosis polymerase chain reaction (TBPCR), etc. Testing for oligoclonal bands lactate may be done in appropriate cases.

Table 5.2.2: Cerebrospinal fluid (CSF) findings in different intracranial infections.

	Pyogenic meningitis	Aseptic meningitis	Tuberculous meningitis	Fungal meningitis
Opening pressure	High	Variable	High	High/variable
Color	Turbid	Clear	Opalescent (cobweb coagulum)	Opalescent
Cells/per mm^3	>1,000	<100	100–500	100–500
Differential count	Predominant PMN	Lymphocytes	Lymphocytes	Lymphocytes
Protein	High	Normal	High to very high	High
Glucose	Very low	Normal	Low	Low

(PMN: polymorphonuclear leukocytes)

Magnetic Resonance Imaging

Magnetic resonance imaging (MRI) is the investigation of choice in febrile encephalopathy.[11] CT scan is recommended, if facilities for urgent MRI are not available or when the general condition of the child is unstable. The important findings on MRI which help in diagnosis include the following:

- *Herpes simplex encephalitis:* Asymmetric involvement of both gray and white matter of temporal lobe, insula, basi-frontal lobe with swelling and necrosis **(Fig. 5.2.1)**
- *Japanese encephalitis:* In addition to cortical involvement, involvement of thalamus and basal ganglia is characteristic **(Fig. 5.2.2)**
- *Zoster encephalitis:* Thalamic basal ganglia and insular hyperintensity **(Fig. 5.2.3)**
- *Respiratory virus encephalitis* (e.g. influenza, parainfluenza, adenovirus, respiratory syncytial virus): Abnormalities in the thalamus or basal ganglia MRI in H1N1 encephalitis **(Fig. 5.2.4)**
- *Enterovirus 71 encephalitis:* Hyperintense T2 and FLAIR lesions in the midbrain, pons, and medulla
- *Rabies*: Midline rhombencephalitis, involves hippocampus, hypothalamus, dorsal midbrain, medulla, spinal cord and basal ganglia, predominantly gray matter is involved
- *Tuberculous meningitis*: Hydrocephalus, intense meningeal enhancement especially at the base, tuberculomas with ring enhancement
- *Meningitis:* Diffuse meningeal enhancement, subdural empyema/effusion, infarcts, hydrocephalus

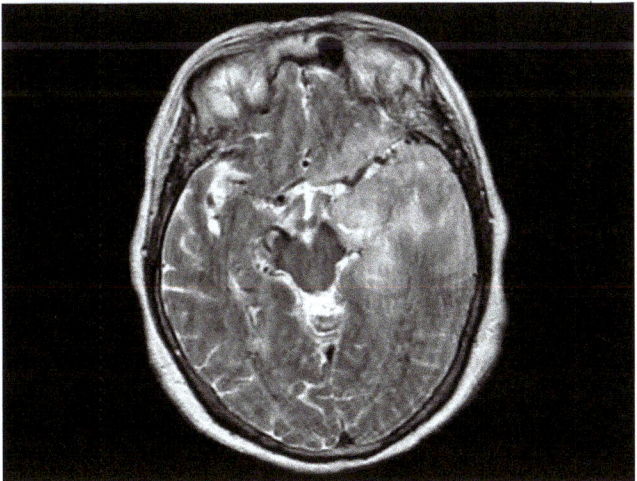

Fig. 5.2.1: Frontotemporal hyperintensity in herpes simplex encephalitis.

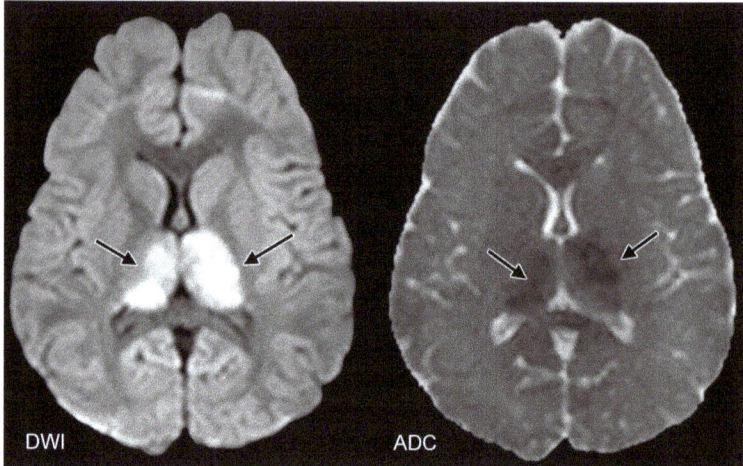

Fig. 5.2.2: Japanese encephalitis: MRI—Symmetrical, T2- and FLAIR—hyperintense signal in both thalami with matching restricted diffusion (DWI—hyperintense, ADC—hypointense)
(DWI: diffusion-weighted imaging; ADC: actual apparent diffusion coefficient; FLAIR: fluid-attenuated inversion recovery)

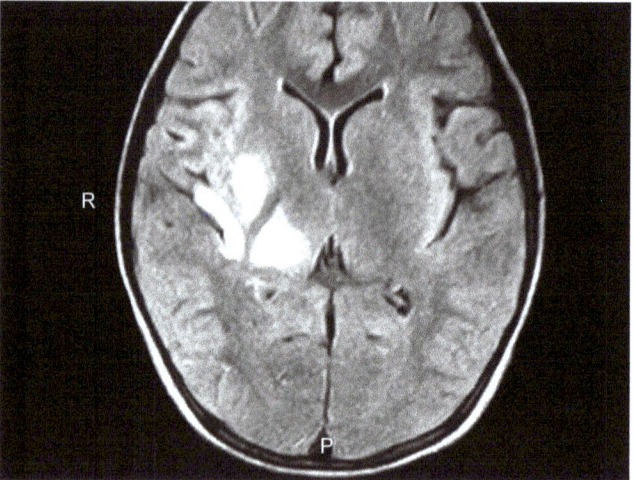

Fig. 5.2.3: Thalamic basal ganglia and insular hyperintensity in a case of zoster encephalitis with arterial ischemic stroke.

- *HIV:* Diffuse brain atrophy, basal ganglia calcification, evidence of opportunistic infection, progressive multifocal leukoencephalopathy
- *Acute disseminated encephalitis:* Predominant white matter involvement of paraventricular white matter, deep gray matter, cerebellar peduncles ± spinal cord **(Fig. 5.2.5)**
- *Autoimmune limbic encephalitis:* Medial temporal lobe involvement

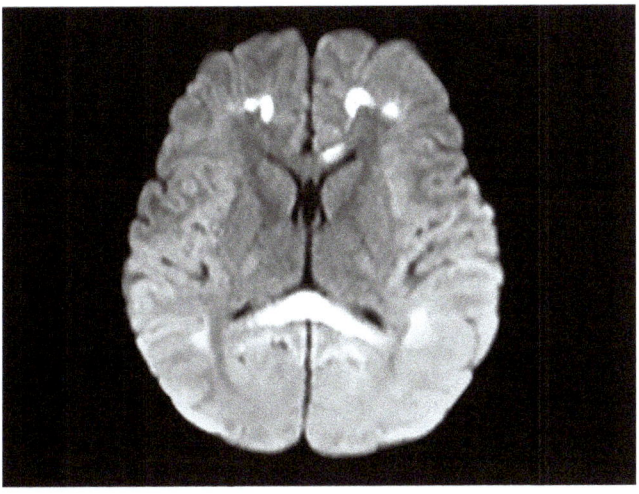

Fig. 5.2.4: Boomerang sign (hyperintensity of splenium) in H1N1 encephalitis.

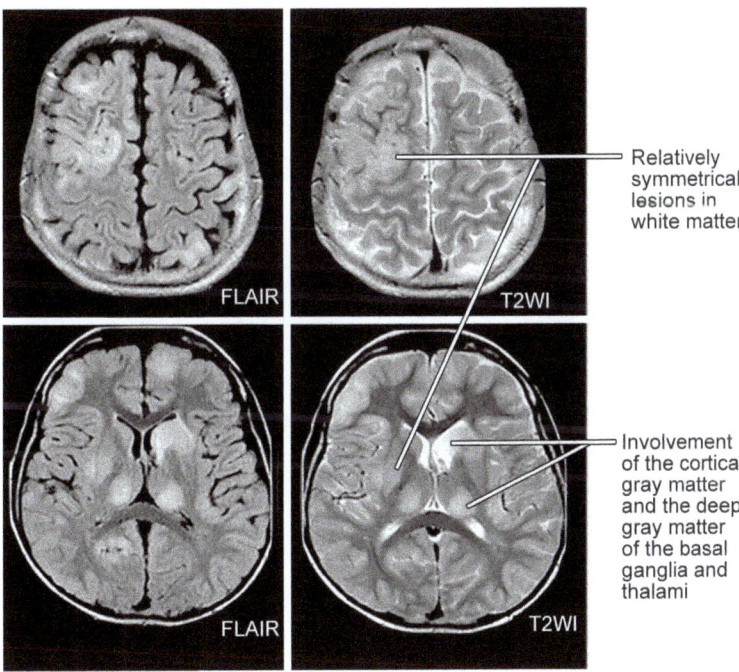

Fig. 5.2.5: Acute disseminated encephalomyelitis (ADEM).

- *Reye's encephalopathy:* Diffuse brain edema
- *Leigh's disease:* Involvement of caudate, putamen and brainstem.
- *Nipah virus:* Focal subcortical and deep white matter and gray matter lesions; small hyperintense lesions in the white matter, cortex, pons and cerebral peduncles.

Electroencephalogram

EEG may be helpful in some situations in arriving at a diagnosis. These include:
- Helpful in identifying nonconvulsive status epilepticus, which aids in management
- Diffuse slowing is the common finding in all encephalopathies
- Focal slowing and periodic lateralized epileptiform discharges (PLEDs), if present are more in favor of herpes simplex encephalitis (HSE)
- Triphasic waves in metabolic encephalopathies.

Polymerase Chain Reaction

Confirmation of diagnosis using polymerase chain reaction (PCR) has high degree of sensitivity and specificity in viral encephalitis. CSF should not be mixed with blood and should be sufficient in quantity for doing PCR. The PCR may be negative early in the course of HSE and after 10 days of treatment PCR. Never stop acyclovir if the result of first PCR is negative. If EEG and imaging support the diagnosis, repeat LP after 72 hours, and repeat PCR. PCR is also useful in diagnosis of tuberculous meningitis.

Clinical and lab findings for differentiating various causes of AFE are given in **Table 5.2.3.**

When the following infections with nonviral pathogens are suspected specific testing is required:
- *M. pneumoniae*
- *L. monocytogenes*
- *Mycobacterium tuberculosis*
- *Borrelia burgdorferi* (Lyme disease)
- *Rickettsia rickettsii* (scrub typhus).

■ EMERGING ENCEPHALITIDES

One condition that must be specially considered is Nipah encephalitis.

Nipah Virus Encephalitis

Nipah virus in humans causes a range of infections from subclinical infection to acute respiratory infection and encephalitis. The mortality rate ranges from 40 to 75%. The infection is transmitted from infected pigs and bats. Person to person spread can also occur. Infected people develop fever, myalgia, vomiting, sore throat followed by drowsiness, and neurological signs which indicate acute encephalitis. Encephalitis and seizures progress to coma in 24 to 48 hours. Some people may also have atypical pneumonia and ARDS. Treatment is limited to supportive care and antiviral agent ribavirin. Twenty percent of the survivors are left with neurological sequelae.

Table 5.2.3: Clinical and lab findings for differentiating various causes of AFE.	
Disease	*Diagnostic criteria*
Pyogenic meningitis	AFE ± meningeal + culture of compatible microorganisms from CSF or presence of ≥2 of the following CSF abnormalities: (i) polymorphonuclear leukocytosis (ii) glucose <40 mg/dL or 50% of blood sugar (iii) bacteria seen by Gram staining
Cerebral malaria	AFE with malaria parasite demonstrated on blood film/positive malaria antigen test
Viral meningoencephalitis	AFE + CSF pleocytosis with lymphocyte predominance (>5 cells/mm³) and absence of bacteria on Gram stain and culture with no other alternative diagnosis identifiable
Tubercular meningitis	Clinical case definition of tuberculous meningitis devised by Doerr et al.[12] • Abnormal neurological signs and/or symptoms, and two or more of the following • Discovery of adult source patient with contagious TB who had significant contact with child • Presence of Mantoux (5 tuberculin units) skin test reaction • Cerebrospinal fluid abnormalities without evidence of other infectious cause • Abnormalities on cranial computed tomography consistent with central nervous system TB
Enteric encephalopathy	AFE + evidence of Salmonellosis (positive blood culture or positive Widal test)
Japanese encephalitis	AFE + positive CSF/serum IgM antibody against JE virus ± typical neuroimaging
Measles encephalopathy	AFE + physician-diagnosed measles within the last 1 month with no other alternative diagnosis identifiable
HIV encephalopathy	AFE + HIV ELISA/HIV DNA PCR positive with no other alternative diagnosis identifiable
HSV encephalitis	AFE + positive CSF HSV PCR ± typical neuroimaging
Varicella encephalitis	AFE + positive CSF VZV PCR ± typical neuroimaging
H1N1 encephalopathy	AFE + H1N1 PCR positive respiratoty tract infection within 5 days of ILI symptom onset with no other alternative diagnosis identifiable
Dengue encephalopathy	AFE + positive NS1 antigen or dengue IgM with no other alternative diagnosis identifiable

(AFE: acute febrile encephalopathy; HSV: herpes simplex virus; CSF: cerebrospinal fluid; JE: Japanese encephalitis; PCR: polymerase chain reaction; VZV: Varicella zoster virus; ILI: influenza like illness; TB: tuberculosis)

Muzaffarpur Encephalopathy

The incident in Muzaffarpur, Bihar is an encephalopathy, which was metabolic, i.e., due to hypoglycemia. The toxin that is attributed is methylene cyclopropyl glycine in litchi fruit, which is similar to the toxin methylene cyclopropyl alanine seen in unripe ackee fruit and both of them belong to the same family. The heavy consumption of unripe litchi with no other meals predisposes the malnourished children to the risk of hypoglycemia, encephalopathy and death.

Sepsis-associated Encephalopathy

Sepsis-associated encephalopathy (SAE) is a diffuse brain dysfunction secondary to extracranial infection without overt nervous system infection. The pathophysiology includes vascular damage, endothelial activation, and breakdown of the blood brain barrier, altered brain signaling, brain inflammation, and apoptosis. Manifestations of SAE range from mild symptoms like malaise, concentration deficits or deep coma. It is difficult to make an accurate diagnosis due to the use of sedatives in critically ill patients. Thus, SAE is a diagnosis by exclusion of direct infection of CNS. Management of SAE is the treatment of the underlying infection and symptomatic treatment for delirium and seizures. SAE may be present in early stages of sepsis, even before the diagnosis of sepsis is made.

Some AES like situation can be due to invasion of the pathogens into CNS, as with dengue fever, chikungunya, scrub typhus and leptospirosis. In such instances, it is to be considered as a complication of the primary disease, and not as acute encephalitis.

Febrile Infection-related Epilepsy Syndrome

Febrile infection-related epilepsy syndrome (FIRES) is a refractory status epilepticus state that occurs in previously healthy child between the ages of 3 and 15 years due to unknown etiology. They present with a nonspecific fever that is followed by prolonged status epilepticus. FIRES evolve as a biphasic illness, with an acute phase of seizure for a few weeks, followed by the chronic status phase. The FIRES is difficult to manage and is often unresponsive to usual antiepileptic drugs. Immune modulation therapies, ketogenic diet and anesthetic drugs like ketamine may benefit the patient.

GLOBAL WATCHLIST OF ACUTE ENCEPHALITIS SYNDROMES

Global watch for viral epidemics and warning given by WHO periodically should be considered in the investigation of an acute encephalitic syndrome. Several additional diseases either emerging or reemerging are considered recently for inclusion in the priority list of WHO. These include:
- Crimean-Congo hemorrhagic fever (CCHF)
- Ebola virus disease and Marburg virus disease
- Lassa fever

- Middle East respiratory syndrome coronavirus (MERS-CoV) and severe acute respiratory syndrome (SARS)
- Nipah and henipaviral diseases
- Rift Valley fever (RVF)
- Zika, arenaviral hemorrhagic fevers other than Lassa fever, chikungunya, highly pathogenic coronaviral diseases other than MERS and SARS, emergent nonpolio enteroviruses (including EV71, D68) and severe fever with thrombocytopenia syndrome (SFTS).

To conclude all those who have fever and cerebral dysfunction do not have acute infectious encephalitis. All acute-onset CNS diseases of children do not constitute one syndrome. It can be due to encephalitis, encephalopathy and meningitis but also CNS complications of systemic diseases, brain abscess, subarachnoid hemorrhage, etc. No single syndrome can explain all these clinical presentations. Every clinical situation must be explored according to the recent governmental and public health protocols for individual and community. Most of these are medical emergencies and must be diagnosed promptly by utilizing clinical, lab and epidemiological features. Early diagnosis and expert management are required for saving life and preserving brain functions.

■ CLINICAL PEARLS

Etiological diagnosis of encephalitic syndrome is important for the individual treatment plan and for the public health perspective. The knowledge about the etiological spectrum of febrile encephalopathy across different geographic regions as well as for different age groups is a necessity for protocol development at the regional level.

Provisional diagnosis (without sophisticated tests) can be made with clinical features and epidemiological evidence:
- Lumbar puncture should be part of the routine sepsis work-up in infants
- Paradoxical irritability—An infant who is quiet at rest but who cries when moved or comforted may have meningeal irritation
- A cranial CT scan is not always required before lumbar puncture is performed
- Indications for CT scan prior to lumbar puncture include:
  - Altered level of consciousness
  - Papilledema
  - Focal neurological deficits, and/or focal seizure
- Antigen tests on CSF are useful in patients who have been pretreated with antibiotics and in those cases where the Gram's stain and CSF culture are negative
- For diagnosis of eosinophilic meningitis:
  - Hematoxylin and eosin staining, or Leishman staining of the patient's CSF is needed

- Eosinophilia in the CSF, either greater than 10 eosinophils/mm^3 or greater than 10% of the total CSF leukocytes
- Mumps virus and lymphocytic choriomeningitis virus are two of the few viral etiologies of aseptic meningitis with a decreased CSF sugar
- Migraine may be associated with a CSF lymphocytic pleocytosis, and aseptic meningitis may be associated with migraine-like attacks
- Fungal meningitis—Suspect a fungal infection in neutropenic patients with persistent fever
- Triad of ophthalmoplegia, somnolence, and ataxia is diagnostic of brainstem encephalitis
- Encephalopathy is the most common neurological manifestation of dengue fever.

■ REFERENCES

1. World Health Organization. R & D Blueprint. List of Blueprint priority diseases. Available at https://www.who.int/blueprint/priority-diseases/en/ accessed on October 22, 2019.
2. Lyons JL. Viral meningitis and encephalitis. Continuum (Minneap Minn). 2018;24(5):1284-97.
3. John TJ, Verghese VP, Arunkumar G, et al. The syndrome of acute encephalitis in children in India: need for new thinking. Indian J Med Res. 2017;146(2):158-61.
4. Baldwin KJ, Cummings CL. Herpesvirus infectious of the nervous system. Continuum (Minneap Minn). 2018;24(5):1349-69.
5. Sharma S, Mishra D, Aneja S, Kumar R, Jain A, Vashishtha VM for the Expert Group on Encephalitis, Indian Academy of Pediatrics. Consensus Guidelines on Evaluation and Management of Suspected Acute Viral Encephalitis in Children in India. Indian Pediatr. 2012;49:897-910.
6. Granerod J, Tam CC, Crowcroft NS, et al. Challenge of the unknown. A systematic review of acute encephalitis in non-outbreak situations. Neurology. 2010;75(10):924-32.
7. Bansal A, Singhi S, Singhi P, et al. Non-Traumatic coma in children. Indian J Pediatr. 2005;72:467-73.
8. Karmarkar SA, Aneja S, Khare S, et al. A study of acute febrile encephalopathy with special reference to viral etiology. Indian J Pediatr. 2008;75:801-5.
9. Kumar R, Tripathi S, Tambe JJ, et al. Dengue encephalopathy in children in Northern India: Clinical features and comparison with non-dengue. J Neurol Sci. 2008;269:41-8.
10. Janowsky AB, Hunstad DA, Central nervous system infections. In: Kliegman RM, St. Geme JW, Blum NJ, Shah SS, Tasker RC, Wilson KM, Behrman RE (Eds). Nelson Textbook of Pediatrics. 21st edn, Reed Elsevier; 2019. Ch 621-622, Ebook pp. 12522-73.
11. Modi A, Atam V, Jain N, et al. The etiological diagnosis and outcome in patients of acute febrile encephalopathy: A prospective observational study at tertiary care center. Neurol India. 2012;60:168-73.
12. Doerr CA, Starke JR, Ong LT. Clinical and public health aspects of tuberculous meningitis in children. J Pediatr. 1995;127:27-33.

CHAPTER 6

CARDIOLOGY

6.1 Managing Congestive Cardiac Failure in Children
Sanjay Khatri

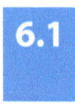

6.1 MANAGING CONGESTIVE CARDIAC FAILURE IN CHILDREN

Sanjay Khatri

■ INTRODUCTION

Heart failure (HF) in children is a clinical and pathophysiological syndrome that results from ventricular dysfunction, volume or pressure overload, either alone or in combination.[1] As a complex clinical syndrome, HF is characterized by typical symptoms and signs associated with specific circulatory, neurohormonal, and molecular abnormalities.

Acute heart failure: It is the structural or functional alteration in the heart that occurs in minutes to hours followed by congestion, malperfusion, tachycardia, and hypotension.[2]

Chronic heart failure: It is a progressive clinical and pathophysiological syndrome caused by cardiovascular and noncardiovascular abnormalities that result in characteristic signs and symptoms, including edema, respiratory distress, growth failure, and exercise intolerance, and is accompanied by circulatory, neurohormonal, and molecular derangement.[3]

Advanced heart failure: These patients have clinically significant circulatory compromise and require special care, including consideration for continuous inotropic therapy, mechanical circulatory support, or heart transplantation.

End-stage heart failure: It is the final common pathway of all forms of heart disease and may lead to heart–lung transplantation.

There are also other nomenclatures of heart failure. These may be described as "compensated HF" or "decompensated HF" depending upon whether end-organ perfusion is maintained.

Heart failure can also be described as "systolic HF" with reduced ejection fraction, HF with preserved systolic function, which is synonymous with "diastolic HF", and combined systolic and diastolic HF.

The term "high output HF" is often used to describe cardiac or extracardiovascular conditions leading to volume overload and congestion.

■ ETIOLOGY

The two most common causes of pediatric HF are congenital heart disease (CHD) and cardiomyopathies.[4] **Tables 6.1.1 and 6.1.2** present various precipitating factors of the above two causes. The various causes of CHD as per age of onset are presented in **Table 6.1.3**.

Table 6.1.1: Precipitating factors of congenital heart disease (CHD).

Cyanotic Heart Disease

Pressure overload
- Aortic stenosis
- Coarctation of aorta
- Interrupted aortic arch
- Pulmonary stenosis
- Pulmonary vein stenosis

Volume overload
- Left to right shunt
- Mitral regurgitation
- Aortic regurgitation

Both volume and pressure overload
- Hypoplastic left heart
- Single ventricle physiology

Ischemia
- Coronaries anomalies

Table 6.1.2: Precipitating factors of cardiomyopathy.

Cardiomyopathy

Primary cardiomyopathy
- Dilated cardiomyopathy
- Hypertrophic cardiomyopathy
- Restrictive cardiomyopathy
- LV noncompaction cardiomyopathy

Secondary cardiomyopathy
- Inflammatory—myocarditis
- Drugs or toxin related—doxorubicin, iron overload
- Infection—HIV, rheumatic fever
- Arrhythmias—tachyarrhythmia, congenital heart block
- Nutritional deficiency—carnitine deficiency
- Endocrine—thyrotoxicosis
- Storage disease—Pompe disease
- Mitochondrial myopathies
- Neuromuscular disorder

(HIV: human immunodeficiency syndrome; LV: left ventricular)

■ PATHOPHYSIOLOGY

An "index event", regardless of the cause, produces an initial reduction of cardiomyocyte contractility in HF. The initial injury results in a reduction in cardiac output that is, in turn, countered by two major "compensatory mechanisms".

The first of these mechanisms is the activation of the sympathetic nervous system (SNS), resulting in increased release and decreased uptake of norepinephrine, with peripheral vasoconstriction to maintain (by increasing systemic vascular resistance) mean arterial pressure and organ perfusion. Enhanced catecholamine levels, however, at the cellular level, the compensatory gain in cardiac excitation-contraction coupling mediated by sympathetic stimulation ultimately becomes unsuccessful, as the sustained leak of calcium from the sarcoplasmic reticulum leads to depletion of intracellular calcium that leads to further cardiomyocyte injury,

Table 6.1.3: Causes of congestive heart failure resulting from congenital heart disease.

Age of onset	Causes
At birth	• Volume overloaded lesions • Severe TR/PR • Large systemic AV fistula • HLHS
First week	• PDA in small preterm • TGA • Obstructed TAPVC • Severe AS/PS
1–4 weeks	• Large VSD/PDA in preterm • Severe COA • AV canal defects • All defects listed previously
4–6 weeks	Large VSD/PDA in term babies
6 weeks to 3 months	ALCAPA

(HLHS: hypoplastic left heart syndrome; TR: tricuspid regurgitation; PR: pulmonary regurgitation; TAPVC: total anomalous pulmonary venous connection; AS: aortic stenosis; PS: pulmonary stenosis; VSD: ventricular septal defect; PDA: patent ductus arteriosus; COA: coarctation of aorta; ALCAPA: anomalous left coronary artery from pulmonary artery; AV: arteriovenous; AV: atrioventricular)

dysfunctional intracellular signaling, and cardiomyocyte death ultimately impairs contractility and progress to heart failure.

The second important "compensatory" mechanism is the stimulation of the renin-angiotensin-aldosterone system (RAAS), consisting of increased circulating levels of renin, angiotensin II, and aldosterone.

Renin is responsible for cleaving angiotensinogen in angiotensin I, which is converted into angiotensin II by the angiotensin-converting enzyme (ACE). Angiotensin II is a potent vasoconstrictor that preserves end-organ perfusion.

Aldosterone causes salt and water retention, resulting in increased preload and then cardiac output according to the Frank–Starling mechanism. However, the elevation of both aldosterone and angiotensin II promotes cardiac fibrosis and apoptosis. These mechanisms may temporarily contribute to circulatory stability, but over time become maladaptive and promote the progression of HF. **Flowchart 6.1.1** shows the pathophysiology of chronic heart failure.

On the other hand, there are several peptides, such as the natriuretic peptides (NPs), bradykinin, and adrenomedullin that help to ameliorate all the harmful effects of SNS and RAAS by attenuating vasoconstriction, sodium retention, and retarding cardiac and vascular remodeling. NPs are coupled to, and activate, guanylyl cyclase A, which increases the intracellular concentrations of the second messenger, cyclic guanosine monophosphate.

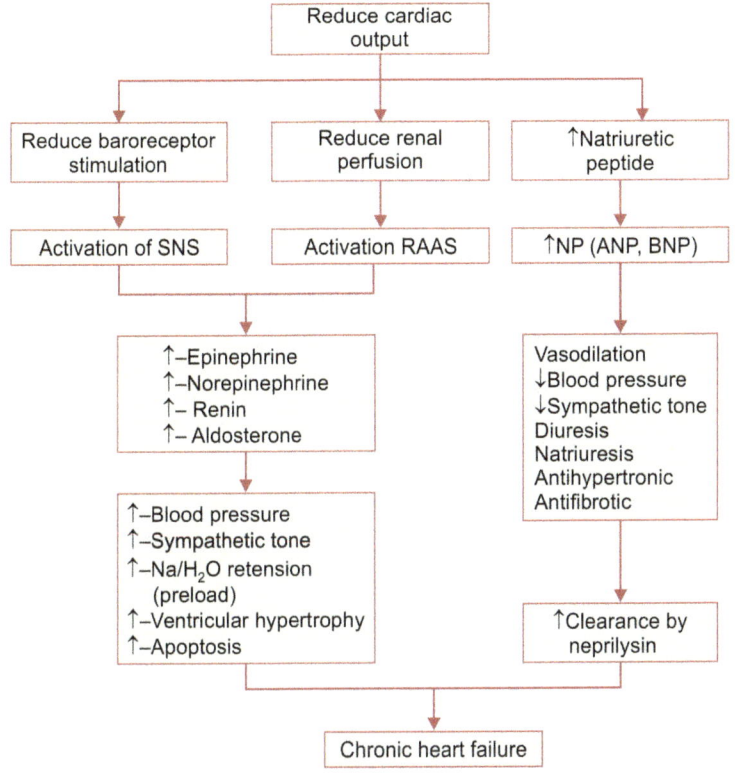

Flowchart 6.1.1: Pathophysiology of chronic heart failure.

(NP: natriuretic peptide; ANP: atrial natriuretic peptide; BNP: B-type natriuretic peptide; RAAS: renin-angiotensin-aldosterone system; SNS: sympathetic nervous system)

The latter, in turn, activates protein kinase G, leading to vasorelaxation, natriuresis, and diuresis. Atrial NP and B-type natriuretic peptide (BNP) also inhibit renin secretion and aldosterone production and attenuate cardiac and vascular remodeling, apoptosis, ventricular hypertrophy, and fibrosis.[5] Normally, these compensatory actions are not sufficient to prevent or stop HF development because NPs are readily destroyed by an enzyme, neprilysin. Neprilysin levels are increased in chronic HF, and, thus, the clearance of these neuropeptides is accelerated. In addition, RAAS is responsible in mediating renal hyporesponsiveness to NPs, which facilitates progression of HF.[6]

■ CLINICAL PRESENTATION

The clinical picture of HF is directly related to age; **Table 6.1.4** describes the age-related specific signs and symptoms due to HF.

In general, the symptoms of HF depend upon whether there is congestion due to chronic right HF or hypo-perfusion due to acute left HF.

Table 6.1.4: Common signs and symptoms of heart failure in children.[7]

Infants	Toddlers
• Growth failure • Persistent tachypnea • Hepatomegaly • Respiratory distress	• Respiratory distress • Poor appetite • Deceased activity • Hepatomegaly
School age	*Adolescents*
• Fatigue • Exercise intolerance • Poor appetite • Hepatomegaly • Orthopnea	• Chest pain • Dyspnea • Pain abdomen, nausea/vomiting • Hepatomegaly • Orthopnea

Signs and symptoms of chronic right HF:
- Elevated jugular venous pressure
- Pleural effusion
- Ascites
- Pedal edema
- Abdominal discomfort
- Hepatomegaly.

Signs and symptoms of acute left HF include:
- Dyspnea
- Orthopnea
- Rales on auscultation due to pulmonary edema
- Dizziness
- Fatigability
- Nausea, vomiting, abdominal pain, and feeding intolerance.

When right HF is acute, it can present with hypoperfusion, tachycardia, and hypotension. Similarly, when left HF is chronic, it can present with signs and symptoms of chronic congestion. Right HF is associated with left HF and is a predictor of increased morbidity and mortality. **Table 6.1.5** shows NYHA and modified Ross classification of heart failure in children.

■ DIAGNOSTIC APPROACH

The first step in diagnostic approach to pediatric heart failure (PHF) is history, physical examination, and then a battery of investigations.[9]

History

Chest pain, dyspnea, palpitation, syncope, dizziness, fatigue, edema, feed pattern, abdominal pain, vomiting, loss of appetite, prior cardiac surgery or intervention, family history of cardiomyopathy or sudden cardiac death (SCD).

Table 6.1.5: New York Heart Association (NYHA) and modified Ross classification of heart failure (HF) in children.[8]

Modified Ross classification of HF in children < 6 years	NYHA classification of HF in children > 6 years
Class I: Asymptomatic	Class I: Asymptomatic
Class II: Mild tachypnea or diaphoresis with feeding in infants; dyspnea on exertion in older children	Class II: Slight or moderate limitations of physical activity
Class III: Marked tachypnea or diaphoresis with feeding in infants. Prolonged feeding times with growth failure; Marked dyspnea on exertion in older children	Class III: Marked limitation of physical activity
Class IV: Symptoms such as tachypnea, retractions, grunting, or diaphoresis at rest	Class IV: Symptoms at rest

Physical Examination

One should look for rhythm (tachy- or bradyarrhythmias), gallop rhythm, respiratory distress, edema, hypotension, and hepatomegaly.

Investigations

Blood investigations are summarized in **Table 6.1.6**.

Chest X-ray

To evaluate cardiac size and pulmonary edema, Kerley lines, pleural effusion.

Electrocardiogram

To look for arrhythmia, ischemia, and left bundle branch block (LBBB). Sinus tachycardia is common in acute heart failure.

Echocardiography

The echocardiogram is the most useful, widely available, and low-cost test for patients with PHF. Echocardiography provides immediate data on cardiac morphology and structure, chamber volumes/diameters, wall thickness, ventricular systolic/diastolic function, and pulmonary pressure. These data are crucial to make the correct diagnosis and to guide appropriate treatment.[10]

Cardiac Magnetic Resonance Imaging

Cardiac magnetic resonance imaging (MRI) is indicated to study complexities. It also helps in the diagnosis and risk stratification of specific forms of cardiomyopathy.[11]

Table 6.1.6: Blood investigations.

Tests	Rationale
Complete blood count	• To assess anemia, which may cause or aggravate heart failure • WBC count to rule out any infective etiology
Serum electrolyte	• Hyponatremia reflects on expansion of extracellular fluid volume in the setting of a normal total body sodium • Hypokalemia can be result of prolonged use of diuretics
Renal function tests	Elevated BUN and BUN/creatinine ratio are seen in decompensated heart failure
Liver function tests	Congestive hepatomegaly is often associated with impaired hepatic function, which is characterized by the elevation of AST, ALT, LDH, and other liver enzymes. Hyperbilirubinemia (both direct and indirect) is related to acute hepatic venous congestion and is common with severe heart failure. Elevated ALP and prolongation of the PTT time can be seen. In children with long-standing heart failure and poor nutritional status, hypoalbuminemia results from hepatic synthesis impairment
Arterial blood gas analysis	For electrolytes and lactates, degree of hypoxemia, elevated lactate level seen in patients with decompensated heart failure as a result of deceased tissue perfusion
Troponin I CPK-MB	Useful, if clinical scenario is suggestive of an ischemic process (postsurgical or intervention) or myocarditis
Natriuretic peptides (NT pro-BNP/BNP)	Natriuretic peptide levels correlate closely with NYHA/Ross classification of heart failure and with ventricular filling process
Thyroid function tests	Both severe hyperthyroidism and hypothyroidism can cause heart failure

(ALT: alanine aminotransferase; AST: aspartate aminotransferase; LDH: lactate dehydrogenase; ALP: alkaline phosphatase; BNP: B-type natriuretic peptide; BUN: blood urea nitrogen; PTT: partial thromboplastin time)

Cardiac Catheterization

Despite advances in noninvasive diagnostic techniques, cardiac catheterization is presently indicated for:
- Accurate evaluation of pressure gradients in patients with complex valve diseases
- Evaluation of hemodynamic parameters (pulmonary and systemic vascular resistance, cardiac output, and cardiac index) in Fontan patients or during pretransplant screening.[12] **Flowchart 6.1.2** shows the diagnosis and management of acute heart failure in children.

Flowchart 6.1.2: Diagnosis and management of acute heart failure in children.

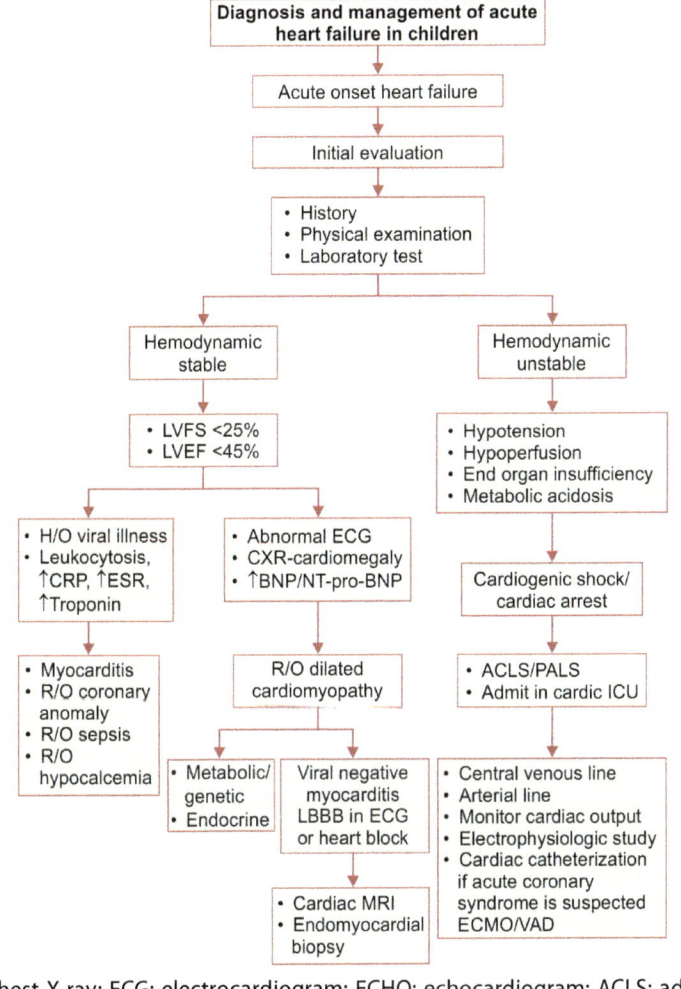

(CXR: chest X-ray; ECG: electrocardiogram; ECHO: echocardiogram; ACLS: advanced cardiac life support; PALS: pediatric advanced life support; ICU: intensive care unit; ECMO: extracorporeal membrane oxygenation; VAD: ventricular assist device; MRI: magnetic resonance imaging; CRP: C-reactive protein; ESR: erythrocyte sedimentation rate; LVFS: left ventricular fractional shortening; LVEF: left ventricular ejection fraction; LBBB: left bundle branch block; BNP: B-type natriuretic peptide; R/O= rule out; H/O: history of)

■ TREATMENT OF HEART FAILURE

Treatment of heart failure depends upon the underlying cause and age of the child.

Goals of the treatment are:
1. Correct the underlying cause
2. Control of symptom and disease progression
3. Improve the functional status and quality of life.

Correct the Underlying Cause

When possible, the causes of HF must be corrected through different approach:
- Corrective treatment should be performed in CHDs (surgical or intervention)
- Electrolyte imbalance such as hypocalcemia must be treated aggressively as hypocalcemic dilated cardiomyopathy (DCM) is one of the reversible causes of severe LV dysfunction.
- Acute viral myocarditis with severe LV dysfunction should be treated with early initiation of IV immunoglobins.

Control of Symptoms and Disease Progression

General Measures

In infants, nutritional support must ensure a caloric intake of about 150 kcal/kg/day. This is achieved using dietary supplements, preferring small and frequent meals that are better tolerated.[13]

In children and adolescents, current recommendations suggest that 25–30 kcal/kg/day is a reasonable target for most patients.

Carbohydrates should not exceed 6 g/kg/day and lipids should not exceed 2.5 g/kg/day. The provision of essential amino acids is necessary in the critically ill.

Evidence suggests that 1.2–1.5 g/kg/day of protein is needed.

Nutritional supplementation is required in HF secondary to metabolic and mitochondrial diseases (such as carnitine and ubiquinone).

In acyanotic CHD patients or in patients with cardiomyopathies, ventilatory support with oxygen must be initiated when oxygen saturation (SaO_2) < 90%.

On the contrary, in patients with cyanotic CHD, oxygen has little effect in raising SaO_2 and is not indicated.[14]

Reduction of salt intake is recommended in all patients with edema and fluid retention. Restriction of fluids is indicated in patients with edema unresponsive to diuretic therapy or hyponatremia.

Medical Therapy

Goals of acute HF management in children are to improve hemodynamics and prevent progression.

Current management includes stabilization with intravenous inotropes/vasopressors, mechanical ventilation, treatment of arrhythmia, and progression to mechanical support, if needed.

Despite the lack of sufficient randomized prospective studies, angiotensin-converting enzyme inhibitors (ACEIs) are first-line and β-receptor antagonists are second-line therapies in children, while diuretics should only be used to achieve a euvolemic status.

ACE inhibitors: They block the conversion of angiotensin I to II and activate bradykinin and kallidin, cause vasodilation and natriuresis, reduce afterload ACE inhibitors, and prevent, attenuate, or possibly reverse the pathophysiological myocardial remodeling.[15]

Indications:
1. Heart failure due to ventricular dysfunction
2. Significant valvular regurgitation (even without heart failure)
3. Heart failure secondary to large left to right shunts.

According to recent guidelines of The International Society of Heart and Lung Transplantation on the management of pediatric HF, ACE inhibitors are recommended in all patients with HF and left ventricular systolic dysfunction.[16]

Currently ACEI therapy is recommended as the first-line treatment for heart failure.

Therapy with ACE inhibitors should be started at low doses with a subsequent uptitration to the target dose with careful monitoring of blood pressure, renal function, and serum potassium.

Classification: ACEIs are classified into three classes:
1. Captopril is the active form of the drug and it is metabolized in liver
2. *Enalapril and ramipril*: These are pro-drugs and are metabolized to the active form.
3. *Lisinopril*: It is excreted without being metabolized by the kidney.

Captopril: The starting dose is 0.1 mg/kg/dose; it is gradually increased to 0.5–1 mg/kg/dose three times a day (increase after every 4 to 5 doses). Maximum dose is 2 mg/kg/dose. BP and renal parameters should be monitored when uptitrating the dose.

Enalapril: It is longer acting and given twice daily. The dose is 0.1–0.5 mg/kg/dose twice a day. The initial dose may be smaller. Monitoring is as for captopril.

Ramipril and lisinopril are other ACEIs; both are commonly used for hypertension. The doses for heart failure in children are not defined.
Side effects:
- Hypotension—it usually occurs in the initial phase (4 or 5 doses) and recovers after reduction of the dose.
- Cough is the most troublesome side effect. It is due to increased levels of bradykinin.

β-blockers: β-blockers are now an accepted therapy in the pediatric population. β-blockers antagonize the deleterious effects of chronic sympathetic myocardial activation and can reverse left ventricular remodeling and improve systolic function.[17] Carvedilol has vasodilatory, antioxidant, antiproliferative, and anti-apoptotic properties, reversing cardiac remodeling.

Recent reports seem to show that the addition of β-blockers to the standard therapy may be useful in patients with left ventricular systolic dysfunction. In addition, a recent Cochrane Database of Systematic Reviews on β-blockers for children with congestive HF was published. Seven studies of a total of 420 children were included in the review and the authors conclude that the current available data suggest children with HF might benefit from β-blocker treatment. Low-dose therapy should be started in stable patients with a progressive uptitration to the target dose.

Dosages:
- *Metoprolol*: 0.2–0.4 mg/kg/day initially and gradually increases to a maximum of 1 mg/kg/day in two divided doses.
- *Carvedilol*: 0.1 mg/kg/day in two divided doses and increases at 1–2 weekly intervals to 1 mg/kg/day with a maximum of 2 mg/kg/day.
- *Side effects*: Bronchospasm, bradycardia, heart block, hypotension, hyperglycemia, and dizziness.

Diuretics: Diuretics therapy plays a crucial role in the treatment of pediatric patients with HF. The benefits of diuretic therapy include reduction of systemic, pulmonary, and venous congestion but do not change the long-term outcome.[18]

Spironolactone may exert additional beneficial effects by attenuating the development of aldosterone-induced myocardial fibrosis and catecholamine release.

Diuretics from different groups can be combined for greater efficacy:
- *Loop diuretics*: Act on the ascending limb of loop of Henle, resulting in Na, K⁺, chloride, and water excretion. Examples include furosemide and torsemide.
- *Thiazides*: These drugs act at the distal convoluted tubule and also result in Na, K⁺, and chloride excretion. Examples include hydrochlorothiazide and metolazone.
- *Aldosterone antagonists*: These drugs act primarily by competing for intracellular aldosterone receptors in the distal tubule. The excretion of water and Na is increased, while K⁺ excretion is spared. Examples include spironolactone and eplerenone.

Potential complications of diuretic therapy include electrolyte abnormalities (hyponatremia, hypo- or hyperkalemia, and hypochloremia) and metabolic alkalosis. Electrolyte balance should be carefully monitored, especially during aggressive diuretic therapy, as the failing myocardium is more sensitive to arrhythmias induced by electrolyte imbalance.

Dosages:
- *Furosemide*:
  - *Oral*: 1–2 mg/kg every 12 hours, maximum of 4 mg/kg/day
  - *Intravenous*: 1 mg/kg/dose up to 3–4 times a day
  - *Continuous IV infusion*: 1–4 mg/kg/day.

- *Hydrochlorothiazide*: 2 mg/kg/day in two divided doses.
- *Metolazone*: 0.1 mg/kg dose BID up to maximum 20 mg/day.

Inotropes: Digoxin is a digitalis glycoside. It inhibits the sodium–potassium adenosine triphosphatase (Na-KATPase), increasing the intracellular calcium levels, thereby increasing the contractile state of the myocardium (positive inotropic effect). Inhibition of Na-K-ATPase also reduces sympathetic flow from the central nervous system and reduces the renal absorption of sodium in the kidney. This leads to suppression of renin secretion from the kidneys.[19] It increases the vagal tone, thereby increasing the refractory period and slowing the conduction through the sinus node and the atrioventricular node. Digoxin is the main oral inotropic drug used in HF in children and is indicated in symptomatic patients with left and/or right ventricular systolic dysfunction.

Very narrow toxic to therapeutic ratio; most common side effects are conduction disturbances (atrioventricular block). Its role in heart failure secondary to left to right shunt lesions, where systolic function of the myocardium is preserved, is not well defined.

The use of intravenous inotropes should be reserved for patients with a severity of cardiac output resulting in compromised vital organ perfusion (hypotensive acute/decompensated HF). Although increased inotropy results in improved cardiac output and blood pressure, the final result is increased myocardial oxygen consumption and demand. The failing myocardium has a limited contractile reserve and hemodynamic collapse can occur with high dose.

Sympathomimetic amines: Dopamine and dobutamine have been shown to be effective inotropes and vasopressors in neonates, infants, and children with circulatory failure. These drugs increase cardiac output and decrease systemic and pulmonary vascular resistance; however, they can induce tachycardia/tachyarrhythmia with a mismatch between myocardial oxygen delivery and the requirement. Therefore, we reserve the use of these drugs only for patients with low cardiac output despite other therapies.

Phosphodiesterase type III inhibitors: This class of drugs incorporates amrinone, enoximone, milrinone, and olprinone, of which milrinone, the strongest and shortest acting with the best control, is the most commonly used in pediatric intensive care. Type III inhibitors have vasodilatory and inotropic actions (inodilator effect) and improve diastolic ventricular relaxation (lusitropic effect). Additional effects include anti-ischemic effect on myocardium and inhibition of proinflammatory cytokines. Milrinone represents the first choice of therapy in patients with moderate/severe ventricular dysfunction with hypoperfusion symptoms.

Calcium sensitizer: Levosimendan inotropic agents play an important role in treating acute decompensation of patients with heart failure due to left ventricular systolic dysfunction. Levosimendan is a new positive inotropic agent having ATP-dependent potassium-channel opening and calcium-sensitizing effects, which increases cardiac contractility and performance along with vasodilatatory action without increasing myocardial oxygen demand and is with neutral effects on heart rhythm.[20] It is 98% bound to plasma proteins and completely metabolized prior to excretion. Wide range of levosimendan doses has been reported in critically ill patients with doses differing significantly between studies (bolus 0–24 µg/kg, continuous infusion 0.05–0.2 µg/kg/min).

Vasodilators: Vasodilators administered intravenously (nitroglycerin and nitroprusside) or orally (hydralazine and nifedipine) are indicated only in cases of:
- Hypertensive acute HF refractory to treatment (β-blockers and ACE inhibitors)
- Severe valve regurgitations in patients intolerant to ACE inhibitors.

Promising new drugs:
- *Ivabradine*:
1. Negative chronotropic effect on the sinoatrial node.
2. The clinical use of ivabradine is predicated on its mechanism of action on sinoatrial nodal tissue where it selectively inhibits the funny current (*If*) and results in a decrease in heart rate.[21]
3. It is distinct from other pharmacological agents known to have benefit in heart failure with reduced ejection fraction in that it does not target the neurohormonal system.
   The use of ivabradine was associated with fewer HF hospitalizations and deaths from HF.
   It is indicated for treatment of stable symptomatic heart failure due to DCM in children aged ≥ 6 months, who are in sinus rhythm with an elevated heart rate < 6 months: safety and efficacy not established ≥ 6 months.
   - <40 kg (oral solution):
     - *Initial*: 0.05 mg/kg PO BID with meals
     - Assess patient at 2-week intervals and adjust dose by 0.05 mg/kg to target HR reduction of at least 20%, based on tolerability
     - *Maximum dose aged 6 months to <1 year*: Not to exceed 0.2 mg/kg BID
     - *Maximum dose aged ≥1 year*: 0.3 mg/kg BID; not to exceed 7.5 mg BID.
   - ≥40 kg (oral tablets):
     - *Initial*: 2.5 mg PO BID with meals
     - Assess patient at 2-week intervals and adjust dose by 2.5 mg to target HR reduction of at least 20%, based on tolerability; not to exceed 7.5 mg BID.

- *Neprilysin inhibitors (NIs) and angiotensin II receptor blocker (ARB) inhibitors*: Neprilysin catalyzes the degradation of NPs. NPs are produced in response to volume overload and cardiac dysfunction, and exert a beneficial response in HF. Sacubitril is a prodrug, and its active metabolite inhibits neprilysin, thus allowing NPs to persist longer and promote vasodilation, diuresis, and natriuresis, as well as prevent cardiac hypertrophy.
- *Sacubitril:* It is the first Food and Drug Administration (FDA)-approved NI. Sacubitril is combined with *valsartan*, an ARB that acts on the renin-angiotensin-aldosterone system and prevents vasoconstriction and decreases both aldosterone secretion and renal reabsorption of sodium.

Sacubitril/valsartan is FDA-approved drug to reduce the risk of cardiovascular death and hospitalization in patients with chronic HF (NYHA class II-IV) with reduced ejection fraction.

The PARADIGM-HF [Prospective Comparison of Angiotensin Receptor Antagonist (Valsartan) and Neprilysin Inhibitor (Sacubitril) with Angiotensin-converting Enzyme Inhibitor (Enalapril) to determine Impact on Global Mortality and Morbidity in Heart Failure) trial has demonstrated that sacubitril/valsartan is superior to enalapril in reducing the risks of both sudden cardiac death and death from worsening heart failure.[22] This novel combination of drugs, sacubitril/valsartan, is also shown to reduce the risk of hospitalization and the progression of heart failure in adults. However, the benefit of sacubitril/valsartan in pediatric heart failure patients is under evaluation and various studies are going on this.

Device Therapy

Medical therapy has improved the survival and quality of life of children with HF; however, there are still a significant proportion of patients with poor prognosis due to the progression of the disease or sudden cardiac death. These patients are candidates for device therapy.[23] The two main devices used in patients with heart failure are:
1. Implantable cardioverter defibrillator (ICD)
2. Cardiac resynchronization therapy (CRT).

Implantable cardioverter defibrillator: In HF patients, ICD has a key role in preventing sudden cardiac death due to ventricular arrhythmias. Based on data from observational studies, accepted indications for ICD implantation in PHF are:
- Secondary prevention of sudden cardiac death in patients with aborted cardiac arrest or in patients with a previous episode of ventricular tachycardia determining hemodynamic instability.
- Unexplained syncope in patients with surgically repaired CHDs.
- Patients with severe left systolic ventricular dysfunction (left ventricular ejection fraction < 35%).

Cardiac resynchronization therapy: Left ventricular dyssynchrony is that in failing hearts, left ventricular function is affected not only by a depressed contractile status of the myocardium, abnormal loading conditions, or both, but also by a disturbed synchronicity of the myocardial walls.[24] Late activation of some segments leads to a slower rise in systolic pressure and delayed left ventricular ejection and also to slower relaxation and delayed left ventricular filling.

This pathophysiological condition is the assumption that CRT, through biventricular pacing, improves the pattern of contraction of the left ventricle. Despite the lack of randomized clinical trials, retrospective studies demonstrated the utility of CRT in pediatric patients with:

- Dilated cardiomyopathy, complete LBBB, and severe reduction of left ventricular systolic function (left ventricular ejection fraction < 35%)
- Third-degree atrioventricular block requiring the implantation of a pacemaker in DDD modality in patients with mild/moderate systolic dysfunction (left ventricular ejection fraction < 55%)
- CHDs with double-ventricle physiology with systemic left with severe reduction of systolic function.

In patients with single ventricle physiology, evidence supporting CRT is limited to a few studies. There are controversial results about the efficacy of CRT in patients with isolated right ventricle dysfunction.

Mechanical Circulatory Support and Heart Transplantation

Medical therapy has improved the survival and quality of life of children with HF; however, there are still a significant proportion of patients who have poor outcomes and need advanced HF therapy including:

- Continuous intravenous inotropes
- Mechanical support, and/or
- Heart transplantation.

Heart transplant offers prolonged survival for children with end-stage HF; however, cardiac transplantation is a last resort, given the limited availability of donor organs, complicated management, and associated morbidity and mortality. The waitlist mortality is less than the transplantation rate (17% vs 63%).

Mechanical circulatory support systems should be used in children with decompensated HF who cannot be stabilized with medical therapy alone to unload the failing ventricle and maintain end-organ perfusion.

The AHA guidelines are for recommendations for use of mechanical circulatory support, device strategies, and patient—adults. However, there are no published guidelines for determining the mechanical circulatory support in children with HF.

Extracorporeal membrane oxygenation (ECMO): ECMO is the preferred means of mechanical support in infants and children where myocardial failure which can be either uni- or bi-ventricular and associated with respiratory insufficiency or pulmonary hypertension.

Extracorporeal membrane oxygenation facilitates ventricular recovery by reducing myocardial wall tension, increasing coronary perfusion pressure, and providing adequate systemic perfusion with oxygenated blood.[25]

Patients who presented with acute fulminating myocarditis can be successfully managed with ECMO. They may present with full cardiac arrest, low cardiac output state, or with hemodynamically unstable dysrhythmias including ventricular tachycardia or heart block.

Extracorporeal membrane oxygenation has been shown to be associated with high waitlist mortality and poor post-transplant survival. This is particularly true for infants < 1 year of age, for those with a diagnosis of complex CHD, and for patients with renal insufficiency.

When a patient is placed on ECMO, it is important that discussion should be done with the family in detail in every aspect.

If no recovery of myocardial function occurs within 2-3 days, listing for cardiac transplant or withdrawal from support must be considered.

Ventricular assist device (VAD): VADs have progressively gained popularity as a therapy for pediatric heart failure in recent times, and its primary use is as a bridge to heart transplant until a donor heart becomes available. The VAD consists of a specialized pump, which takes over the function of the heart and allows the heart to rest and regenerate, if it can.[26] Types of VAD include right VAD, left VAD, and biventricular assist device, of which left ventricular assist device (LVAD) is the most commonly used. The types of VAD available are:
- *Transcutaneous VAD*: This type has the pump and circuit located outside the body and the patient is essentially confined to the hospital, if placed on this type of device.
- *Implantable VAD*: This device has the pump located inside the body with an external portable battery. The patient can be fully mobile when placed on this type of device.

Pediatric VADs offer specific advantages over ECMO, including reduced anticoagulation requirements, decreased use of blood products, decreased risk of systemic thromboembolic complications and inflammatory response, longer duration of support, increased mobility, participation in rehabilitation, and the possibility of hospital discharge.

Complications of VADs include infection, bleeding, device malfunction, and neurologic injury in children.

The use of short-term VADs in children with decompensated HF has demonstrated longer survival to transplant compared to ECMO.

The smallest devices currently approved for children are for those with a body surface area of at least 0.7 m². Smaller devices are under development.

Heart transplantation: It is an accepted treatment for patients with refractory HF. Although controlled trials have never been conducted, there is a consensus that cardiac transplantation significantly increases survival, functional capacity, and quality of life. In recent years, the outcome of pediatric transplantation has continued to improve. The most recent data from the International Society of Heart and Lung Transplantation demonstrate that the median survival is 19.7 years for infants, 16.8 years for children 1–5 years, 14.5 years for children 6–10 years, and 12.4 years for children 11–17 years of age at the time of transplantation.[27]

In infants younger than 12 months, which account for about 23% of pediatric cardiac transplant, hypoplastic left heart syndrome (HLHS) is the most common indication followed by dilated cardiomyopathy.

In children, cardiomyopathies (dilated and restrictive) account for about 60% of cases.

■ CONCLUSION

Pediatric HF is a complex clinical syndrome resulting from diverse primary and secondary causes and shared pathways of disease progression. Unlike adults, PHF is commonly due to structural heart disease and reversible conditions, thus lending it amenable to definitive therapy or short-term aggressive therapy.

Treatment of pediatric HF has evolved over the past decade to meet the growing demands and challenges in the care of this complex group of patients. The ultimate goal is to find a readily available, affordable, easily administered, and safe therapy. While the general principles of management are similar to those in adults, there is a lack of randomized clinical trials and international guidelines for PHF. The emerging evidence from the recent studies in pediatric HF and a collaborative multidisciplinary approach will likely to improve the outcomes of children with HF in future.

■ REFERENCES

1. Kirk R, Dipchand AI, Rosenthal DN, et al. The international Society of Heart and Lung Transplantation Guidelines for the management of pediatric heart failure: Executive summary. J Heart Lung Transpl. 2014;33(9):888-909.
2. Mebazaa A. Acute heart failure deserves a log-scale boost in research support. Call for Multidisciplinary and universal actions. JACC Heart Fail. 2018;6(1):76-9.
3. Hsu DT, Pearson GD. Heart failure in children: part I: history, etiology, and pathophysiology. Circ Heart Fail. 2009;2(1):63-70.
4. Hinton RB, Ware SM. Heart failure in pediatric patients with congenital heart disease. Circ Res. 2017;120(6):978-94.

5. Das BB. Plasma B-type natriuretic peptides in children with cardiovascular diseases. Pediatr Cardiol. 2010;31(8):1135-45.
6. Braunwald E. The path to an angiotensin receptor antagonist-neprilysin inhibitor in the treatment of heart failure. J Am Coll Cardiol. 2015;65(10):1029-41.
7. Das BB. Current state of pediatric heart failure. Children (Basel). 2018;5(7): pii: E88.
8. Ross RD. The Ross classification for heart failure in children after 25 years: a review and an age-stratified revision. Pediatr Cardiol. 2012;33(8):295-300.
9. Masarone D, Valente F, Rubino M, et al. Pediatric heart failure: a practical guide to diagnosis and management. Pediatr Neonatol. 2017;58(4):303-12.
10. Goldberg SJ, Valdes-Cruz LM, Sahn DJ, et al. Two-dimensional echocardiographic evaluation of dilated cardiomyopathy in children. Am J Cardiol. 1983;52(10): 1244-8.
11. Mitchell FM, Prasad SK, Greil GF, et al. Cardiovascular magnetic resonance: diagnostic utility and specific considerations in the pediatric population. World J Clin Pediatr. 2016;5(1):1-15.
12. Feltes TF, Bacha E, Beekman 3rd RH, et al. Indications for cardiac catheterization and intervention in pediatric cardiac disease: a scientific statement from the American Heart Association. Circulation. 2011;123(22):2607-52.
13. Meltzer JS, Moitra VK. The nutritional and metabolic support of heart failure in the intensive care unit. Curr Opin Clin Nutr Metab Care. 2008;11(2):140-6.
14. Balfour-Lynn IM, Primhak RA, Shaw BN. Home oxygen for children: who, how and when? Thorax. 2005;60(1):76-81.
15. Momma K. ACE inhibitors in pediatric patients with heart failure. Paediatr Drugs. 2006;8(1):55-69.
16. Kirk R, Dipchand AI, Rosenthal DN, et al. The International Society for Heart and Lung Transplantation Guidelines for the management of pediatric heart failure: executive summary. J Heart Lung Transplant. 2014;33(9):888-909.
17. Hussey AD, Weintraub RG. Drug treatment of heart failure in children: focus on recent recommendations from the ISHLT Guidelines for the Management of Pediatric Heart Failure. Paediatr Drugs. 2016;18(2):89-99.
18. Hood Jr WB, Dans AL, Guyatt GH, et al. Digitalis for treatment of congestive heart failure in patients in sinus rhythm. Cochrane Database Syst Rev. 2004;(2):CD002901.
19. Faris R, Flather M, Purcell H, et al. Current evidence supporting the role of diuretics in heart failure: a meta-analysis of randomised controlled trials. Int J Cardiol. 2002;82(2):149-58.
20. Angadi U, Westrope C, Chowdhry MF. Is levosimendan effective in paediatric heart failure and post-cardiac surgeries? Interact Cardiovasc Thorac Surg. 2013;17(4):710-4.
21. Swedberg K, Komajda M, Böhm M, et al. Ivabradine and outcomes in chronic heart failure (SHIFT): a randomised placebo-controlled study. Lancet. 2010;376(9744):875-85.
22. Shaddy R, Canter C, Halnon N, et al. Design for the sacubitril/valsartan (LCZ696) compared with enalapril study of pediatric patients with heart failure due to systemic left heart ventricle systolic dysfunction. Am Heart J. 2017;193: 23-34.

23. Motonaga KS, Dubin AM. Cardiac resynchronization therapy for pediatric patients with heart failure and congenital heart disease a reappraisal of results. Circulation. 2014;129(18):1879-91.
24. Cecchin F, Frangini PA, Brown DW, et al. Cardiac resynchronization therapy (and multisite pacing) in pediatrics and congenital disease: five years' experience in a single institution. J Cardiovasc Electrophysiol. 2009;20(1):58-65.
25. Adachi I, Fraser Jr CD. Mechanical circulatory support for infants and small children. Semin Thoracic Cardiovasc Surg Pediatr Card Surg Annu. 2011;14(1):38-42.
26. Lorts A, Zafar F, Adachi I, et al. Mechanical assist devices in neonates and infants. Semin Thorac Cardiovasc Surg Pediatr Card Surg Annu. 2014;17(1):91-5.
27. Dipchand AI, Kirk R, Edwards LB, et al. The Registry of the International Society for Heart and Lung Transplantation: Sixteenth Official Pediatric Heart Transplantation Report-2013; focus theme: age. J Heart Lung Transplant. 2013;32(10):979-88.

CHAPTER 7

PULMONOLOGY

7.1 Diagnosis and Management of Bronchial Asthma
NC Gowrishankar

7.1 DIAGNOSIS AND MANAGEMENT OF BRONCHIAL ASTHMA

NC Gowrishankar

■ INTRODUCTION

Asthma is a heterogeneous disease, which is characterized by chronic inflammation of the airways with respiratory symptoms manifesting as cough, wheeze, chest tightness, and breathlessness, varying over time and in intensity along with variable airflow limitation.[1] Usually, the diagnosis of asthma is made clinically. Further insights have shown that "asthma" is an umbrella term having different subtypes based on the underlying pathophysiological process. Whatever may be the subtype, documentary evidence of airflow limitation along with bronchodilator reversibility needs to be done wherever possible, before starting treatment. This is reiterated by almost all the recent guidelines on diagnosis and management of asthma.

■ POINTERS FOR DIAGNOSIS

Asthma is a clinical diagnosis. The qualifying features to make a diagnosis of asthma include recurrent episodes of respiratory symptoms of wheeze, cough, chest tightness or breathlessness, nocturnal cough, trigger-induced symptoms, activity-induced symptoms, relief of symptoms with bronchodilators and a family or personal history of atopy. The diagnosis of asthma cannot be made by a single test. Apart from a good history and thorough clinical examination (normal at the time of examination when asymptomatic), tests of lung function and markers of airway inflammation need to be done wherever possible for a diagnosis of asthma.

Tests that measure markers of airway inflammation by direct invasive methods require bronchoalveolar lavage and brush biopsy. In view of the invasive nature, it is not feasible in day-to-day practice. Another method is to document airway hyper-responsiveness by bronchial provocation (challenge) test. This can be done by either direct stimuli (methacholine and histamine) or by indirect stimuli (adenosine monophosphate, exercise, mannitol, and hypertonic aerosol).

Skin prick test usually helps to identify whether a child with respiratory symptoms suggestive of asthma is atopic or not. This is easy to perform and rapid, but should be done with standardized extracts by an experienced person. Atopic status can also be determined by estimating specific immunoglobulin E (IgE) by immunocap method in blood. This is very helpful in children who are not cooperative for skin tests and if there is a risk of anaphylaxis.

Tests of Lung Function

Spirometry

Spirometry plays a key role in the diagnosis of asthma by demonstrating reversible airflow obstruction. It is also very helpful in evaluating children with asthma who present with isolated symptoms such as persistent cough and exercise intolerance besides atypical presentations and also in monitoring the effectiveness of therapeutic interventions. Usually, children above the age of 5 years are able to do spirometry. The quality of spirometry results depends on the ability of the child to do a forced expiratory maneuver followed by a maximal inspiration. The result of this maneuver is a flow–volume loop with volume in the X-axis and flow in the Y-axis. The main advantage is that it can be performed in an office setting. The reliability of the results depends on the experienced technician who can devote time and effort to each child in an appropriate atmosphere to get a good spirometry recording. Spirometry measures flow and volume of the air entering and leaving the lungs. The lung volumes and capacities depend on age, height, weight, gender, and altitude. When performed correctly, it gives an accurate assessment of the forced vital capacity (FVC), forced expiratory volume in the first second (FEV1) and the FEV1/FVC ratio. There are robust predicted values based on height, age, sex, and ethnic origin, allowing assessment of the individual's measured performance against their predicted "normal" values.

Dynamic lung volumes [FVC, FEV1, and forced expiratory flow at 25-75% of forced vital capacity (FEF25-75)] are valuable to assess the response to treatment. A decrease in FEV1 is seen in those with suspected asthma. If reduced FEV1 is present along with reduced FEV1/FVC (normal above 0.9), it indicates expiratory airflow limitation. An increase in FEV1 by ≥12% of the predicted value, following inhalation of salbutamol 200–400 µg indicates a positive bronchodilator test **(Fig. 7.1.1)**.[2] The bronchodilator test may be negative during viral respiratory tract infection and acute severe exacerbation.

The concave shape of the flow–volume loop gives the indication that the individual has expiratory airflow obstruction even without looking at the other parameters. It is important to note that a normal lung function test does not exclude the diagnosis of asthma especially in milder forms; performing the tests when the child is symptomatic may document expiratory airflow limitation.

Maximal mid-expiratory flow also known as forced expiratory flow (FEF25-75) initially thought as a very sensitive indicator of small airway obstruction and also a better indicator of response to bronchodilator than both FEV1 and FVC has not been found to be precise, as it is a highly variable measure, which may be readily influenced by the expiratory time as well as FVC. Spirometry is recommended by Global Initiative for Asthma (GINA),

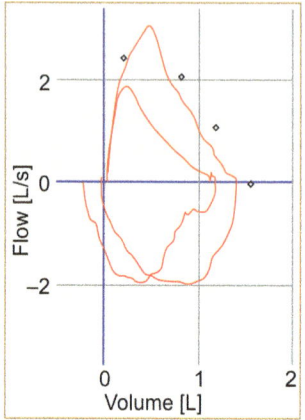

Parameter	Pred	LLN	Pre Best Trial 11	%Pred	Post Best Trial 4	%Pred	%Chg
FEV1 [L]	1.35	1.05	0.89*	66	1.25	92	40*
FEV1/FVC	0.905	0.769	0.769*	85	0.909	100	18
FEF25[L/s]	–	–	1.55	–	2.95	–	91
FEF25-75 [L/s]	1.80	0.79	0 75*	42	1.67	93	123
FEF75 [L/s]	1.07	0.26	0.37	34	0.79	74	115
PEF [L/s]	2.44	–	1.87	77	3.07	126	64
FIVC[L]	1.52	1.14	1.40	92	1.42	93	1
FEV3 [L]	1.14	–	1.14	100	1.38	121	21
FEV6 [L]	–	–	1.16	–	1.38	–	19
FVC (L)	1.52	1.14	1.16	76	1.38	90	19*

Fig. 7.1.1: Spirometry: significant postbronchodilator response. (FEV: forced expiratory volume; FEF: forced expiratory flow; FIVC: forced inspiratory vital capacity; FVC: forced vital capacity)
*Significant postbronchodilator change

British Thoracic Society (BTS), Canadian Thoracic Society (CTS), Spanish Guideline on the Management of Asthma (GEMA), Australian Asthma Handbook (AAH), and National Institute for Health and Care Excellence (NICE) in children of 6 years and above. GINA and BTS do not recommend spirometry in under-5 wheezers.

Impulse Oscillometry

Impulse oscillometry (IOS) helps to assess lung function in younger children who may not be able to do a forced expiratory maneuver needed for spirometry. It is a variant of the forced oscillation technique (FOT). It is a very simple test to perform where the child needs to have normal breathing for 20 seconds. The respiratory resistance and respiratory reactance are measured at multiple frequencies in both IOS and FOT, but the values are not identical. Both instruments detect obstruction in small airways as in asthma much better than spirometry but FOT has a better temporal resolution than IOS.[3]

The basis of this test rests on the principle that if there is an obstruction, the airway caliber decreases leading to increase in resistance. IOS measures the pulmonary resistance to the airflow by the large and small airways noninvasively and identifies whether the site of obstruction is in large (proximal) or small (distal) airways. Pressure waves of different frequencies travel to different distances in the lung. Low-frequency pressure waves (5 Hz) travel to the distal airways while higher frequency waves (20 Hz) travel till the proximal airways. The pressure transducer produces pressure waves with different frequencies of 3–35 Hz, which are transmitted to the airways through the mouthpiece. The resulting pressure oscillations and flow are measured at the mouth and impedance is calculated. R5 is the measure of total airway resistance, while R20 is the resistance of large airways. The difference between R5 and R20 represents the resistance of the smaller airways.

Impulse oscillometry needs only tidal breathing and thus obviates the need for cooperation from the child, especially younger ones. The interest in IOS increased, as it was shown to detect peripheral airway impairment early, which is associated with nocturnal asthma and exacerbations including fatal asthma. In children whose asthma symptoms are well under control, an abnormal IOS is a pointer of worsening of asthma. Even when spirometry and fraction of exhaled nitric oxide (FeNO) are normal, an abnormal IOS is an indicator of losing their control of asthma in the subsequent 8–12 weeks, which cannot be predicted by FeNO or spirometry. Children below 5 years of age with wheezing when subjected to IOS show an increase in the resistance and a decrease in the reactance. Hence, IOS helps not only in the diagnosis of asthma but also in predicting poor control during treatment.

Biomarkers

Though many biomarkers are used in research, blood eosinophils and FeNO are the two biomarkers commonly used **(Table 7.1.1)**.

Fraction of Exhaled Nitric Oxide

It can be measured during normal tidal breathing with a single breath and constant expiratory flow. It is expressed as parts per million (ppm) in exhaled breath. If the levels are above 50 ppm, eosinophilic inflammation in airway is likely to be present, but is less likely if less than 20 ppm. A note of caution needs to be added, as there are conditions, which can increase and decrease the values of FeNO. Those with primary ciliary dyskinesia and cystic fibrosis

Table 7.1.1: Investigations and biomarkers in asthma.

Methods	Potential for clinical application and significance in airway inflammation
Bronchoalveolar lavage and biopsy	Cellular and tissue component analysis
Sputum	Cellular component analysis
Fraction of exhaled nitric oxide (FeNO)	• Helper T cell subset 2 (Th2) inflammation • Response to inhaled corticosteroids
Exhaled breath temperature	Airway inflammation
Exhaled breath condensate	• Patient phenotyping and prediction of therapy response • Airway inflammation—prostanoids, leukotriene B4 (LTB4) • Oxidative stress—8-isoprostane, hydrogen peroxide, and 3-nitrotyrosine
Volatile organic compounds	• Early asthma diagnosis, patient stratification, and phenotyping • Biochemical pathways, endotype clusters, and prediction of exacerbation

show lower values of FeNO, while those with atopy and respiratory infections may show higher values. The BTS guideline advises the use of FeNO to find the evidence for eosinophilic inflammation, while NICE guideline recommends to use it in children with a probability of having asthma as a diagnostic tool along with other investigations like spirometry.[4] FeNO is recommended by GINA, GEMA, and BTS (for 3–4 years) in under-5 wheezers; but in children of 6 years and above, it is recommended by NICE and BTS (for eosinophilic asthma) but not by GINA.[5]

Eosinophils

Eosinophils in blood (>300 cell per mm^3) and sputum are important markers to predict if a child or adult with asthma will show a response to treatment with inhaled corticosteroid. Though this was identified decades ago, it still holds good. Sputum eosinophilia can predict exacerbations too. But in management of asthma, both blood and sputum eosinophilia tests are still underutilized.[6]

Exhaled Breath Temperature

This can be used to for the detection of airway inflammation and remodeling. The temperature of exhaled breath increases with airway inflammation and decreases with treatment with anti-inflammatory agents.

Exhaled Breath Condensate

It can be done with tidal breathing. It is collected by cooling the exhaled air by contact with either a condenser or cold surface. Apart from water, the condensate contains both nonvolatile molecules like cytokines and proteins and volatile but unstable molecules like hydrogen peroxide. The levels of these molecules are supposed to reflect that of the lining fluid of the airway. Though noninvasive and good for measuring biomarkers of asthma, the process of collection, preservation, and analysis has not been standardized.[7]

The levels of 8-isoprostane formed by arachidonic acid peroxidation are higher in exhaled breath condensate (EBC) of asthmatic children. The inflamed airways also release hydrogen peroxide, which can be measured in EBC and their levels are higher in those with asthma. A product of nitric oxide, 3-nitrotyrosine, is also formed in increased amounts during oxidative stress and elevated levels have been found in the EBC of asthmatic children.

Volatile organic compounds (VOC) analysis in EBC has been used to differentiate children with asthma and those without asthma. Also, it has been found that the profile of VOC in EBC is different in children with preschool wheeze compared to those without wheeze. These are exciting avenues for future research, as the measures of these biomarkers can help not only to diagnose asthma but also for identifying different endotypes in asthma.

Bronchial Provocation Tests

An objective way of measuring the airway responsiveness is to measure 20% fall in FEV1 over a set period of time after exposing the airway to histamine or methacholine in increasing concentrations by using a hand-held atomizer or breath-activated dosimeter or nebulizer. Methacholine challenge is an FDA (Food and Drug Administration)-approved direct stimulus test. Bronchial hyper-reactivity is present, if FEV1 falls below baseline with increasing concentration. Bronchial provocation tests are not recommended by GINA in under-5 wheezers, but recommended in children of 6 years and older by GINA, BTS, AAH, and CTS. A negative test makes a diagnosis of asthma unlikely.[5]

The GINA and GEMA recommend allergen sensitization tests in under-5 wheezers. GINA, GEMA, and BTS also recommend these tests for those who are 6 years old and above, but adds that this is not conclusive.[5]

■ MANAGEMENT

Managing a child with asthma has undergone a major change from the initial days where bronchodilator alone was the only treatment, followed by introduction of the oral anti-inflammatory drug corticosteroid till late 1980s, followed by introduction of inhaled corticosteroid (ICS) more recently. ICS has remained as the cornerstone in the treatment of children with asthma. With greater insights in the pathophysiology of asthma, it has been observed that though ICS is the most effective in eosinophilic inflammation, long-acting beta-2 agonists and long-acting antimuscarinic agents as well as drugs, which are effective against other mediators in airway inflammation such as leukotrienes, IgE, interleukin-6 (IL-6), interleukin-4 (IL-4), and interleukin-5 (IL-5), may also have role in those with poor control of symptoms.

The aims of the treatment are not only to reduce the airway inflammation and risk for acute exacerbations but also to reduce mortality in asthma. It may not be appropriate to just prescribe inhaled medication in children with asthma and remains complacent. Management is incomplete without looking for and treating comorbid conditions and trying to modify or reduce indoor air pollution wherever possible including first-hand and second-hand smoking, so that there is a risk reduction for acute flare-up in asthma.

The inhaled medications are of two types—controller and reliever. The term "controller medication" is often used interchangeably as "preventer medication" but controller medication is the apt term as till now there are no medications, which can prevent airway inflammation. Beclomethasone, budesonide, and fluticasone are the controller drugs available in India. Ciclesonide with a novel mechanism of action has not gained much attention and is unavailable in India, while mometasone has not been promoted much in pediatric asthma. Among the controller medications, fluticasone has the least bioavailability of less than 1% due to its nearly complete first pass mechanism.

Reliever medications are those that are used to relieve the broncho-constriction. Short-acting beta-2 agonists (SABAs) include salbutamol and levosalbutamol. Though formoterol, a long-acting beta-2 agonists (LABAs), exerts its bronchodilator action within 30 minutes, it is not the drug of choice for acute asthma in emergency room or intensive care setting. Other drugs used as reliever medications along with SABA are systemic corticosteroids and ipratropium.

Inhaled Corticosteroid

Inhaled corticosteroid forms the cornerstone in the management of asthma. The anti-inflammatory action is by downregulating the proinflammatory proteins and reducing the chemotactic mediators. Both genomic and nongenomic mechanisms play their part **(Table 7.1.2)**.[8] By their action on airway vasculature, which peaks in about 30 minutes after inhalation, ICS enhances the inhaled bronchodilator action by reducing their clearance from the airway when both bronchodilators and ICS are administered simultaneously. In addition, ICS also increases the beta-2 adrenergic receptor expression. ICS also increases the translocation of glucocorticoid

Table 7.1.2: Inhaled corticosteroids—mechanisms of action.

Characteristics	Genomic	Nongenomic
Action	Cytoplasmic glucocorticoid receptor-alpha	Membrane-bound/by cytoplasmic glucocorticoid receptor/direct interaction with airway vasculature
Onset	Hours to days	Seconds to minutes
Effects	• Selective switch off in multiple activated inflammatory genes • Trans-repression by reversal of histone acetylation • Increasing mRNA degradation and hence blocking production of pro-inflammatory cytokines • Increasing the synthesis of anti-inflammatory proteins	• Suppressing increased microvascular permeability and plasma leakage into the airway lumen • Acutely suppressing airway hyper-perfusion in dose-dependent manner • Inhibiting remodeling process (only long-term therapy in a dose-dependent manner)

receptors (GRs) into the nucleus β2-agonists. ICS as monotherapy is superior to leukotriene receptor antagonists (LTRAs) alone when starting therapy in asthma, while a combination of ICS and long-acting beta-2 agonists (LABAs) is superior to increasing the dose of ICS alone or addition of LTRA to ICS while stepping up therapy.

Potential Adverse Effects

Though uncommon, oropharyngeal candidiasis, dysphonia, and pharyngitis are the local side effects, while altered growth velocity, reduced bone mineral density, hypothalamic-pituitary-adrenal (HPA) axis suppression, adrenal crisis, osteoporosis, cataracts and glaucoma are systemic adverse effects. However, these are uncommon.[9]

Inhaled Corticosteroid Formulations

Beclomethasone dipropionate is a prodrug, which gets converted in lungs (97%) by esterases to beclomethasone-17-monopropionate. Another prodrug, ciclesonide, also gets converted in lungs to its active form desisobutyrylciclesonide, which has a very high GR-binding affinity. ICS becomes more potent, if the affinity of ICS to GR increases wherein the anti-inflammatory action becomes intense and so also the chance for side effects. Among the available ICS formulations, fluticasone furoate has a higher potency than fluticasone propionate, beclomethasone, and budesonide. The first pass metabolism is the mechanism whereby the concentration of a drug is greatly reduced before it reaches the systemic circulation. Fluticasone furoate has highest first pass effect, while beclomethasone has the lowest.

Dose of Inhaled Corticosteroid

The ideal dose will be the one that will give the child good control of asthma symptoms. The dose of ICS formulations as recommended by GINA, 2019 is given in **Table 7.1.3 and 7.1.4** while **Table 7.1.5** show the available ICS, ICS-LABA combinations in India and the available strengths.

Table 7.1.3: Inhaled corticosteroids (ICS) dose in under 5 years old (GINA, 2019).

Age	ICS and daily dose
Under 5 years	• Beclomethasone 100 µg (≥5 years) • Fluticasone propionate 50 µg (≥4 years) • Budesonide (nebulized) 500 µg (≥1 years)

(GINA: Global Initiative for Asthma)

Table 7.1.4: Inhaled corticosteroids (ICS) and dosage in older children and adolescents (GINA, 2019)*.

ICS	Low dose (µg)	Medium dose (µg)	High dose (µg)
Children 6–11 years:			
Beclomethasone dipropionate (HFA)	50–100	>100–200	>200
Fluticasone propionate (DPI)	100–200	>200–500	>500
Budesonide (DPI)	100–200	>200–400	>400
Adolescents and adults (12 years and older):			
Beclomethasone dipropionate (HFA)	100–200	>200–400	>400
Fluticasone propionate (DPI)	100–250	>250–500	>500
Budesonide (DPI)	200–400	>400–800	>800

(GINA: Global Initiative for Asthma)
*Not a table of equivalence but of estimated clinical comparability.

Table 7.1.5: Available inhaled corticosteroid (ICS) preparations in India.

Drug	pMDI (µg)	Rotacaps (µg)	Respules
Beclomethasone	100, 200	100, 200, 400	—
Budesonide	100, 200	100, 200, 200	0.5 mg
Fluticasone propionate	50	—	0.5 mg, 2 mg
ICS/LABA	—	—	—
Formoterol/budesonide	6/100, 6/200, 6/400	6/100, 6/200, 6/400	20/500 µg, 20/1000 µg
Salmeterol/fluticasone propionate	25/50, 25/125, 25/250	50/100, 50/250, 50/500	—

(LABAs: long-acting beta-2 agonists; pMDIs: pressurized metered dose inhalers)

Devices for Inhaled Corticosteroid

The delivery of ICS can be done in the following ways—pressurized metered dose inhalers (pMDI) with or without valve spacers, nebulizers (jet and ultrasonic), dry powder inhalers or breath actuated devices. Among the devices available, pMDI with valve spacers are widely used in children.

For a successful asthma management, the followings need to be addressed diligently: (1) correctly diagnosing asthma, (2) choosing the correct drug and dosage and (3) delivering the medication correctly with appropriate device. If any of the above is not right then the management becomes suboptimal or symptoms do not get controlled.

A proper delivery of the inhaled medications in asthma is essential. A valved-holding chamber helps to deliver the inhaled medications properly in children, as tidal breathing is enough to get the medications delivered to the lower airways. Younger children less than 5 years would need a facemask with the valved-holding chamber. A static-free holding chamber made of static-free material would be easy to maintain. It is necessary to demonstrate the method of giving the inhaled medication with holding chamber with or without mask to both the child and caregiver. Though this may appear trivial, an incorrect method of using pMDI with holding chamber appears as an important reason for poor control of asthma symptoms in most children. To minimize the side effects of ICS, it is necessary to inform the child and caregivers to rinse the mouth after use of medication every time and wash the face too, if facemask is used. Drugs other than ICS, their dosages, and side effects are given in **Table 7.1.6**.[10]

How to Start Treatment?

Different guidelines give conflicting versions of when to start treatment. Any child who is 6 years of age and above, with daytime asthma symptoms, has the need to take a reliever more than twice a month, with night awakening due to asthma symptom at least once a month, or has limitation of activity, needs to be started on ICS. Recent GINA, 2019 guidelines advise the use of low-dose ICS-LABA from step 3 not only in adolescents but also in children between 6 years and 11 years in view of partial or poor control of asthma.

The need for the introduction of ICS-LABA combination has dawned on the researchers after the audit of deaths due to asthma, where most of those who died had only mild asthma. The usage of SABA alone has been found to be more compared to usage of ICS or ICS-LABA in these patients who had died. Lancet Commission on asthma has suggested the use of low-dose ICS-rapid onset β_2-agonist combination inhaler as the default reliever option, so that patients with episodic symptoms and airway inflammation are more likely to receive ICS at a critical time, though they acknowledge that this needs to be tested in more studies.[11]

Table 7.1.6: Other anti-asthma drugs and side effects.[11]

Drugs	Action	Dosages	Side effects
Leukotriene receptor antagonist—Montelukast		4 mg (<5 years) 5 mg (6–14 years) 10 mg (>15 years)	Irritability, aggressiveness, and sleep disturbances
Monoclonal antibodies—Anti-IgE—omalizumab-recombinant, DNA-derived, humanized IgG monoclonal antibody	Bind selectively to human IgE on surface of mast cells and basophils; for use in 6 years or older when symptoms not controlled by ICS	6 to <12 years: 75–375 mg SC, 2–4 weekly ≥12 years: 150–375 mg SC, 2–4 weekly	Injection site reactions, viral infections, sinusitis, headache, and pharyngitis
Mepolizumab—humanized kappa monoclonal antibody specific for interleukin-5	Binds to IL-5 and prevents IL-5 from binding to receptor on eosinophil surface—12 years or older in eosinophilic inflammation	100 mg SC—4 weekly	Headache and injection site reactions
Benralizumab—humanized monoclonal antibody (IgG1/kappa-class)—IL-5 alpha subunit of basophils and eosinophils	Add-on maintenance drug in severe asthma—age 12 years or older with eosinophilic phenotype	30 mg SC every 4 weeks for first 3 doses followed by every 8 weeks	Injection site reactions, conjunctivitis, blepharitis, oral herpes, keratitis, and eye pruritus
Dupilumab—inhibits IL-4 receptor alpha, blocks IL-4 and IL-13 signaling	Reduces cytokine-induced inflammatory response—moderate-to-severe asthma—age 12 years or older with eosinophilic phenotype or oral corticosteroid-dependent asthma	<60 kg: 400 mg SC once, followed by 200 mg SC every other week	

(ICS: inhaled corticosteroid; IgE: immunoglobulin E; SC: subcutaneous; IgG: immunoglobulin G)

In children, till recently, the first step of asthma management in most of the guidelines is to give only a reliever, which is SABA, and when the child's symptoms increase, the next step is to give a controller, which has to be given daily. The use of inhaled SABA at the first step as needed gives relief not only to the child but also to the caregivers, as they are able to see the relief of the child's symptoms. When symptoms become more frequent requiring a step-up of therapy to ICS use daily, the parents who are used to seeing relief within a short time after giving inhaled SABA are less convinced and prepared to accept in view of the previous experience with relief from SABA. Many continue to be overdependent on SABA, which increases the risk for exacerbations and poor control. This allows the airway inflammation and remodeling to progress leading their children to grow as adults with increased risk for decreased lung function.

Knowledge gained from studies in adults with asthma has revealed that even in those with intermittent asthma, inflammation of airways starts at a very early stage but at a lower intensity, and when ICS is introduced early, they have better control of asthma.[12] It has also been found that not only the need for rescue steroids is reduced by half but also the daytime and nighttime symptoms are decreased by intermittent use of ICS when symptoms start in children with frequent wheeze.[13]

It has also been demonstrated in a study from Brazil that when beclomethasone was used intermittently, it reduced the frequency of exacerbations significantly but to a lesser degree when compared with daily ICS, suggesting that intermittent ICS can be used as an alternate regimen in those with mild persistent asthma.[14]

For persistent asthma in children less than 5 years of age, regular daily ICS reduces the frequency of asthma exacerbation. Even in those children who had intermittent asthma symptoms or viral induced wheeze, ICS started at the first sign of respiratory infection intermittently for 7-10 days was found to be effective in reducing the risk for severe exacerbations.[15,16]

Assessment of Symptom Control

Many symptom control tools are available and assessment of control by scoring methods helps to differentiate different levels of control. These include childhood asthma control test (c-ACT) and asthma control questionnaire (ACQ). The asthma control assessment by GINA is simple and easy to use **(Table 7.1.7)**.[1]

It is important for the pediatrician to get details about asthma control from both the child and caregivers who would help in the proper management of asthmatic children. If the symptoms are well controlled for at least 3 months, stepping down of ICS is recommended. If symptoms are under partial control, it is necessary not only to check the correctness of inhalation technique but also to identify and manage comorbid conditions. If symptoms are uncontrolled, in addition to the above, one needs to find out other issues for uncontrolled symptoms including smoking as well as indoor and outdoor air pollution.

Table 7.1.7: Assessment of asthma control.

Characteristics	Level of control		
	Well controlled	Partly controlled	Uncontrolled
Daytime asthma symptoms more than twice/week (Yes/No)	None of these	1–2 of these	3–4 of these
Any night waking due to asthma (Yes/No)			
Reliever needed for symptoms more than twice/week (Yes/No)			
Any activity limitation due to asthma			

Adjusting Treatment

Step-up

If symptom control is not adequate as evidenced by c-ACT/ACQ, after diligently checking for compliance to treatment and inhaler technique, the ICS dose may be stepped up. But if the child's symptoms are not controlled in 8-12 weeks, the dose needs to be brought down to previous level and other controller options or add-on therapy needs to be considered. Always it is necessary not to step up hastily without looking at probable factors responsible for poor control.

Step-down

If symptoms of asthma are well controlled at least for a 3-month period, stepping down the dose of ICS should be done but with a note of caution to the child and caretakers that this measure is a therapeutic trial. If ICS alone is used, the dose of ICS needs to be reduced by 25–50%. But one must be cautious while stepping down, if there are risk factors for exacerbation. If ICS-LABA combination has been the inhaled medication used, it needs to be reduced to once daily dose.

Follow-up

It is advisable to have a follow-up in 3-4 weeks after starting controllers. It helps the clinician to check and reiterate the correct inhalation technique and to find out the response to treatment, which may start within days of starting the controller medication. After the initial visit, it is ideal to have follow-up every 8–12 weeks wherein the compliance to treatment and inhaler technique needs to be checked. If symptoms are under good control, step-down can be planned.

Comorbid Conditions

Obesity

Obesity-related asthma may be a distinct phenotype. Control of asthma symptoms becomes much more complicated in obese children as airway inflammation is different along with sleep-disordered breathing and poor stamina. In those who are obese, airway inflammation is mediated by interleukin-6 and may have bad outcome too. If symptoms are not controlled in these children, with obesity being a proinflammatory state, it is advisable to do FeNO and eosinophil measurement in blood before planning an increase in ICS dose.[17] Interventions starting from lifestyle modification along with exercise to make them lose atleast 5–10% of body weight can bring their asthma symptoms under good control.

Allergic Rhinitis

It is an independent risk factor for the development of asthma. Though early identification and proper treatment of allergic rhinitis do not prevent asthma, correct management does bring about short-term control of asthma symptoms.

Gastroesophageal Reflux Disease

Most of the times, the symptoms of gastroesophageal reflux disease (GERD) and asthma overlap with each other. Triggering an inflammatory response in the airway due to microaspiration may be the reason for aggravation of asthma symptoms. Treatment with proton-pump inhibitors does not seem to bring about control of asthma symptoms in children with poor control although children with severe GERD symptoms need to be treated.

Management of Wheeze Under 5 Years of Age

The first and foremost is to make sure that the child's wheeze is not due to any other condition as investigations to suggest asthma in under 5 years of age are minimal and not available in all places. The following suggest that the etiology of wheeze is due to conditions other than asthma: moist cough, failure to thrive, oil in stool, recurrent sinopulmonary infection and dextrocardia, rhinitis from early infancy, clubbing, cyanosis, hypoxemia, and cardiac murmurs.

Many children under 5 years of age do wheeze with viral respiratory infections and are asymptomatic between episodes. They can be termed as episodic wheezers. The management of these children is symptomatic using pMDI and spacers or nebulizer for delivery of SABA. It is advisable to use oxygen (wherever feasible) to drive the nebulization, if SABA is delivered by nebulizer. There is no role for LTRA and ICS in management of children who are episodic wheezers.

Children under 5 years of age with wheeze who have interval symptoms in-between acute episodes are "multiple-trigger wheezers" and their management varies. The acute episodes need inhaled SABA either through pMDI with spacer or nebulizer. To control the interval symptoms and to reduce the frequency of acute exacerbation, a trial of ICS is advised for 8–12 weeks. This must be considered as a therapeutic trial only, as confirming a diagnosis of asthma is difficult in this age group. Trial is stopped at the end of 8–12 weeks. If the child's symptoms become well controlled during the treatment trial and appear again frequently after stopping ICS, this child may be considered to have asthma, which can get reinforced if child has personal atopy and either of the parents have atopy or asthma. In this situation, the child is presumed to have asthma and started on long-term ICS as in any other older child with asthma to get the symptoms under control and looking out for possible adverse effects too because of the younger age.

Resarch has shown that the classification of under 5 wheezers as episodic and multi-trigger type are not water tight compartment as episodic wheezer can move to multi-trigger type and vice versa. In view of this, many has questioned the continued usage of this classification. But from a practitioners point of view, this classification atleast helps to manage under 5 child with wheeze to a reasonable extent wherein investigations to guide proper management are still lacking.

Leukotriene receptor antagonist does not appear to be superior or having an equivalent efficiency when compared to ICS in multi-trigger wheezers.[5] Also, it has been shown that the relief of symptoms is better in those under-5 wheezers who have concomitant allergic rhinitis.

Recently, it has been shown that beneficial effects of ICS in under-5 wheezers are seen in those where eosinophilic inflammation is the main underlying factor. But given the many different phenotypes in under-5 wheezers, who would benefit with ICS, can never be found with confidence in clinical practice, as doing bronchoalveolar lavage (BAL) and brushing from the airways in under-5 wheezers is difficult in most of the places in India. A clue to diagnosis of asthma and responsiveness for ICS can be found with modified asthma predictive index (mAPI) **(Table 7.1.8)**.[18]

Modified asthma predictive index may be used in children ≤3 years old and is deemed positive in a child who had four episodes of wheezing and has in addition at least one major or two minor criteria. Also in under-5 wheezers with positive mAPI, who are boys, with emergency room (ER) visits or hospitalization for asthma in recent past or had sensitization to an aeroallergen, treatment with ICS leads to more symptom-free days and less frequent exacerbations.[19] Also, a positive mAPI can pick up children at risk of

Table 7.1.8: Modified asthma predictive index.

Characteristics	Features
Primary	≥4 wheezing episodes in a year
Secondary	
At least one major: • Parental physician-diagnosed asthma • Physician-diagnosed atopic dermatitis • Allergic sensitization to at least one aeroallergen	*At least two minor:* • Wheezing unrelated to colds • Eosinophils ≥4% in circulation • Allergic sensitization to milk, egg, or peanuts

asthma persisting in school age, which helps the clinician when dealing with under-5 wheezers not only to identify children at risk of asthma persisting in school age but also plan to formulate prevention strategies. Hence, in under-5 wheezers, a positive mAPI can make the clinician to advise parents about the possibility of developing school-age asthma and to follow-up the child carefully and institute treatment, if they present with frequent symptoms after therapeutic trial with ICS.

To summarize, children under 5 years of age with wheeze with evidence of atopy or allergic sensitization, a therapeutic trial of ICS is given, while in those with no evidence of atopy or allergic sensitization, the treatment options are intermittent ICS, daily ICS, or LTRA. For those with severe intermittent wheezing but are asymptomatic in-between with a positive mAPI, episodic high-dose ICS is effective. It has also been found that if azithromycin is given intermittently early during episodes of respiratory tract infections, the risk of severe episodes is decreased.[19]

In a recent study, addition of tiotropium by SoftMist inhaler to children aged 1–5 years with persistent asthmatic symptoms in spite of ICS treatment was found to have decreased flare-up when compared to placebo apart from being safe in this age group. Biologicals have not been approved for use in under-5 wheezers.[19]

Acute Episode: Management

The term acute exacerbation of asthma or flare-up has been used for acute asthma. These terms are very mild, and the new terminology suggested by Bush et al. is "acute lung attack". This is because of the fact that most often it leads to impaired airway growth apart from development of school-age atopic asthma.[20] Acute asthma is defined as a progressive increase in the symptoms of shortness of breath, cough, wheeze or chest tightness, and progressive decrease in lung function.[1] But the "2018 Lancet Commission on Asthma" had stressed the need for objective assessment like oxygen saturation and lung function, though unbiased biomarkers for acute asthma are still not elucidated.

The mainstay of treatment in acute lung attack is providing oxygen with tight-fitting face mask or nasal prongs to maintain $SpO_2 \geq 94\%$, inhaled SABA using pMDI and valved-holding chamber for mild-to-moderate severity and using oxygen to run the nebulizer, if severe. Ipratropium bromide is added, if response to inhaled SABA is not satisfactory. The early use of corticosteroids reduces the need for hospital admission, if administered in ER.

A fivefold increase in the dose of maintenance ICS has not reduced the need for systemic steroids or hospital admission when given at the first sign of uncontrolled symptoms. Two doses of dexamethasone at the dose of 0.6 mg/kg/day have shown no difference in the outcome of symptoms and quality of life at day 7 when compared to 5 day course of prednisolone. Also, systematic review on the use of dexamethasone orally or intramuscularly in acute asthma has shown that, apart from no difference in revisits to emergency department when compared to prednisolone, two doses of oral dexamethasone (second dose 24–48 after first) have been found to have reduced emesis compared to prednisolone. Single-dose dexamethasone, though has equivalent improvement, does show a need for additional corticosteroids.[21]

Intravenous (IV) magnesium sulfate has been found to be of use in older children (6 years and above), if they remain symptomatic after 1 hour of intensive conventional therapy with inhaled SABA and oxygen. But in under-5 wheezers, IV magnesium sulfate has not been found to be an effective additional agent to treat the acute exacerbation. The plausible reason is a different type of pathophysiology (inflammation) in the airway.[22] Systematic review on the use of nebulized magnesium sulfate in acute asthma has not been shown to be beneficial in children with acute asthma.[23]

In school-age children, acute lung attacks occur in the backdrop of respiratory allergy, but most often are precipitated by bacterial infection. The altered immune response as evidenced by airway eosinophilia and elevated IL-5 implies that the acute lung attack will be responsive to oral corticosteroids. But the same cannot be said in under-5 wheezers, as little information is available on the type of inflammatory response in acute lung attacks. The indirect evidence for the same is obtained by the variable response to corticosteroids and IV magnesium sulfate as well in these children suggesting that the inflammatory response might not be predominantly eosinophilic in the airways. Another evidence to substantiate this comes from the study of azithromycin in acute lung attacks, which reveals that children who receive azithromycin from the time of onset of symptoms have reduced duration of symptoms compared to placebo. The reason may be that azithromycin apart from its other properties has antineutrophilic property too. In view of this finding, inappropriate use of azithromycin would definitely lead to antimicrobial resistance while the use of oral corticosteroid in acute lung attack may not also be always right as the type of underlying inflammation, eosinophilic or neutrophilic, is still not clearly known.[20]

Device

Breath-enhanced nebulizers using one-way valves system have been shown to improve deposition of inhaled medications in adults, especially in acute care settings. But in children, conventional jet nebulizer-delivered SABA is better than breath-enhanced nebulizers as evidenced by improvements in FEV1.[24]

■ WHERE ARE WE NOW?

Research in asthma in India is lagging when compared to the developed countries. The availability of the basic lung function testing has been limited to major cities. Also, IOS has been limited to very few centers in India. Most of the government district hospitals and almost all the community healthcare centers lack lung function testing facilities. Testing for biomarkers is also difficult. The inhaled controller medication in government facilities for needy children is often unavailable. Also, most, if not all, government hospitals do not provide holding chamber and face mask for the delivery of inhaled medication. There is a big felt need by the pediatric medical community for the government to act and rectify the roadblocks, so that any child in our country whether he/she is in metropolitan cities or living in villages has free access to inhaled medications and valved-holding chambers.

■ WHAT IS THE WAY FORWARD?

Asthma needs to be defined better. It is an umbrella term comprising many conditions, which has similar presentation, especially in children under 5 years of age. The biomarkers, which can play a vital role in diagnosis and guide therapy, must be fast-tracked from research laboratory to practice, which can help the clinician to improve the quality of care given to every asthmatic child. The mindset of pediatrician handling a child with asthma should change from just relieving the symptoms by SABA to providing as needed controller therapy with inhaled corticosteroids therapy.

■ CONCLUSION

Asthma has to be diagnosed objectively. The commonly used lung function test—spirometry—can be done for children above 5 years of age. The need for simple tests, which can be done by younger children, is still elusive but research in biomarkers as an alternative should be able to bridge this gap. More insight on the type of airway inflammation in under-5 wheezers can help in choosing the appropriate treatment plan as not all of them have eosinophilic inflammation. Inhaled corticosteroids are the mainstay in the treatment but only a correct technique will help in the proper delivery of the medication into the airway. New GINA, 2019 guidelines have suggested the use of ICS in combination with SABA from step 1 in view of the presence of airway inflammation even with the first episode, which was suggested by Lancet Commission on asthma in 2018. Combination maintenance and reliever therapy is a major step forward, though approval for LABA in younger children is still awaited. Before adding on drugs for either partly controlled or uncontrolled symptoms, one must ensure that the delivery of inhaled medication is correct along with elimination of triggers wherever possible. Available results from the use of biologicals in that small subset of children of 6 years and above with severe asthma have shown promising results. The future of treatment in asthma should start from what type of asthma is present in this child based on the type of airway inflammation so that the treating pediatrician will know if ICS would work or one should resort to use of other medications including early use of biologicals to modify not only the course of asthma but also improve the quality of life and lung health as well.

■ REFERENCES

1. GINA Committees. (2019). Global strategy for asthma management and prevention. [online] Available from https://ginasthma.org/wp-content/uploads/2019/06/GINA-2019-main-report-June-2019-wms.pdf. [Last accessed December, 2019].
2. Mulholland A, Ainsworth A, Pillarisetti N. Tools in asthma evaluation and management: when and how to use them? Indian J Pediatr. 2018;85(8):651-7.
3. Brashier B, Salvi S. Measuring lung function using sound waves: role of the forced oscillation technique and impulse oscillometry system. Breathe (Sheff). 2015;11(1):57-65.
4. Pijnenburg MW. The role of FeNO in predicting asthma. Front Pediatr. 2019;7:41.
5. Kaplan A, Hardjojo A, Yu S, et al. Asthma across age: Insights from primary care. Front Pediatr. 2019;7:162.
6. Sonntag HJ, Filippi S, Pipis S, et al. Blood biomarkers of sensitization and asthma. Front Pediatr. 2019;7:251.
7. Ferraro V, Carraro S, Bozzetto S, et al. Exhaled biomarkers in childhood asthma: old and new approaches. Asthma Res Prac. 2018;4(1):1-7.
8. Hossny E, Rosario N, Lee BW, et al. The use of inhaled corticosteroids in pediatric asthma: update. World Allergy Organ J. 2016;9(1):26.
9. Ye Q, He XO, D'Urzo A. A review on the safety and efficacy of inhaled corticosteroids in the management of asthma. Pulm Ther. 2017;3(1):1-8.
10. Benard B, Bastien V, Vinet B, et al. Neuropsychiatric adverse drug reactions in children initiated on montelukast in real-life practice. Eur Respir J. 2017;50(2): pii: 1700148.
11. Pavord ID, Beasley R, Agusti A, et al. After asthma: redefining airways diseases. Lancet. 2018;391(10118):350-400.
12. Chung LP, Paton JY. Two Sides of the Same Coin?—Treatment of chronic asthma in children and adults. Front Pediatr. 2019;7:62.
13. Chong J, Haran C, Chauhan BF, et al. Intermittent inhaled corticosteroid therapy versus placebo for persistent asthma in children and adults. Cochrane Database Syst Rev. 2015;(7):CD011032.

14. Camargos P, Affonso A, Calazans G, et al. On-demand intermittent beclomethasone is effective for mild asthma in Brazil. Clin Transl Allergy. 2018;8:7.
15. Kaiser SV, Huynh T, Bacharier LB, et al. Preventing exacerbations in preschoolers with recurrent wheeze: a meta-analysis. Pediatrics. 2016;137(6). pii: e20154496.
16. Sobieraj DM, Baker WL, Weeda ER, et al. Intermittent Inhaled Corticosteroids and Long-Acting Muscarinic Antagonists for Asthma. Rockville (MD): Agency for Healthcare Research and Quality (US); 2018. [online] Available from https://www.ncbi.nlm.nih.gov/books/NBK499563. [Last accessed December, 2019].
17. Bush A. Management of asthma in children. Minerva Pediatr. 2018;70(5):444-57.
18. Chang TS, Lemanske Jr RF, Guilbert TW, et al. Evaluation of the modified asthma predictive index in high-risk preschool children. J Allergy Clin Immunol. 2013;1(2):152-6.
19. Kwong CG, Bacharier LB. Management of asthma in the preschool child. Immunol Allergy Clin North Am. 2019;39(2):177-90.
20. Saglani S, Fleming L, Sonnappa S, et al. Advances in the aetiology, management, and prevention of acute asthma attacks in children. Lancet Child Adolesc Health. 2019;3(5):354-64.
21. Abaya R, Jones L, Zorc JJ. Dexamethasone compared to prednisone for the treatment of children with acute asthma exacerbations. Pediatr Emerg Care. 2018;34(1):53-8.
22. Pruikkonen H, Tapiainen T, Kallio M, et al. Intravenous magnesium sulfate for acute wheezing in young children: a randomised double-blind trial. Eur Respir J. 2018;51:1701579.
23. Su Z, Li R, Gai Z. Intravenous and nebulized magnesium sulfate for treating acute asthma in children: A systematic review and meta-analysis. Pediatr Emerg Care. 2018;34(6):390-5.
24. Gardiner MA, Wilkinson MH. Randomized clinical trial comparing breath-enhanced to conventional nebulizers in the treatment of children with acute asthma. J Pediatr. 2019;204:245-9.e2.

CHAPTER 8

ALLERGY AND IMMUNOLOGY

8.1 Recent Advances in Diagnostic Modalities of Pediatric-allergic Diseases
Remesh Kumar R, Krishna Mohan R

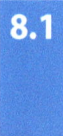

8.1 RECENT ADVANCES IN DIAGNOSTIC MODALITIES OF PEDIATRIC-ALLERGIC DISEASES

Remesh Kumar R, Krishna Mohan R

■ INTRODUCTION

The prevalence and incidence of allergic diseases is definitely on a rise, both in the developed and developing nations, especially in the pediatric age group. *Allergy* is defined as an abnormal clinical reaction towards substances which are harmless to most individuals. The typical allergic reaction is an IgE-mediated response resulting from activation of TH2 pathway (instead of TH1 pathway). Even though used interchangeably, the terms 'Atopy' and 'Allergy' are not the same. 'Atopy' is only an increased tendency to produce specific IgE to common environmental allergens.

■ DIAGNOSIS OF ALLERGIC DISORDERS

The term *allergen* refers to an antigen that can trigger an allergic reaction. Allergens can sensitize the immune system via respiratory tract (aeroallergens), gastrointestinal tract (food allergens) or skin (contact allergens). A thorough history including details of clinical features, trigger factors, family history, environment history, diet history and medication history along with a focused clinical examination are important in making a diagnosis of any allergic disease.

Various *in-vitro* and *in-vivo* tests are available to help diagnosis of allergic disease and identification of the allergen(s). However, it is very important to remember that, in fact, all *allergy tests* can detect *only sensitization* and cannot diagnose *allergy* as allergy is a clinical syndrome and the diagnosis is mainly clinical. Sensitization does not mean that patient has clinical allergy. All those in whom sensitization is demonstrated need not have allergic symptoms. But those with sensitization however, have an increased risk of developing clinical allergy in their life time.

Clinical Relevance of Identifying the Allergens

- Helps in the targeted avoidance of the relevant exposure which has better outcome than untargeted allergen avoidance measures.
- Helps in selecting the patients for allergen immunotherapy
- Identification of a seasonal pattern especially in case of pollens, which would help to start controller therapy before the anticipated onset of symptoms.

■ *IN-VITRO* SCREENING TESTS

The presence of IgE specific for a particular allergen can be documented *in-vitro* by the measurement of allergen-specific IgE (sIgE) levels in the serum. The presence of allergen specific IgE is correctly interpreted as evidence that the patient is sensitized to that allergen and may react upon exposure. The likelihood of clinical reactivity is influenced by the degree of positivity, the allergen in question, and the patient's clinical history. The first test for documenting the presence of sIgE was called the radio-allergosorbent test (RAST) because it used a radiolabeled anti-IgE antibody.

Nowadays, this has been replaced by an improved generation of automated enzymatic sIgE immunoassays. These assays use solid phase supports to which allergens of an individual allergen extract are bound. A small amount of the patient's serum is incubated with the allergen-coated support. The allergen-coated support bound to the patient's sIgE is then incubated with enzyme-labeled antibodies (Ab) against IgE. After incubation, unbound enzyme labeled anti-IgE is washed away. The bound complex is then incubated with a fluorescent substrate. After stopping the reaction, the fluorescence of the eluate is measured. The higher the fluorescence, the more specific IgE is present in the sample.

There are different *in-vitro* diagnostic systems available such as Immunocap, Immulite, Hytec, etc. Quantification of the specific IgE is expressed as kUa/L (Kilo units of antibody/liter). ImmunoCAP specific-IgE detects IgE antibodies in the range 0–100 kUA/L. In clinical practice, 0.35 kUA/L has commonly been used as a cut-off.

The sensitivity and specificity of immunoassays vary with the system being used and the quality of the allergen. Overall, sensitivity ranges from 60–95% and specificity from 30–95%.

Proper selection of antigens for testing should be based upon patient's detailed history. *In-vitro* allergy tests done as broad panels without considering the patient's history, local environment and allergen exposure will lead to false positive results. This is important, especially in food allergy. Food allergy panel testing often results in misdiagnosis of food allergy, which leads to unnecessary dietary restrictions and malnutrition.

Multi-Allergen IgE Antibody Screening Assays

Here the test is done using a mixture of most common allergens rather than individual allergens. These are screening tests which help to differentiate between atopic and non-atopic patients. Phadiatop is a commonly used multi-allergen IgE screening test.

IN-VIVO SCREENING TESTS

Allergy skin testing is an important *in-vivo* test for detecting the allergen specific IgE. It is done by introducing a very small quantity of allergen into the epidermis by pricking or puncturing. The introduced allergen will link up with the mast cell bound specific-IgE antibodies, if present. This leads to release of chemical mediators, causing a wheal and flare reaction.

Indications of Allergy Skin Testing

- Allergic rhinitis
- Allergic conjunctivitis
- Allergic asthma
- Suspected food allergy
- Insect bite venom allergy
- Suspected drug allergy
- Suspected latex allergy.

Contraindications of Allergy Skin Testing

- Recent anaphylaxis
- Severe eczema
- Severe uncontrolled asthma
- Dermographism, as it gives false positive results.

Procedure

Prick test (epicutaneous test) can be performed on the volar surface of forearm or upper back. Skin testing areas should be at least 5 cm from the wrist and 3 cm from the antecubital fossa. There should be at least 2–2.5 cm gap between each applied allergen to avoid false positive reaction between adjacent skin test sites.

The test should be performed only after cleaning the skin properly. A small lancet or 25/26-gauge needle is used to pierce through a drop of allergen extract placed over the prepared skin. Always make sure that only good quality allergen extracts are used. Skin is pierced at an angle of 45–60°. The needle should be lightly pressed into the epidermis and then lifted creating a break in the epidermis without causing bleeding. After 15–20 minutes, the pricked site should be looked for wheal and flare. A 3-mm or more wheal diameter is taken as positive. Glycerinated buffered saline and histamine are used as negative and positive control respectively.

Prick-to-Prick Test

This is used in diagnosis of food allergy. The commercially obtained food extracts are less reliable as the heat labile proteins are destroyed during preparation. The lancet/needle is inserted into the suspected fresh food, and then the patient's skin is pricked immediately.

Intradermal Skin Tests

Intradermal tests are more sensitive than the prick tests. But they are only done, if the epicutaneous test is negative, and there is high clinical suspicion based on history. The allergen extracts used for intradermal testing are 100- to 1000-fold less concentrated than extracts used in epicutaneous tests. A small amount of allergen extract (0.01–0.02 mL) is injected into the dermis of the arm using 25–27-gauge needles. Intradermal tests are never done with food allergens because of the risk of anaphylaxis.

Medications to be Avoided before Allergy Skin Testing

Antihistamines, both H1 and H2 blockers should be discontinued for 3 days, Fexofenadine for 5–7 days, Loratidine and Cetrizine for 7 days. Tricyclic anti-depressants should be discontinued for 7 days as they have anti-histaminic effects. Beta-blockers increase the risk of allergic reactions, and hence they should be discontinued for 1–2 days.

Advantages of *In-vitro* Tests Compared to Skin Tests

- It poses no risk to the patient of an allergic reaction. The risk of an allergic reaction in response to skin testing in patients with very severe allergic reactions even to minute number of allergens, although small, may not be acceptable.
- It is not affected by medications the patient may be taking.
- It is not dependent upon skin integrity or affected by skin disease.
- The skin of infants less than 12 months old may not yet fully reflect their allergic sensitivities. In contrast, immunoassays are valid for infants as young as six weeks of age and can be performed on capillary blood samples.
- *In-vitro* testing may be better for patients with certain skin conditions, such as severe and widespread atopic dermatitis or dermographism.
- More convenient for the patient.

■ COMPONENT-RESOLVED DIAGNOSTICS

Component-resolved diagnostics (CRDs) is a testing method that helps in more specific identification of the allergen to which a patient's specific-IgE reacts. This involves microarray testing using recombinant allergens and antigenic components of major allergens and nano-biologic techniques to assess the precise antigenic epitopes to which a patient's IgE binds. CRDs can be effectively used to diagnose food and inhalant sensitization and as a means of predicting cross-reactivity between food and pollen allergens. ImmunoCAP ISAC, is a commercially available example of CRD which allows for detection of IgE against more than 100 individual components derived from more than 50 allergen sources.

ORAL FOOD CHALLENGE FOR FOOD ALLERGY

Double-blind, placebo-controlled food challenge (DBPCFC) is the gold standard of diagnosing an IgE-mediated food allergy. Open challenges or single-blind challenges, whereby a placebo dose is introduced into the succession of true allergen doses, may be considered if DBPCFC is not feasible. Food challenge involves ingesting multiple doses of a food spaced out over time to minimize the risk of severe reactions. Patients are then observed for clinical reactions, with medications to treat allergic reactions readily available in the clinic. The challenge is ideally done in the presence of a specialist well trained in treating allergic reactions.

TESTS FOR ANAPHYLAXIS

The clinical diagnosis of anaphylaxis can sometimes be supported by documentation of elevated concentrations of serum or plasma total tryptase or plasma histamine. Elevations of these mediators are transient; it is important to obtain blood samples for measurement soon after the onset of symptoms.

FRACTIONAL CONCENTRATION OF EXHALED NITRIC OXIDE (FeNO)

Nitric oxide (NO) is an endogenous messenger molecule, which is widespread in the human body including upper and lower airways. In bronchial epithelium, it is formed by activity of the enzyme inducible nitric oxide synthase (INOS). Under normal conditions, bronchial epithelial cells continuously produce low levels of nitric oxide synthase. This is upregulated by interleukin 4 (IL-4) and 13 (IL-13) and stimuli after allergen exposure in atopic individuals. NO regulates vascular and bronchial tone and facilitates coordinated beating of ciliated epithelial cells. Measuring NO in exhaled air is a new and revolutionary opportunity for differential diagnosis and monitoring of patients with airway disease.

Measurement of exhaled NO is a good indicator of airway inflammation. The levels are raised during asthma exacerbation and reduced to normal following treatment with steroids. So FeNO measurement helps in detection of eosinophilic inflammation and also in determining corticosteroid response (**Table 8.1.1**).

Table 8.1.1: Interpretations of FeNO test.

Inference	Children	Adults
Eosinophilic inflammation unlikely	<20 ppb	<25 ppb
Unclear, to be interpreted with clinical history	20–35 ppb	25–50 ppb
Eosinophilic inflammation likely, usually steroid responsive	>35 ppb	>50 ppb

(ppb: parts per billion)

■ TESTS USED FOR RESEARCH PURPOSES

Basophil Tests

Basophils as well as mast cells express the high affinity receptor for IgE on the cell surface and are activated when this IgE encounters enough specific allergen. Mast cells are seen in tissues, while basophils circulate in the blood, making them more accessible to collection and study. Several techniques have been developed to examine basophil responses to allergens.

Basophil Histamine Release Test

Basophil histamine release test measures the release of histamine from human peripheral blood basophils incubated with allergen.

Other tests of basophil function following incubation with allergen include, release of leukotriene C4 and measurement of the level of activation via expression of surface proteins by flow cytometry.

Eosinophil cationic protein levels: Eosinophil cationic protein (ECP) is an eosinophil-specific mediator that can be measured in bodily fluids to estimate the extent of eosinophil activation.

■ CONCLUSION

The diagnosis and management of pediatric allergy is revolutionized with the advent of variety of allergy tests, both for allergen identification as well as supportive investigations. It is a clinical dilemma for a practitioner to make a judicious selection between these tests. No single test is complete in itself. The diagnosis is largely dependent upon a detailed history, and physical examination assisted with the appropriate investigations. This is extremely important while choosing *in-vitro* allergen panels and various other allergy tests available. Customizing appropriate test to the individual patient is very important.

BIBLIOGRAPHY

1. Ballardini N, Nilsson C, Nilsson M, Lilja G. ImmunoCAP Phadiatop Infant: a new blood test for detecting IgE sensitisation in children at 2 years of age. Allergy. 2006;61:337-43.
2. Bousquet J, Heinzerling L, Bachert C, Papadopoulos NG, Bousquet PJ, Burney PG, et al. Global Allergy and Asthma European Network; Allergic rhinitis and its impact on asthma. Practical guide to skin prick tests in allergy to aeroallergens. Allergy. 2012;67:18-24.
3. Chinthrajah RS, Tupa D, Prince BT, Block WM, Rosa JS, Singh AM, et al. Diagnosis of food allergy. Pediatr Clin North Am. 2015;62(6):1393-408.
4. Christopher DJ, Ashok N, Ravivarma A, Shankar D, Peterson E, Dinh PT, Vedanthan PK. Low potency of Indian dust mite allergen skin prick test extracts compared to FDA approved extracts: A double-blind randomized control trial. Allergy Rhinol (Providence). 2018;9:2152656718796746. doi: 10.1177/2152656718796746. eCollection 2018 Jan-Dec.
5. Gupta N. Allergy in a Nutshell. A handbook, 1st edn. New Delhi; Jaypee Brothers Medical Publishers, 2019.
6. Hamilton RG, Franklin Adkinson Jr. N. In-vitro assays for the diagnosis of IgE-mediated disorders. J Allerg Clin Immunol. 2004;114:213-25.
7. Shreffler WG. Microarrayed recombinant allergens for diagnostic testing. J Allergy Clin Immunol. 2011;127:843-9.
8. Vedanthan PK, Mahesh PA, Christopher DJ. Allergy screening tests: Role in the assessment of childhood allergy. Indian J Pract Pediatr. 2013;15(3):206-11.
9. Williams PB, Barnes JH, Szeinbach SL, Sullivan TJ. Analytic precision and accuracy of commercial immunoassays for specific IgE: establishing a standard. J Allergy Clin Immunol. 2000;105:1221-30.

CHAPTER 9

GASTROENTEROLOGY

9.1 Inflammatory Bowel Disease
Surender Kumar Yachha, Moinak Sen Sarma

9.1 INFLAMMATORY BOWEL DISEASE

Surender Kumar Yachha, Moinak Sen Sarma

■ INTRODUCTION

Inflammatory bowel disease (IBD) is a chronic inflammatory condition of the gastrointestinal (GI) tract and classified into two main subtypes—Crohn's disease (CD) and ulcerative colitis (UC). Approximately, 10–20% cases remain as unclassified IBD at presentation and later evolve into either of the two subtypes. Worldwide, the incidence of IBD in children is increasing, more so in CD. Large population-based studies have shown an incidence of 1.2–11.8 cases per 100,000 predominantly in the West. Tertiary referral centers in India report growing incidence with average age of presentation as 10–11 years.[1] Younger age groups of IBD is now increasingly common and reported in neonates as well.

Being an immune-mediated disease, there is a complex interaction of innate and adaptive immunity, gut bacteria, genetic predisposition, and environmental factors. Genome-wide association studies have revealed >200 genetic loci responsible for the pathogenesis of IBD. These genes that code for proteins modify the body's immunity. IBD2 locus on chromosome 12 is identified in UC. *NOD2/CARD15* gene on chromosome 16 increases the risk of CD and is associated with ileal disease, younger age onset, and penetrating phenotypes. Genetics is a very important risk factor for IBD and up to 19–41% children in the West may have an affected family member with IBD. Concordance in monozygotic twins is as high as 50%. Having a first-degree relative with IBD increases the risk about 30-fold.[2]

■ DISEASE DISTRIBUTION

Crohn's disease involves all layers (mucosa, submucosa, muscular layers, and serosa) of gastrointestinal tract (GIT). Hence, it is a "transmural" inflammation. It can involve any part or all parts of GIT (pan-enteric). In UC, the inflammation is limited to the colonic mucosa only. Primary differentiation of CD and UC based on the extent is summarized in **Table 9.1.1**.

■ CLINICAL FEATURES

Children with CD present with abdominal pain, diarrhea (with or without blood), and constitutional symptoms (fever and anorexia). In contrast, children with UC present with bloody diarrhea. Growth failure and weight loss are attributable to CD in West. However, in developing countries, the growth parameters are affected in all types of IBD, as referral is late. **Table 9.1.2** summarizes the clinical, histologic, and endoscopic differences

Table 9.1.1: Disease distribution in inflammatory disease.

Ulcerative colitis		Crohn's disease	
Site of involvement	*% of cases*	*Site of involvement*	*% of cases*
Pancolitis	50–90	Ileocolonic disease	50–70
Left side colitis (up to splenic flexure)	10–40	Small bowel	10–15
Distal colitis (proctitis/ proctosigmoiditis)	5–20	Associated: • Upper gastrointestinal • Perianal disease	 30–40 20–25

Table 9.1.2: Differentiation between Crohn's disease and ulcerative colitis.

Parameters	*Crohn's disease*	*Ulcerative colitis*
Distribution	• Entire gastrointestinal (GI) tract • Transmural inflammation • Discontinuous lesions	• Colon only • Mucosal disease • Continuous involvement
Bloody diarrhea	Less common	Common
Abdominal pain	Common	Less common
Growth failure	Common	Less common
Perianal disease	Present (abscess, tags, fistulae: **Figure 9.1.1A**)	Absent
Histopathology	• Noncaseating ill defined (<300 microns) granuloma (throughout GI tract) • No goblet cell dysplasia • Focal discontinuous crypt architectural distortion • Focal discontinuous chronic inflammation • Focally enhancing gastritis (biopsy of stomach) • Pyloric gland metaplasia (terminal ileum)	• No granuloma • Widespread crypt architectural distortion • Diffuse inflammatory infiltrate • Basal plasmacytosis • Goblet cell depletion • Crypt abscess • Paneth cell metaplasia
Endoscopy **(Figs. 9.1.1B to E)**	• Deep irregular serpiginous or aphthous ulcers • Normal intervening mucosa (skip lesion) • Ileal involvement, rectal sparing (60%) • Internal fistulae	• Diffuse superficial ulceration • Granularity, loss of vascular pattern, and friability • Rectal involvement and ileal sparing (unless backwash ileitis)

between UC and CD. Extraintestinal manifestations **(Table 9.1.3)** are seen in 25-30% children with IBD. They can precede, follow, or occur concurrently

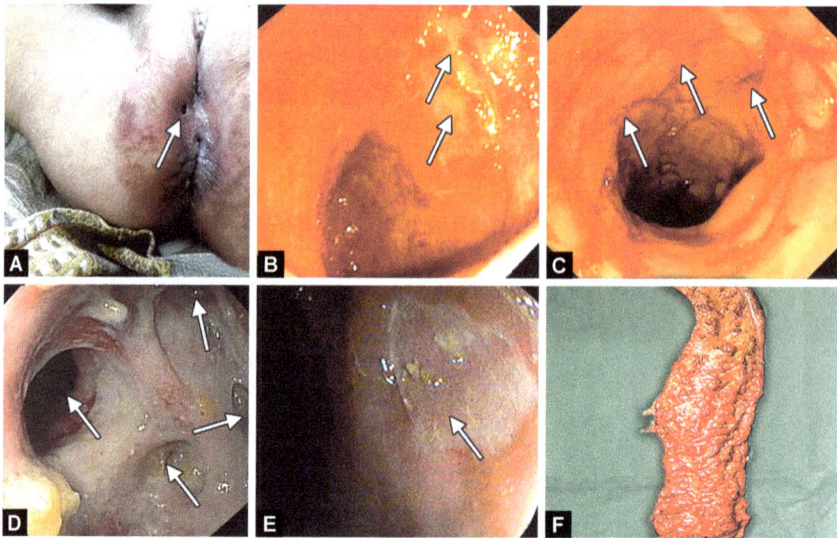

Figs. 9.1.1A to F: (A) Perianal fistula in infantile Crohn's disease (CD); (B) Superficial ulcers in ulcerative colitis (UC); (C) Linear serpiginous ulcers in CD; (D) Multiple internal fistulae of colon to small bowel; (E) Ileal ulcer in CD; (F): Colectomy specimen in acute severe ulcerative colitis showing large areas of ulcerated colonic mucosa with areas of pseudopolyps.

Table 9.1.3: Extraintestinal manifestations in inflammatory bowel disease.

System	Extraintestinal manifestation
Joints	• Nondeforming arthritis (large joints > small joints) and arthralgia • Enthesitis • Sacroiliitis • Ankylosing spondylitis *(HLA-B27 positive)*
Skin/oral cavity	• Oral ulcers • Pyoderma gangrenosum • Erythema nodosum • Alopecia areata • "Metastatic" Crohn's disease (ulcers and granulomatosis of penis, vulva, and labia)
Eye	• Uveitis • Episcleritis
Liver/biliary tract	• Primary or autoimmune sclerosing cholangitis • Autoimmune hepatitis • Pancreatitis • Cholelithiasis • Fatty liver • Asymptomatic hypertransaminasemia • IgG4 cholangiopathy
Bones	Osteopenia and osteoporosis
Coagulation	Venous thrombosis (portal vein, hepatic vein, and mesenteric veins)
Kidneys	Renal stones (oxalate)

(IgG4: immunoglobulin G4)

with the intestinal disease and may be related/unrelated to activity of the intestinal disease. Of all the extraintestinal manifestations, arthralgia/arthritis is most common manifestation seen in 15–17% cases.[1-4]

■ DIAGNOSIS

The initial evaluation of a child with suspected IBD includes a detailed clinical, family, and treatment history in the past. A complete examination is mandatory with growth charting and perianal examination for fistulae, tags and fissures. Laboratory tests may reveal anemia and thrombocytosis (67%), low serum albumin, high erythrocyte sedimentation rate (ESR), and raised C-reactive protein (CRP) in 40–60% of cases. ESR and CRP are reliable indicators of ongoing inflammation or active disease in IBD.

Fecal inflammatory markers such as fecal calprotectin are popular in the West for screening of IBD. However, it has many fallacies, especially in developing countries. Fecal calprotectin may not sufficiently rise in early stage of disease. It has poor specificity and may be otherwise raised in intercurrent gastrointestinal infections (bacterial, parasitic, *Helicobacter pylori* infection, and small bowel bacterial overgrowth).

Markers like antineutrophil cytoplasmic antibody (ANCA) positivity are seen in two-thirds of UC and <20% of CD patients. Anti-*Saccharomyces cerevisiae* (ASCA) antibody positivity is found in more than half of CD patients and is uncommon in UC patients. Because there is overlap between CD and UC, none of these tests can discriminate absolutely between the two conditions. The use of antibodies is complementary and ancillary in the diagnosis of IBD. They may have a role in prognostication of the disease and help in IBD-U to gauge the anticipated progression. ASCA-positive CD patients are likely to have ileal involvement and greater need for surgery in future. ANCA-positive CD patients have left colonic disease, sparing of terminal ileum, and lesser need for surgery.

Table 9.1.4 summarizes the diagnostic modalities available for IBD. Upper gastrointestinal (UGI) endoscopy, colonoscopy, and small bowel imaging are mandatory for mapping of disease and confirmation of diagnosis in all cases.[5] Biopsies from endoscopically involved and uninvolved sites at the onset are essential.

■ TREATMENT

General Management

Classification of severity of disease is done by pediatric ulcerative colitis activity index (PUCAI) and pediatric Crohn's disease activity index (PCDAI). While PUCAI takes consideration of grading of clinical parameters (abdominal pain, rectal bleeding, stool number, consistency, nocturnal awakening, and

Table 9.1.4: Diagnostic modalities used in inflammatory bowel disease.

Diagnostic modality	Importance
• Colonoscopy with ileal intubation • Multiple biopsies from diseased and non-diseased sites (pancolonic) • UGI endoscopy with biopsies	• Most important to differentiate UC vs CD • To look for granulomas
• Small-bowel imaging • Barium enteroclysis, CT or MR enteroclysis	• For small bowel strictures fistula (Crohn's disease) • Extramural complications may be seen in CT/MRI
MRI pelvis	Fistula, pelvic, and genitourinary abscess (Crohn's disease)
Capsule endoscopy	Ideal to evaluate small-bowel involvement after excluding intestinal stricture that may result in retention of capsule. Disadvantage: biopsies cannot be taken
Enteroscopy	Limitation of not being able to pass bigger diameter enteroscopes in younger children

(UGI: upper gastrointestinal; CT: computed tomography; MRI: magnetic resonance imaging; UC: ulcerative colitis; CD: Crohn's disease)

daily activity), PCDAI is a much more elaborate grading that incorporates clinical as well as laboratory parameters (hematocrit, ESR, and albumin), examination (height, weight, abdominal tenderness, perirectal disease, and extraintestinal manifestations). Both the indices are important for assessing response to therapy.[6,7]

The goal of treatment is to control inflammation, mucosal healing, improve growth, and ensure a good quality of life by using therapeutic regimens that are least toxic. Ensuring proper nutrition with caloric supplementation [~120% of RDA (recommended dietary allowance)] is necessity for children with IBD. Calcium and vitamin D supplementation should be given, as these children are at an increased risk of osteoporosis. As IBD is a chronic disease with remissions and exacerbations, proper counseling of both the patient and family at diagnosis is essential.

Drugs

The main drugs used for IBD are listed in the **Tables 9.1.5 and 9.1.6**. There are two phases of therapy: induction and maintenance.

Steroids have a central role, as these are the most commonly used induction agent in moderate-to-severe UC and in all severities of CD and IBD-U.

Table 9.1.5: Drugs used in inflammatory bowel disease (IBD) (first-line therapy).

Drug	Dosage and route	Indication	Main side effects
Sulfasalazine or 5-aminosalicylic acid or mesalamine (active moiety of sulfasalazine)	• 40–60 mg/kg/d oral • 50–100 mg/kg/d oral • Enema	• Anti-inflammatory (local action) in mild UC and maintenance • Enema in mild left-sided colonic disease	• Folate deficiency • Pancreatitis • Steven–Johnson syndrome • Hepatotoxicity • Oligospermia (with sulfa-salazine)
Prednisolone	1–2 mg/kg oral	• Induction therapy (first-line) in all types of IBD	• Cushingoid facies • Hypertension • Glaucoma • Cataract • Bone fractures • Hyperglycemia • Growth impairment
Thiopurines: Azathioprine (AZA) 6-Mercaptopurine (active moiety of AZA)	2–3 mg/kg/d oral 1–2 mg/kg/d oral	• Frequent relapses* • Steroid dependence# • Steroid resistance% • Maintenance in moderate to severe disease	• Myelosuppression • Hepatotoxicity • Pancreatitis

Frequent relapses: 2–3 relapses per year.
#*Steroid dependency:* Initial remission but recurrence while tapering or inability to stop steroids in 14–16 weeks of initiation.
%*Steroid resistance:* Nonresponse to optimal doses of oral steroids within 7–14 days of initiation and good compliance.
(UC: ulcerative colitis)

Prednisolone is started as 2 mg/kg (maximum 40 mg/day and 60 mg/day in case of unsatisfactory response in older children) for 2-4 weeks followed by gradual tapering over 6-8 weeks by which time clinical remission is observed in the majority cases. Toxicity of steroids must be monitored from time to time (every 2-3 weeks) with mandatory examination of blood pressure, intraocular pressure, and cataract formation. Steroid enema may have an adjunct role, if there is suboptimal response to mesalamine enema in mild UC.

In cases of UC with steroid dependence, relapse, or steroid refractory course and invariably in all cases of CD, *azathioprine* (1-2 mg/kg) is added on for maintenance. Azathioprine is a steroid-sparing agent, which takes approximately 2-3 months for optimal action. On azathioprine, regular monitoring of blood counts for bone marrow suppression and liver

Table 9.1.6: Drugs used in inflammatory bowel disease (IBD) (second-line therapy).

Drug	Dosage and route	Indication	Main side effects
Methotrexate	15 mg/m² IM weekly	• Steroid sparing • Refractory disease and/or intolerant to thiopurines	• Hepatotoxicity • Myelosuppression • Folate deficiency
Cyclosporine	2–4 mg/kg/d IV infusion followed by 5–8 mg/kg/d oral	Rescue therapy for maximum 4 weeks in severe refractory UC	• Nephrotoxicity • Hypertrichosis • Gum hyperplasia • Hypertension
Tacrolimus	0.1 mg/kg oral		• Paresthesia
Biological agents (infliximab, adalimumab)	• Infliximab 5 mg/kg IV at 0, 2, 6 weeks and thereafter 8 weekly • Adalimumab 2.4 mg/kg first dose followed by 1.2 mg/kg second dose followed by 0.6 mg/kg every 2 weekly	• Fistuling CD • Perianal disease • Severe disease not responding to immunomodulators	• Infusion reaction • Autoimmunity • Demyelination • Psychiatric problems • Flare infections • Hepatosplenic T-cell lymphoma
Thalidomide	1.5–2.5 mg/kg oral	Refractory CD and intolerant to biological agents (very selective group)	• Irreversible peripheral neuropathy • Agitation • Hallucination

(UC: ulcerative colitis; CD: Crohn's disease, IM: intramuscular, IV: intravenous)

transaminases for hepatotoxicity is required. Second-line agents are used in select situations.

Patients who are steroid resistant and thiopurine intolerant are invariably considered for biologicals. *Infliximab* (human source) and *adalimumab* have been used with response rates of 50–60% to achieve remission. Biologicals are used, if there is a fistulizing disease or severe perianal disease at the onset. Adalimumab has a better safety profile (lesser infusion reactions) as compared to infliximab and can be used if antibodies to infliximab have developed leading to infliximab nonresponse. Biologicals may be combined with immunomodulators in severe disease. In developing countries, biologicals can only be started once tuberculosis is ruled out. Biologicals are anti-TNF (tumor necrosis factor) alpha agents that may reactivate a dormant tubercular focus and allow the mycobacteria to disseminate. Biologicals are also contraindicated in the presence of active suppurative infections. *Vedolizumab* is a gut-specific biological that is presently not marketed widely in India. It is reserved in cases which are refractory to infliximab and adalimumab. High cost of biologicals and unaffordability in developing countries are a major limiting factor.

Biosimilar is a new term that denotes drugs pharmacologically near-similar to human source biologicals. These drugs are thought to be equally efficacious and are promoted to reduce cost of therapy.

Additionally, for perianal fistulizing CD, *antibiotics* (ciprofloxacin 20 mg/kg, metronidazole 10–20 mg/kg, or rifaximin 10–30 mg/kg) for 4–6 weeks have shown good short-term response. In mild-to-moderate nonfistulizing, nonstricturing CD, exclusive *enteral nutrition* with polymeric, semielemental, or elemental formulations may be used for 6–8 weeks for induction of remission, followed by a maintenance first-line immunomodulator. *Oral 5-aminosalicylic acid (5-ASA)* has a role in induction of remission in mild UC and maintenance phase of mild-to-moderate UC. Topical 5-ASA may be used in localized left-sided UC. 5-ASA has limited role in CD. The algorithm for management of UC and CD are shown in **Flowcharts 9.1.1 and 9.1.2**.[6,7]

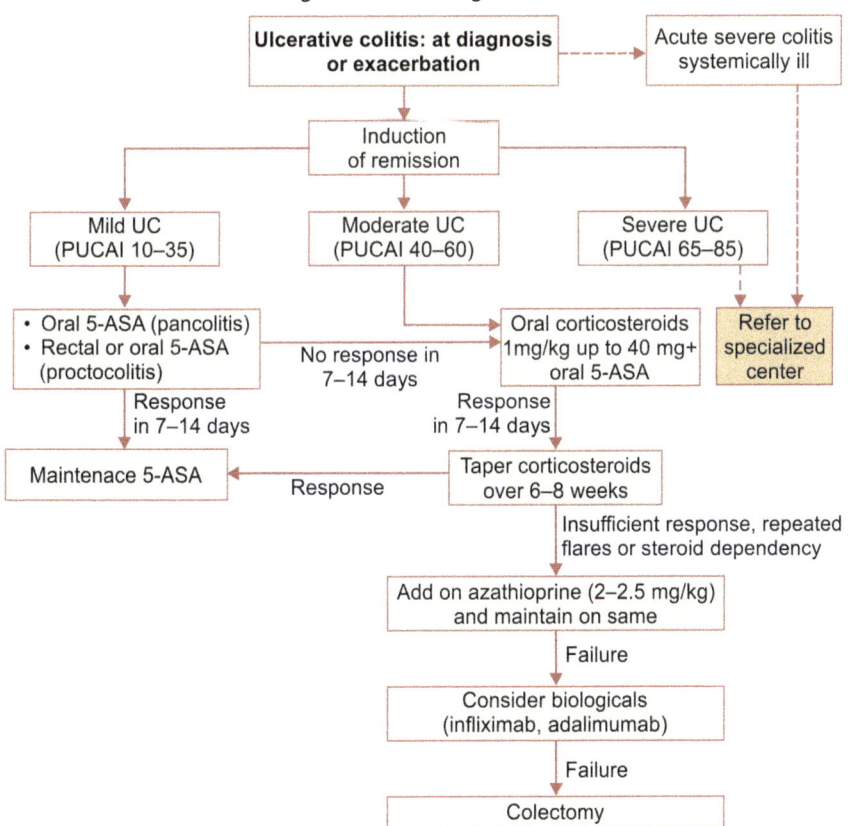

Flowchart 9.1.1: Algorithm for management of ulcerative colitis.

(UC: ulcerative colitis; PUCAI: pediatric ulcerative colitis activity index; 5-ASA: 5-aminosalicylic acid)

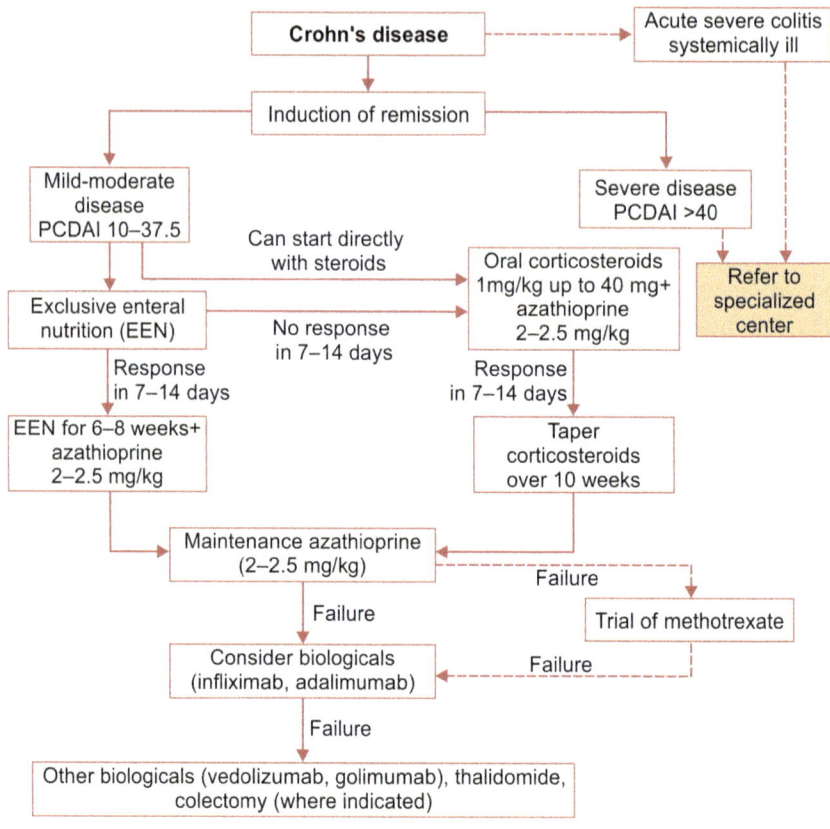

Flowchart 9.1.2: Algorithm for management of Crohn's disease.

(PCDAI: pediatric Crohn's disease activity index)

Surgery

In IBD, cumulative risk of surgery increases with duration of disease (CD: 18%, 27%, and 32% at 1, 5, and 10 years, respectively; and UC: 8% and 20% at 1 and 5 years, respectively). Surgery is indicated in UC patients with severe acute colitis refractory to medical disease **(Fig. 9.1.1F)**. Uncontrolled hemorrhage, perforation, toxic megacolon, abscesses, and obstruction are the other indications for surgery. Proctocolectomy is curative in UC. However, creating an ileal pouch for fecal continence is performed with caution in an adolescent girl due to reduced chances of fecundity later in adulthood. Since surgery is not curative in CD, its role is limited. Surgery is considered only in patients who have biological-refractory disease, fibrotic strictures causing symptoms, nonhealing fistulae, and colon diversion procedures (to induce remission). Risk of adenocarcinoma colon is 8% after 20 years of disease in pediatric UC and should be suspected with new onset of symptoms after years of remission or features of large bowel obstruction and occult GI blood loss.[3,4,6,7]

SPECIAL SITUATIONS

Acute Severe Colitis

Approximately, 18-25% of UC may experience acute severe symptoms (PUCAI >65) at any point of time during their disease course. This may happen at onset or on follow-up with relapse. In relapse settings, the patient is usually refractory to oral steroids. In acute severe colitis, it is mandatory to rule out and appropriately treat associated infections such as *Clostridium difficile* (stool toxin assay and passage membranes per rectum), *Cytomegalovirus* (deep colonic ulcers, immunohistochemistry, and inclusion bodies in colonic biopsies), concurrent fungal infections (stool for fungal hyphae), and infective colitis (stool culture for *Shigella*, enterohemorrhagic *Escherichia coli*, etc.). Toxic megacolon should be routinely looked for in a patient with severe colitis. Considering the case as a steroid refractory state, intravenous methylprednisolone 1-1.5 mg/kg/day should be started. If there is failure of response to methylprednisolone then second-line rescue therapy with IV cyclosporine/oral tacrolimus or infliximab must be considered. Both cyclosporine and infliximab are equally efficacious with similar response (75-80%) for remission. Cyclosporine is given for 3-4 months but therapy with infliximab is indefinite. Infliximab has lower future colectomy rates than cyclosporine. Failure of second-line therapy is an indication for colectomy. Colectomy is also indicated, if, during the course, the patient develops perforation, hemorrhage, or nonresponsive toxic megacolon.[8]

Toxic Megacolon

Toxic megacolon is a complication seen in the setting of acute severe UC. It is to be diagnosed, if transverse colon diameter in an erect X-ray abdomen is >40 mm (<10 years of age) and >56 mm (>10 years of age) with evidence of systemic toxicity (fever, tachycardia, dehydration, dyselectrolytemia, altered sensorium, and hypotension or shock). Intravenous antibiotics, correction of electrolyte imbalance, and supportive therapy are required in such cases. Failure of medical management is an indication for emergency colectomy.[8]

Early-onset Inflammatory Bowel Disease

Recently, pediatric IBD has been reclassified into various age groups in relation to onset of disease: neonatal (<28 days), infantile (<2 years), very early (2-6 years), early (6-10 years), and pediatric (10-17 years). Older children with IBD have polygenic inheritance like adults. IBD starting <2 years of age comprises <5% of all pediatric IBD and requires detailed immunological workup for immunodeficiencies of monogenic inheritance. Some of the notable genetic defects associated with the infantile onset IBD are IL (interleukin)-10, IL-10 receptor A, IL-10 receptor B, ADAM-17, XIAP, TTC7A (apoptotic enterocolitis), IPEX syndrome, atypical severe combined immunodeficiency (Omenn syndrome), Wiskott–Aldrich syndrome, agammaglobulinemia, hyperimmunoglobulin M (hyper-IgM) syndrome, common variable immunodeficiency (CVID), and chronic granulomatous disease. These diseases are primary immunodeficiencies, which manifest as recurrent infections and IBD. They may have significant family history, associated autoimmunity, and atypical features on endoscopy and histology. The very early-onset, infantile, and neonatal IBDs have marked poor prognosis. They have severe course, fistulizing disease, and resistance to biological therapy and often require colectomy or colonic diversion. Allogeneic hematopoietic stem cell transplants (HSCT) have shown to produce 80% remission in those who do not respond to standard therapy. Due to the significant risk associated with HSCT, including graft-versus-host disease and severe infections, it is important to determine the genetic basis for each patient's VEOIBD (very early-onset IBD) before selecting HSCT as a treatment approach.[9]

■ DIFFERENTIAL DIAGNOSIS OF IBD

Abdominal Tuberculosis

In developing countries, tubercular small-bowel obstruction and colitis are close differential diagnosis and possibly more common than IBD. Hence, while working up for IBD, simultaneous evaluation for tuberculosis is mandatory. The pointers favoring tuberculosis are shown in **Table 9.1.7**. Basic workups required are chest X-ray, Mantoux test, and computed tomography (CT) enterography. In select scenarios and high index of suspicion, high-resolution CT (HRCT) chest is required. Circular transverse ulcers are commonly seen in tubercular colitis. Tissue biopsies should be also processed for tuberculosis-polymerase chain reaction (TB-PCR), ZN stain, TB culture, and GeneXpert/

Table 9.1.7: Pointers favoring tuberculosis.

Clinical	Contact history, peripheral lymphadenopathy, disseminated disease (pulmonary, central nervous system), and abdominal lump
Laboratory	Mantoux positivity and low SAAG ascites (lymphocyte predominant ± high-adenosine deaminase)
Imaging	Necrotic, calcified or conglomerate abdominal lymph nodes, peritoneal thickening, pericardial effusion, lung involvement (military, bronchiectasis, and mediastinal lymph nodes), and calcified space occupying lesions in brain
Histopathology	Caseating large well-defined granulomas (>300 microns size)
Microbiology	Acid-fast bacilli in Ziehl–Neelsen (ZN) stain, culture positivity, or positive GeneXpert/line probe assay

(SAAG: serum-ascites albumin gradient)

Line probe assay. Interferon gamma release assay is not recommended due to poor sensitivity. Occasionally, it is very difficult to differentiate despite thorough workup and hence a trial and response to at least 8–12 weeks of antitubercular therapy (ATT) is required.

Bovine Milk Allergy, Multiple Food Protein Allergy, and Eosinophilic Colitis

This is to be considered in setting of infantile IBD. Temporal correlation with introduction of bovine milk or soy, colonic aphthous ulcers, and eosinophilic infiltration of colonic biopsies are features of allergic etiology.

Acquired Immunodeficiency Syndrome

Presentation may mimic IBD colitis. It is suspected in the presence of recurrent urinary, sinopulmonary, or dermatological infections (extensive scabies and dermatophytoses), hepatosplenomegaly, generalized lymphadenopathy, thrombocytopenia, and hypergammaglobulinemia.

■ LONG-TERM ISSUES IN PEDIATRIC IBD

Bone density and linear growth (on steroids), nutrition (due to anorexia, recurrent pain abdomen, small-bowel strictures, and malabsorption), immunizations (live vaccines contraindication on immunosuppression), drug compliance (due to polytherapy, affordability of biologicals, and adolescence), psychosocial issues (due to cosmetic stigmata of surgery and recurrent infections), school absenteeism (recurrent hospital admissions), fertility potential (due to drug toxicity and colectomy), and cumulative cancer risks are some of the long-term issues prevailing in IBD.[2-4]

■ REFERENCES

1. Sathiyasekaran M, Bavanandam S, Sankaranarayanan S, et al. A questionnaire survey of pediatric inflammatory bowel disease in India. Indian J Gastroenterol. 2014;33(6):543-9.
2. Sauer CG, Kugathasan S. Pediatric inflammatory bowel disease: highlighting pediatric differences in IBD. Gastroenterol Clin North Am. 2009;38(4):611-28.
3. Gower-Rousseau C, Dauchet L, Vernier-Massouille G, et al. The natural history of pediatric ulcerative colitis: a population-based cohort study. Am J Gastroenterol. 2009;104(8):2080-8.
4. Vernier-Massouille G, Balde M, Salleron J, et al. Natural history of pediatric Crohn's disease: a population-based cohort study. Gastroenterology. 2008;135(4):1106-13.
5. Levine A, Koletzko S, Turner D, et al. ESPGHAN revised porto criteria for the diagnosis of inflammatory bowel disease in children and adolescents. J Pediatr Gastroenterol Nutr. 2014;58(6):795-806.

6. Turner D, Ruemmele FM, Orlanski-Meyer E, et al. Management of paediatric ulcerative colitis, Part 1: Ambulatory Care-An Evidence-based Guideline From European Crohn's and Colitis Organization and European Society of Paediatric Gastroenterology, Hepatology and Nutrition. J Pediatr Gastroenterol Nutr. 2018;67(2):257-91.
7. Ruemmele FM, Veres G, Kolho KL, et al. Consensus guidelines of ECCO/ESPGHAN on the medical management of pediatric Crohn's disease. J Crohns Colitis. 2014;8(10):1179-207.
8. Turner D, Ruemmele FM, Orlanski-Meyer E, et al. Management of Paediatric Ulcerative Colitis, Part 2: Acute Severe Colitis-An Evidence-based Consensus Guideline From the European Crohn's and Colitis Organization and the European Society of Paediatric Gastroenterology, Hepatology and Nutrition. J Pediatr Gastroenterol Nutr. 2018;67:292-310.
9. Uhlig HH, Schwerd T, Koletzko S, et al. The diagnostic approach to monogenic very early onset inflammatory bowel disease. Gastroenterology. 2014;147(5):990-1007.e3.

CHAPTER 10

HEPATOLOGY

10.1 Spectrum of Hepatitis B in Children
Malathi Sathiyasekaran, Ganesh Ramaswamy

10.2 Pediatric Liver Transplantation
Smita Malhotra, Anupam Sibal

10.1 SPECTRUM OF HEPATITIS B IN CHILDREN

Malathi Sathiyasekaran, Ganesh Ramaswamy

■ INTRODUCTION

Hepatitis B virus (HBV) infection remains a universal public health problem associated with significant morbidity and mortality. The worldwide prevalence ranges from <2% to >8%. There is a changing epidemiology due to various reasons including travel and migration, improved socioeconomic status, stringent screening of blood and transplant donors, universal immunization policies, adoption programs, screening of contacts, vaccination of those who are hepatitis B surface antigen (HBsAg) negative, and introduction of antiviral therapy. However, the disease is still rampant in high-risk individuals including adolescents due to unsafe habits such as intravenous (IV) drug usage, and shared shaving and tattooing practices.

Hepatitis B virus is a complex, dynamic DNA virus with a propensity to progress to chronic hepatitis, cirrhosis, end-stage liver disease, and hepatocellular carcinoma (HCC). Vertical transmission (VT) is a unique problem seen in children. The disease may take several years to manifest; and it has to be curbed effectively to reduce the burden of HBV infection. The integration of the HBV with the host DNA makes it difficult to cure HBV infection with the available anti-viral therapy. Several guidelines including the "Andaman Statement", which is "India specific", have been published, which provide a uniform standard of care. At present, universal immunization program with the HBV vaccine forms the cornerstone to prevent this morbid infection.

■ EPIDEMIOLOGY

Hepatitis B virus is prevalent worldwide and approximately one-third of the world's population demonstrates serological evidence of infection. The estimated global prevalence in 2015 was 3.5% with about 257 million people with chronic HBV infection and 887,000 deaths.[1] Annually, there are almost 2 million new infections in children younger than 5 years, mostly through mother-to-child transmission and horizontal transmission (HT) in early life. The true prevalence in India in 2007 from a meta-analysis in nontribal populations was 2.4% (95% CI: 2.2–2.7%) and 15.9% (CI: 11.4–20.4%) in tribal populations.[2] A more recent estimate is 1.46% (95% CI 1.44–1.47) indicating that the present prevalence of chronic hepatitis B (CHB) in the general population in India may lie between 1.4% and 2.7%.[3]

VIRAL CHARACTERISTICS

Hepatitis B virus is a hepatotropic DNA virus belonging to the Hepadnaviridae family **(Fig. 10.1.1)**. Three types of viral particles are visualized in the serum by electron microscopy. Two noninfectious viral particles comprise the surface antigen (HBsAg) and are represented as 20-nm spheres and 200 × 22-nm filaments. HBV is the only virus, which produces superfluous protein coat (HBsAg) that is thus used for screening. The infectious HBV virion (Dane particle) is a spherical, double-shelled structure, 42 nm in diameter, consisting of a lipid envelope containing HBsAg that surrounds an inner nucleocapsid composed of hepatitis B core antigen (HBcAg) and nonstructural antigen HBeAg. The viral genome is an incomplete, relaxed double-stranded DNA. There are more than 10 HBV genotypes, A to J, which have a specific geographic distribution and a subtle difference in the severity, occurrence of HCC, and response to therapy. In India, genotypes A and D are common and D is considered less favorable than A, though this is controversial. The biomarkers associated with HBV are hepatitis B surface antigen (HBsAg), core antigen (HBcAg), envelope antigen (HBeAg), and the corresponding antibodies—anti-HBs, anti-HBc (IgG, IgM), and anti-HBe. The DNA polymerase is represented by the viral HBV DNA.

Transmission of Virus

The incubation period for HBV infection is 60–180 days and is spread through parenteral route. In India, transmission occurs both by VT and HT and the latter is more predominant. VT plays a very important role in pediatric population. HBV is spread through blood, blood products, and body fluids

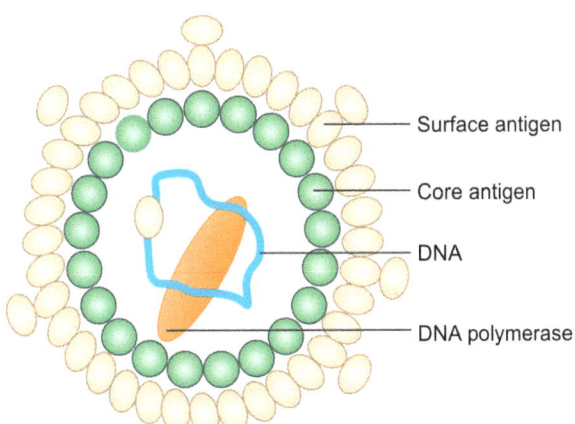

Fig. 10.1.1: Diagrammatic representation of hepatitis B virus.

(vaginal secretions, semen, nasopharyngeal secretions, sweat, saliva, tears, and breastmilk). The risk of HBV infection to the neonate by VT is higher, if the mother has a high viral load and is HBsAg and HBeAg positive (58–90%) compared to if she was only HBsAg positive (5–20%).[4,5] HBV is very infectious and can survive outside the body for at least 7 days and 0.00002 mL of infected blood is enough to contract an infection.

Life Cycle of HBV

The hepatitis B virus enters the hepatocyte and exits as virions in the order of attachment or fusion of the virion to the hepatocyte. During entry into the cell, the outer coat is removed. This is followed by a crucial step in the nucleus of the hepatocyte where the relaxed circular DNA (rcDNA) is converted to covalently closed circular DNA (cccDNA). Subsequent steps take place in the hepatocyte cytoplasm where the cccDNA, which is the template for pregenomic RNA (pgRNA) directs synthesis of mRNA and viral DNA. Reverse transcription follows and core proteins are formed. The virion is then directed into two pathways, viz. the genomic amplification pathway, which redelivers rcDNA into nucleus and the virion assembly pathway, which directs the mature virions to endoplasmic reticulum followed by the exit of the virion.

■ PATHOGENESIS

Hepatitis B is a noncytopathic virus that causes injury predominantly by immune-mediated process. The severity of hepatocyte lysis reflects the degree of immune response. The elimination of virus-infected hepatocyte is dependent on the recognition by cytotoxic T lymphocytes of viral determinants in association with HLA protein on the infected cell.

■ PATHOLOGY

There are no histopathological changes, which are specific for HBV-related chronic hepatitis or cirrhosis. Chronic inflammatory cells, bridging fibrosis, and nodules may be seen depending on the stage of the disease. The necroinflammation and the degree of fibrosis are used in scoring and are useful when clear-cut criteria are not met for initiating treatment.

Viral Biomarkers in Serum and Their Interpretation (Fig. 10.1.2)

Hepatitis B Surface Antigen and Antibody

The HBsAg appears 6 weeks after exposure to infection and usually disappears by 6 months. The persistence of this antigen for more than 6 months indicates chronicity. HBsAg is positive in both acute and chronic infections and is used as a simple screening test. Quantitative HBsAg (qHBsAg) correlates

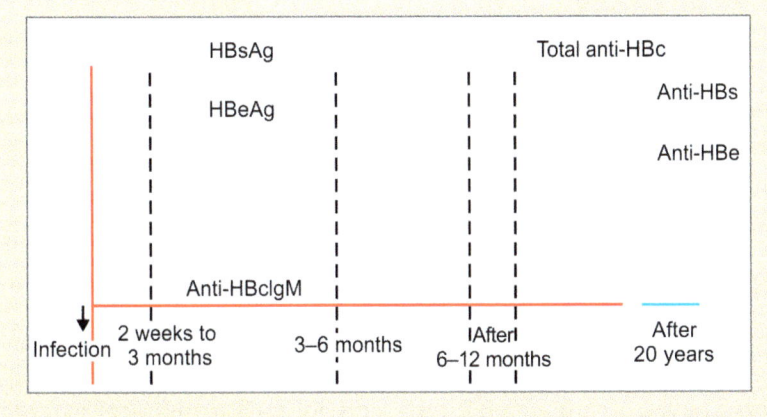

Fig. 10.1.2: Biomarkers in hepatitis B viral infection. (HBsAg: hepatitis B virus surface antigen; HBeAg: hepatitis B virus envelope antigen; HBcIgM: hepatitis B core immunoglobulin M)

with cccDNA and is considered as a marker of infected cells. It is useful for monitoring therapy of CHB. Hepatitis B surface antibody (anti-HBs) is a protective antibody and is detected soon after HBsAg clears from serum. This persists lifelong though the titers may decrease. It is present in both—following recovery from a natural infection (anti-HBc +ve) and after an effective vaccination (anti-HBc −ve). The recommended protective titer is >10 mIU/mL. The annual natural HBsAg clearance is 0.6% per year with VT but is higher (1–2%) with HT.

Hepatitis Envelope Antigen and Antibody

Hepatitis B envelope antigen appears soon after HBsAg and is a marker of infectivity and active viral replication. It usually disappears by 6 weeks and persistence of this antigen >6 weeks indicates progression to chronicity. It is detected in wild virus infection; however, it is not present in pre-core mutant infection. An infant born to an HBsAg and HBeAg +ve mother has a 90% chance of acquiring the infection. Anti-HBe is not a protective antibody. In the management of HBeAg +ve CHB, the seroconversion of HBeAg +ve to anti-HBe +ve is considered a good response to therapy. The annual natural HBeAg clearance is better in HT (5–15%), whereas it is around 3% in VT.[6]

Hepatitis Core Antigen and Antibody

Hepatitis core antigen (HBcAg) is not detected in the serum but is seen in the liver as a ground glass hepatocyte. Anti-HBc is also not a protective antibody, but is a useful marker in serodiagnosis. Anti-HBc IgM indicates recent infection and anti-HBc IgG (measured as total) indicates past infection.

Hepatitis B Virus DNA

Hepatitis B virus DNA represents the viral DNA polymerase and indicates active viral replication. The levels differ depending on the stage of infection. The levels can fluctuate and flare spontaneously. HBV DNA level measurement is essential for diagnosing the stage of chronic infection, and for the decision to treat and subsequent monitoring of patients. Their high levels correlate with occurrence of HCC.

■ NATURAL HISTORY OF HBV INFECTION (FIG. 10.1.3)

The clinical course of chronic HBV infection is influenced by the age at primary infection, gender, transmission route, HBV genotype, and environmental factors. The risk of chronicity is inversely proportional to the age of acquisition of the virus. In neonates and children less than 1 year of age, the incidence of chronicity is as high as 90%; by the age of 1–5 years, it decreases to 30%; and in a child more than 5 years of age, it is around 10%, which may decrease to even 2%. CHB may progress to cirrhosis, HCC, end-stage liver disease, and death, if not treated adequately. Liver transplantation has significantly changed the natural history of chronic HBV infection.[3] It has been estimated that 3–5% and 0.01–0.03% of children with chronic infection develop cirrhosis and HCC, respectively, before adulthood.[7]

■ CLINICAL PRESENTATION

The spectrum of hepatitis B infection is shown in **Flowchart 10.1.1**. The majority of children with HBV infection are asymptomatic and incidentally detected to have hepatomegaly, elevated transaminases, or HBsAg positivity.

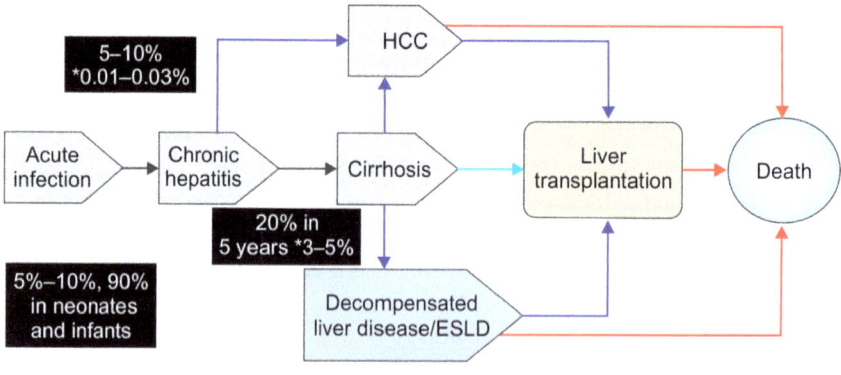

Fig. 10.1.3: Natural history of hepatitis B virus infection. (ESLD: end-stage liver disease)

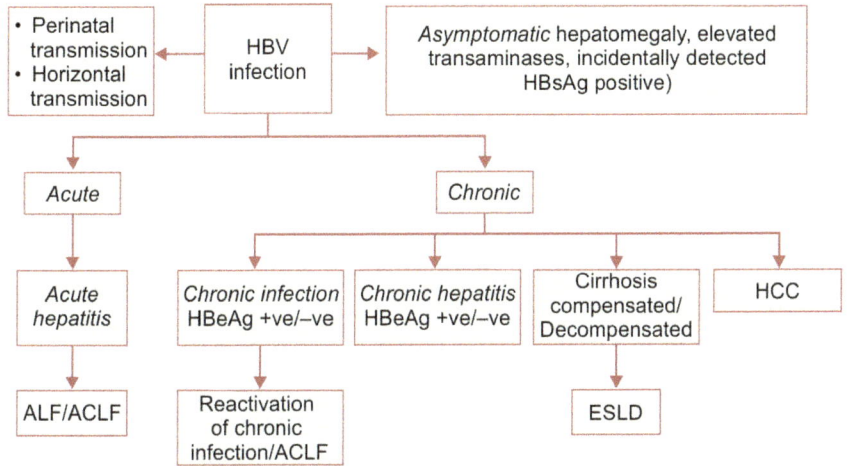

Flowchart 10.1.1: Spectrum of hepatitis B virus (HBV) infection.

(ACLF: acute-on-chronic liver failure; ALF: acute liver failure; ESLD: end-stage liver disease; HCC: hepatocellular carcinoma)

The spectrum of symptomatic HBV infection includes acute hepatitis, acute liver failure, reactivation of chronic hepatitis, HBeAg-positive or -negative CHB, compensated and decompensated cirrhosis, end-stage liver disease, and HCC.

Acute Viral Hepatitis B

Hepatitis B virus is present in 10–15% of children with acute viral hepatitis (AVH) in India. The majority is anicteric or may be asymptomatic. Symptomatic AVHB infection is characterized by three phases, viz. prodromal phase, icteric phase, and convalescent phase. During prodromal phase, children develop fever, intense fatigue, anorexia, nausea, and myalgia, which last for a few days. Biochemically serum bilirubin and alanine aminotransferase (ALT) levels rise and serologically HBsAg and anti-HBc IgM are positive with high HBV DNA being detectable. The icteric phase, which lasts for 1–2 weeks, is heralded by onset of jaundice or high-colored urine and may be seen in 25% during which viral levels decrease. During convalescence, jaundice resolves but constitutional symptoms may last for weeks or months. During this phase, HBsAg is cleared followed by the disappearance of detectable HBV DNA. In addition to the hepatic manifestations, there are other immune-mediated extrahepatic manifestations such as maculopapular or urticarial rash, migratory arthritis, serum sickness like syndrome, polyarteritis nodosa, glomerulonephritis, aplastic anemia, and papular acrodermatitis of childhood or Gianotti–Crosti syndrome. Less than 10% of infants born to HBeAg-positive mothers develop acute hepatitis. The illness will resolve and progression to chronic hepatitis depends on the age of the child. A small percentage will advance into acute liver failure.

Acute Liver Failure

The HBV-related acute liver failure (ALF) is uncommon (1%) in infants and children and is associated with a high mortality (>40%) without liver transplantation. The child with ALF usually presents with fever, abdominal pain, vomiting, and jaundice, followed by altered sensorium and encephalopathy. HBsAg and HBV DNA levels generally fall rapidly as liver failure develops, and some patients are HBsAg negative by the time ALF sets in. Patients with ALF due to HBV should be monitored in hepatic ICU and referred for liver transplant. The majority of neonates born to HBsAg-positive mothers are asymptomatic, but rarely around 8–12 weeks of age, they could present with ALF when the mother is HBsAg positive and HBeAg negative.

Reactivation of Chronic Hepatitis B

It is difficult to differentiate AVHB from reactivation of CHB and it requires a high index of suspicion. In the presence of high HBV DNA (>2 × 10^4 IU/mL), underlying liver disease should be investigated by liver biopsy, endoscopy, and/or imaging. The degree of liver failure often depends on the severity of acute insult and the stage of underlying chronic liver disease. Mutations in the HBV genome, immunosuppressive therapy, and viral or drug-induced injury are common causes of reactivation. The use of a potent oral nucleo(t)side analog (NA) is necessary as soon as possible in patients with CHB reactivation. Liver transplantation benefits those with liver failure secondary to severe acute exacerbation. Granulocyte colony-stimulating factor (GCSF) has been found beneficial.

Chronic HBV Infection

Chronic HBV infection is a dynamic disease and reflects the interaction between viral replication and the host immune response during the various stages. The natural history is schematically classified into five immunological phases depending on HBeAg status, transaminase level, HBV DNA level, and presence or absence of inflammation on biopsy.
1. The immune-tolerant phase (IT)
2. Immune-reactive phase (HBeAg-positive CHB)
3. Low replicative or inactive carrier
4. Reactivation (HBeAg-negative CHB)
5. HBsAg clearance.

Single determination of viral markers or transaminases may not reflect the actual phase of infection.[8,9] These phases are of variable duration, may or may not be sequential, and may not be seen in all individuals with HBV infection.

Immune-tolerant Phase

This is the first phase of chronic HBV infection in which the host immune system is in a state of tolerance to HBV. The duration of the immune tolerant phase is variable and may last for more than 20 years in those who acquire HBV by VT; whereas, it is short in those who are infected by HT. The IT phase is characterized by the presence of HBsAg, HBeAg, high level of serum HBV DNA (200,000 IU/L), and normal or slightly elevated ALT levels. Liver biopsy shows normal histology or minimal histological changes. Antiviral treatment is ineffective and not recommended in the immune-tolerant phase.

Immune-reactive Phase (HBeAg-positive CHB)

This is the second phase and characterized by presence of HBsAg and HBeAg, high (>20,000 IU/L), fluctuating, or gradually decreasing serum HBV DNA (compared to IT phase) levels, and persistent or intermittent ALT elevation. Liver histology shows active necroinflammation since the host immune system begins to recognize HBV as a target and attacks the infected hepatocytes. The longer the duration of this phase, the higher the chance of progressing to cirrhosis and HCC. Treatment is recommended in this phase.

Spontaneous HBeAg seroconversion: ALT flares may predict HBeAg seroconversion and though it may appear to be a favorable response, the active necroinflammation during seroconversion can also cause liver injury and increase the risk of both cirrhosis and HCC. The rate of spontaneous HBeAg seroconversion is less than 2% per year among those aged 3 years or less and 4–5% per year in older children.[6,10] In children who were mainly infected through HT, the rate of spontaneous HBeAg seroconversion was 14–16% per year during the first 10 years of follow-up. However children infected horizontally show higher spontaneous HBeAg seroconversion, 14–16% per year during the first 10 years of follow-up.[10]

Inactive Carrier State

This is the third phase where the virus is in a low-replicative state and seroconversion of HBeAg to anti-HBe occurs. It is characterized by the presence of HBsAg, absence of HBeAg, the presence of anti-HBe, persistently normal ALT levels, and low serum HBV DNA levels (<2,000 IU/mL). Liver histology shows minimal inflammation and minimal fibrosis. The term inactive carrier state is a misnomer, since there is always potential for disease flare and progression to HCC, as the HBV had already integrated into the hepatocyte.

HBeAg-negative Immune Reactivation Phase

The reactivation phase is the fourth phase and is also called *HBeAg-negative/anti-HB-positive CHB*. Some patients even after HBeAg seroconversion develop significant HBV replication and progress to liver injury. The reactivation phase is usually characterized by the presence of precore mutants or variants in the basal core promoter regions that impair HBeAg expression. In this phase, with low rates of spontaneous disease remission, anti-HBe is present with elevated or fluctuating ALT levels and detectable serum HBV DNA (>2,000 IU/mL). The liver histopathology shows moderate or severe necroinflammation with fibrosis. Reactivation of viral replication may at times induce the reversion back to the HBeAg-positive state. In children with chronic HBV infection, 4–5% develop HBeAg-negative CHB after achieving HBeAg seroconversion.

HBsAg Clearance Phase

This phase is characterized by serum being negative for HBsAg and positive for antibodies to HBcAg (anti-HBc), with or without detectable antibodies to HBsAg (anti-HBs). This phase is also known as *occult HBV infection*. In this phase, ALT and HBV DNA are usually normal or undetectable, respectively; however, HBV DNA (cccDNA) can be detected frequently in the liver. If HBsAg loss occurs before the onset of cirrhosis, the risk of progression to cirrhosis, decompensation, and HCC is less than if cirrhosis has already set in. HBV reactivation may occur with immunosuppression in these patients.

The terminologies such as immune tolerant, immune active HBeAg-positive CHB, immune active HBeAg-negative CHB, inactive carrier, and HBsAg clearance have been changed. The recent classification is based only on HBeAg positive or negative and presence of infection or disease **(Table 10.1.1)**.[9]

■ COMPLICATIONS

The main complications are cirrhosis, decompensated liver disease, end-stage liver disease, and HCC. HBV constitutes 20–30% of pediatric chronic liver disease (CLD) in India. The incidence is decreasing with widespread universal immunization. The child may present with fever, loss of appetite, lethargy, prolonged jaundice, and gastrointestinal (GI) bleed. In decompensated liver disease, the liver is usually firm with splenomegaly and ascites.

Hepatocellular Carcinoma

Hepatocellular carcinoma has been described in children both with vertical and HT. Around 0.01–0.03% of patients with CHB develop HCC during childhood (32 per 100,000 person/year). These are more likely to be males (70%)

Table 10.1.1: Phases of chronic hepatitis B virus (HBV) infection.

	HBeAg-positive Chronic infection	HBeAg-positive Chronic hepatitis	HBeAg-negative Chronic infection	HBeAg-negative Chronic hepatitis	HBsAg-negative Chronic infection
HBsAg	High	High/intermediate	Low	Low/Intermediate	Negative Anti HBc+
HBeAg	Positive	Positive	Negative	Negative	Anti HBs±
HBV DNA	>10^7 IU/mL	10^4–10^7 IU/mL	<2,000 IU/mL*	>2,000 IU/mL	Undetectable cccDNA+
ALT	Normal	Elevated	Normal	Elevated**	Normal
Liver disease	None/minimal	Moderate/severe	None	Moderate/severe	
Old terminology	Immune tolerant	Immune reactive HBeAg +ve hepatitis	Inactive carrier	HBeAg-negative chronic hepatitis	HBsAg clearance/Occult HBV

(ALT: alanine aminotransferase; cccDNA: covalently closed circular DNA; HBsAg: hepatitis B virus surface antigen; HBeAg: hepatitis B virus envelope antigen)
Note:
*HBV DNA levels >2,000–20,000 IU/mL may be present without features of chronic hepatitis.
**Persistently or intermittently.

with cirrhosis (80%) and those who have undergone early seroconversion. The necroinflammation during seroconversion is severe enough to cause cirrhosis and HCC. The risk of developing HCC is higher in patients with one or more factors that relate to the host [cirrhosis, chronic hepatic necroinflammation, older age, male sex, African origin, alcohol abuse, chronic coinfections with other hepatitis viruses or human immunodeficiency virus (HIV), diabetes or metabolic syndrome, active smoking, positive family history] and/or to HBV properties (high HBV DNA and/or HBsAg levels, HBV genotype C > B, and specific mutations). The above factors seem to affect the progression to cirrhosis in untreated CHB patients.

■ EVALUATION OF CHILDREN WITH CHRONIC HEPATITIS B

The basic evaluation before definitive therapy includes a detailed history whether asymptomatic or symptomatic. If symptomatic, history of jaundice, fluid retention, loss of weight or appetite, GI bleed, urine output, sensorium, blood transfusions, surgery, recurrent needle pricks, IV drug abuse, tattoos, liver disease in the family, death related to liver disease and HCC should be obtained. A thorough clinical examination including icterus, digital clubbing, palmar erythema, abdomen (liver size, spleen, free fluid, and presence of veins), and other systems is essential. Investigations should include complete blood counts, biochemical tests of the liver, prothrombin time, creatinine and sugar, ultrasound of abdomen, and upper GI endoscopy. Liver biopsy is preferable prior to initiating therapy in CHB. This may be useful when the transaminases are normal or fluctuating and there is family history of liver disease.

SERODIAGNOSIS

The combination of various biomarkers helps in the accurate diagnosis of the stage of the disease.

- *Acute hepatitis B:* Acute HBV is diagnosed by the presence of HBsAg, HBV DNA by polymerase chain reaction (PCR), and anti-HBc immunoglobulin M (IgM).
- *Acute liver failure due to HBV:* The presence of HBsAg, anti-HBc IgM, and prolonged prothrombin time in a child with no known pre-existing liver disease.
- *Acute-on-chronic liver failure*: The presence of raised bilirubin, elevated transaminases, coagulopathy, ascites with or without encephalopathy in a child who is known to be HBsAg positive or has features suggestive of chronic disease such as firm liver. The viral markers are HBsAg positive, anti-HBc IgM, and high HBV DNA.
- *Chronic hepatitis B:* The various phases are designated by the combination of HBsAg, HBeAg, HBV DNA viral load, and transaminase level. Histopathology may be essential before the onset of therapy **(Table 10.1.1)**.

MOTHER-TO-CHILD TRANSMISSION

Transmission from mother to infant either vertical or horizontal is an important mode of viral spread. The course of illness is more severe when the infection is acquired during delivery. The incidence of HBsAg positivity in pregnant women in India is about 0.9–1.1% and VT occurs in 45.2%.[4,5] The risk of transmission is higher, if mother is HBsAg and HBeAg positive (58–90%), whereas it is 5–20%, if HBsAg positive and HBeAg negative. Screening for HBsAg in the first trimester of pregnancy is therefore strongly recommended by all liver societies. Most of the transmission occurs during the perinatal period at the time of delivery from the placental blood and cervical secretions. This forms the basis of active immunization with birth dose of vaccine along with HBIG given preferably within 24 hours.

In spite of adequate precaution to administer post-exposure prophylaxis (PEP), 3–9% of infants acquire infection. The plausible explanations for this may be the prenatal spread of infection because of:
- A breach in the placental barrier
- Placental infection and trans-placental and transmission of HBV
- HBV-DNA exists in oocytes of infected females and sperms of HBV-infected males, and
- Intrauterine (IU) transmission from vaginal secretions.

Though several mechanisms have been proposed, they are not sufficient to recommend cesarean section, as the mode of delivery in all HBsAg-positive pregnancy. Similarly, though natal spread can occur from breastmilk, in India, it is not necessary to withhold breastfeeding; however, the infant should be immunized and also administered HBIG.

■ MANAGEMENT OF HBV INFECTION

Since the spectrum of HBV infection spreads from acute disease to chronic disease, the recommended treatment protocols differ in the various groups.[10,11]

Goals of Therapy in Chronic HBV Infection

The goals of therapy are to attain HBeAg seroconversion, HBV DNA suppression, and ALT normalization and, at the same time, to arrest the necroinflammation, prevent decompensation, reverse fibrosis, prevent cirrhosis, HCC, and death. Since HBV integration occurs very early in infection and there is no method to detect, suppress, or eradicate cccDNA, it seems impossible to cure HBV infection with the available therapy. The goal is, therefore, to suppress the viral replication as long as possible.[3]

Since active HBV replication is the key driver of liver injury and disease progression, sustained viral suppression is of paramount importance. The primary aim is to permanently suppress the HBV viral replication thereby decreasing infectivity and pathogenicity, which results in reduced hepatic necroinflammation.

Medications

The medications approved in pediatric chronic HBV infection are interferon (IFN), both conventional and pegylated, antiviral nucleoside analogs (lamivudine or entecavir), or nucleotide analogs (tenofovir).[8]

Interferon

Interferon-alpha and peginterferon-alpha act as immune modulators and can be administered for a finite period of 6 months. This is the only drug associated with higher rates of HBsAg loss when compared with nucleoside or nucleotide analogs. It is not a child friendly drug, since it has to be given as injections. Children tolerate the drug better than adults yet there are several side effects. IFN therapy is not recommended in infants or pregnant women and is contraindicated in decompensated cirrhosis, uncontrolled psychiatric disease, severe cytopenia, severe cardiac disease, or uncontrolled seizures.

Dosage of IFN-alpha-2b in children >1 year of age is 6 million units/m^2 thrice a week, PEG IFN-alpha-2a >3 years of age 180 μg/1.73 m^2 once a week.[8]

Nucleos(t)ide Analogs

These are prodrugs and need intracellular activation before they can exert their therapeutic action. They are highly effective in inhibiting the HBV replication. HBV DNA polymerase is their main target of action. Lamivudine was the first antiviral to be introduced but the main drawback with this drug was the high incidence of YMDD mutations. Hence, it is no longer recommended in the treatment. Entecavir and tenofovir are very effective and are associated with a very low drug resistance. Entecavir can be used in children >2 years of age at a dose of 0.015 mg/kg/day for children weighing 10–30 kg and 0.5 mg, if the weight is more than 30 kg.[12] Tenofovir disoproxil fumarate is used at a dose of 300 mg/day in children >2 years and tenofovir alafenamide 25 mg in children >12 years of age.[8] These drugs have minimal side effects, have no contraindications, and can safely be prescribed in all stages of chronic liver disease. The rate of HBsAg seroconversion is very minimal. The duration of treatment is still debatable; ideally, it should be continued till HBsAg seroconversion. In HBeAg-positive CHB, the end point suggested is to continue for 1 year after HBeAg seroconversion; whereas, the recommended treatment for HBeAg-negative CHB is for lifelong.[13]

Acute Hepatitis B

The treatment of acute HBV is largely supportive and close monitoring for acute liver failure, extrahepatic complications, and chronic hepatitis forms the cornerstone in management. Once child recovers, repeat HBsAg after 6 months. If HBsAg is negative, then child has seroconverted; check anti-HBs status and if positive then child is seroprotected. If HBsAg continues to be positive, child has progressed to chronic hepatitis.

Severe Acute Hepatitis and ALF

American Association for the Study of Liver Diseases (AASLD), European Association for the Study of Liver (EASL), and Asian Pacific Association for the Study of the Liver (APASL) recommend antiviral therapy for severe acute hepatitis and ALF.[7,14,15] The criteria for severe acute hepatitis include coagulopathy INR > 1.5, or a protracted course (i.e. persistent symptoms > 4 weeks) or marked jaundice (total bilirubin > 3 mg/dL or direct bilirubin > 1.5 mg/dL); APASL defines it as serum bilirubin > 10 mg/dL, encephalopathy, or ascites. Early antiviral therapy with highly potent nucleoside analogs can prevent progression to ALF, liver transplant, or death. This is not seen, if therapy is initiated late in the course of severe acute hepatitis B or in patients with already manifested acute liver failure and advanced hepatic encephalopathy.

Reactivation of Chronic Hepatitis B

The use of a potent oral nucleo(t)side analog early in the course of the disease either entecavir or tenofovir is necessary in patients with CHB reactivation. Liver transplantation benefits those with liver failure secondary to severe acute exacerbation.

Chronic Hepatitis B

Those children with CHB either HBeAg-positive or HBeAg-negative CHB with persistently elevated transaminases (minimum more than 3 months) should be treated as per the present recommendations of European Society for Paediatric Gastroenterology, Hepatology and Nutrition (ESPGHAN) and APASL. The algorithms recommended by APASL in 2015 for management of HBeAg-positive and HBeAg-negative CHB are shown in **Flowcharts 10.1.2 and 10.1.3**.[15]

Cirrhosis

For those with cirrhosis either compensated or decompensated cirrhosis, antivirals should be given irrespective of the level of serum transaminases and HBV DNA. In children with decompensated cirrhosis in addition should be referred for liver transplantation. The details are shown in **Table 10.1.2**.

Immune Tolerant of HBeAg-positive Infection

In this phase, the transaminases are normal but the HBV DNA is very high. At present, there is no definite treatment for this phase. Recent studies with entecavir and PEG/IFN for up to 48 weeks rarely led to loss of HBeAg with sustained suppression of HBV DNA levels in children in the immune tolerant phase of HBV infection, and treatment was associated with frequent adverse events.[16] The recommendation for IT phase HBeAg positive or HBeAg negative is to monitor every 3 months. Liver biopsy is advised, if ALT is persistently elevated or there is family history of HCC or cirrhosis. Treat, if moderate to severe inflammation or significant fibrosis is present on liver biopsy.

Inactive Carrier or HBeAg-negative Infection

Monitor ALT regularly once in 3 months for 1 year, if normal then every 6–12 months thereafter. Liver biopsy is advised, if ALT > 2 UL/N. Treatment is initiated, if biopsy shows moderate/severe inflammation or HBV DNA > 2,000 IU/L.

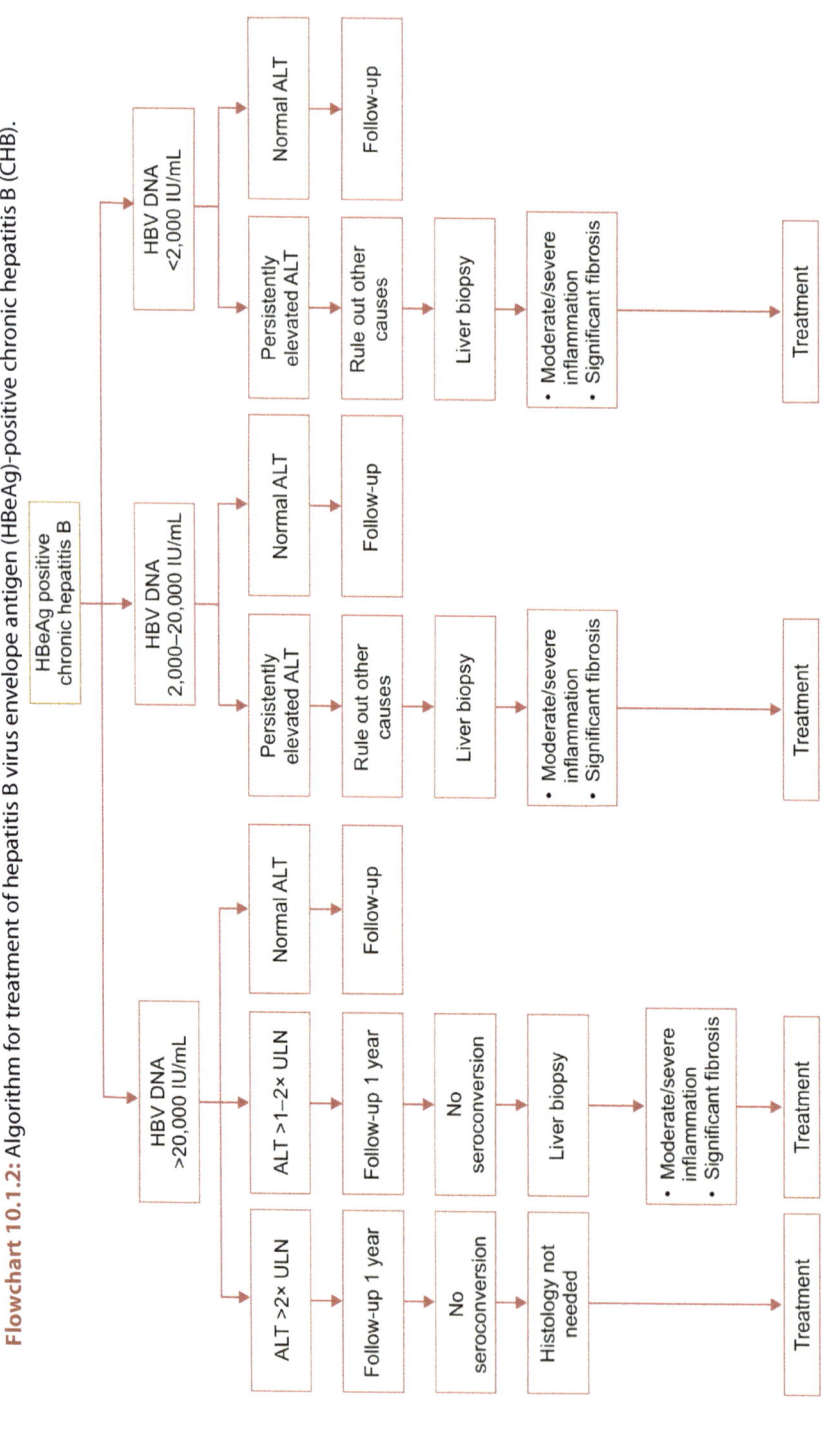

Flowchart 10.1.2: Algorithm for treatment of hepatitis B virus envelope antigen (HBeAg)-positive chronic hepatitis B (CHB).

(ALT: alanine aminotransferase; HBV: hepatitis B virus)

Source: Adapted from Asian Pacific Association for the Study of the Liver (APASL), 2015.

Flowchart 10.1.3: Algorithm for hepatitis B virus envelope antigen (HBeAg)-negative chronic hepatitis B (CHB).

```
                    HBeAg-negative
                   chronic hepatitis B
                    /              \
            HBV DNA              HBV DNA
           >2,000 IU/mL         <2,000 IU/mL
          /      |      \          /        \
  Persistently Persistently Normal  Persistently Normal
  elevated ALT elevated ALT  ALT   elevated ALT  ALT
       |           |          |         |          |
   ALT >2× ULN  ALT >1–2× ULN           ALT >ULN
       |           |          |         |          |
   Histology    Rule out   Follow-up  Rule out  Follow-up
   not needed   other                 other
                causes                causes
                   |                     |
               Liver biopsy         Rule out other
                   |                   causes
           • Moderate/severe       • Moderate/severe
             inflammation            inflammation
           • Significant fibrosis  • Significant fibrosis
       |           |                     |
   Treatment   Treatment             Treatment
```

(ALT: alanine aminotransferase; HBV: hepatitis B virus)
Source: Asian Pacific Association for the Study of the Liver (APASL), 2015.

Table 10.1.2: Indications for treatment of chronic hepatitis B.

Disease	HBeAg	ALT level	HBV DNA	Liver histology	Treatment
HBeAg-positive CHB	Positive	Persistently elevated >6 m	>2,000 IU/mL	Moderate/severe inflammation/fibrosis	IFN/NA
HBeAg-negative CHB	Negative	Persistently elevated >6 m	>2,000 IU/mL	Moderate/severe inflammation/fibrosis	IFN/NA
Compensated cirrhosis	Any	Any	Detectable	Cirrhosis	NA
Decompensated cirrhosis	Any	Any	Detectable	Not done	NA

(ALT: alanine aminotransferase; HBeAg: hepatitis B virus envelope antigen; IFN: interferon; NA: nucleo(t)side analog)

Special Situations

There are some situations where antivirals are prescribed in spite of normal transaminases. Children who are HBsAg positive and are on chemotherapy or immunosuppression irrespective of HBV DNA levels should be started on antivirals and continued for 12 months after the cessation of therapy. The others include those with glomerulonephritis due to HBV infection and prevention or treatment of recurrent HBV infection after liver transplantation [recipients of a liver graft from an anti-hepatitis B core antigen (anti-HBc) positive donor and presence of coinfections (HBV/HIV, HBV/HCV, and HBV/HDV)].

■ PREVENTION OF HBV

General Measures

If the child is HBsAg positive, it is crucial to follow some simple measures such as covering open wounds and scratches, cleaning blood spills with detergent or bleach and avoid sharing toothbrushes, or unsafe IV drug use. They should refrain themselves from donation of blood or organs. However, they can participate in all activities including sports. They should not be deprived of admissions in schools and not be isolated from other children. They can share food and utensils. Other comorbid states such as obesity, alcohol, and intravenous drug usage should be avoided to prevent further liver damage. They should receive hepatitis A vaccination, as it triggers decompensation in those with chronic HBV infection.

Active Immunization

This forms the cornerstone in preventing the transmission of HBV.

Newborns and infants: If mother is HBsAg negative, WHO recommends administration of first dose hepatitis B vaccine 10 μg within 24 hours after birth for newborn infants followed by subsequent doses at 6, 10, and 14 weeks. Presently combination vaccines containing DTP, HIB (*Haemophilus influenzae* type B), and IPV (inactivated polio vaccine) are widely used.

Older children, adolescents: The recommended schedule is 20 μg at 0, 1, and, 6 months for children more than 12 years.

If mother is HBsAg positive: The first dose of hepatitis B vaccine along with hepatitis B immune globulin (0.5 mL) is administered within 12 hours after birth followed by subsequent doses at 6, 10, and 14 weeks. Postvaccination testing for HBsAg and anti-HBs should be done at 9–18 months. If the child is positive for anti-HBs then the child is seroprotected. If the infant is positive for HBsAg, detailed re-evaluation is necessary.

Antiviral Therapy for Mother

Around 10% of infants born to HBsAg- and HBeAg-positive mothers acquire infection in spite of vaccine and HBIG. Antiviral therapy is recommended to decrease the viral load and decrease the mother-to-child transmission. Tenofovir is given during the antenatal period in the last trimester from 26 weeks to 28 weeks and continued for 12 weeks after delivery. Mothers with a high viral load more than 10^7 copies/mL, or those with previous sibling with HBV infection and >10^6 copies/mL are candidates for treatment.

Post-liver Transplant

All patients on the transplant waiting list with HBV-related liver disease should be treated with NA. Combination of hepatitis B immunoglobulin (HBIG) and a potent NA is recommended for the prevention of HBV recurrence. HBIG can be discontinued and a potent NA continued in low-risk individuals. HBsAg-negative patients receiving livers from donors with evidence of past HBV infection (anti-HBc positive) are at risk of HBV recurrence and should receive antiviral prophylaxis with an NA.

■ CONCLUSION

Hepatitis B virus infection is an important cause of acute and chronic liver disease morbidity and mortality in children and adolescents. Understanding the viral dynamics is essential for precise and proper evaluation and therapy. Quantification of HBV DNA is vital in the management of the illness. At present, immunoprophylaxis to prevent VT and universal immunization are the only ways to curb this devastating highly contagious disease. There are several lacunae, which need to be answered and worked up such as identifying biomarkers to predict progression of disease, effective drugs for the immune tolerant phase, methods to diagnose and eradicate cccDNA, and more effective immunoprophylaxis to prevent VT.

■ REFERENCES

1. World Health Organization. (2019). Hepatitis B. [online] Available from https://www.who.int/news-room/fact-sheets/detail/hepatitis-b. [Last accessed December, 2019].
2. Batham A, Narula D, Toteja T, et al. Systematic review and meta-analysis of prevalence of hepatitis B in India. Indian Pediatr. 2007;44(9):663-74.
3. Arora A, Singh SP, Kumar A, et al. INASL position statements on prevention, diagnosis and management of hepatitis B virus Infection in India: The Andaman Statements. J Clin Exp Hepatol. 2018;8(1):58-80.
4. Dwivedi M, Misra SP, Misra V. Seroprevalence of hepatitis B infection during pregnancy and risk of perinatal transmission. Indian J Gastroenterol. 2011;30(2):66-71.

5. Pande C, Sarin SK, Patra S. Prevalence, risk factors and virological profile of chronic hepatitis B virus infection in pregnant women in India. J Med Virol. 2011;83(6):962-7.
6. Chang MH, Hsu HY, Hsu HC, et al. The significance of spontaneous hepatitis B e antigen seroconversion in childhood: with special emphasis on the clearance of hepatitis B e antigen before 3 years of age. Hepatology. 1995;22(5):1387-92.
7. Wen WH, Chang MH, Hsu HY, et al. The development of hepatocellular carcinoma among prospectively followed children with chronic hepatitis B virus infection. J Pediatr. 2004;144(3):397-9.
8. Indolfi G, Easterbrook P, Dusheiko G, et al. Hepatitis B virus infection in children and adolescents. Lancet Gastroenterol Hepatol. 2019;4(6):466-76.
9. European Association for the Study of the Liver. EASL 2017 Clinical Practice Guidelines on the management of hepatitis B virus infection. J Hepatol. 2017;67(2):370-98.
10. Bortolotti F, Guido M, Bartolacci S, et al. Chronic hepatitis B in children after e antigen seroclearance: final report of a 29-year longitudinal study. Hepatology. 2006;43(3):556-62.
11. Sokal EM, Paganelli M, Wirth S, et al. Management of chronic hepatitis B in childhood: ESPGHAN clinical practice guidelines: consensus of an expert panel on behalf of the European Society of Pediatric Gastroenterology, Hepatology and Nutrition. J Hepatol. 2013;59(4):814-29.
12. Jonas MM, Chang MH, Sokal E, et al. Randomized, controlled trial of entecavir versus placebo in children with hepatitis B envelope antigen-positive chronic hepatitis B. Hepatology. 2016;63(2):377-87.
13. Komatsu H, Inui A, Fujisawa T. Pediatric hepatitis B treatment. Ann Transl Med. 2017;5(3):37. doi: 10.21037/atm.2016.11.52 PMCID: PMC5326647.
14. Terrault NA, Bzowej NH, Chang KM, et al. AASLD guidelines for treatment of chronic hepatitis B. Hepatology. 2016;63(1):261-83.
15. Sarin SK, Kumar M, Lau GK, et al. Asian-Pacific clinical practice guidelines on the management of hepatitis B: a 2015 update. Hepatol Int. 2016;10(1):1-98.
16. Rosenthal P, Ling SC, Belle SH, et al. The Hepatitis B Research Network (HBRN) Combination of entecavir/peginterferon alfa-2a in children with HBeAg-positive immune tolerant chronic hepatitis B virus. Hepatology. 2019;69(6):2326-37.

10.2 PEDIATRIC LIVER TRANSPLANTATION

Smita Malhotra, Anupam Sibal

■ INTRODUCTION

One of the marvels of modern medicine has been the evolution of liver transplantation (LT) as an established therapy in the last 5 decades. Ever since the first attempt in 1963 by Dr Thomas Starzl, his first success after 7 failed attempts in 1967 in a 3-year-old boy with biliary atresia,[1] to the current worldwide experience and acceptance, LT has come a long way. In the US alone, over 750,000 liver transplants have been performed of which about 54,000 have been in children.[2] In the 80s and 90s, LT in India seemed unthinkable till the first successful pediatric liver transplant in 1998 at Indraprastha Apollo Hospital, Delhi.[3] The progress was slow over the next decade due to scarcity of trained personnel, poor awareness among primary care doctors, reservations regarding donor safety, and the huge financial implications. By 2007, 318 LTs had been performed in India.[4] However, the last decade has seen a phenomenal growth with the advent of multiple liver transplant centers. Presently, about 1,500 liver transplants are performed in India yearly with about 10% being in children. The growth has primarily comprised living donor liver transplant (LDLT) though cadaveric donation is picking up, primarily in the Southern part of the country. As per the provisions of the Indian Human Organ Transplant Act (HOTA), foreign patients can be offered a cadaveric transplant only if no suitable organ recipient is available in India. Hence, these patients are only candidates for LRLT further contributing to this pool.

The establishment of every new LT program requires authorization from a regional health body after evaluation of infrastructure and expertise. To maintain transparency and prevent any irregularities, authorization committees have been set up in all states. Every LT has to be approved by the authorization committee that screens all documents and interviews the family members to establish relationship proof and ensure that donation is voluntary.

India is now an important regional center for LT in South East Asia, more so for pediatric LT. Many of the neighboring countries have either not yet set up transplant units or are in the fledgling phase running predominantly adult programs. Pediatric LT carries its own set of challenges due to the smaller diameter of vessels requiring greater surgical expertise along with the need for specialized pediatric intensive care and usually a longer duration of postoperative hospital stay. Many of these countries have very few pediatric hepatologists with expertise in post-transplant care, thus necessitating a thorough coordination with the transplant unit for follow-up once the families travel back to their native countries.

■ INDICATIONS

Pediatric indications are very different from adults with cholestatic liver diseases, especially biliary atresia forming a major cohort. They can be broadly classified into:
- Primary liver disorders leading to end-stage liver disease that includes cholestatic disorders and acute and chronic hepatitis
- Acute liver failure
- Metabolic disorders including those that cause liver cirrhosis and others that do not cause liver injury, but LT corrects the metabolic error

- Secondary liver disease as part of systemic illness, and
- Liver tumors.

The indications are tabulated in **Box 10.2.1**.

Box 10.2.1: Indications for liver transplant.

A. *Primary liver disorders with cholestasis/hepatitis resulting in liver failure:*
  - Extrahepatic biliary atresia
  - Intrahepatic biliary hypoplasia (syndromic and nonsyndromic bile duct paucity)
  - Progressive familial intrahepatic cholestasis
  - Sclerosing cholangitis
  - Caroli's disease
  - Congenital hepatic fibrosis
  - Total parenteral nutrition (TPN)-associated cholestasis
  - Inborn errors of bile acid synthesis
  - Infectious hepatitis
  - Choledochal cyst
  - Aagenaes syndrome (hereditary cholestasis with lymphedema)
  - Neonatal hepatitis
  - Autoimmune hepatitis
  - Chronic hepatitis B and C

B. *Secondary liver disease:*
  - Cystic fibrosis
  - Sclerosing cholangitis secondary to Langerhans cell histiocytosis
  - Mucopolysaccharidosis (isolated reports)
  - Budd–Chiari syndrome

C. *Metabolic disorders*:
  - Wilson's disease
  - Alpha-1 antitrypsin deficiency
  - *Disorders of amino acid metabolism*: Tyrosinemia, urea cycle defect, MMA, PPA, MSUD
  - *Disorders of carbohydrate metabolism*: Galactosemia, fructosemia, and GSD
  - *Disorders of lipid metabolism*: Familial hypercholesterolemia, lipidoses (Gaucher, Niemann–Pick, Wolman, cholesteryl ester storage disease)
  - Neonatal hemochromatosis
  - *Disorders of bilirubin metabolism*: Crigler–Najjar type 1
  - Primary hyperoxaluria (liver kidney transplant)
  - Selected defects of mitochondrial function

D. *Liver tumors:*
  - Hepatoblastoma
  - Hepatocellular carcinoma
  - Hemangioendothelioma
  - Fibrolamellar carcinoma

(MMA: methylmalonic acidemia; PPA: propionic acidemia; MSUD: maple syrup urine disease; GSD: glycogen storage disease)

Liver Transplantation: When, Where and How?

The most important questions in LT are: When? Where? How? The pediatrician needs to identify children who may benefit from LT and refer them to a transplant center even if LT is not required immediately. Late referral when complications of advanced liver disease have set in adversely affects the morbidity and mortality. Moreover, busy transplant centers have considerable experience in managing liver disorders and a joint care with them helps pediatricians in management of complications, nutritional optimization before LT, improving diagnosis, and suggesting alternate therapies that are less morbid. For example, children with biliary atresia with good synthetic function but refractory portal hypertension may benefit from a shunt surgery. Similarly, children with Alagille syndrome with intractable pruritus and xanthomas may be helped with biliary diversion. Many centers actively help with fund raising and connecting with social support groups. Donor optimization also may require time, as metabolic syndrome and fatty liver are very common in the Asian population.

Children with chronic liver disease are candidates for LT in case of decreased synthetic function, persistent uncorrectable coagulopathy, refractory ascites, refractory portal hypertension with hypersplenism, hepatic encephalopathy, growth retardation despite adequate nutrition, recurrent cholangitis or spontaneous bacterial peritonitis, development of hepatorenal or hepatopulmonary syndrome, and debilitating pruritus nonresponsive to optimal medication. In patients of sclerosing cholangitis secondary to Langerhans cell histiocytosis, LT is feasible only after complete eradication of the primary disease. Patients with cystic fibrosis also are considered for LT on a case-to-case basis depending on the status of other body organs.

A few pediatric liver conditions have a natural course as clearly defined as for biliary atresia. Those babies who either did not undergo a Kasai surgery or the ones in whom it was unsuccessful will decompensate between 6 months and 18 months of age and are candidates for LT in infancy. SPLIT data indicates that this single disease results in 41% of pediatric transplants performed and 65% performed in children under the age of 1 year.[5] Anicteric post-Kasai babies may still require LT in case of recurrent cholangitis, refractory portal hypertension, development of hepatopulmonary syndrome, or portopulmonary hypertension. Progressive fibrosis occurs as part of natural course of disease despite adequate biliary drainage after a successful Kasai surgery and LT will be required when end-stage liver disease develops eventually.[6,7]

In pediatric acute liver failure (PALF), there are no clearly defined scoring systems that adequately predict need for LT. The King's College criteria have been used to guide therapy but have been questioned as they are derived from a largely adult cohort and carry poor sensitivity.[8] Factor V levels <20% and INR >4 have also been variably used though none are absolute; additional variables like lactate are being assessed.[9] Etiology is a very important prognostic indicator as spontaneous recovery is more likely in paracetamol poisoning, acute viral hepatitis and ischemic hepatitis in contrast to autoimmune hepatitis, Wilson's disease, indeterminate PALF, and hemophagocytic histiocytosis.[10] The New Wilson's Index is a score based on five common laboratory criteria and a value of >11 in patients presenting with acute liver failure due to Wilson's disease carries high mortality.[11] Every effort should be made to arrive at an etiological diagnosis though the rapid progression may not always provide an adequate time window to do so. Timely referral before development of advanced encephalopathy and/or multiorgan failure is imperative. This also offers the opportunity for better intensive care, diagnostic evaluation, and specific therapy thus improving the chances of recovery without LT.

Metabolic disorders are an important indication for LT, the most common being Wilson's disease. Any unexplained mortality due to acute or acute-on-chronic liver failure warrants family screening for Wilson's disease, as definitive therapy is available. Wilson's disease presenting with acute decompensation and hepatic encephalopathy has an almost 100% mortality and emergency LT is lifesaving. Alpha-1 antitrypsin deficiency is relatively rare in our population.[12] An important group of metabolic disorders are those that do not cause liver cirrhosis, but LT is curative as it corrects the liver-based metabolic error. However, it does not reverse the neurologic damage that has already occurred. Hence, children with Crigler–Najjar syndrome should be transplanted before kernicterus sets in.[13] Urea cycle defects with severe derangements in ammonia and organic acidemias with repeated episodes of metabolic crisis warrant early LT. Primary hyperoxaluria is a disorder of oxalate excess and accumulation in the body including kidneys due to liver-based enzymatic defect in oxalate metabolism. LT should be performed before development of renal failure, or else a combined or sequential liver kidney transplant is required. Livers from patients with maple syrup urine disease (MSUD) and familial hypercholesterolemia may be donated to cirrhotic patients, as they are structurally and functionally normal apart from an enzyme deficiency that may be compensated by other body tissues to sustain function. Such domino transplants have been successfully reported from India.[14]

Hepatoblastoma is the most common primary liver tumor requiring LT when adequate surgical resection after prior shrinkage by neoadjuvant chemotherapy is not feasible as in multifocal tumors and large ones occurring in the central part of the liver and encroaching all sectors with tumor invasion of hepatic veins and portal vein. Lung metastases that are amenable to chemotherapy or surgical resection do not constitute a contraindication to LT. Post-transplant neoadjuvant chemotherapy also improves survival. Rescue LT for tumor recurrence after initial surgical resection is a relative contraindication, as it carries a bad prognosis.[15] Hepatocellular carcinoma (HCC) is exceedingly rare in children apart from in those with diseased livers, especially metabolic disease such as tyrosinemia. Pediatric HCC is very poorly responsive to chemotherapy and when disease is confined to the liver, LT is indicated. Hemangioendotheliomas are benign tumors of infancy that usually regress with age. Large ones may occasionally cause acute liver failure (ALF) when LT may be required.

Contraindications to Liver Transplantation

Conditions where outcome is expected to be dismal constitute contraindications to a transplant **(Box 10.2.2)**. Additionally, when a very a poor quality of life is expected post-transplant as in advanced neurological injury, it is prudent to not offer transplantation. All efforts must be made to explore alternate therapies that may delay or subvert need for transplantation. Parameters to be assessed in a thorough pretransplant evaluation are tabulated in **Box 10.2.3**.

■ TYPES

Deceased Donor LT

Deceased donor LT (DDLT) is liver transplanted after donation from brain-dead donor. This is the most common modality in the West where organ allocation is made based on criteria that define disease severity and prioritize listing for LT.

Living Donor LT

Transplanted liver segment comes from a living donor who undergoes partial hepatectomy to provide the graft, usually right hemi-liver for adults

---

Box 10.2.2: Contraindications to liver transplantation (LT).
- Severe systemic sepsis
- Multiorgan failure
- Severe cardiopulmonary disease, portopulmonary hypertension unresponsive to medical therapy
- Extrahepatic malignancy
- Severe structural brain damage
- Uncontrolled AIDS
- Mitochondrial disorders, valproate-associated liver failure
- Uncorrectable congenital anomalies affecting multiple organs
- Niemann–Pick disease type C
- Alper's syndrome

> **Box 10.2.3:** Pretransplant evaluation.
>
> - Confirm indication, rule out contraindications
> - Detect and treat any active infections
> - Cardiopulmonary and renal assessment
> - Detect any associated anomalies that need to be addressed before LT (e.g. cardiac and vascular anomalies in Alagille syndrome)
> - *Assess and optimize nutrition*: MCT-rich normal protein diet, may use special formulas in cholestasis, nasogastric feeds, and total parenteral nutrition
> - Optimize bone health
> - Dental care, exclude and address caries
> - Complete age appropriate vaccinations, and prepone live vaccines (at least 3 weeks before LT)
> - Vaccinate family members
> - Psychosocial assessment and preparation of recipient and donor
> - Guide on social and logistical support including on avenues for financial support
>
> (LT: liver transplantation; MCT: medium-chain triglyceride)

and left lateral for children. This subverts the need to be on a waiting list and overcomes shortage on the donor pool.

LDLT has the advantage of providing a donor graft before morbid complications of decompensation have set in, ensuring good quality of the graft based on stringent donor evaluation and minimization of time lost in graft preservation. However, as a healthy individual is subjected to a major surgery, donor safety must be ensured, and any coercion prevented especially of dependent family members. The donor is thus almost always a blood relative as altruistic donation is subject to strict screening and permitted only in exceptional circumstances. A blood group compatible donor is preferred as results in ABO incompatibility are inferior.

Donation after Cardiac Death

Donation after cardiac death (DCD) is not yet practiced in our country; here, donor liver is retrieved after cardiac activity has ceased.

Donor Selection Criteria

The donor selection criteria broadly followed are given in **Table 10.2.1**.

Technical Variations

Split Liver Transplantation

The cadaveric donor liver is split into two recipients, usually one adult who receives the right lobe segment and the left lateral one is transplanted into a pediatric recipient. However, the donor liver may also be split into two adults.

Table 10.2.1: Donor selection criteria.	
Cadaveric donor	Living donor
Age <40 years	Age 18–55 years
Donation after brain death	BMI <27 Asians, <30 Middle East
Trauma as cause of death	No comorbidities
No communicable disease	Remnant liver volume >30%
Disease-free liver	Hepatic steatosis <30%, ideal <10%
No or minimal hepatic steatosis	No smoking or oral contraceptive pills for 6 weeks preprocedure

(BMI: body mass index)

Auxiliary Partial Orthotopic LT

This is a technique where the native liver is retained, and a partial liver graft is implanted alongside. This provides a chance for recovery of the native liver as in ALF[16] and is also useful in metabolic disorders[17] where a partial graft corrects the error.

Monosegment Liver Transplantation

In neonates and small children, the required graft size is very small and the discrepancy in donor and recipient size is overcome by using reduced left lateral segments.[18]

Dual Graft LDLT

Dual grafts from two donors are used to attain combined graft sufficiency while, at the same time, preserving adequate residual liver volume in the donors.[19]

Domino Liver Transplantation

In domino transplantation, the explanted liver from a patient who undergoes LT is transplanted to another recipient. This is feasible in a few metabolic disorders that do not cause liver injury including MSUD, familial hypercholesterolemia, and familial amyloidotic polyneuropathy.

■ TRANSPLANT OPERATION

Transplant surgery has three main phases beginning with the recipient hepatectomy where the native liver is removed. The recipient inferior vena cava (IVC) is retained in the now almost universally adopted piggyback technique, the donor IVC is anastomosed side to side to it in the next anhepatic phase. In this phase, the patient is without a functioning liver as the graft placement and the vascular anastomosis are done in this phase. The third final phase is that of neoperfusion when the graft gets reperfused. The biliary anastomosis is done in this phase. As the duct sizes are comparable and compatible, older children undergo a duct-to-duct anastomosis. Due to recipient-donor duct size disparity in younger children and in those with biliary tree anomalies like in biliary atresia and sclerosing cholangitis, the donor duct is implanted in a Roux-en-Y limb.

■ COMPLICATIONS

Major complications include bleeding, primary graft nonfunction, rejection, vascular complications, biliary complications, and infections. Systemic sepsis, renal failure, fluid imbalance, and pulmonary complications are more likely in the early postoperative period. The major complications are listed in **Box 10.2.4**.

> **Box 10.2.4:** Complications.
>
> - Primary nonfunction
> - Hepatic artery thrombosis, stenosis, pseudoaneurysm, or hemorrhage
> - Portal vein thrombosis and stenosis
> - *Biliary complications*: Leak, biloma, anastomotic, and nonanastomotic biliary stricture
> - *Rejection*: Acute, chronic, and antibody mediated
> - *Sepsis*: Bacterial, viral, and fungal
> - *Late graft dysfunction*: De novo autoimmune hepatitis and graft fibrosis
> - *Disease recurrence*: Autoimmune hepatitis, primary sclerosing cholangitis, PFIC 2, and primary biliary cirrhosis
> - *Late effects of immunosuppression*: Metabolic syndrome and renal dysfunction
> - Post-transplant lymphoproliferative disorder (PTLD)
> - Psychosocial issues
>
> (PFIC: progressive familial intrahepatic cholestasis)

Primary Graft Nonfunction

This exceedingly rare but catastrophic early complication manifests in the first few hours after transplant with increasing lactate levels and worsening coagulopathy and liver functions with failure of the patient to arouse after withdrawal of sedation. Failure of aggressive management leads to early graft loss and need for immediate retransplant. Exact etiology remains unknown but ischemia/reperfusion injury, hyperacute rejection, and/or suboptimal donor graft quality are postulated reasons.[20]

Vascular Complications

Both arterial and venous complications are more common in pediatric LT as compared to adults.[21]

Hepatic artery thrombosis (HAT) with an incidence of 5–8% occurring equally in LDLT and DDLT is a dreaded complication that may lead to graft loss due to massive hepatic necrosis. As the bile ducts are supplied by the hepatic artery, HAT also leads to biliary complications. Early HAT occurs within 30 days of LT and is the most common cause of graft loss in pediatric LT. Late HAT presents after 30 days in a less catastrophic manner and has a lower incidence. Presentations of HAT include increased bilirubin and transaminases, bile leak, hepatic abscess, fever, sepsis, and graft failure. Later presentations include bilomas and biliary strictures. Monitoring with serial liver function test (LFT) and Doppler ultrasound helps in early diagnosis that is confirmed by CT/MR angiography. Management strategies include endovascular radiological intervention as first line, secondly open surgical revascularization, and finally retransplantation.[22] Other arterial complications include hepatic artery stenosis, hepatic artery pseudoaneurysm, and hepatic artery hemorrhage.

Venous complications may involve the caval/hepatic vein or portal vein. *Portal vein thrombosis (PVT)* occurs in 5–10% cases and is more frequent in pediatric LT, LDLT, and split LT. Portal vein hypoplasia in biliary atresia makes these babies at particular risk of PVT. Narrow caliber of the portal vein, size disparity between recipient and donor, presence of thrombus pretransplant, large portosystemic collaterals, and use of cryopreserved venous conduits are predisposing factors. Early PVT is more common and presents as graft dysfunction that may rapidly progress to multiorgan failure. Later manifestations include ascites, splenomegaly, and upper gastrointestinal (GI) bleed. Early thrombectomy and portal vein reconstruction may be required to prevent graft loss. Other strategies include systemic anticoagulation, catheter-based thrombolytic therapy by percutaneous radiological intervention with or without stent placement to portosystemic shunting (TIPS). Retransplant may be required in unresolvable cases.[22] Stenosis ratio >50% or a portal velocity ratio >3:1 defines portal vein stenosis that may even be asymptomatic.

Outflow obstruction may occur due to kinking, stenosis, or thrombosis of the hepatic veins or the inferior vena cava. Clinical presentation is analogous to Budd-Chiari syndrome and angioplasty with stent placement is therapeutic.

Biliary Complications

Biliary complications with either duct-to-duct or Roux-en-Y anastomoses occur in 10–30% of pediatric liver transplant recipients.[20] Bile-stained abdominal drains are an indicator of bile leaks that occur early in the post-transplant phase and may either resolve spontaneously or require surgical intervention. These occur due to technical errors including graft handling, preservation, surgical technique, and ischemia. HAT must always be excluded.

Biliary stenosis/strictures occur more insidiously and require a high index of suspicion as the deranged liver functions may be attributed to sepsis/rejection. Late complications presenting more than 90 days of LT are classified as anastomotic or nonanastomotic strictures. They may present years after LT with increased gamma-glutamyl transpeptidase (GGTP) and alkaline phosphatase, recurrent cholangitis, and dilatation of intrahepatic biliary radicles on ultrasound or magnetic resonance cholangiopancreatography (MRCP). Endoscopic stricture dilation with stent placement helps but surgical revision of anastomosis or hepaticojejunostomy may be required.[23]

Rejection

Acute cellular rejection (ACR) occurring in the first few weeks of transplant has been reported with incidence ranging from 20% to 50% despite immunosuppression.[21] Increasing liver enzymes especially GGTP, leukocytosis with eosinophilia may develop before clinical features of fever, diarrhea, or jaundice manifest. These features of leukocytosis, fever, and cholestasis may make differentiation from infection difficult. Confirmation is by liver biopsy that shows the classical histological features of endothelial inflammation, portal triad lymphocytic infiltration with bile duct injury, and hepatocellular damage that are objectified by the Banff grading and rejection activity index. Increased immunosuppression with short-course corticosteroids, increased drug dosage to attain higher target levels, or addition of another immunosuppressant may be required.

Chronic rejection is uncommon and causes progressive ductopenia. Chronic ductopenic rejection (CDR) is defined as duct loss in >50% of portal tracts regardless of timing and reversibility. It may occur as early as 2–5 weeks post-transplant though the usual timing is from 6 weeks to 6 months. Resistant unresolving CDR may require retransplant; however, the rate of graft loss is <2%.[24]

Antibody-mediated rejection (AMR) is uncommon and causes graft dysfunction and acute tissue injury due to C4d antibody deposition in the presence of HLA-specific donor antibodies. AMR is difficult to treat and may cause early or late graft injury.

Infections

Systemic immunosuppression predisposes the LT recipient to opportunistic infections or reactivation of latent infections. Children with prolonged or complicated postoperative course are at higher risk. Though bacterial infections constitute the majority, fungal and viral infections are also common. Prophylactic antibiotics should be discontinued early to prevent emergence of resistant bacterial and fungal infections. *Pneumocystis carinii* infection is rare as sulfamethoxazole prophylaxis is routinely used. Infants and young children who are *Epstein-Barr virus* (*EBV*) and *Cytomegalovirus* (*CMV*) naïve are at particular risk of these viral infections and most units use prophylactic antivirals in the initial postoperative phase with regular screening to detect early infection. Post-transplant lymphoproliferative disorder (PTLD) may develop in *EBV*-naïve recipients and is related to viral load and degree of immunosuppression. As live vaccines are contraindicated, post-transplant seronegative unprotected children may develop varicella on exposure and should receive VZIG (varicella zoster immune globulin) within 96 hours and oral acyclovir should be started. If disease occurs, isolation and IV acyclovir should be instituted immediately as post-transplant chickenpox carries high morbidity and mortality.

Late Allograft Dysfunction

Late acute rejection and chronic rejection that occur insidiously or due to unresponsive acute rejection occur most commonly due to inadequate immunosuppression or poor drug compliance especially in adolescence. They cause progressive cholestasis and require aggressive immunosuppression to prevent graft loss. AMR may also cause late graft dysfunction.

Recurrent or de novo autoimmune hepatitis also presents similarly and is characterized by presence of nonorgan-specific autoantibodies and characteristic histological changes. All patients transplanted for autoimmune hepatitis need a meticulous follow-up with a very conservative approach to withdrawal or decrease in immunosuppression to prevent disease recurrence. Other diseases that may recur are primary sclerosing cholangitis and rarely, PFIC type 2.

De novo autoimmune hepatitis may occur in any graft and occurs in recipients not transplanted for autoimmune hepatitis. Risk factors for its occurrence are yet not clearly known but patients on single drug immunosuppression, those in whom steroids have been discontinued and those with acute rejection, were found to have a higher incidence. Most of them responded to prednisolone with or without mycophenolate.[25,26] Protocol biopsies in pediatric LT recipients done on follow-up have shown that chronic hepatitis with progressive fibrosis occurs in asymptomatic individuals[27] and is a risk factor for cirrhosis and autoantibody production.

■ IMMUNOSUPPRESSION

The immediate goal post-transplant is preventing acute or hyperacute graft rejection that is attained by intensive prophylactic immunosuppression in the perioperative period. This induction phase is followed by the maintenance phase that is less intense and involves progressive tapering of drugs over time as required to preserve long-term graft function with minimal side effects. The commonly used immunosuppressants with their doses and major side effects are outlined in **Table 10.2.2**.

Table 10.2.2: Commonly used immunosuppressants.

Agent	Dose	Side effects
Corticosteroids Induction: Methylprednisolone Maintenance: Prednisolone	10–20 mg/kg/day for 3–5 days Rapid taper of oral prednisolone to 0.2–0.3 mg/kg/day once daily	Impaired wound healing Hypertension Hyperlipidemia Hyperglycemia Cushingoid syndrome Metabolic syndrome Peptic ulcers Myopathy Osteoporosis Growth delay Cataracts
Antithymocyte globulin (ATG) Nonspecific T cell-depleting antibody	Induction with 1.5 mg/kg/day for 7–14 days	Fever Chills Hypotension (CK release syndrome)
Alemtuzumab Anti-CD52 T and B cell depleting antibody	Induction with 4 doses: 0.3 mg/kg each Before and after LT, day 3, and day 7	Mild CK release syndrome Pancytopenia
Basiliximab Nondepleting antibody: IL-2 receptor blocker	Induction with two IV doses day 0 and 4 <35 kg: 10 mg >35 kg: 20 mg	Well tolerated Rarely hypersensitivity reactions
Cyclosporine Calcineurin inhibitor	10–15 mg/kg/day in two divided doses first 2 weeks, then 4–12 mg/kg/day Target trough levels (ng/mL): 0–3 months: 200–250 3–12 months: 150–200 >12 months: 50–100	Nephrotoxicity Neurotoxicity Hyperkalemia Gingival hyperplasia Hirsutism Metabolic syndrome
Tacrolimus Calcineurin inhibitor	0.1–0.2 mg/kg/day in two divided doses Target trough levels (ng/mL): 0–3 months: 10–12 3–12 months: 8–10 >12 months: 5–7	Nephrotoxicity Neurotoxicity Hemolytic uremic syndrome Hyperkalemia Metabolic syndrome
Mycophenolate mofetil Antimetabolite	10–15 mg/kg/dose, maximum 1 g/dose Twice daily	GI symptoms: diarrhea, pain abdomen, nausea Cytopenias

Contd...

Contd...

Agent	Dose	Side effects
Azathioprine Antimetabolite	1–2 mg/kg/day once daily	Hepatotoxicity Bone marrow suppression
Sirolimus (Rapamycin) mTOR inhibitor	Not approved for LT Off-label use: Loading 3 mg/m² day 1, then 1–2 mg/m²/day Trough level 4–10 ng/mL	Concerns about HAT not substantiated Mouth ulcers Proteinuria Pneumonitis Impaired wound healing
Everolimus mTOR inhibitor	0.75 mg twice daily Trough level 3–8 ng/mL	Cytopenia Hyperlipidemia Impaired wound healing Proteinuria

(HAT: hepatic artery thrombosis; LT: liver transplantation; mTOR: mammalian target of rapamycin)

Induction Phase

Induction immunosuppression mostly involves use of high-dose steroids perioperatively to prevent graft rejection. Steroids are the only agent useful for both induction and maintenance immunosuppression, high-dose IV forms for the former and oral doses for the latter.

Steroid-free induction agents are antibody based and include lymphocyte nondepleting agents such as the IL-2R blocker basiliximab, or lymphocyte depleting, such as the polyclonal antibody rATG or the monoclonal anti-CD25 blocker alemtuzumab. Their primary indications are either to delay introduction of calcineurin inhibitors (CNIs), especially in patients with renal dysfunction, or to minimize steroid use.

Maintenance Phase

Maintenance phase is administered to all LT recipients and agents include corticosteroids, CNIs cyclosporine (CSA) and tacrolimus (TAC), antimetabolites mycophenolate (MMF) and azathioprine (AZT), and mammalian target of rapamycin (mTOR) inhibitors sirolimus and everolimus. CNI introduction has been the cornerstone of improved LT outcomes and most initial triple drug regimens involve TAC, MMF, and steroids that taper to TAC monotherapy by the 2nd year of LT.[28] TAC is superior to CSA, as rejection episodes are fewer and cosmetic side effects are lesser. Doses range from 0.1 mg/kg/day to 0.15 mg/kg/day orally given twice daily and are modulated based on trough levels that ranges between 10 ng/mL and 15 ng/mL early after transplant. Major CNI side effects are nephrotoxicity, neurotoxicity, metabolic syndrome, and hyperkalemia. Longitudinal monitoring of renal function is

> **Box 10.2.5:** Long-term post-transplant care.
>
> - Regular monitoring of liver function at increasingly spaced intervals as per time since LT
> - Monitor growth velocity
> - Monitor for persistent hepatic osteodystrophy, risk of fractures, and scoliosis
> - Assess school performance and attendance
> - Assess for psychosocial issues and mental health
> - Ensure compliance with IS
> - Sports and normal physical activity allowed after 2–3 months
> - Prevent infections with food hygiene, handwashing, and other measures
> - Live vaccines contraindicated, do not administer OPV to household contacts
> - Vaccinate with recombinant and killed vaccines including influenza and pneumococcus
> - Assess renal function, monitor for metabolic disease and diabetes
>
> (IS: immunosuppression; LT: liver transplantation)

mandatory. Most programs follow a policy of gradual steroid weaning and withdrawal within 3-6 months post-LT. However, patients transplanted for autoimmune hepatitis and primary sclerosing cholangitis need continuation of steroids in minimal possible doses. Use of sirolimus and everolimus in pediatric LT has remained largely limited as rescue agents for rejection or to minimize TAC side effects. Sirolimus has been shown to be useful in hepatoblastoma and PTLD to prevent tumor recurrence.[29]

Immunosuppressive drugs can affect growth, development, and learning, and serial assessments of these parameters must be made on long-term follow-up **(Box 10.2.5)**. Metabolic syndrome in childhood is an important risk factor for cardiovascular disease in adulthood. Obesity, hypertension, and diabetes may be caused by immunosuppression and appropriate interventions, and drug modifications should be done in a timely manner.

■ OUTCOMES

Excellent steadily improving outcomes of pediatric LT are being reported, as long-term follow-up data is now available across many centers all over the world. A retrospective cohort study of all consecutive patients undergoing isolated LT between 2000 and 2015 at The Hospital for Sick Children (SickKids) in Toronto, Canada has reported overall 1-, 5-, and 10-year patient survivals for the entire cohort as 95%, 90%, and 86%, respectively and overall 1-, 5-, and 10-year graft survival was 92%, 86%, and 79%, respectively.[30] 1-, 5-, and 10-year patient survival rates after LDLT (97%, 94%, and 94%) were significantly higher than after DDLT (92%, 87%, and 80%). Data from Japanese Liver Transplant Society, the largest pediatric LDLT cohort in the world comprising 2,224 recipients over a 21-year period, demonstrate 5- and 20-year patient survival rates of 85.4% and 79.6%, respectively.[31]

Blood-type incompatibility, recipient age, etiology of liver disease, and transplant era were found to be significant predictors of overall survival. Best survivals were reported in cholestatic liver disease including biliary atresia, the leading indication for LT in the cohort. Similar to the Japanese registry, data from the European registry has been equally encouraging.[32] SPLIT database analyses have reported 1-year graft survival of 94% and 10-year survival of 88%.[33] Data from 250 pediatric LDLT recipients, performed at Cliniques Universitaires Saint-Luc between July, 1993 and June, 2012, has reported 10-year survival of 93.2%.[34] There has been a steady learning curve with better outcomes attained in the last decade. In a cohort of 200 children from a single center, the overall patient survival rates before 2003 at 1, 5, and 10 years were 86.4%, 79.5%, and 78.4%, respectively; whereas after 2003, they were 95.4% and 95.4% at 1 and 5 years, respectively.[35]

In addition to surgical complications, infection remains the most serious threat perioperatively and also later, as recipients are on immunosuppression. Incidences of 1.36 episodes and 1.57 episodes per patient have been reported in two similar studies.[36,37] Data from SPLIT registry that included 2,291 children over an 11-year period reported that severe infectious complications occurred in 52% of patients within 15 months after LT. Infection caused more deaths than rejection (5.5% vs 0.6% of patients, p < 0.001).[38] Surgical complications include biliary complications (14–20.6%), HAT (6%–10.7%), and portal vein complications (stenosis or thrombosis, 4–9.1%). Acute cellular rejection is the most frequent histological abnormality (29.5–48.7%). Chronic rejection has a lower incidence, at 2–3.4%; whereas in pediatric liver transplants, overall rejection is reported at 5%.[35] PTLD has also been described with an incidence of 2.4–11.3%.

Outcomes reported from India are equally commendable. Mohan et al.[39] have reported their experience of 200 pediatric LDLT over a 12-year period where overall 1-year survival rate was 94% and 5-year actuarial survival was 87%, with no statistically significant difference between children weight <10 kg versus >10 kg. At a median follow-up of 2 years and 3 months, Sibal et al. reported patient survival of 88% in 50 pediatric liver transplants over a 5-year period.[40] Excellent results have also been reported in younger children. 100% survival for both graft and recipient in infants with weight less than 7.5 kg was reported in 2010.[41] Sepsis constitutes a major challenge and leading cause of mortality in our patients as reported in various series.[39,40,42]

As in the West, Indian series also report cholestatic liver disease as the most common indication followed by metabolic disorders. The first LT for Crigler–Najjar syndrome in India was performed in 2008.[13] Combined liver kidney transplants[43] and domino transplants[14] are also being successfully performed in India. Successful auxiliary LT for ALF has also been reported from India.[16] India being a predominantly patriarchal society, increasing numbers of fathers as liver donors reflect on the increasing confidence in the modality in our country.[44] Though southern part of the country has reported steady rise in DDLT, LDLT continues to be the predominant modality more so in children.[45]

◼ ONGOING CONCERNS

Studies on long-term morbidities after transplant and effects of immunosuppression are lacking from our country. LT requires lower immunosuppression compared to other organs. Moreover, Indian patients have been shown to do well on lower immunosuppression, as infections are more common in our scenario.[46] Regimens vary across different programs, but corticosteroids remain the induction agents of choice with dual agent regimens including calcineurin inhibitors and renal-sparing mycophenolate for the 1st year with the aim to come down to a single agent by the 2nd year.

Many skeptics believe that LT means trading one disease for another. The SPLIT database analysis has revealed that the ideal triad of normal growth, stable allograft function on single-agent immunosuppression, and an absence of immunosuppression-related complications are achieved in only about a third of recipients 10 years after LT.[33] Though children with LT have lower health-related quality of life compared to normal individuals, these impairments are comparable, if not better, to those of children with other chronic health conditions.[33,47] The chances of attaining *prope tolerance*, i.e. almost immune tolerant state where the recipient is alive with first allograft with no ongoing rejection episode on tacrolimus monotherapy with trough levels less than 3 ng/mL, 3-year post-LT survivals are maximum in the pediatric age group, especially in infants. Studies indicate that almost 20% pediatric patients may attain such immune tolerance.[48,49] Many of our patients are doing well on minimal immunosuppression and long-term data from leading programs needs to be reviewed to compute numbers. Lack of a database has been a big disadvantage and with the formation of the Indian Liver Transplant Registry, more data should be available in the coming years.

◼ REFERENCES

1. Starzl TE, Iwatsuki S, Van thiel DH, et al. Evolution of liver transplantation. Hepatology. 1982;2(5):14-36.
2. US Department of Health and Human Services; Organ Procurement and Transplantation Network. (2019). Data. [online] Available from https://optn.transplant.hrsa.gov/data. [Last Accessed December, 2019].
3. Poonacha P, Sibal A, Soin AS, et al. India's first successful pediatric liver transplant. Indian Pediatr. 2001;38(3):287-91.

4. Kakodkar R, Soin A, Nundy S. Liver transplantation in India: its evolution, problems and the way forward. Natl Med J India. 2007;20(2):53-6.
5. McDiarmid SV, Anand R, Lindblad AS. Studies of pediatric liver transplantation: 2002 update. An overview of demographics, indications, timing, and immunosuppressive practices in pediatric liver transplantation in the United States and Canada. Pediatr Transplant. 2004;8(3):284-94.
6. Malhotra S, Sibal A, Bhatia V, et al. Living related liver transplantation for biliary atresia in the last 5 years: Experience from the first liver transplant program in India. Indian J Pediatr. 2015;82(10):884-9.
7. Safwan M, Ramachandran P, Reddy MS, et al. Living donor liver transplantation for biliary atresia—an Indian experience. Pediatr Transplant. 2016;20(8):1045-50.
8. McPhail MJ, Wendon JA, Bernal W. Meta-analysis of performance of Kings's College Hospital Criteria in prediction of outcome in non-paracetamol-induced acute liver failure. J Hepatol. 2010;53(3):492-9.
9. Bernal W. Lactate is important in determining prognosis in acute liver failure. J Hepatol. 2010;53(1):209-10.
10. Squires RH Jr, Shneider BL, Bucuvalas J, et al. Acute liver failure in children: the first 348 patients in the pediatric acute liver failure study group. J Pediatr. 2006;148(5):652-8.
11. Dhawan A, Taylor RM, Cheeseman P, et al. Wilson's disease in children: 37-year experience and revised King's score for liver transplantation. Liver Transpl. 2005;11(4):441-8.
12. Arora NK, Arora S, Ahuja A, et al. Alpha 1 antitrypsin deficiency in children with chronic liver disease in North India. Indian Pediatr. 2010;47(12):1015-23.
13. Guru FR, Sibal A. Liver transplant for Crigler-Najjar syndrome. Indian Pediatr. 2010;47(3):285-6.
14. Mohan N, Karkra S, Rastogi A, et al. Living donor liver transplantation in maple syrup urine disease. Case series and world's youngest domino liver donor and recipient. Pediatr Transplant. 2016;20(3):395-400.
15. Otte JB. Progress in the surgical treatment of malignant liver tumors in children. Cancer Treat Rev. 2010;36(4):360-71.
16. Shanmugam NP, Al-Lawati T, Kelgeri C, et al. Auxiliary liver transplantation for acute liver failure. Indian Pediatr. 2016;53(1):67-9.
17. Shanmugam NP, Perumalla R, Gopinath R, et al. Auxiliary liver transplantation: a form of gene therapy in selective metabolic disorders. J Clin Exp Hepatol. 2011;1(2):118-20.
18. Enne M, Pacheco-Moreira L, Balbi E, et al. Liver transplantation with monosegments. Technical aspects and outcome: a meta-analysis. Liver Transpl. 2005;11(5):564-9.
19. Xu Y, Chen H, Yeh H, et al. Living donor liver transplantation using dual grafts: Experience and lessons learned from cases worldwide. Liver Transpl. 2015;21(11):1438-48.
20. Kamath BM, Olthoff KM. Liver transplantation in children: update 2010. Pediatr Clin North Am. 2010;57(2):401-14.
21. Spada M, Riva S, Maggiore G, et al. Pediatric liver transplantation. World J Gastroenterol. 2009;15(6):648-74.

22. Piardi T, Lhuaire M, Bruno O, et al. Vascular complications following liver transplantation: A literature review of advances in 2015. World J Hepatol. 2016;8(1):36-57.
23. Anderson CD, Turmelle YP, Darcy M, et al. Biliary strictures in pediatric liver transplant recipients—early diagnosis and treatment results in excellent graft outcomes. Pediatr Transplant. 2010;14(3):358-63.
24. European Association for the Study of the Liver. EASL clinical practice guidelines: liver transplantation. J Hepatol. 2016;64(2):433-85.
25. Vukotic R, Vitale G, D'Errico-Grigioni A, et al. De novo autoimmune hepatitis in liver transplant: State-of-the-art review. World J Gastroenterol. 2016;22(10):2906-14.
26. Venick RS, McDiarmid SV, Farmer DG, et al. Rejection and steroid dependence: unique risk factors in the development of pediatric posttransplant de novo autoimmune hepatitis. Am J Transplant. 2007;7(4):955-63.
27. Evans HM, Kelly DA, McKiernan PJ, et al. Progressive histological damage in liver allografts following pediatric liver transplantation. Hepatology. 2006;43(5):1109-17.
28. Wiesner RH, Fung JJ. Present state of immunosuppressive therapy in liver transplant recipients. Liver Transpl. 2011;17 Suppl 3:S1-9.
29. Jimenez-Rivera C, Avitzur Y, Fecteau AH, et al. Sirolimus for pediatric liver transplant recipients with post-transplant lymphoproliferative disease and hepatoblastoma. Pediatr Transplant. 2004;8(3):243-8.
30. Kehar M, Parekh RS, Stunguris J, et al. Superior outcomes and reduced wait times in pediatric recipients of living donor liver transplantation. Transplant Direct. 2019;5(3):e430.
31. Kasahara M, Umeshita K, Inomata Y, et al. Long-term outcomes of pediatric living donor liver transplantation in Japan: an analysis of more than 2200 cases listed in the registry of the Japanese Liver Transplantation Society. Am J Transplant. 2013;13(7):1830-9.
32. Adam R, Karam V, Delvart V, et al. Evolution of indications and results of liver transplantation in Europe. A report from the European liver transplant registry (ELTR). J Hepatol. 2012;57(3):675-88.
33. Ng VL, Alonso EM, Bucuvalas JC, et al. Health status of children alive 10 years after pediatric liver transplantation performed in the US and Canada: report of the studies of pediatric liver transplantation experience. J Pediatr. 2012;160(5):820-6.
34. Gurevich M, Guy-Viterbo V, Janssen M, et al. Living donor liver transplantation in children: surgical and immunological results in 250 recipients at Universite Catholique de Louvain. Ann Surg. 2015;262(6):1141-9.
35. Oh SH, Kim KM, Kim DY, et al. Clinical experience of more than 200 cases of pediatric liver transplantation at a single center: improved patient survival. Transplant Proc. 2012;44(2):484-6.
36. Bouchut JC, Stamm D, Boillot O, et al. Postoperative infectious complications in paediatric liver transplantation: a study of 48 transplants. Paediatr Anaesth. 2001;11(1):93-8.
37. Kim JE, Oh SH, Kim KM, et al. Infections after living donor liver transplantation in children. J Korean Med Sci. 2010;25(4):527-31.
38. Shepherd RW, Turmelle Y, Nadler M, et al. Risk factors for rejection and infection in pediatric liver transplantation. Am J Transplant. 2008;8(2):396-403.

39. Mohan N, Karkra S, Rastogi A, et al. Outcome of 200 pediatric living donor liver transplantations in India. Indian Pediatr. 2017;54(11):913-8.
40. Sibal A, Malhotra S, Guru FR, et al. Experience of 100 solid organ transplants over a five-yr period from the first successful pediatric multi-organ transplant program in India. Pediatr Transplant. 2014;18(7):740-5.
41. Kaur S, Wadhwa N, Sibal A, et al. Outcome of live donor liver transplantation in Indian children with bodyweight 7.5 kg. Indian Pediatr. 2011;48(1):51-4.
42. Varghese J, Gomathy N, Rajashekhar P, et al. Perioperative bacterial infections in deceased donor and living donor liver transplant recipients. J Clin Exp Hepatol. 2012;2(1):35-41.
43. Narasimhan G, Govil S, Rajalingam R, et al. Preserving double equipoise in living donor liver-kidney transplantation for primary Hyperoxaluria Type 1. Liver Transpl. 2015;21(10):1324-6.
44. Bhatia V, Sibal A. Are fathers catching up with mothers in liver donation? Indian Pediatr. 2013;50(1):158.
45. Narasimhan G. Living donor liver transplantation in India. Hepatobiliary Surg Nutr. 2016;5(2):127-32.
46. Varghese J, Reddy MS, Venugopal K, et al. Tacrolimus related adverse effects in liver transplant recipients: its association with trough concentrations. Indian J Gastroenterol. 2014;33(3):219-25.
47. Limbers CA, Neighbors K, Martz K, et al. Health-related quality of life in pediatric liver transplant recipients compared with other chronic disease groups. Pediatr Transplant. 2011;15(3):245-53.
48. Mazariegos GV, Sindhi R, Thomson AW, et al. Clinical tolerance following liver transplantation: long term results and future prospects. Transpl Immunol. 2007;17(2):114-9.
49. Miloh T, Barton A, Wheeler J, et al. Immunosuppression in pediatric liver transplant recipients: Unique aspects. Liver Transpl. 2017;23(2):244-56.

CHAPTER 11

NEPHROLOGY

11.1 Urinary Tract Infections
Pankaj Deshpande

11.1 URINARY TRACT INFECTIONS

Pankaj Deshpande

■ INTRODUCTION

"Urinary tract infection (UTI)" is a subject that raises much debate. It is one of the areas where the pendulum of recommendations has swung back and forth. Where the focus seemed to be on more investigations and terminating every "bug", recent years have seen a much-needed movement toward understanding that all "bugs" may not be UTIs and a barrage of tests may not be needed for everyone!

Urinary tract infections are one of the common infections seen in the pediatric outpatient department (OPD) and some children with UTI may be sick enough to need admission to the hospital. While various studies show different numbers, the general figure of 6–8% of children having UTI in childhood is agreed upon. In a 2008 systematic review, approximately 7% of children 2–24 months of age presenting with fever without a source and 8% of children 2–19 years of age presenting with possible urinary symptoms were diagnosed with a UTI.[1] One should, however, note that "positive urine culture" that is considered as evidence of UTI is not necessarily considered a gospel today. Hence, the numbers may vary depending on the criteria used for diagnosis of UTI. Contamination of urine samples leading to positive diagnosis of UTI is a major problem while looking at these numbers.

There is no doubt that repeated episodes of acute pyelonephritis may damage the kidney parenchyma and lead to long-term problems. Hence, diagnosis and treatment of UTIs along with prevention of long-term consequences are the aim of ideal management of UTIs.

The major problems that UTIs can lead to are:
- Sepsis, especially in babies less than 3 months of age, which could be life-threatening
- *Renal dysfunction:* If large parts of renal parenchyma are damaged
- *Hypertension:* Presence of parenchymal damage/"scars" can potentially cause hypertension
- *Preterm labor:* UTIs in pregnancy can precipitate preterm labor.

■ CLINICAL FEATURES

The presenting features in a child are the most important aspect of diagnosis of UTI. The temptation to label any infection as UTI because a focus is not found along with inappropriate focus on investigations has led us astray!

In neonates and very young babies, UTI may present only with fever. Poor feeding, lethargy, irritability, and occasionally prolonged jaundice may also be seen along with it.

In infants and younger children, the only presenting feature may be fever without any evident focus. A high index of suspicion in such children will allow for the diagnosis of UTI early. Urinary symptoms like dysuria, even if present may not be articulated well and hence, are likely to be missed. Persistent crying while voiding or increased frequency of voiding with small volumes may be seen in some children. Associated features may include vomiting, lethargy, and straining to void.

Urinary tract infection involving the upper tracts leads to pyelonephritis and carries major risk of damage to the kidneys. UTI involving the lower urinary tract is usually limited to the bladder and while there may be many symptoms, the risk for kidney damage is limited. However, in neonates, infants, and young children, it is impossible to differentiate between upper and lower UTIs based on symptoms. It is therefore recommended to consider every UTI in this age group to be upper UTI.

In older children and adolescents, the symptoms will vary, based on whether it is a lower or upper UTI. Lower UTI will present mainly with urgency, frequency, and dysuria while upper UTI is more likely to have high-grade fever (> 38°C), vomiting, loin pain and back or abdominal pain, and a general sick look.

In these conditions where UTI is suspected, a urine sample is asked for to diagnose UTI. A fair number of older children and adolescents present to the OPD with only abdominal pain and neither fever nor dysuria. These children are unlikely to have UTI and an inappropriately collected urine sample often misleads the clinician.

The presence of turbid or milky urine should also lead one to suspect UTI. However, in the absence of any urinary symptoms and fever, if such urine examination is normal, one should realize that there may be a different cause for the turbidity and not subject these children to antibiotic therapy. Other causes may include either mucus, especially with inadequate fluid intake in the child, amorphous phosphates, or severe hypercalciuria. Similarly, change in odor of urine or color is not diagnostic of UTI unless supported by evidence in the form of a urine examination. These are mistakenly believed to be UTIs and treated with antibiotics.

■ DIAGNOSIS

The most crucial aspect after clinical features is not just the urine tests but advice regarding when and how to do the tests.

One of the forgotten aspects is that a urine test should be done in a child only when we suspect a urine infection. This means that a urine test would be done only in a child presenting with fever having no cause or focus or presenting with urinary symptoms suggestive of a UTI like dysuria or frequency. In all other cases, the urine test loses significance in terms of diagnosis of a UTI.

Thus, a child clearly presenting with a cough or an upper respiratory infection should not have urine tests done. In such cases, as we shall discuss later, pyuria is often present and does not indicate a UTI. Similarly, in an asymptomatic child, any urine test done for diagnosis of UTI carries no significance. Thus, surveillance samples in children who have had a prior UTI carry no meaning and should not be advised. One should also bear in mind that a urine test may be asked for as the child presents with a fever with no focus but by the time the urine test result is available, there may be a florid cough or some other focus that is evident. The urine test in such cases is likely to reveal pyuria but does not indicate a UTI.

On routine microscopy, presence of greater than 10 white blood cells (WBC)/microliter in an noncentrifuged sample of urine is considered significant pyuria though many centers report the number of WBC per high power field and more than 5 in a centrifuged urine sample is significant pyuria.[2] Significant pyuria may be seen in any fever, dehydration, urinary calculi, or any form of nephritis. So, it is not exclusive to UTIs. The "pus" cells are inflammatory cells and will be seen in inflammation present anywhere in the body. Hence, a severe cough may also be the reason for pyuria as may be appendicitis.

The diagnosis of UTI hinges on the urine culture as most literature has been telling us. Unfortunately, focus only on urine culture without the aspect of when and how to do it leads to erroneous results that cause more grief and harm. The urine culture has to be sent when we suspect a urine infection. Similar to the microscopy, it means that there should be fever without focus or urinary symptoms. A positive urine culture in asymptomatic children does not mean a urine infection. While a study of children with bronchiolitis showed positive urine cultures without a UTI,[3] the differentiating feature between a UTI and asymptomatic bacteriuria (ASB) is the presence or absence of urinary symptoms.[4]

The next important task for the clinician is to explain how the urine has to be collected. Without this advice, the urine samples collected lose significance and cannot be relied upon to provide the accurate clinical answers. Once ascertained that the clinical features justify a urine sample, the genital area should be washed with normal soap and water. Bag urine samples are not recommended for the high contamination rate that is associated with them. In a study, the contamination rate was as high as 63%.[5]

There are several methods to collect urine:
- *A mid-stream urine sample*: The initial urine is discarded, and the middle part of the urine is collected. Ideally, every urine sample to be sent for urine culture should be a mid-stream urine sample. This may be an arduous task even in adults. Hence, a clean catch urine sample is acceptable in children.
- *A clean catch urine sample:* When the baby passes urine either on appropriate stimulation or involuntarily, it is collected in a bottle.

- *Catheter sample:* A urinary catheter is inserted ensuring strict asepsis and the urine sample is collected.
- *Suprapubic aspirate:* The bladder is an abdominal organ till 5 years of age. Hence, inserting a needle attached to a syringe just above the pubic symphysis to collect urine is remarkably safe with virtually no complications and avoids all possibilities of contamination. As it is an invasive procedure, there seem to be few takers for this method in OPD practice.

Once the urine sample is collected, it needs to be sent to the laboratory immediately. It should be plated within an hour. A delay of greater than 1 hour with the sample in room temperature causes growth of contaminant organisms thereby invalidating the urine culture report. If such a delay is anticipated, the sample should be kept in the refrigerator at 4°C. Often, the laboratory advises the parents to collect the first morning urine sample for a child and thus, it is not uncommon to find that the urine sample may be collected early morning (like 6 am) and the sample is then provided to the laboratory on the way to work at 8 am with the urine sample sitting in room temperature and carried in the pocket. Unless an effort is made to communicate and educate the parents and understand their difficulties, the desired urine sample is unlikely to come by.

While collecting the urine sample in girls, it is also important to ensure that there is no vulval redness. In the presence of vulval redness, both the microscopy and urine culture may be abnormal with no real evidence of a UTI. The presenting features of vulval redness are similar to UTI. There will be urgency, frequency of voiding along with dysuria. One of the important points to note is that the pain is present not only during voiding but often throughout the day. The common worsening factor for this symptom is repeated washing. Emollient creams are required to treat this condition.[6]

Depending on the method used for urine collection, the results of urine culture need to be interpreted. A growth of a single organism with more than 100,000 colony forming units (CFU)/mL is considered significant in a mid-stream or clean catch urine sample. However, recent studies and recommendations indicate that only a positive urine culture in the absence of pyuria is not enough to diagnose a UTI. The logic and understanding is that in the presence of an active infection, one would expect inflammation and hence, a significant pyuria.[7] The absence of pyuria raises the question of ASB again. So, merely because a urine culture is positive, one should not label a child as having a UTI. Several studies have highlighted this aspect. On comparison of mid-stream urine samples with suprapubic aspirates in children with suspected symptoms, only 34% of children with a positive urine culture on mid-stream urine sample had positive diagnosis of UTI on suprapubic aspirate.[8] This clearly shows how high the contamination rate is and therefore relying on only urine culture may be fallacious. Another study concluded that only 25% of positive urine cultures in 335 patients were actual UTIs while the rest were ASB or contamination. Unfortunately, all received antibiotics and hence the authors argued that antimicrobial use was inappropriate as only urine cultures were being chased.[9]

In a urine catheter sample, the risk of contamination is lower and hence any growth of a single organism greater than 10,000 organisms/mL is considered significant. One should remember that this is for a sample taken when the urinary catheter is inserted and removed for the purpose of collecting a sample. Again, as mentioned above, care has to be taken that UTI does not develop after the catheterization. An indwelling urine catheter present in patients, especially in intensive care may be used for a sample in such patients but sometimes a biofilm develops in such catheters and hence, cautious interpretation of the results obtained is warranted.

In the case of a suprapubic aspirate, any growth is considered significant, as there is no possibility of contamination in such a sample. It should be noted that periurethral flora is the cause of contamination and as suprapubic aspirate obtains urine from the bladder, this is obviated.

Conditions like detrusor instability or irritable bladder, where children have frequency, urgency and daytime wetting are often misdiagnosed as UTI. Similarly, hypercalciuria or renal calculi with the presence of pyuria are also mistakenly treated as UTI. Clear evidence of UTI should be the sole basis for prescribing antibiotics and this would go a long way in preventing antibiotic resistance in bacteria. Similarly, mere presence of "bacteria" in a routine urine examination usually reflects contamination, especially with no symptoms of UTI and absence of significant pyuria.

One of the newer modalities that one can use in the clinics is a urine "dipstix" or "multistix". The presence of leukocytes can be detected by means of the leukocyte esterase enzyme on the dipstix. Mere presence of leukocytes has the same possibilities as pyuria on a routine microscopy and cannot be labeled as UTI. Conversion of nitrate-to-nitrite by bacteria is used as a basis to have the nitrite test on dipstix. A positive test, especially with positive leucocytes, is a strong predictor of a UTI. However, one should be aware of false positive nitrite test also. If the urine sample is not fresh, growth of contaminant organisms may lead to a positive nitrite test. Similarly, repeated exposure to air of the multistix makes a false positive test more likely. A false negative test is likely if the urine has not been in the bladder long enough. Once these factors are kept in mind, the multistix can be an important tool for early detection of the possibility of UTI. A urine culture must still be sent to confirm UTI.

■ ETIOLOGY

Most of the urine infections are ascending infections. This means that the urethra is the site of entry for the causative organisms and they then spread the infection to the bladder and kidneys. Normal periurethral flora present usually prevents infections. However, under disturbed conditions, the same organisms may cause a UTI or allow pathogenic bacteria to take hold in the urethra thus causing a UTI.

Gram-negative organisms are the common cause of UTIs. *Escherichia coli* is the most common organism causing UTIs. *Proteus, Klebsiella,* and *Pseudomonas* are the other organisms seen often. Infections with enterococci are also being seen frequently at present. Gram-positive organisms like *Staphylococcus* can also cause UTIs and in such cases, obstructive problems in the urinary tract are seen commonly associated with it.

The recent worry is ESBL organisms (extended-spectrum beta-lactamase organisms). They show resistance to the common antibiotics used. While it was believed that it was seen commonly in children in hospitals as a nosocomial infection, community UTIs are being seen with ESBL organisms because of widespread and rampant use of antibiotics, even when they are not indicated. However, the mere presence of resistant organisms on urine culture need not set off panic alarms in clinicians, as we shall discuss later in therapy.

Urinary tract infections with organisms other than bacteria can also present difficulties in diagnosis and treatment. Fungal infections with organisms like *Candida* are seen especially in immunocompromised hosts, in children on long and multiple courses of antibiotics in hospital and even in normal neonates or babies up to 3 months of age. Development of fungal balls can cause obstruction in the urinary tract and treatment needs to be aggressive with surgical intervention in such babies.

Viral cystitis is far more common and may occur in normal children also. The typical example is viral hemorrhagic cystitis by adenovirus or enteroviruses.

■ TREATMENT

Antibiotics

It is clear that the mainstay of immediate treatment of an acute UTI is antibiotic therapy. But certain simple rules need to be remembered. The foremost among them is that when a UTI is suspected on the basis of significant pyuria, urine culture has to be sent immediately before any antibiotics are started. This sounds logical and simple. In practice, it seems to be done much lesser number of times than needed. Often, one dose of an antibiotic is already administered before urine culture is sent. It may be due to many reasons that include lack of awareness, microscopy result available in evening and culture sent next morning, inability to collect a sample and so on.

If a culture is not done before starting antibiotics, there are different problems encountered. Firstly, a negative culture will not rule out a UTI as antibiotics have already been administered. Secondly, diagnosis of UTI cannot be made with certainty. More importantly, if the child remains symptomatic after 48–72 hours of initial therapy, the lack of an appropriate urine culture report makes it impossible to determine as to which antibiotic should be used to eliminate the UTI. Hence, a urine culture before starting antibiotics is a must for appropriate diagnosis and therapy. It will also allow one to confidently state that there is no evidence of UTI, if the urine culture is negative and helps to stop antibiotics unless the other infection causing the symptoms warrants it.

Urine culture showing growth of a small number of organisms (nonsignificant level to diagnose UTI) is not considered a UTI. So, growth of 1,000 or 10,000 organisms in midstream or clean catch sample do not indicate a UTI and should not be treated as UTI.

In most children, an oral antibiotic is the first choice of an antibiotic. The antibiotic used should take into consideration the local practices and organisms commonly seen. We should also realize that rampant use of amoxicillin and cotrimoxazole in the past have rendered them useless for treating most UTIs at present as the organisms are resistant to them. This also carries a lesson for us, as we cannot afford to lose more antibiotics in this manner, as there are hardly any newer antibiotics on the horizon.

The antibiotic used commonly is a third-generation cephalosporin, cefixime in the dose given in the table below **(Table 11.1.1)**.[10] Other antibiotics used are also given in the table. Quinolones are not necessarily the first choice but may be used when the choice is limited bearing in mind the adverse effects on cartilage in growing children. If the child can tolerate oral medications, does not have vomiting, is not very sick looking, then oral therapy remains the therapy of choice. The fever and symptoms usually settle down within 48–72 hours.

If the child is sick looking or toxic, has persistent vomiting, is unable to tolerate oral antibiotics, then parenteral antibiotics [intravenous (IV) antibiotics] have to be used. The choice of antibiotic is as per the table given **(Table 11.1.2)**.[10] One of the common errors done is prescribing a combination of two antibiotics. That is unnecessary and a single antibiotic is as effective. If an injectable cephalosporin is used, changing to an oral cephalosporin is easier when the change to an oral antibiotic is made. Once the fever

Table 11.1.1: Oral antibiotics for urinary tract infection (UTI).	
Cefixime	10 mg/kg/day in 2 divided doses
Co-amoxiclav	35 mg of amoxicillin in 2 doses
Ciprofloxacin	10–20 mg/kg/day in 2 divided doses
Ofloxacin	15–20 mg/kg/day in 2 divided doses
Cephalexin	50 mg/kg/day in 3 doses

Table 11.1.2: Intravenous antibiotics for urinary tract infection (UTI).

Ceftriaxone	75–100 mg/kg/day in 1–2 doses
Amikacin	10–15 mg/kg/day in a single dose
Gentamicin	5–6 mg/kg/day in a single dose
Co-amoxiclav	35 mg/kg/day of amoxicillin in 2 doses

settles and the symptoms abate and the child can tolerate oral food well, the antibiotic can be changed to an oral one. This helps to reduce hospital stay. If an aminoglycoside is used, this option becomes limited and hence, parenteral therapy may have to be continued for at least 7 days. Single daily doses of aminoglycosides with appropriate dose can also be used in such cases. It is also important to remember that aminoglycosides cause ototoxicity and renal toxicity. Hence, it has to be given slowly and estimation of serum creatinine has to be done at 48 hours of therapy with aminoglycosides if therapy is to be continued with the same agent. The other option, though not ideal is to switch to a sensitive cephalosporin to complete the course. In neonates and babies less than 3 months of age, parenteral therapy is the preferred route of administration.

In cases where upper UTI is suspected, a total course of 14 days (IV and oral together) is recommended. In infants and babies, where it is generally prudent to consider every UTI as upper UTI, 14 days therapy is given. In children treated as outpatients where the child is not sick-looking, a total of 7–10 days may suffice.

The urine culture report is available after 48–72 hours of starting therapy. If the child has shown a clinical response, the antibiotic sensitivity report has no significance. By clinical response, we mean the absence of fever, symptoms abated (like dysuria), and the child looking better with no vomiting. In such a case, even if the organism isolated shows resistance to the antibiotic that has been started, there is absolutely no need to change the agent. A 14-day course of the same antibiotic should be completed. This is because the *in vitro* and *in vivo* sensitivities may not always match as high concentration of the antibiotic can be achieved in the urine. As mentioned earlier, if the culture shows a nonsignificant growth, it should not be labeled as a UTI. If there has been no clinical response till the culture report has become available, then the child often needs admission to be given the appropriate antibiotic to which the organism shows sensitivity.

If there is no clinical response in 48–72 hours, there should be a renewed look into the reasons for a poor response. These include the presence of obstruction that would preclude good drainage and response, development of an abscess in the renal parenchyma, a different infection (not a UTI), or infection with a resistant organism. Resistant organisms like ESBL organisms may need carbapenems like meropenem to eradicate them. Meropenem is used in the dose of 10-20 mg/kg per dose three times a day for at least 7-10 days.

After the course of antibiotics is complete, it is important to note that a urine culture does not have to be repeated. In fact, repeating a urine culture in an asymptomatic patient leads to a spiraling downward trend of multiple antibiotics to get rid of a nonexistent UTI. Similarly, if the microscopy is repeated, chasing every pus cell to eliminate it is a pointless exercise that will only increase antibiotic resistance. Similarly, rechecking of urine at specific intervals is to be avoided. Contaminated samples and ASB are a bane in asymptomatic patients and they are best left alone.

Fungal infection needs a prolonged course of antifungal therapy for at least 4 weeks and in many cases, 6 weeks. The presence of fungal balls causing obstruction may need drainage procedures and instillation of antifungal agents like amphotericin in the ureters. It should be noted that fluconazole achieves good urinary concentration while amphotericin concentration in the urine is not high enough though the systemic and blood levels are very good.

Viral cystitis usually needs only symptomatic therapy and it resolves in 7-10 days. It is a fearful period for the parents as they can see gross hematuria and clots on regular basis for many days. Reassurance has to be given to them.

It should also be noted that often, a lack of identifying the source of infection leads one to look at the urine report and latch on to innocent aspects to label it as a UTI. Presence of blood and protein without pyuria is not indicative of a UTI. Similarly, turbidity, haziness without pyuria does not make it a UTI. Let us all take care to not throw antibiotics in such cases as the easy way out.

■ PREVENTION

The only aspect that remains in constant focus for UTIs, unfortunately, is imaging and antibiotic therapy. As mentioned earlier, it is recurrent episodes of acute pyelonephritis that can lead to renal damage. Thus, it would make far greater sense to focus on aspects that help in preventing further UTIs.

Constipation has been shown to be one of the major factors in repeated UTIs.[11] It causes incomplete voiding and hence urinary stasis in the bladder and therefore, predisposes to UTIs. Unless this history is elicited, the child has a high risk of repeated UTIs. It should also be borne in mind that constipation treatment is not only for a few days. It can take weeks and months for the children to establish a regular pattern of passing soft stools and therapy should be continued for that length of period. Encouraging fiber and fruit in the diet along with fluids, of course, goes hand in hand with this treatment.

The bladder has good defense mechanisms and one of the foremost is voiding urine regularly that eliminates any bacteria that may otherwise be present in the bladder. Infrequent voiding can therefore lead to UTIs. This is usually associated with constipation. A child should void at least six to eight times in the daytime. That flushes the bladder and prevents UTIs.

The third arm of this problem is inadequate fluid intake. This not only causes constipation but also leads to infrequent voiding, thereby leading to UTIs. Constant encouragement is required to ensure that the child has the requisite amount of fluids. In infants, at least a liter of fluid (including milk) is recommended, while in older children at least 1.5 liters of fluid daily help in regular voiding. A different variety of fluids may be tried like fruit juices. However, fizzy drinks and drinks like tea and coffee are not recommended as they cause bladder stimulation and may lead to detrusor instability.

Adequate hygiene has to be advised and yet, "over-hygiene" is detrimental. Repeated washing after every void causes vulval redness in many girls with sensitive skin and they get diagnosed as having UTIs. That is to be avoided. Washing during a bath and after stools is advised along with emollient creams in such cases.

Children are quite engrossed in play activities and hence reluctant to go to void urine despite having the urge to do so. Apart from irregular voiding, this also leads to a situation where the child runs out quickly from the bathroom so that he/she does not miss a moment of "fun" outside. This again predisposes to UTI due to urinary stasis. This can be objectively assessed on ultrasound examination of the kidneys and bladder. A postvoid residue of greater than 20 mL in children greater than 3 years of age is a risk factor for further UTIs. Children have to be encouraged to do double voiding. This would mean that after the child voids, the child voids again after a gap of 30 seconds or a minute. This ensures complete bladder emptying. To make it "fun", one can advise the child to sing his/her favorite song after the first void and on completion of the song, void again!

Apart from these measures, simple issues like use of a cotton underwear, avoiding bubble baths helps in preventing urethritis. Parents should also be counseled that children do not get UTIs from dirty toilets. That is often the reason given for infrequent voiding.

It is estimated that at least one-third to half the children with an episode of UTI develops a repeat UTI.[12] For clinical purposes, frequent or recurrent UTIs are said to be present when the child has at least two episodes of UTIs in 6 months despite adequate measures to prevent UTIs. UTIs occurring years apart do not qualify for a radical change in management but need a relook at the risk factors again.

Circumcision has been noted to reduce UTIs significantly. A study showed that circumcision reduced 90% of recurrent UTIs.[13] It is also noted that circumcised children have a lower incidence of UTIs. However, that is not sufficient grounds for subjecting every child to a circumcision. The risk factors that affect bladder bowel function mentioned above should be addressed and if UTIs keep occurring despite that, circumcision can be offered. Use of steroid creams like diprovate for a short period (fortnight) also helps in treating physiological phimosis that many children display.

■ RADIOLOGY

Radiological investigations in a child with UTI are done with the aim of determining, if any risk factor can be identified that would lead to further UTIs and/or renal damage. The Working Group of the Royal College of Physicians in 1991 was entrusted with the task of formulating a strategy of investigations for a child with UTI. The reason it was constituted was because there was no uniformity in investigating UTIs and every center seemed to be doing a different set of investigations including tests like IV pyelograms (IVPs). They came up with a set of investigations that were recommended for every child who had a proven UTI.

It was clear that younger children and infants were at more risk of renal damage and hence they were subjected to the maximum investigations. With increasing age, the suggested number of investigations was reduced. It should be noted that all were not in favor of so many investigations, but the consensus was that these are required. **Table 11.1.3** provides the recommendations.

Clinical considerations have been taken into account in these recommendations. Thus, when a 3-year-old child presents with a UTI, ultrasound scan and dimercaptosuccinic acid (DMSA) are strongly recommended but micturating cystourethrogram (MCUG) can also be done, if the clinical scenario demands it. This would include an abnormal ultrasound or repeated proven UTIs, etc. Similarly, a DMSA scan in a child of 8 years is left to the clinical discretion. These recommendations have provided the much-needed uniformity in investigating UTIs and avoiding tests like IVPs. The trend at present, worldwide, seems to be that even these investigations are far too many and much debate has been generated on whether some of these can and should be avoided. With a realization that some children have renal dysplasia and not all changes are secondary to UTIs, focus has shifted back to appropriate diagnosis of UTI and minimal investigations.

It is important not just to know what investigations are to be done but the timing when they are to be done and what they can show.

Table 11.1.3: Radiological tests for urinary tract infection (UTIs) in children.

Age	Investigations recommended
Less than 1 year	US scan, DMSA scan, and MCUG
1–6 years	US scan and DMSA scan
More than 6 years	US scan

(DMSA: dimercaptosuccinic acid; MCUG: micturating cystourethrogram; US: ultrasound)

The ultrasound scan of the kidneys and bladder is recommended for every child who has a proven UTI. The anteroposterior diameter (AP) of the renal pelvis should be insisted upon. Any diameter that is greater than 10 mm is significant. Conversely, though the impression may say dilatation of the renal pelvis, if the diameter is less than 10 mm, it is not significant. Similarly, the prevoid and postvoid volumes are predictors for further UTIs in children greater than 3 years of age. Very often these are not mentioned in the report. Hence, the request for ultrasound should include a request for both these.

An ultrasound scan is done as soon as possible. This would mean that it should be done while the child is admitted in an inpatient and within a week, if the child is being treated as an outpatient. Dilatation of the ureters, small/hypoplastic kidneys, renal calculi, cysts in the kidneys, and bladder thickness all convey important messages. Beware of the bladder thickness. Often an ultrasound scan reports saying that the bladder wall is thickened suggesting cystitis **(Fig. 11.1.1)**. Never get misled by this! Diagnosis of UTI, as clearly outlined earlier is based on urine reports. Often the bladder thickness is more because the prevoid volume is low and in a collapsed state, the bladder wall appears thicker (like a collapsed balloon). Unless the bladder is full, commenting on bladder thickness may be fraught with errors **(Fig. 11.1.2)**.

One of the common finding is "hypoechoic areas" in the kidney parenchyma suggestive of a collection or abscess and the recommendation for a computed tomography (CT) scan. If the child has clinically improved, the chances of an abscess are very low and these actually represent parenchymal changes in the kidneys secondary to the infection. They do not improve immediately and may take up to 2 months to resolve completely. There is no urgency of a CT

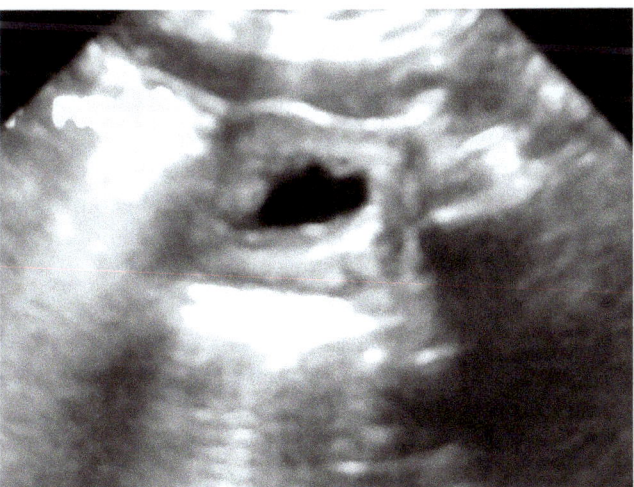

Fig. 11.1.1: Bladder reported as thick-walled suggesting "cystitis".

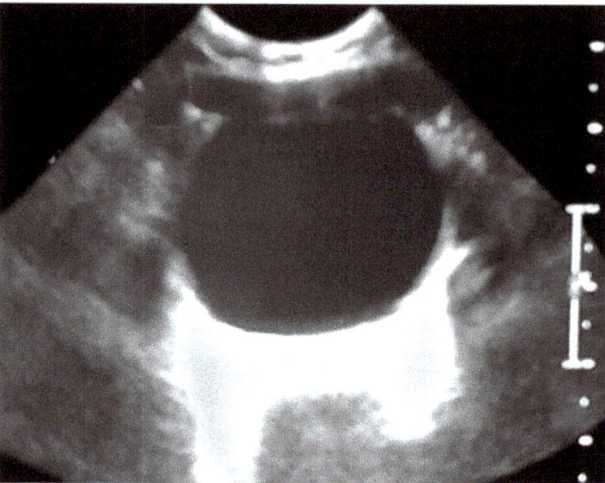

Fig. 11.1.2: The same bladder, when full showing normal walls.

scan in such patients. If the child continues to have high-grade fever, is toxic, then search for an abscess can be considered.

Subtle changes on ultrasound scan like loss of corticomedullary junction or increased echogenicity of the kidneys, especially in follow-up ultrasound a few months later may indicate renal dysplasia and need to be kept under observation.

Dimercaptosuccinic acid scan should be done at least 4–6 months after the episode of UTI. One needs to understand the principle involved in a DMSA scan. The radioactive material is "picked up" by functioning nephrons and the gamma camera can then "see" these areas on the scan. Thus, only functioning nephrons will be seen. After an episode of pyelonephritis, where the kidney parenchyma has been involved, there are changes seen in the uptake, which can revert to normal in about 6 months. Thus, a DMSA done soon after a UTI (acute DMSA) is likely to show abnormalities that can become normal in 6 months. A repeat DMSA then becomes necessary. We are interested in the long-term outcome and follow-up of children who show permanent changes on DMSA, not acute resolving ones. Hence, the prudent course of action is to do DMSA 6 months after a UTI so that only permanent abnormalities can be seen.

The other common error made is to label all changes on DMSA as scarring. As explained above, DMSA only shows areas of reduced uptake. Thus, renal dysplasia where the kidneys have formed abnormally will also have an abnormal uptake. This cannot be labeled as scarring. A typical scar on DMSA is a wedge-shaped defect in otherwise normal kidneys. The other changes where the uptake is diffuse, or the kidneys look like amorphous blobs are not scarring but renal dysplasia. A single UTI cannot damage the kidney to such an extent that the function drops dramatically, and it looks like an amorphous blob! This appearance is present from birth and would have been present if the DMSA had been done before the UTI also. The basic presumption that all kidneys are completely normal on DMSA before the UTI is fallacious and should be rectified.

Figures 11.1.3 and 11.1.4 show how acute changes resolve in 6 months though it was reported as scarring on the first DMSA scan.

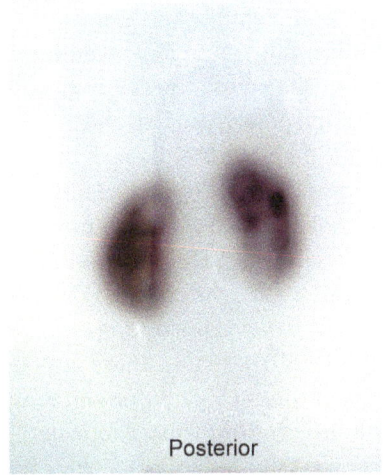

Fig. 11.1.3: Dimercaptosuccinic acid done 10 weeks after a UTI, reported as scarring in both kidneys.

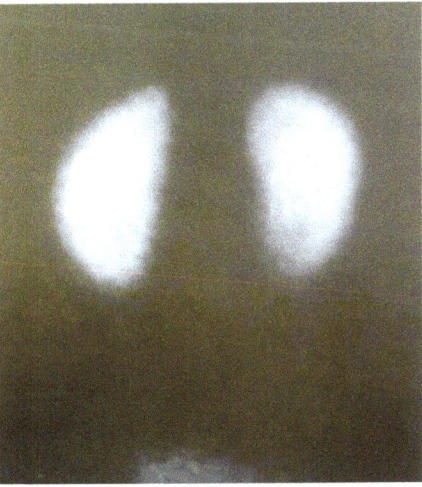

Fig. 11.1.4: Dimercaptosuccinic acid of same child 6 months later, normal kidneys with no scarring.

Micturating cystourethrogram has been given enormous importance beyond what is required. Fortunately, recent literature has revisited this area and tried to bring some sanity to the proceedings. The younger the child, more the risk of renal damage and hence MCUG is recommended in every infant who has a proven UTI. However, just demonstrating vesicoureteric reflux (VUR) does not mean the end of the world or that all questions are answered. The important thing for clinicians to note is that MCUG should be done under proper antibiotic cover. Too many children develop UTIs after an MCUG, which is inexcusable and avoidable.

Vesicoureteric reflux is of 5 grades and primary VUR (not due to causes like posterior urethral valves and neurogenic bladder) is what is being talked about in UTIs. Grade 1 to 3 is where the reflux remains in the ureters and does not go beyond the renal pelvis. Grade 4 and 5 are associated with severe dilatation and tortuosity of the ureters and reach the renal pelvis and calyces. Whatever grade VUR is seen, it is present from birth. So, when it is detected in an 11-month-old baby or a 3-year-old girl, remember they have lived with it from birth and not suffered UTIs! VUR worsens a UTI by increasing the risk of pyelonephritis but is rarely ever the cause of UTIs. VUR can be present in normal persons also and a study done a long-time ago suggested that 1% of the population may have VUR.[14] Thus, there are changes that cause UTI and then VUR can worsen the UTI. These are precisely the factors, which were discussed earlier in prevention. Thus, if repeated UTIs are prevented by adopting simple measures, VUR is no longer a clinical problem and trying to "fix" every VUR is then pointless. Just because VUR is present, does not mean the kidneys are damaged!

There are specific indications for doing MCUG in UTIs:
- Proven UTIs in infants
- Repeated UTIs in children despite adequate simple measures to prevent UTIs
- Abnormalities on ultrasound scan (like dilatation) and sometimes on DMSA scan.

Of course, MCUG has to be done in conditions like urethral obstruction in posterior urethral valves, neurogenic bladder, etc.

While MCUG can be done soon after a UTI, the risk that the UTI may not have cleared is higher and hence it is better done 4 weeks after the UTI episode under appropriate antibiotic cover.

■ PROPHYLAXIS

Using a small dose of an antibiotic to prevent repeated UTIs has been an age-old practice. Recent data from studies suggest that this practice can be changed. In children with VUR, prophylactic agents were used so that they would be taken at bedtime to prevent bacteria from gaining a foothold in the bladder, as most children will not void through sleep.

The premise was that infants and children diagnosed with any grade of VUR were at increased risk for recurrent UTIs and therefore required antibiotic prophylaxis to prevent UTIs and long-term sequelae like hypertension and renal failure.[14] For ethical reasons that absence of prophylactic agents may harm the kidneys and other reasons, very few studies actually assessed the outcome and as UTI definitions were not stringent, it was incorrectly presumed that prophylaxis was highly beneficial.

The American Academy of Pediatrics Subcommittee on UTIs had published guidelines in 2011. Their meta-analysis of six studies for children less than 24 months of age did not show a significant benefit of antibiotic prophylaxis, either in infants without VUR or in those with grades I-V VUR.[7] If one reviews the Cochrane meta-analysis of 12 studies or recent studies like the Randomized Intervention for Children with Vesicoureteric Reflux (RIVUR trial) along with older studies like Montini et al. or PRIVENT trial, it is generally noted that the results are varied as there was heterogeneity in the study design for all. There was a small benefit noted but it was noted that prophylactic antibiotics would have to be prescribed for long periods in many children (2 years for nine children) to prevent recurrent UTIs in 1 child.[15,16] More importantly, all trials found a similarly low rate of worsening of renal scarring in both cases and controls. This would beg the question about how effective prophylaxis really is, as there seems no evidence of it preventing renal scarring or long-term sequelae.

Based on these observations, it is clear that prolonged use of prophylaxis as was being done in the past (till the child was 5 or 7 years old, so called beyond the age of scarring) is no longer recommended or useful. Prolonged use of prophylaxis comes with its own problems.

The foremost among them being that taking medications regularly on a daily basis is an impossible task for many people, especially children. In fact, studies regarding whether prophylaxis was being taken were done by analyzing the urine samples to detect the antibiotics, it was clear that more than 25% had poor compliance.[17] So what use are the prophylactic antibiotics if they are not being taken at all? Apart from the possible adverse effects, the risk of which is minimal, the more difficult problem remains of bacteria developing resistance to these antibiotics because of prolonged exposure. Clearly, we do not want this.

Hence, prophylaxis is not necessarily recommended for VUR in all cases. For the Indian scenario, one could use prophylaxis till the child is 1-year-old or for a period of 6 months–1 year from the last UTI. If there are no further UTIs, prophylaxis can be stopped. It is also worth noting that as children get older, it becomes easier to diagnose UTIs and hence prophylaxis really has no role then. This is because diagnosing UTIs and treating them promptly are likely to be reducing the risk factors for renal damage considerably.

With regards to which prophylactic agent should be used, the ideal agent should be cheap, easy to use and not change the periurethral flora. Only trimethoprim and nitrofurantoin satisfy all these criteria. In the absence of trimethoprim as a single agent, cotrimoxazole can be used in the dose of 2 mg/kg/day of the trimethoprim component. Similarly, nitrofurantoin can be given as a bedtime dose of 1-2 mg/kg/day. Unfortunately, nitrofurantoin is quite unpalatable, and children tend to have vomiting with that agent.

If both agents cannot be used, cephalexin can be used in the dose of 15 mg/kg/day as a single dose. Cephalosporins tend to change the periurethral flora and hence, the risk of developing UTI with severely pathogenic organisms remains.

Prophylaxis can also be used in children after the first episode of UTI till all investigations are complete and till the risk factors for repeat UTI like constipation are treated. In fact, by treating bowel bladder problems and using the simple measures mentioned in prevention earlier, most UTIs can be prevented.

There is no need to rotate prophylactic agents. This implies that the previous advice about changing prophylactic antibiotics so that one antibiotic is given for 1 month and another for the next month is no longer recommended.

■ LONG-TERM OUTCOME

Recent data suggest that even recurrent UTIs in otherwise normal kidneys do not lead to long-term problems in the kidneys even if there may be minor scarring.[18]

Our focus on VUR and UTIs has probably diverted our attention from the real issue of kidney function. Recent data from the end-stage kidney disease statistics has started realizing that kidney failure may be due to abnormally formed kidneys (meaning renal dysplasia and inadequate nephron number). Thus, the category of reflux nephropathy has started shrinking as the correct diagnosis of renal dysplasia is being made in such children. Though renal function may be adequately supported in younger children, during puberty, the rapid growth phase, the renal function drops, leading to renal failure.

Subtle changes on ultrasound (loss of CM differentiation), and diffuse reduced uptake on DMSA scan may be the only clue for diagnosis, as symptoms will appear too late [when glomerular filtration rate (GFR) is less than 20 mL/min].

More importantly, regular monitoring of the renal function with a serum creatinine, urine protein/creatinine ratio, and a blood pressure done annually are mandatory. It is surprising to see how few children seem to have these tests done regularly. The creatinine should be interpreted in terms of estimated glomerular filtration rate (eGFR) with the modified Schwartz formula:

eGFR = 0.5 × height of the child in cm/serum creatinine in mg/dL.

Values should be more than 80 in children more than 2 years of age.

Proteinuria may also not be evident on a routine urine test as specific gravity and pH change the protein reading in a semiquantitative assay. Hence, a urine protein/creatinine ratio is required, and though normal values should be less than 0.5 (both protein and creatinine in mg/dL), values above 1 are dangerous for the kidneys. Heavy proteinuria on a persistent basis is the single most lethal factor in decreasing renal function.

In children with renal dysplasia, surgical treatment of VUR or trying to fix VUR in any way will not change the outcome. Hence, it is imperative that we diagnose the children with this condition.

Renal dysplasia would mean that the number of nephrons is not normal though the kidneys may look normal on ultrasound scan. Oligohydramnios provides an important early clue for diagnosis. When the nephron number is low, in early stages (infancy and early childhood), the nephrons provide adequate function but when the body size increases, especially in the rapid growth phase of puberty, the kidneys can no longer provide function that is sufficient for the entire body. Consequently, chronic kidney disease ensues. Regular monitoring of renal function by the modified Schwartz formula applied to serum creatinine, monitoring of an early morning urine protein/creatinine ratio and blood pressure will help to diagnose renal dysplasia and take adequate measures to preserve and prolong kidney function. These tests should be done at least once a year till the child is past puberty at least.

■ CONCLUSION

Urinary tract infections are common in children. The most important aspect of UTI is appropriate diagnosis. Only in the presence of symptoms suggestive of UTI, a urine sample should be sent. Adequate explanation about urine collection should be given to the parents failing which the urine results may lead to erroneous diagnosis and management. Antibiotics in confirmed UTI should be for a period of 14 days in suspected pyelonephritis and 7-10 days in UTIs managed on an outpatient basis in older children.

Instead of jumping into radiological tests, the goal of prevention of further UTIs should be achieved by addressing issues like constipation, bowel bladder disturbances, adequate fluid intake, and regular voiding. Radiological tests should be done at the appropriate time (ultrasound soon after a UTI, DMSA 6 months later) and care should be taken not to get misled by conclusions provided by these tests. VUR on MCUG does not need surgical treatment always. Prophylaxis with a small dose of antibiotics is used for a short duration like 6 months to a year and not for 5-7 years as in the past.

Finally, the most important aspect is monitoring of renal function by serum creatinine (applying the modified Schwartz formula), a urine protein/creatinine ratio, and regular blood pressure readings done at least once a year.

■ REFERENCES

1. Shaikh N, Morone NE, Bost JE, et al. Prevalence of urinary tract infection in childhood: a meta-analysis. Pediatr Infect Dis J. 2008;27(4):302-8.
2. Robinson JL, Finlay JC, Lang ME, et al. Urinary tract infection in infants and children: Diagnosis and management. Pediatric Child Health. 2014;19(6):315-25.
3. Ralston S, Hill V, Waters A. Occult serious bacterial infection in infants younger than 60 to 90 days with bronchiolitis: a systematic review. Arch Pediatr Adolesc Med. 2011;165(10):951-6.
4. Trautner BW, Grigoryan L. Approach to a positive urine culture in a patient without urinary symptoms. Infect Dis Clin North Am. 2014;28(1):15-31.
5. Al-Orifi F, McGillivray D, Tange S, et al. Urine culture from bag specimens in young children: are the risks too high? J Pediatr. 2000;137(2):221-6.
6. Fischer GO. Vulval disease in pre-pubertal girls. Australas J Dermatol. 2001;42(4):225-34.
7. Subcommittee on Urinary Tract Infection, Steering Committee on Quality Improvement and Management, Roberts KB. Urinary tract infection: clinical practice guideline for the diagnosis and management of the initial UTI in febrile infants and children 2 to 24 months. Pediatrics. 2011;128(3):595-60.
8. Krzemień G, Szmigielska A, Artemiuk I, et al. False positive urine cultures in children under two years of age-own research. Dev Period Med. 2014;18(2)203-8.
9. Silver SA, Baillie L, Simor AE. Positive urine cultures: A major cause of inappropriate antimicrobial use in hospitals? Can J Infect Dis Med Microbiol. 2009;20(4):107-11.
10. Bagga A, Babu K, Kanitkar M, et al. Consensus statement on management of urinary tract infections. Indian Pediatr. 2001;38(10):1106-15.
11. Hari P, Bagga A. Antimicrobial prophylaxis for children with vesicoureteral reflux. N Engl J Med. 2014;371(11):1071-2.
12. Paintsil E. Update on recent guidelines for the management of urinary tract infections in children: the shifting paradigm. Curr Opin Pediatr. 2013;25(1):88-94.
13. Bader M, McCarthy L. What is the efficacy of circumcision in boys with complex urinary tract abnormalities? Pediatr Nephrol. 2013;28(12):2267-72.
14. American Academy of Pediatrics, Committee on Quality Improvement. Subcommittee on Urinary Tract Infection. Practice parameter: the diagnosis, treatment, and evaluation of the initial urinary tract infection in febrile infants and young children. Pediatrics. 1999;103(4 Pt 1):843-52.
15. The Rivur Trial Investigators. Antimicrobial prophylaxis for children with vesicoureteral reflux. N Engl J Med. 2014;370(25):2367-76.
16. Robinson JL, Finlay JC, Lang ME, et al. Prophylactic antibiotics for children with recurrent urinary tract infections. Pediatr Child Health. 2015;20(1):45-7.
17. Smyth AR, Judd BA. Compliance with antibiotic prophylaxis in urinary tract infection. Arch Dis Child. 1993;68(2):235-6.
18. Craig JC, Williams GJ. Denominators do matter: it's a myth—urinary tract infection does not cause chronic kidney disease. Pediatrics. 2011;128(5):984-5.

CHAPTER 12

UROLOGY

12.1 Vesicoureteric Reflux
Senthil Ganesh Kamaraj, Uday Bhaskar

12.1 VESICOURETERIC REFLUX

Senthil Ganesh Kamaraj, Uday Bhaskar

■ INTRODUCTION

Vesicoureteral reflux (VUR), a retrograde flow of bladder urine into the upper urinary tract, is one of the most commonly encountered pediatric urological anomalies (1%). Vesicoureteral reflux has been categorized etiologically into primary and secondary.
- *Primary VUR* is thought to represent an abnormal anatomy and function of the ureterovesical junction (UVJ), with a normal bladder and urethra.
- *Secondary VUR* implies an acquired condition as a result of increased intravesical pressure secondary to neurogenic and non-neurogenic bladder dysfunction, or outlet obstruction.

Depending on its severity, VUR leads to pyelonephritis, renal scarring, hypertension, and chronic renal insufficiency (reflux nephropathy) and such sequelae have been the primary concern for diagnostic and therapeutic interventions for VUR.

Because of lack of robust prospective trials the scientific community ends up with treatment options rather than recommendations in most scenarios of reflux management.[1]

■ EPIDEMIOLOGY

Vesicoureteral reflux is diagnosed usually after investigation of either urinary tract infection (UTI) or antenatal hydronephrosis. The *incidence of VUR in children* with UTI is typically around 30–50%, with an even higher incidence in *infants* with UTI.[1]

Of the one of every 500–1200 live births detected to have *antenatal hydronephrosis*, VUR is identified in about 15–38%, with the highest incidence noted in infants with persistent postnatal renal abnormalities.[2]

Male preponderance is seen in infants with VUR diagnosed from antenatal hydronephrosis while *females predominate* with VUR diagnosed after presenting with UTI. *Boys* tend to present at a younger age, and often have more severe degrees of VUR, especially if diagnosed in infancy.

Vesicoureteral reflux appears to be a *heritable disorder* and identical twins have been observed to have a higher incidence.[3] VUR occurs in other siblings of affected children as well (as high as 40–50%). Various studies suggest a dominant inheritance pattern with a variable penetrance. Evidence suggests that different genes act on different families.[4]

Children of African ancestry have a lower rate of VUR than those of Caucasian genetic background (ratio of 3.4 to 1) and girls of Asian ancestry are suggested to be less likely to have scarring associated with reflux than Caucasian girls.[5]

■ PATHOPHYSIOLOGY

The ureterovesical junction (UVJ)[6,7] is anatomically and functionally adapted to allow intermittent passage of the urinary bolus from the ureter into the bladder while preventing the retrograde flow of urine (reflux into the ureters and kidneys).

To achieve these, the ureter enters the bladder detrusor obliquely *(intramural ureter)* and courses beneath a submucosal tunnel of appropriate length *(submucosal ureter)* before opening onto the trigone. This results in the intramural ureter to stay shut during bladder contraction and prevents retrograde flow of urine during. And hence, reflux is prevented **(Figs. 12.1.1A and B)**.

In addition to this, there is an active component of contraction and relaxation at the UVJ as result of functional integration of the inner and outer layers of the ureteric musculature with the trigonal structure and the bladder wall respectively. This allows the ureter to slide freely during filling and emptying and results in active flow of urine from the kidney through the ureter into the bladder **(Fig. 12.1.2)**.

The intravesical ureter (the intramural segment plus the submucosal tunnel) has been estimated to lengthen with age, providing rationale for spontaneous VUR resolution with maturation and the mature length was thought to be achieved by 10–12 years of age.[8,9]

Inadequate trigonal function allows the ureteric orifice to displace laterally and migrate away from the bladder neck during bladder filling, leading to reduction of the intravesical ureteral length.

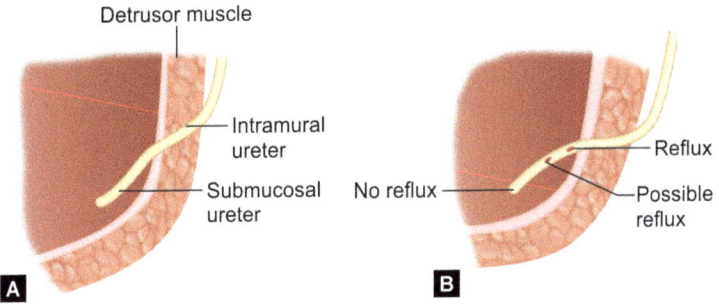

Figs. 12.1.1A and B: (A) *Normal ureterovesical junction (UVJ):* Demonstration of the intravesical ureter (intramural + submucosal); (B) *Refluxing UVJ:* In contrast to nonrefluxing orifice, there is an inadequate length of the intravesical ureter, compromising the flap valve mechanism. The red dots signify the possible levels of termination of the ureter in the trigone.

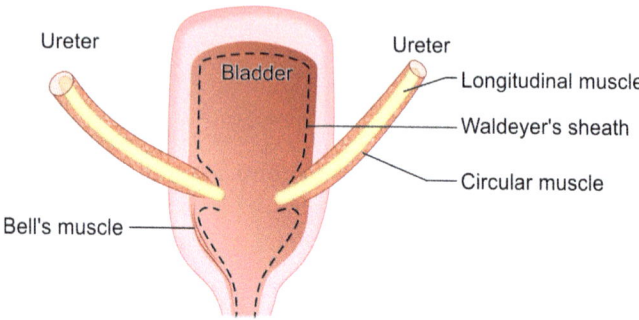

Fig. 12.1.2: Passage of the distal ureter through the ureteral hiatus in the bladder wall. Ureteral inner longitudinal muscle fibers extend into the trigone to form Bell's muscle. The Waldeyer's sheath anchors the distal ureter at the hiatus.

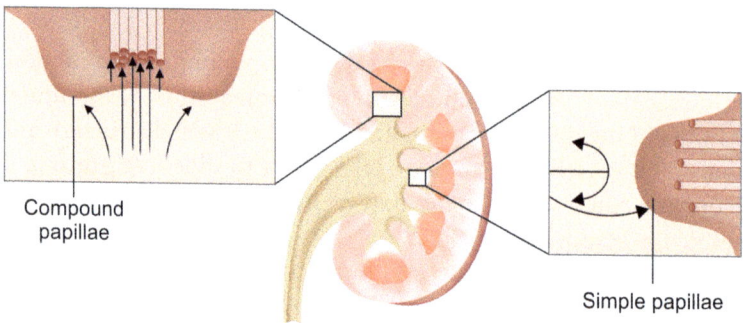

Fig. 12.1.3: *Simple papillae* are the most common type. They have slit-like papillary duct openings on their *convex surface*. These papillae are compressed by increases in pelvic pressure, preventing urine from entering the papillary ducts [intrarenal reflux (IRR)]. *Compound papillae* are formed by the fusion of two or more simple papillae. In compound papillae, some ducts open onto a flat or *concave surface* at less oblique angles. Increased intrapelvic pressure may permit IRR. Compound papillae usually are found in the renal poles.

Of critical importance is the concept of intrarenal reflux (IRR), which has been demonstrated clinically[10] and which is usually inhibited by the oblique entry of the papillary ducts into the papillae of the renal pyramids (simple and compound). Increased intravesical pressure is associated with increased risk of occurrence of IRR, resulting in scarring as does IRR secondary to infection. The usual oblique entry of the papillary ducts onto the surface of simple papillae inhibits IRR **(Fig. 12.1.3)**.

■ CLASSIFICATION

Vesicoureteral reflux is graded from I to V according to the International Grading System.[11] This classification system is based not only on the proximal extent of retrograde urine flow and ureteral and pelvic dilatation, but also on

Table 12.1.1: International Grading System of vesicoureteral reflux.	
Grade I	Reflux into to lower ureter
Grade II	Reflux into the ureter and renal pelvis—undilated collecting system
Grade III	Reflux into the ureter and renal pelvis—moderate dilatation of the collecting system
Grade IV	Moderate dilation of the collecting system and ureter with or without kinking—normal or minimally deformed fornices
Grade V	Gross dilatation and kinking of the ureter. Marked dilatation of the collecting system. Blunted fornices with loss of papillary impression

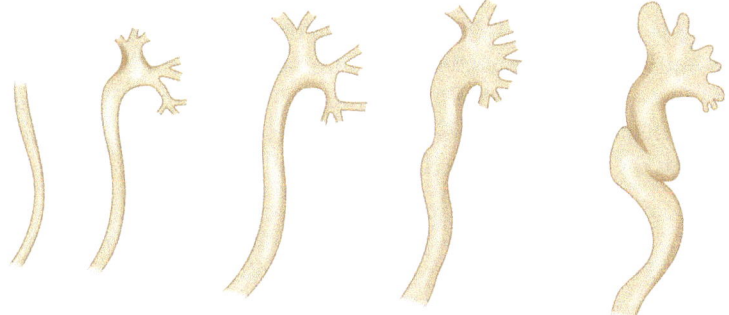

Fig. 12.1.4: Grades of vesicoureteral reflux.

the resultant anatomy of the calyceal fornices. The current classification is shown in **Table 12.1.1 and Figure 12.1.4**.

■ NATURAL HISTORY OF VESICOURETERAL REFLUX

The natural history of VUR is extremely variable and ranges from *Spontaneous resolution; Clinically silent scar formation; Recurrent pyelonephritis; Recurrent pyelonephritis with hypertension and end-stage renal disease (ESRD)* (which is a rarity with current level of awareness amongst pediatric practitioners).

Numerous factors may contribute to the potential for resolution, including the patient's age, the grade of reflux, and the intravesical detrusor filling pressures.

A lower reflux grade correlated with a better chance of *spontaneous resolution*. The chances of reflux resolution are enhanced in *infant males during first year* and to a certain extent through the second year of life. This is in part may be a result of normalization of the high detrusor pressures in normal infant bladders or a heightened degree of trigonal growth in normal infant bladders.

Spontaneous resolution is relatively independent of grade in secondary reflux, implicating management of primary bladder dysfunction as the primary prognostic variable.

Renal injury due to VUR may take the form of focal scarring, generalized scarring with atrophy, and failure of renal growth.[12] As a result, kidneys in patients with VUR should be observed not only for scarring but also for renal growth, typically with serial renal ultrasound. Reflux-induced renal injury is usually a result of the association of VUR with UTI. Renal changes secondary to reflux is most likely in children under the age of 2 years especially in boys.

Secondary reflux can also cause renal injury in the absence of UTI due to the pressure effects from neurogenic bladder and bladder outlet obstruction (BOO).

Rarely patients may not have had an evident prior infection or will have the first recognized infection at or near the time of diagnosis of ESRD. Glomerular lesions play an important role in the progression of reflux nephropathy (RN). There is a clear association between RN, "heavy" proteinuria, and glomerular lesions that resemble focal segmental glomerulosclerosis.[13]

■ DIAGNOSIS AND WORKUP OF A CHILD WITH VESICOURETERAL REFLUX[1,14]

General Evaluation

As VUR and UTIs may affect the overall wellbeing and renal function, measurement of height, weight, blood pressure and serum creatinine in selected cases, history of UTIs, evaluation of bladder symptoms if present would include the primary assessment of a child with reflux and UTI at initial presentation.[1]

Radiologic assessment includes ultrasound, micturating cystourethrogram (MCU) and nuclear imaging [dimercaptosuccinic acid (DMSA) scan].

Evaluation of Bladder Bowel Function (in Toilet-trained Children)

In toilet-trained children, kids with bladder/bowel dysfunction (BBD) may be at a greater risk of UTIs and renal injuries. BBD may include children presenting with lower urinary tract symptoms (such as urgency, frequency, dribbling, voiding postponement. etc.), secondary to abnormal storage and emptying of the bladder (dysfunctional voiders)—abnormal bowel pattern such as constipation and soiling—or a combination of both.

Vesicoureteric reflux may be co-existing or secondary to BBD in these kids. *Focused history taking* would provide adequate documentation as to its existence and can be further confirmed by uroflowmetry and ultrasound examination if necessary.

It is worth mentioning that incidence of UTIs (primary and break through), and failure of treatment (endoscopic or surgical) is higher in kids with BBD.

Bladder/bowel dysfunction if present needs to be effectively addressed and managed before venturing upon any specific line of management in a child with VUR.

Documentation of Urinary Tract Infection

Documentation of true UTI is paramount in the appropriate management of a patient with reflux. Many other variables such as presence of fever, method of collection and transport of the urine specimen, results of urine routine analysis are also responsible for accurate assessment and interpretation of UTI apart from significant bacteriuria on culture.

A *urine specimen in neonates* should be obtained through suprapubic aspiration or catheterization of the bladder. The collection of urine with the use of adhesive bags in the perineal area has a high risk of contamination UTI. Urinalysis does not carry a great significance in neonates and small infants as compared to older kids. Some studies suggest using an enhanced urinalysis to predict UTI in infants, using a hemocytometer cell count and Gram staining on uncentrifuged urine. Results are reported as the number of white blood cells (WBCs) per microliter, a cut-off of 10/mL or more is used to define pyuria.[15]

The diagnosis of a *UTI in older children* is typically based on the presence of pyuria on urinalysis and bacteriuria on urine culture. The sensitivity and negative predictive value of the enhanced urinalysis are higher than those of the standard urinalysis.[16] Currently, these methods are not widely used.

The *gold standard* for diagnosing UTI is positive culture for a single organism. A positive culture is defined as growth of 10,000 or more colony-forming units (CFU) per milliliter if the urine is obtained using suprapubic aspiration, or 100,000 CFU/mL or more if it is obtained through catheterization.[16,17] But about 20% infants with symptomatic UTI show low bacterial counts. Serious consideration of a UTI may be a safer option in infants and especially neonates because they are at high risk for bacteremia, especially when there is high level of suspicion.

Ultrasonography of Kidney, Ureter, and Bladder

The mainstay of *renal imaging* in VUR management is ultrasonography. It is a nonionizing and noninvasive imaging platform, ideally suited for assessment of upper tract (kidneys and renal pelvis) and lower tract (ureters and bladder) and serial follow-up of renal growth and development. Loss of corticomedullary differentiation, or an increase in the overall echogenicity of the kidney, suggests some degree of renal functional impairment. Secondly, it aids in differentiating between primary and secondary reflux in most clinical scenarios. Further, in *reflux nephropathy* imaged by color Doppler ultrasound, renal resistive index measurements derived from blood flow in the inter-lobar and arcuate arteries are significantly increased in the presence of higher grades of reflux and correlate positively with scintigraphy findings from the same renal unit.

Cystographic Imaging

The *gold standard for diagnosis of VUR is the MCU* especially at the initial workup.[1] It permits accurate grading of the severity of VUR, which is important when assessing prognosis and planning treatment.

The grading system is based on extent of filling and dilatation of the ureter, renal pelvis and calyces on filling the bladder with contrast per urethra (*see* **Fig. 12.1.4**).

Recent imaging studies such as *voiding ultrasound and MRI MCU* have promised good results, less invasive and no ionizing radiation. However, the conventional MCU still remains the Gold standard (also allowing concurrent assessment of the bladder and the urethra).

Nuclear cystogram (direct nuclear cystogram—DRCG), which involves suprapubic injection of the tracer (technetium 99) and asking the child to void, is another investigation that can be used to identify and grade VUR in toilet-trained children. Reflux is detected on the Gamma camera images. It is less invasive and involves less ionizing radiation as compared to the conventional MCU. Currently, it plays a role in the follow-up of patients previously diagnosed with VUR on the conventional MCU (**Fig. 12.1.5**).

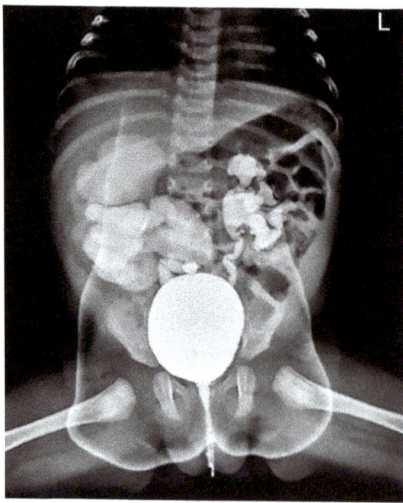

Fig. 12.1.5: Micturating cystourethrogram showing bilateral high-grade reflux.

Renal Scintigraphy

99mTc-labeled DMSA is the most sensitive modality for visualizing scarring and quantifying differential renal function. Because pyelonephritis impairs tubular uptake of radiotracer, these areas will fail to radio emit photons and appear as photopenic regions in the resultant renal cortical images. Even though many such affected areas in the kidney resolve, especially if prompt medical treatment is possible[18] when they persist, irreversible renal damage or scarring is said to have occurred.

One advance in nuclear scintigraphy of the kidneys is single-photon emission computed tomography (SPECT imaging). This approach reconstructs three-dimensional (3D) images of the renal cortical architecture, which can be viewed in any aspect in 360° of rotation **(Fig. 12.1.6)**.

Top-down Approach

The top-down approach is an interesting concept based on the notion that only clinically relevant reflux with potential to cause renal injury is worthy of uncovering, with the critical assumption that VUR in the absence of scintigraphic renal abnormality is unlikely to cause future renal damage. Only a DMSA renal scan is obtained after a febrile UTI, with cystography reserved only for patients with abnormal scintigraphy findings. Children with a negative DMSA scan undergo no further evaluation unless they develop recurrent UTI, in which case a voiding cystourethrography (VCUG) should be obtained.[19]

Associated Anomalies

Vesicoureteral reflux and pelviureteric junction obstruction (PUJO) are two of the most common pathologic conditions in pediatric urology. Thus, it is not

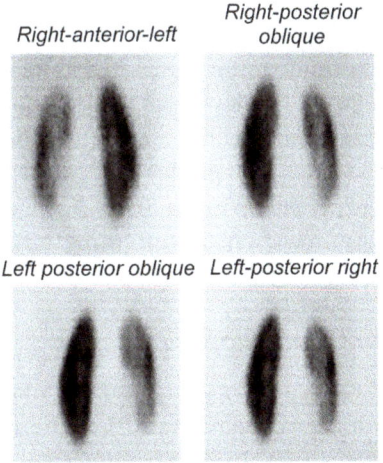

Fig. 12.1.6: Nuclear scan (DMSA) showed reduced tracer concentration and scarring over the right kidney as a result of right high-grade reflux.

unusual that these two conditions co-exist. The incidence of VUR associated with UPJO ranges from 9 to 18%.[20]

Posterior urethral valves and neurogenic bladder are two urological conditions which should be ruled out before confirming the diagnosis of primary VUR. Vesicoureteral reflux is the most common abnormality associated with complete ureteral duplications (duplex kidneys or double moieties).

Bladder diverticula, multicystic dysplastic kidneys (MCDK), megacystis-megaureter association, Prune-Belly syndrome are few other urological conditions associated with VUR. VUR also has been described in association with a number of congenital conditions and syndromes. These include the VACTERL association (Vertebral, Anal, Cardiac, Tracheoesophageal, Renal, and Limb anomalies), CHARGE syndrome (Coloboma, Heart disease, Atresia choanae, Retarded development, Genital hypoplasia, and Ear anomalies), and imperforate anus.

■ TREATMENT OPTIONS FOR A CHILD WITH VESICOURETERIC REFLUX[1,14]

The treatment options are either medical or surgical.

Medical Management

Medical or conservative line of management by means of continuous antibiotic prophylaxis with observation, appropriate imaging and follow-up; and circumcision in boys, is the most widely followed line of management of most patients with VUR, especially uncomplicated, low and intermediate grades of reflux (Grades I, II and III).

This is a result of the understanding that
- Most cases with low grade reflux undergo spontaneous resolution—low grade reflux and reflux in first few years of life as do a lesser percentage of intermediate and high grade reflux
- VUR grades I and II (80%), VUR grades III-V (30-50%)
- Resolution can be expected up to the first 4-5 years of life
- The sequelae of reflux such as inflammation, scarring and renal compromise do not occur if the kids are free of infection.

Role of Continuous Antibiotic Prophylaxis

Many prospective and retrospective studies have confirmed the effectiveness of continuous antibiotic prophylaxis (CAP) in the management of VUR. Recently, few studies negate the absolute benefit in low grade, uncomplicated reflux.

In grades III and IV reflux, and in bigger kids with lower urinary tract dysfunction (LUTD) and all reflux grades antibiotic prophylaxis plays a definite role in preventing further UTIs.

Nevertheless, it may be hard to decide and select patients who do not require CAP. Hence, it may be worthwhile considering CAP in all kids with reflux until they are toilet-trained and confirming absence of LUTD.

Drugs[8] commonly used as CAP:
- *Cephalexin:* 10 mg/kg once daily
- *Ampicillin:* 20 mg/kg once daily
- *Amoxicillin:* 10 mg/kg once daily

In infants over two months:
- Tmp-smx (Trimethoprim-sulfamethoxazole) at 2 mg/kg once daily is the antibiotic of choice
- Nitrofurantoin at 1–2 mg once daily is the other drug most commonly used.[9]

Circumcision[21]

During early infancy circumcision may be considered as part of the conservative approach as it reduces the risk of infection.

It is considered based on an increased risk of UTIs in boys who are not circumcised compared to those who are circumcised.

Surgical Management[1,9,14]

A bird's eye view with regards to indications for surgical intervention in a child with VUR include:
- *Breakthrough febrile UTI*, especially for children over an year of age *while on conservative management*, with emphasis on recent changes on DMSA scan (cortical inflammation, new scars, loss of function).
- *Nonresolving persistent high-grade reflux* in toilet-trained children (especially in girls).
- *Parental preference* for surgical correction in high-grade reflux should be given due consideration.

The two options in surgical management are:
1. Endoscopic (Cystoscopic)—subureteral injection of bulking agents
2. Ureteral reimplantation.

Bulking agents in use are Dextromer/hyaluronic acid (Deflux), polytetrafluoroethylene (PTFE) or Teflon, autologous fat, silicone, etc. Though PTFE is known to give best results it is still not approved for use in kids and Deflux/Dexell are the most widely used.

The reflux resolution rate using bulking agents are as follows:
- 78.5% for grades I and II reflux
- 72% for grade III
- 63% for grade IV
- 51% for grade V

A high recurrence rate of 20% overall is reported. A second injection can be considered if the first treatment was unsuccessful. Failure rates are higher with associated anomalies such as neuropathic bladder, duplicated ureters, etc.

In the Indian scenario, the high cost benefit ratio is prohibitory and use of bulking agents is highly selective as in complicated low and intermediate grade reflux (in lieu of ureteric reimplantation).

Strong Parental Preferences

All the major *surgical techniques* involve the principle of lengthening the intramural ureter by passing the ureter underneath an adequate submucosal tunnel. This can be achieved both extravesically (without opening the bladder) and intravesically (but splitting the bladder and disconnecting and reimplanting the ureter). The most popular method is the Cohen's cross-trigonal reimplantation. Other named techniques are the Politano–Leadbetter technique (suprahiatal reimplantation), Lich–Gregoir (extravesical technique) and the Glenn–Anderson technique.

These operations can be done using laparoscopy and robot-assisted though non-availability of long-term results and long operative times hinder widespread acceptance.

Though excellent success rates (92–98%) are reported, antireflux surgeries should be considered after serious speculation in a child with complicated reflux. This is taking into consideration the long-term complications such as neurogenic bladder, obstructed ureters (secondary to ureteral ischemia), recurrent reflux and difficulty in accessing the ureters endoscopically (say for urolithiasis in future).

■ MANAGEMENT OF VESICOURETERIC REFLUX IN DIFFERENT SUBGROUPS

Urinary Tract Infection and Reflux in Neonates and Small Infants[8]

Urinary tract infection is the most common bacterial infection in the febrile newborns. A strong male preponderance is noted (with UTIs). However, incidence of VUR was equal at 20% among male and female neonates and small infants. Incidence of VUR is lower in preterm neonates than in full-term neonates with UTI.

Approximately 10% of patients with antenatally diagnosed hydronephrosis are found to have VUR on routine postnatal follow-up. Newborns with UTI may present with low-grade fever or none at all (poor feeding, lethargy, vomiting, diarrhea, jaundice). Organisms other than *E. coli* are noted in infants with bacteremia and UTI, if there are associated anatomical anomalies.

All neonates and infants with UTIs should have a renal ultrasound. DMSA scans are done 3-6 months later.

Micturating cystourethrograms are definitely recommended for infants with UTI and USG changes and may be considered for others without USG changes, as a result of poor correlation between severity of VUR and hydronephrosis in small babies.

Infants with bacteremia should be treated with parenteral antibiotics for 10-14 days. After initial treatment with intravenous (IV) antibiotics, oral therapy may be considered in infants.

Continuous antibiotic prophylaxis is recommended for infants with history of reflux and febrile UTIs. In the absence of febrile UTIs, CAP is recommended for grades III-V. It is optional to consider CAP in infants with grades I-II reflux with no febrile UTIs.

Circumcision may be considered in male infants.

Management of VUR in a Child more than one year of Age

- In a child more than one year:
  - BBD has to be ruled out before diagnosing primary VUR[14]
  - Less chances of spontaneous resolution
  - Less morbid acute febrile UTIs as compared to neonates and small infants
- Kids with low-grade reflux can continue to be observed without prophylaxis.
- Girls with persistent intermediate and high-grade reflux can be given a strong consideration for surgical intervention with or without febrile UTIs, especially after completing toilet training.
- Boys with intermediate reflux can still be followed up without surgery or prophylaxis, especially after toilet training.
- Boys with persistent high-grade reflux after toilet training can be considered for surgery if there are recurrent or febrile UTIs or strong parental preferences.
- Symptomatic kids with high-grade reflux, abnormal kidneys, breakthrough infections can be considered for earlier surgical intervention (even before completing toilet training).

Management of BBD if present, constitutes the initial line of management before considering any surgical intervention. Surgical intervention can still be considered in the background of BBD if—persistent febrile UTIs, UTI with onset of new scars, worsening of DMSA scan with nonresolving intermediate/high-grade reflux.

Follow-up Plan for a Child on Observation after Resolution of Vesicoureteral Reflux (Spontaneous or Surgical)[1,14]

Yearly assessment of blood pressure, height and weight, urinalysis for infection and protein up to adolescence. Renal ultrasound can be considered with the general assessment if kidneys or upper tract changes were evident even before surgery.

With occurrence of febrile UTIs, evaluation for recurrent VUR and BBD is recommended. In girls, long-term concerns especially during pregnancy and childbirth (such as hypertension, recurrent UTIs and VUR in the progeny), should be revealed at appropriate age.

Postnatal Screening of Neonates with Prenatal Hydronephrosis[14]

- Reported incidence of VUR in neonates with prenatal hydronephrosis is 16% with higher incidence in female children
- Higher grades are reported in two-thirds of the children
- Higher grade of reflux is reported with renal abnormalities on USG
- Postnatal ultrasound is generally performed after 10–14 days in kids with prenatal hydronephrosis, but are otherwise well. Earlier USG can be performed if there is bilateral upper tract changes with or without bladder changes on the prenatal USG
- MCUG is definitely recommended for kids with high-grade hydronephrosis, or abnormal bladder with or without ureteric dilatation and those developing UTI on observation (with no postnatal hydronephrosis).

Sibling Screening[1,14]

- Prevalence of VUR in siblings is as high as 27%
- Renal ultrasound should be given due to consideration in siblings of children with symptomatic/high-grade reflux
- If there is size asymmetry on ultrasound or there is a febrile UTI, full workup with an MCU and DMSA scan is recommended.

■ CONCLUSION

The overall management of VUR is mostly conservative with surgical therapy reserved for VUR leading on to complications while on medical management (breakthrough UTIs, worsening of renal scarring) and persistent high-grade reflux in girls after completion of toilet training.

Individual reflux has to be managed on its own merit, based on its grade, age and sex of the child, occurrence of UTI, renal scarring and recognizing BBD. Guidelines that are more precise need to be formulated in future based on intensification of scientific research and ongoing review of current available literature.

REFERENCES

1. Radmauyr C (Chair). JMNVC. Vesicoureteric Reflux. EAU Guidlines on Paediatric Urology. ESFP. Urology. EAU Guidelines Office, Arnhem, The Netherlands; 2018.
2. Burge DM, Griffiths MD, Malone PS, et al. Fetal vesicoureteral reflux: outcome following conservative postnatal management. J Urol. 1992;148:1743-5.
3. Kaefer M, Curran M, Treves ST, et al. Sibling vesicoureteral reflux in multiple gestation births. Pediatrics. 2000;105:800-4.
4. Feather SA, Malcolm S, Woolf AS, et al. Primary, nonsyndromic vesicoureteric reflux and its nephropathy is genetically heterogeneous, with a locus on chromosome 1. Am J Hum Genet. 2000;66:1420-5.
5. Howard RG, Roebuck DJ, Yeung PA, et al. Vesicoureteric reflux and renal scarring in Chinese children. Br J Radiol. 2001;74:331-4.
6. Tanagho EA, Pugh RCB. The anatomy and function of the ureterovesical junction. Br J Urol. 1963;35:151-65.
7. Paquin AJJ. Ureterovesical anastomosis: The description and evaluation of a technique. J Urol. 1959;82:573-83.
8. Baracco R, Matoo TK. Diagnosis and management of urinary tract infection and vesicoureteral reflux in the neonate. 2014;41:633-42.
9. Khoury AE, Bagli DJ, Wein AJ (Editor-in-chief). Vesicoureteric Reflux in. Campbell-Walsh Urology, 11th edition. Philadelphia; 2016.
10. Rolleston GL, Maling TM, Hodson CJ. Intrarenal reflux and the scarred kidney. Arch Dis Child. 1974;49:531-9.
11. Medical versus surgical treatment of primary vesicoureteral reflux: report of the International Reflux Study Committee. Pediatrics. 1981;67:392-400.
12. Smellie J, Normand I. Reflux nephropathy in childhood. In: Hodson J, Kincaid-Smith P (Eds). Reflux Nephropathy. New York: Masson; 1979.pp.14.
13. Hinchliffe SA, Kreczy A, Ciftci AO, et al. Focal and segmental glomerulosclerosis in children with reflux nephropathy. Pediatr Pathol. 1994;14:327-38.
14. Peters CA, Skoog SJ, Billy S. Arant, et al, Management and Screening of Primary Vesicoureteral Reflux in Children, American Urological Association Guidelines; 2010.
15. Lin D, Huang F, Chiu N, et al. Comparison of hemocytometer leukocyte counts and standard urinalyses for predicting urinary tract infections in febrile infants. Pediatr Infect Dis J. 2000;19:223-7.
16. Santoro J, Carroll V, Steele R. Diagnosis and management of urinary tract infections in neonates and young infants. Clin Pediatr. 2012;52:111-4.
17. Dayan P, Bennett J, Best R, et al. Test characteristics of the urine Gram stain in infants 60 days of age with fever. Pediatr Emerg Care. 2002;18:12-4.
18. Fernández-Menéndez JM, Málaga S, Matesanz JL, et al. Risk factors in the development of early technetium-99m dimercaptosuccinic acid renal scintigraphy lesions during first urinary tract infection in children. Acta Paediatr. 2003;92:21-6.
19. Preda I, Jodal U, Sixt R, et al. Normal dimercaptosuccinic acid scintigraphy makes voiding cystourethrography unnecessary after urinary tract infection. J Pediatr. 2007;151:581-4.
20. Lebowitz RL, Blickman JG. The coexistence of ureteropelvic junction obstruction and reflux. AJR Am J Roentgenol. 1983;140:231-8.
21. Singh-Grewal D, Macdessi J, Craig J. Circumcision for the prevention of urinary tract infection in boys: a systematic review of randomized trials and observational studies. Arch Dis Child. 2005;90:853-8.

CHAPTER 13

HEMATOLOGY

13.1 Thalassemia Syndromes
MR Lokeshwar, Swati Kanakia

13.2 Nutritional Iron Deficiency Anemia
MR Lokeshwar, Sheikh Minhaj Ahmed

13.1 THALASSEMIA SYNDROMES

MR Lokeshwar, Swati Kanakia

■ INTRODUCTION

Thalassemia syndromes are a heterogeneous group of hematologic disorders characterized by defects in the synthesis of one or more of the globin chains that form the hemoglobin tetramer. This results in reduced or complete absence of production of one or more of the globin polypeptide chains of the hemoglobin molecule leading to imbalance in α and non-α chains of hemoglobin. Depending upon the chains affected, it is named as α- or β-thalassemia. They are single gene disorders inherited in an autosomal recessive manner and represent a major health burden worldwide.

■ HISTORICAL REVIEW

Thomas B Cooley and Pearl Lee first described thalassemia in 1925. During a meeting of the American Pediatric Society, Cooley and Lee presented cases of severe anemia occurring in Italian children with hepatosplenomegaly, growth retardation, and discoloration of skin and sclera, with peculiar bony changes. It was later called as Cooley's anemia.

Whipple and Bradford first used the term *thalassemia* in 1932. The word was taken from the Greek language *"thalassa"* meaning *"sea"* and *"emia"*, meaning anemia around the sea. As it was first described around Mediterranean countries, it was also called as Mediterranean anemia. However, it was soon realized that it also occurs not only around Mediterranean regions but also in South East Asia, Indian subcontinent and Middle East.

In 1938, Mukherjee published the first recorded case of thalassemia in a Hindu boy aged 30 months on east side of Suez at Campbell Medical School and Hospital, Kolkata. Subsequently in 1939, three reports appeared in India by Coelho of two Muslim sisters from Mumbai and another by Napier and Dasgupta from Kolkata. Following these reports, more cases were recognized and reported from other parts of India including Punjab, Delhi, Mumbai, Chandigarh, Bihar, Odisha, Andhra Pradesh, and Rajasthan and other parts. Dr Sukumaran from Mumbai is credited for his pioneering work in the field of diagnosis of thalassemia syndromes in India.

■ EPIDEMIOLOGY

Over 250 million people in the world (1.5% of world population) carry the gene for β-thalassemia, out of which about 40 million are in Southeast Asia and 50% of these (20 million) are in India alone. Nearly 100,000 children are born world over with the homozygous state for thalassemia. Of these, 8,000–10,000

Table 13.1.1: Prevalence of β-thalassemia in various regions and communities of India.

Region	Communities
Northern India, and migrated population	Sindhis and Punjabis, Khatris, Kukrejas
Gujarat	Bhanushalis, Kutchis, Lohanas
Maharashtra	Mahars, Chamars, Buddhas, Navabudhas, Kolis, Agris, Kunbis
Telangana, Karnataka	Reddies, Gowdas, Lingayats, Kurgs
Goa	Goud Saraswats
Others	Muslim and Christian communities

children are born in India. The thalassemia belt stretches across the African continent, the Mediterranean regions, Middle East, Indian subcontinent, Southeast Asia, Thailand, Cambodia, Laos, Vietnam, Malaysia, Singapore, Southern China, and Melanesia.

It is estimated that there are around 65,000–67,000 β-thalassemia patients in our country. The frequency of the trait in general population is 3–18% in northern India and 1–3% or less in the south. **Table 13.1.1** provides the prevalence of β-thalassemia in various regions and communities of India.

■ PATHOPHYSIOLOGY

Thalassemia is an inherited disorder of hemoglobin. The hemoglobin molecule consists of two pairs of amino acid chains. Adult hemoglobin, HbA consists of two pairs of α chains and β chains. HbA2 consists of two pairs of α chains and δ chains. Fetal hemoglobin (HbF) is constituted by two pairs of α chains and γ chains.

In case of β-thalassemia, there is reduced or absent production of β chains, leading to excess α chains with reduced or absent β (non-α) chains **(Flowchart 13.1.1)**. Excess α chains that have no complementary non-α chains with which to pair, form insoluble inclusions that precipitate on the red cell membrane and damages it, leading to premature destruction of red blood cells (RBCs) in bone marrow (ineffective erythropoiesis) and in peripheral circulation, particularly in reticuloendothelial system of spleen (extravascular hemolysis).

Due to reduced production of adult hemoglobin in postnatal life, the normal switch mechanism leading to reduction in β chain synthesis does not occur. This leads to higher fetal hemoglobin (HbF $\alpha^2\gamma^2$) in postnatal life. The precise mechanism controlling the switch from fetal to adult hemoglobin (HbA $\alpha^2\beta^2$) is not fully understood.

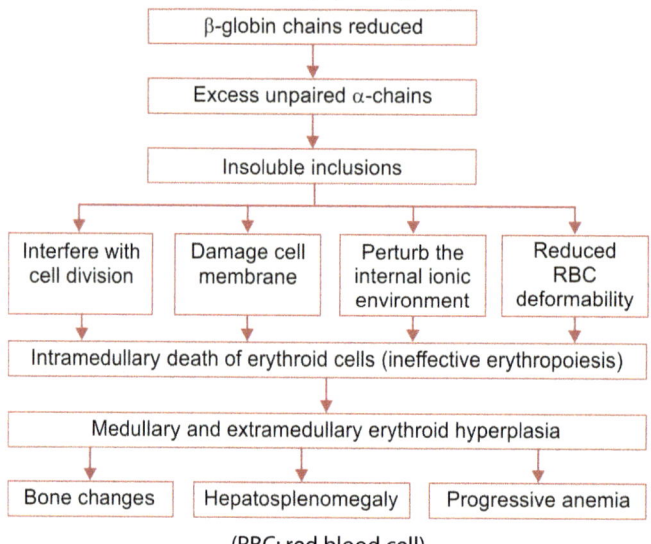

Flowchart 13.1.1: Pathophysiology of β-thalassemia.

(RBC: red blood cell)

Table 13.1.2: Various mutations have been found in the Indian population with β-thalassemia.

Most common mutations in Indian population	Newer mutations
619 bp deletion	Codon 15 (TGG–TAG)
IVS 1-5(G-C)	Codon 4/5 and 6 (ACT CCT GAG–ACA TCT TAG)
IVS 1-1(G-T)	Codon 47/48 (+ATCT)
FS 8/9 (+G)	Codon 55 (+A)
FS 41/42 (-CTTT)	IVS 2-837 (T to G)
	Codon 88 (+T)
	Codon 5 (-CT)
	IVS 1-5 (G-C)

■ MOLECULAR GENETICS

More than 200 mutations have been described that are responsible for thalassemia. The β globin genes are clustered on chromosome 11 and are arranged over approximately 60,000 nucleotide bases. These mutations occur in both introns and exons and outside the coding regions of the genes **(Table 13.1.2)**. Most types of β-thalassemia are due to point mutation affecting the globin gene but some large deletions are also known. However, within

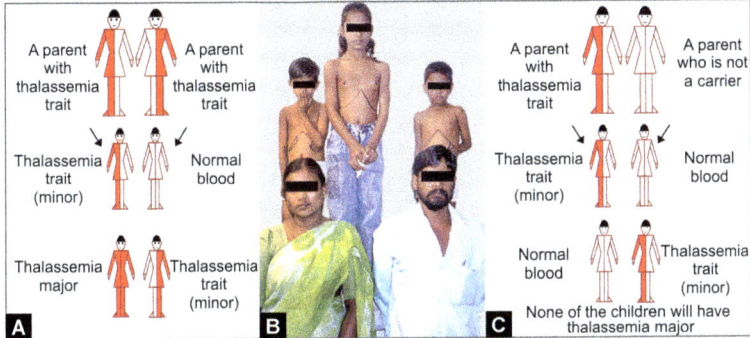

Figs. 13.1.1A to C: *Inheritance of thalassemia major.* 25% inheritance means 25% in each pregnancy (A and C). All the above three children are thalassemia major (B).
Source: Dr MR Lokeshwar, Dr Anupam Sachdev, and Dr Mamta Manglani

each geographical region, few common mutations are responsible for over 90% of β-thalassemia.

Inheritance of Genes

β-thalassemia is inherited in autosomal recessive pattern. If the child inherits one normal and one abnormal gene from each parent, child will have no disease (carrier/minor). If both parents are carriers, i.e. thalassemia minor (single gene affected), there is a 1 in 4 (25%) chance of having a thalassemia major child in each pregnancy. This is depicted in the **Figures 13.1.1A to C**.

■ CLASSIFICATION

Thalassemia is caused by a defect or reduction in Hb chain synthesis due to various mutations of genes, which code for the globin chain. It is characterized by decreased synthesis of one of the polypeptide chains (α or non-α), which form Hb molecule. The α-gene is present on chromosome 16 and β-gene represented on chromosome 11. Thalassemia is classified depending on the deficiency of the type of globin chain of Hb.

- In α-thalassemia, α chain synthesis is affected. They are classified into four different categories depending upon the number of genes affected **(Table 13.1.3)**.
- In β-thalassemia, β-chain is involved. If β chain is absent, it is termed as $β^0$ thalassemia, if partially produced, then $β^+$ thalassemia **(Table 13.1.4)**.

Thalassemia syndromes could be classified into two clinically relevant groups:
1. Transfusion dependent thalassemia (TDT)
2. Nontransfusion dependent thalassemia (NTDT).

Table 13.1.3: Classification of α-thalassemia syndromes.

Syndrome	Clinical features	Hemoglobin pattern	α-globin genes affected
Silent carrier	No anemia, normal red cells	1–2% Hb Bart's ($4\gamma^4$) at birth	1
α-thalassemia trait	Mild anemia, hypochromic microcytic red cells	5–10% Hb Bart's ($4\gamma^4$) at birth	2
Hemoglobin H (HbH) disease	Moderate hypochromic, microcytic anemia	5–30% HbH ($4\beta^4$) red cells	3
Hydrops fetalis	Death in utero caused by severe anemia	Mainly Hb Bart's, small amount of HbH	4

Table 13.1.4: Classification of β-thalassemia.

Syndrome	Clinical features	Hemoglobin pattern	β-globin genes affected
Silent carrier	• Asymptomatic • No anemia	Normal, diagnosed by chain synthesis or identification of mutation	Heterozygous state
Thalassemia trait	• Mild anemia • Hypochromic microcytic red cells	Elevated HbA2 > 3.4%	Heterozygous state
Thalassemia intermedia	• Moderate • Not dependent on blood transfusion for their survival • May require transfusion occasionally	HbF or HbA2 elevated	Homozygous/ double heterozygous state
Thalassemia major	Dependent on regular blood transfusion for survival	HbF markedly elevated	Homozygous state

(HbF: fetal hemoglobin; HbA2: hemoglobin A2)

Nontransfusion dependent thalassemia is a heterogeneous group of thalassemia syndromes, which are characterized by absence of requirement of regular blood transfusion for survival. The three clinical entities, which comprise this group, are:
- β-thalassemia intermedia
- Hemoglobin E β-thalassemia
- α-thalassemia intermedia (Hemoglobin H disease).

Other conditions like hemoglobin S β-thalassemia and hemoglobin C thalassemia may also have similar transfusion requirements.

Hematology

CLINICAL MANIFESTATIONS

Transfusion-dependent Thalassemia (Thalassemia Major)

In India, many children born with thalassemia major die undiagnosed or due to lack of ideal treatment. These children present in early infancy (6–18 months) with progressive pallor, hepatosplenomegaly and bony changes. If untreated, it is invariably fatal during first few years of life **(Figs. 13.1.2A to D)**. Untreated or irregularly treated children develop significant hemolytic facies including frontoparietal bossing with a hot-cross bun appearance of the skull (caput quadratum), depressed bridge of nose, malar prominence and malocclusion of teeth with protrusion of maxillary teeth.

Nontransfusion-dependent Thalassemia

These include forms with varying degrees of clinical manifestations of anemia, hepatosplenomegaly and bony changes who maintain their life fairly comfortably and are not dependent on blood transfusions for their survival and are called thalassemia-intermedia (NTDT). In this heterozygous form (also called thalassemia minor) the patient can lead a practically normal life except for a mild persistent anemia **(Fig. 13.1.3A)**.

The major pathophysiological processes underlying NTDT are ineffective erythropoiesis and peripheral hemolysis. This in turn gives rise to various pathologies like anemia, extramedullary hematopoiesis, hypercoagulability, iron overload, and decreased bone densities. This group, however, does not have a uniform presentation but encompasses highly variable clinical phenotypes. This may present with asymptomatic mild picture with no or occasional requirement of blood transfusion, no or minimal iron overload, and no growth retardation or general debility.

LABORATORY DIAGNOSIS

For a reliable diagnosis of thalassemia, it is advisable to correlate clinical profile and ethnicity of the individual with various laboratory investigations. Hemoglobin electrophoresis is the confirmatory test for diagnosis of most cases of thalassemia syndromes. However, a complete blood count (CBC) including examination of the peripheral blood film (PBF) provides very vital information and is an important primary screen in thalassemia syndromes.

Thalassemia Major and Intermedia

Complete blood count, examination of PBF and a reticulocyte count help in suspecting and identification of hemoglobinopathies. CBC reveals generally severe anemia, a high leukocyte count due to nucleated red cells—also known as a "leukoerythroblastic reaction". White blood cells (WBCs) and platelets may decrease if there is accompanying hypersplenism.

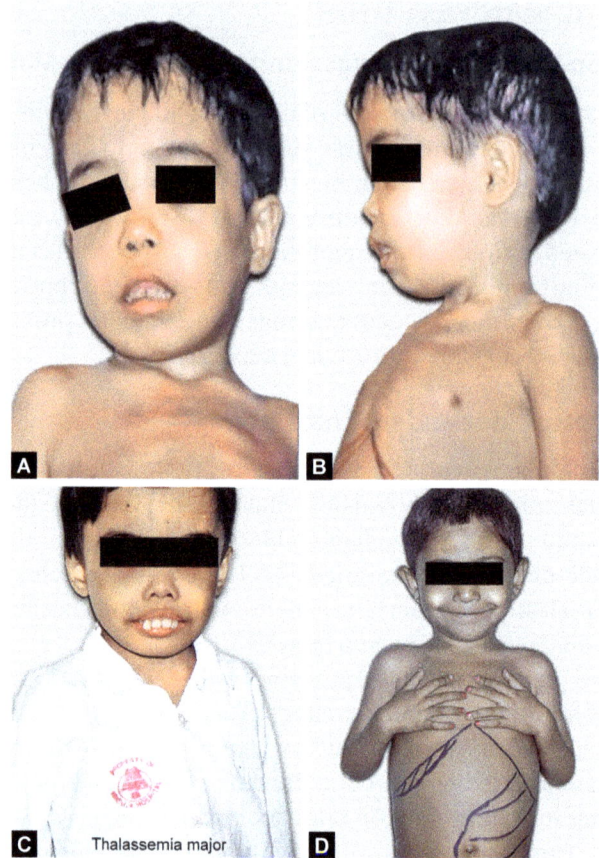

Figs. 13.1.2A to D: Transfusion-dependent thalassemia.

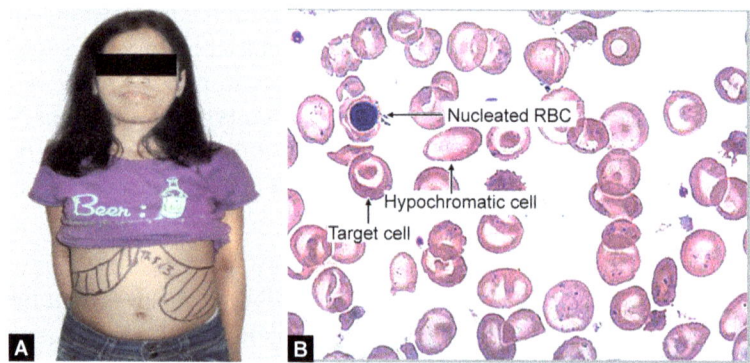

Figs. 13.1.3A and B: (A) Nontransfusion-dependent thalassemia; (B) Peripheral smear in thalassemia showing target cell and normoblasts.

The red cell indices reveal severe hypochromia with microcytosis. There is significant macrocytosis due to relative folate depletion in patients with delayed diagnosis.

The red cell distribution width (RDW) in thalassemia major is significantly high (ranging from 30-40% for a normal value of 12-16%), suggesting a very high degree of anisocytosis.

The PBF (**Fig. 13.1.3B**) shows a striking and characteristic bizarre picture with hypochromic, microcytic and macrocytic red cells, aniso-poikilocytosis, target cells, polychromasia (more common in thalassemia intermedia), basophilic stippling, nucleated red cells and sometimes immature myeloid cells.

Thalassemia Minor

The *CBC* in thalassemia trait is associated with high red cell count relative to hemoglobin concentration and hematocrit, resulting in a marked fall in mean cell volume (MCV), mean cell hemoglobin (MCH) as well as mean cell hemoglobin concentration (MCHC). RDW is normal in thalassemia trait.

Reticulocyte count is generally low to normal in thalassemia major, whereas in thalassemia intermedia, it is increased to 3-6%. The reason for a low reticulocyte count in thalassemia major is significant ineffective erythropoiesis preventing the precursor red cells from maturing to reticulocyte stage to be thrown into peripheral blood. In thalassemia intermedia, since the ineffective erythropoiesis is milder, the reticulocytes are increased in peripheral blood due to the anemia.

Naked-eye Single Tube Red Cell Osmotic Fragility Test for Thalassemia Minor

Many investigators have studied naked-eye single tube red cell osmotic fragility test (NESTROFT), which has a high sensitivity of 95%, but its poor precision, interobserver variability and low specificity has precluded it from becoming a robust test.

Quantitation of Various Hemoglobins

Separation of hemoglobins either by electrophoretic mobility or chromatographic separation is the confirmatory investigation for diagnosis of thalassemia syndromes. Quantitation of various hemoglobins can be done by the following methods:
- Isoelectric focusing
- Microcolumn chromatography
- High performance liquid chromatography (HPLC)
- Both anion and cation exchange HPLC
- Cellulous acetate electrophoresis (**Fig. 13.1.4A**)
- Paper electrophoresis (**Fig. 13.1.4B**).

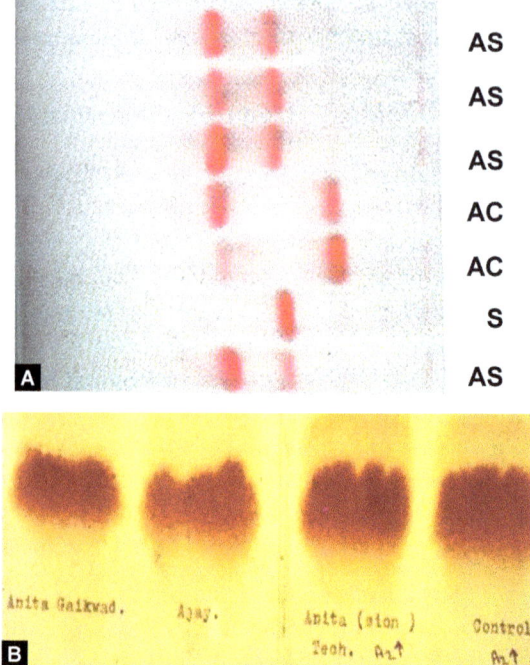

Figs. 13.1.4A and B: (A) Cellulose acetate electrophoresis; (B) Paper electrophoresis.

In non-transfused patients with thalassemia major, hemoglobin pattern reveals 20–100% HbF, 2–7% HbA2, and 0–80% HbA, the quantities varying depending upon the genotype. Thalassemia minor is characterized by elevated HbA2 of more than 3.4% on paper electrophoresis, and more than 4% by certain other methods.

Microcolumn chromatography and HPLC **(Figs. 13.1.5A and B)** by automated machines are now becoming increasingly popular due to the ease of performing the test, less time consumption and greater reliability and reproducibility. It has thus become the gold standard for diagnosis of thalassemia syndromes and other hemoglobinopathies. It generates graphs depicting various abnormal and normal hemoglobins with quantification. HbA2 value of > 9% indicates the presence of a coeluting abnormal hemoglobin such as HbE, HbD Iran and Hb Lepore. Microcolumn chromatography and HPLC are currently used in most laboratories. Hemoglobins are separated graphically and quantified by photometer utilizing sophisticated computer.

Iron Studies

Serum Iron and Transferrin Saturation

Serum iron and transferrin saturation are normal to increased (increased especially in multiply transfused children) in thalassemia major, whereas the

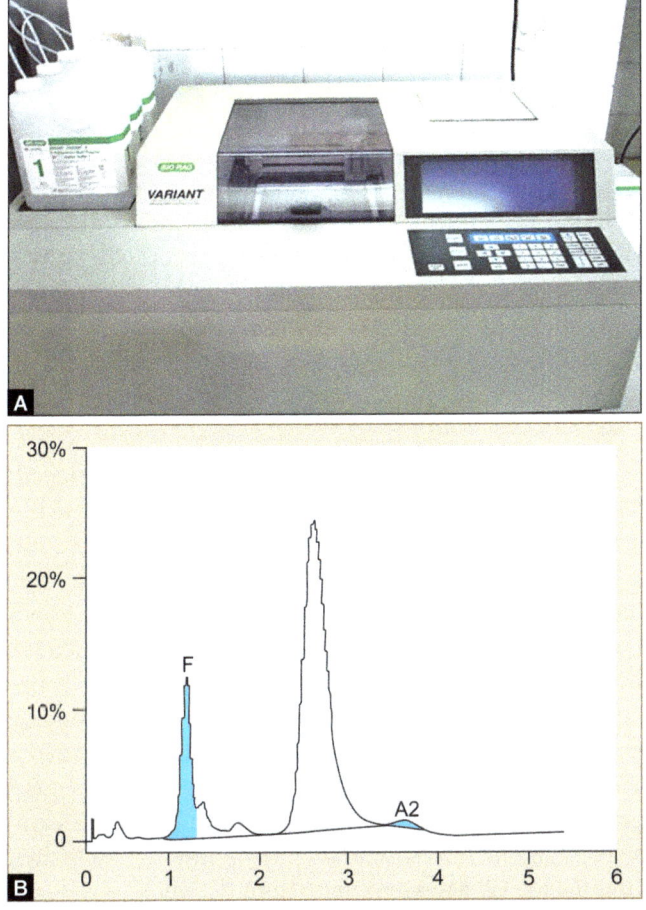

Figs. 13.1.5A and B: (A) Bio-Rad variant machine; (B) Pattern of hemoglobin in thalassemia minor/trait.

total iron binding capacity (TIBC) is decreased. It is generally normal to high even in thalassemia minor. Though iron deficiency is extremely uncommon in thalassemia minor, in our country, due to a high incidence of iron deficiency anemia (IDA), concomitant iron deficiency may be present in children with thalassemia minor. In such patients, serum iron level would be low with reduced transferring saturation and a high TIBC.

Serum Ferritin

Serum ferritin is high in children with thalassemia major and normal to increased or decreased when concomitant iron deficiency associated in those with thalassemia minor. Serum ferritin estimation is used as the most common test for diagnosing iron overload and should be assessed every 3–6 months. In children with thalassemia major, the values of ferritin are proportionate to iron overload. Serum ferritin can be affected by various clinical situations—it may be elevated in acute infections as an acute phase reactant, in chronic diseases and chronic inflammatory disorders, etc.

Liver Iron Concentration

Liver iron concentration (LIC) provides a reliable estimate of total body iron stores. Liver biopsy with iron measurement by atomic absorption spectroscopy is considered the gold standard of LIC and the best predictor of total body iron. Any level above 7 mg/g of dry liver tissue is indicative of significant iron overload. Levels above 15 mg/g are associated with cardiac iron overload. It is an invasive procedure and difficult to perform repeatedly.

Liver and Cardiac Iron Imaging by MRI

Use of *magnetic resonance imaging* (MRI) has generally replaced the more invasive liver biopsy. Liver and cardiac iron imaging by MRI are the standard of care. Spin echo (R2) and gradient echo (R2*) are the two most widely used MRI techniques. MRI-R2* method is more sensitive and suited to measure the relatively low heart iron concentration. Cardiac iron is typically measured with T2* images with electrocardiogram gating, and this technique is widely available and highly reproducible. Results are usually presented in milliseconds with T2* of greater than 20 ms being adequate. Mild cardiac iron overload is defined as T2* of 10–20 ms and severe cardiac overload is less than 10 ms. In a large study nearly half of patients with T2* less than 6 ms developed heart failure within 1 year. Cardiac iron monitoring should begin by age of 10 years of age. Cardiac MRI should then be monitored annually. High-risk patients should have T2* assessed every 6 months whereas well-chelated low risk patients may have assessment spaced to every 2 years.

Newer Noninvasive Methods

Superconducting quantum interference device (SQUID) is a noninvasive method of estimating liver iron and has proven to be more accurate than serum ferritin in quantifying the total body iron overload. *Biometric liver susceptometry or spectrometry* uses SQUID. At present SQUID remains reserved for experimental purpose and few machines are available worldwide.

Bone Marrow Examination

Bone marrow examination is not indicated for the diagnosis of thalassemia major but if done, it shows normoblastic erythroid hyperplasia with *excessive iron on iron staining with Prussian blue.*

Radiological Findings

These include widening of medulla due to bone marrow hyperplasia, thinning of the cortex and trabeculations and fracture are seen in long bones, metacarpals and metatarsals.

Periodic Tests for Organ Dysfunctions

While diagnosis of thalassemia major can be achieved by the tests, it is also mandatory to do baseline screening of various parameters as shown in **Table 13.1.5**.

■ TREATMENT AND COURSE

Management of Thalassemia Major

The management of thalassemia has undergone tremendous changes over the last five decades. If untreated, patients of thalassemia major die by the age of 3-4 years due to severe anemia. With transfusion therapy alone, patients

Table 13.1.5: Routine monitoring for individuals with thalassemia.

Test	Frequency of monitoring
Alpha and beta globin genotyping	Once at diagnosis
High resolution HLA typing	Once
Growth parameters height, weight, head circumference	Every 3–6 months
Tanner staging and menstrual assessment	Every 6 months starting at 8–10 years
Complete blood count	Every 6 months if no transfusion/every 3–5 weeks if on transfusion
Comprehensive biochemistry panel	Every 6 months
Iron panel	Every 6 months
Serum ferritin	Every 3 months (monthly if on aggressive chelation)
Echocardiogram	Annually starting at 10–14 years
TSH and free T4	Annually starting at 6 years
Fasting glucose	Annually starting at 10 years
Hormonal profile	Annually starting at 10 years
Vitamin D, serum calcium, PTH	Annually starting at age of 10 years
Bone density by DEXA scan	Annually starting at 10 years

(DEXA: dual-energy X-ray absorptiometry; HLA: human leukocyte antigen; PTH: parathyroid hormone; TSH: thyroid stimulating hormone)

Table 13.1.6: Management of thalassemia.

S. No.	Management
1.	Confirmation of diagnosis
2.	*Transfusion therapy*: Packed red cell transfusion
3.	Management of complications of transfusion
4.	*Iron overload*: Removal of iron with iron chelating agents
5.	*Hypersplenism*: Role of splenectomy
6.	*Transfusion transmitted infections*: Hepatitis B and C HIV, *Yersinia* species, malaria, CMV
7.	Gallstones and leg ulcers
8.	*Curative treatment*: Bone marrow transplantation
9.	*Future treatment*: Pharmacologic manipulation of HbF/Gene therapy
10.	Prevention of the disease by antenatal diagnosis and genetic counseling

(HbF: fetal hemoglobin; CMV: cytomegalovirus; HIV: human immunodeficiency virus)

with thalassemia major children die due to cardiac complications (related to iron overload) as early as 10–12 years of age.

However, with the advent of chelation therapy as well as better screening procedures for transfusion-related infections as well as leuko-depletion through prestorage or bedside filtration and better facilities at outdoor transfusion centers, the lifespan of these children have improved considerably. If no complications occur, they live for an almost normal span with an improved quality of life.

Management of thalassemia involves a multidisciplinary therapeutic team approach and should be preferably done at a comprehensive thalassemia children care center with outdoor transfusion facilities. The team should include pediatric hematologist, general pediatrician/s, dedicated nurses, transfusion medicine specialist, physiotherapist, endocrinologist, psychologist and social worker.

The major principles of management of thalassemia are detailed in **Table 13.1.6**.

Transfusion Therapy in Thalassemia

The goals of transfusion in thalassemia management are:
- To obviate anemia
- To reduce hepatosplenomegaly by reducing ineffective erythropoiesis
- To reduce hemolytic faces
- To improve tissue oxygenation
- To improve growth.

Various transfusion regimens used in thalassemia management over years are shown in **Table 13.1.7**.

Initiation of Transfusion Therapy

Before embarking on a lifelong transfusion therapy, it is essential to establish the diagnosis. DNA analysis will help to know the severity of thalassemia as well as would help in prenatal diagnosis for future pregnancies. One can ascertain the diagnosis of thalassemia intermedia by observing the rate of fall of hemoglobin without transfusions. If the hemoglobin drops to below 7 g/dL without transfusion, in the absence of any concurrent illness, it is imperative to put the child on a regular transfusion program. If the child maintains hemoglobin above 7 g/dL, the diagnosis of thalassemia intermedia has to be considered.

A goal of pretransfusion Hb of 9.5–10.5 g/dL is highly recommended which can be achieved with every 3–5 weekly transfusions because this level suppresses ineffective erythropoiesis and relieves symptoms of anemia allowing for normal growth. Higher pretransfusion Hb levels may be needed for patients with heart complications **(Table 13.1.8)**.

Whenever possible, complete genotype of the red cells should be recorded. This will help to prevent red cell alloimmunization following repeated transfusions. However, this is not feasible in India and the alternative to this is Coomb's cross-match for each transfusion to prevent alloimmunization.

Table 13.1.7: Various transfusion regimens (progress in transfusion therapy).

Year of regimen	Transfusion regimen	Pretransfusion Hb
1960s	Palliative	Hb to 8.5 g/dL (Wolman et al.)
1970s	Hyper transfusion	Hb 10–12 g/dL (Piomelli et al.)
1980s	Super transfusion	Hb > 14 g/dL (Propper et al.)
2005	Moderate transfusion	Hb 9–10.5 g/dL (European regimen)

Table 13.1.8: Monitoring of transfusion.

Test	Frequency of monitoring
Red blood cell genotype	Once at start of transfusion
Pretransfusion CBC	Every 3–5 week
Transfusion history including (volume transfused, presence of red cell antibody)	Every 3–5 week
Triple H (HIV/HBsAg/HCV)	Annually

(HCV: hepatitis C virus; HBsAg: hepatitis B virus surface antigen; HIV: human immunodeficiency virus; CBC: complete blood count)

Extended red cell antigen typing that includes C, c, E, e and Kell antigen will reduce the incidence of red cell alloimmunization to a very low level compared to only routine ABO and RH(D) screening. The most ideal way to transfuse a thalassemic child is using group and type specific packed red cells that are compatible by direct antiglobulin test. The hematocrit should be standardized to 65–75%. It is ideal to use prestorage leuko-depleted blood and these facilities are not easily available. However, the next best is to use leuko-depleting filters at bedside, but they are also costly. An alternative to this is use of triple saline washed red cells in cold centrifuge.

The red cells should be fresh, not more than 4–5 days old to maintain adequate levels of 2,3-DPG. Various other methods of leuko-depletion are available, including use of frozen red cells (highly expensive and impractical in developing countries).

Rate of Transfusion

These red cells should be transfused, 10–15 mL/kg, at the rate of 3–4 mL/kg/hour every 2–4 weeks to maintain the hemoglobin. Patients with cardiac decompensation should be given red cells at the rate of not more than 1–2 mL/kg/hour.

The new form of transfusions recommended include nucleic acid amplification tested packed cell transfusion (NAAT) which is given as 10–15 mL kg of leuko-reduced, irradiated, cross matched, negative for cytomegalovirus (CMV), human immunodeficiency virus (HIV), hepatitis C virus (HCV) and hepatitis B surface antigen (HbsAg).

Daycare Transfusion Center

Transfusions are preferably given on an outdoor basis at daycare transfusion centers and hence no hospitalization is required. Children are more comfortable with the familiar staff members of the daycare center. There is less school absenteeism and parents lose fewer workdays. The cost of the hospital stay is almost five times less. There is no threat of contacting infections from other patients in the wards in hospitals. Parents and children are happy to be with other children and parents and they get a chance to discuss common issues of thalassemia management.

Management of Complications of Transfusion Therapy

A major problem encountered in the management of thalassemia is iron overload. Regular red cell transfusions to maintain hemoglobin and increased iron absorption from gastrointestinal (GI) tract due to ineffective erythropoiesis and consequent low hemoglobin in irregularly transfused children is responsible for iron overload.

Transfusion-related Complications

These include iron overload and chelation therapy and transfusion transmitted infections. Two factors contribute to iron overload in a thalassemic child: (1) enhanced GI absorption of iron and (2) transfusional siderosis.

Chelation Therapy

Iron chelation should be initiated after age of 2 years when there is evidence of significant iron overload as evidenced by need for 10-20 transfusions, serum ferritin >1,000 ng/mL and LIC > 5-7 mg/g dry weight. The goal is to reduce the iron store and maintain at low ferritin level of < 1,000-1,500 ng/mL. The standard available chelators used are discussed here.

Desferrioxamine

Desferrioxamine (DFO) is a hexa-dentate chelator and cannot easily mobilize iron from intracellular compartment due to its high molecular weight. It slowly binds iron to form ferrioxamine and does not bind with iron from transferrin. One gram of DFO binds 93 mg of iron. Dose is 20-50 mg/kg/day for 6 night/week subcutaneously over 8-10 hours. DFO is the gold standard therapy and is the most effective and safe iron chelator. DFO has not become popular particularly in the developing countries and is preferred by only 10-15% of thalassemia patients in our country. This is mainly due to its high cost and the need for continuous subcutaneous injection over 6-8 hours with the Desferal pump.

The indications to start chelation therapy include:
- Serum ferritin level > 1,000-3,000 ng/mL or above.
- More than 15-20 transfusions
- Hepatic iron concentration > 3.2 mg/g dry weight.

In recent times, methods of administration have improved with better, more convenient smaller, lighter infusion pumps with LCD display. Balloon pumps, prefilled syringes of Desferal are available though they are prohibitively costly.

Intravenous (IV) Desferal can be given particularly in those with very high iron overload through port-a-caths (central line). The dose for IV DFO is 50-100 mg/kg body weight. Indications for IV DFO include very high ferritin levels, presence of cardiac complications, associated pregnancy and prior to stem cell transplantation. Rarely, it is given in patients with persistent local reactions at injection sites.

Toxicity due to DFO is minimal and there is no tachyphylaxis. Local pain, indurations, irritability and redness may occur. Other toxicities include visual abnormality due to cataract, and high frequency sensory-neural hearing loss. Delayed linear growth is accompanied by skeletal abnormalities such as short trunk, sternal protrusion and genu valgum.

As the auditory and visual toxicities are reversible, yearly slit-lamp examination and audiometry are mandatory to detect them early.

Role of Vitamin C

Ascorbic acid deficiency increases insoluble iron (hemosiderin). Vitamin C helps in conversion of hemosiderin into ferritin from which iron can be chelated. High doses of vitamin C can lead to increased free radical reaction and lipid peroxidation resulting in tissue damage and rapid cardiac decompensation and even death. Addition of vitamin C 100 mg daily prior to DFO therapy increases iron excretion. Nearly 60% of DFO chelated iron is excreted in urine and 40% in stool.

Oral Chelators

Deferiprone (L1) or 1,2-dimethyl-3-hydroxypyridin-4-one (Kelfer)

This is a water soluble, bidentate molecule. It mobilizes iron from transferrin, ferritin and hemosiderin. It is used orally and is less expensive. Deferiprone/L1 has a better protective effect on myocardial tissue. Dose is 75–100 mg/kg/day given TDS orally. Side effects of Deferiprone (DFP) include GI symptoms like nausea and vomiting, pain in abdomen and diarrhea, arthropathy and neutropenia or agranulocytosis.

Deferasirox (Asunra, Desirox, Defrijet, Desifer)

Deferasirox is able to mobilize iron from both the hepatocellular and reticuloendothelial source. It has ability to prevent myocardial cell iron uptake and removes iron directly from myocardial cells, the liver cells, the intracellular labile iron pool and the surface of reticuloendothelial cells where iron is handed over to transferrin. Iron is excreted predominantly in the bile and hence in the feces. The drug is given orally as a single dose preferably in the morning on empty stomach. The recommended dose ranges from 20 mg/kg/day to 30 mg/kg/day once daily. Adverse events include GI disturbances causing abdominal pain, nausea, vomiting, diarrhea and occasionally constipation, headache, fever, anxiety, and sleep disorders. Hearing loss has been reported. Nephropathy in patients with compromised renal function can be life-threatening. Regular monitoring of CBC, liver functions, renal functions, urine protein estimation and annual audiometry and ophthalmic examination is required.

Combination Therapy

Combination therapy may be beneficial for some patients with severe iron overload. Additive and synergistic effects of combination of iron chelators have been explained by the shuttle hypothesis. Bidentate (L1) or tridentate ligand with access to a variety of tissues acts as a "shuttle" to mobilize the iron from tissue compartments to the bloodstream, where most exchanges with a larger hexadentate (DFO) "sink". The sink binds this iron irreversibly, promoting its excretion. Experiments using a desferrioxamine-chelatable iron (DCI) assay showed that simultaneous administration of L1 and DFO produced shuttling of iron from L1 (shuttle) to DFO (sink). Clinical studies using DFO and L1 in combination have confirmed this hypothesis. Several other combinations exhibiting shuttle mechanism have been tried with success—hydroxybenzyl-ethylenediamine-diacetic acid (HBED) and L1 as well as ICL670A and DFO (in experimental cells).

The dose of DFO is 50 mg/kg/day as overnight subcutaneous infusion through pump for 2 days a week and deferiprone at 50 mg/kg/day orally in three divided doses for rest of the 5 days a week. In case of cardiac failure DFO can be given at a dose of 80 mg/kg/day along with DFP.

Chelators in Nontransfusion-dependent Thalassemia

In NTDT, deferasirox therapy should be started at a dose of 10 mg/kg/day. Monitor iron overload status using LIC after 6 months of initiation. Consider dose escalation to 20 mg/kg/day in patients with LIC >7 mg Fe/g dry weight or serum ferritin level >1,500–2,000 ng/mL. Chelation should be discontinued at serum ferritin <300 ng/mL and/or LIC < 5 mg/g dry weight of liver. The Thalassemia International Federation guidelines do not recommend the use of other chelators like deferoxamine and deferiprone for management of iron overload in NTDT **(Table 13.1.9)**.

Table 13.1.9: Monitoring for adverse effects of iron chelation.

Test	Frequency of monitoring
All chelators	
Visual acuity	Annually
Audiology examination	Annually
Deferasirox	
Urinalysis for proteinuria	Every 3 months
Liver function testing	Every 2 weeks × 2 months after initiation then monthly
Renal function test including electrolytes	Monthly
Deferiprone	
Complete blood count	Prior to transfusion
Liver function testing	Every 3 months

Newer Chelators

Newer iron chelators being studied in animals as well as in humans are discussed in brief here.

Hydroxybenzyl-ethylenediamine-diacetic Acid

Hydroxybenzyl-ethylenediamine-diacetic acid was able to clear radiolabeled iron when administered parenterally and that it remained active after oral administration, however further evaluation in both iron-loaded primates and humans revealed that the oral activity was too small to be of value in the treatment of iron overload.

Deferitin

This is another oral iron tridentate chelator belonging to ferrothiocin class.

Pyridoxal Isonicotinoyl Hydrazone

It is a tridentate chelator with selectivity for iron comparable to that of DFO, and their analogs.

Desferrithiocin

Desferrithiocin (DFT) caused kidney damage in rats on prolonged oral DFT. The damage was believed to be due to toxic effects of the Fe^{3+} complex, ferrithiocin. One of its analogs, 4-OH-desaza-desmethyl-desferrithiocin, appears to be less toxic while remaining biologically active as an orally administered iron chelator in animal studies.

GT56-252

GT56-252 is a novel orally available iron chelator derived from DFT that forms a 2:1 complex with Fe_3. The compound was well-tolerated, with no related serious adverse clinical events, laboratory abnormalities or changes in the electrocardiogram (ECG). Further studies are in progress to define the effect of GT56-252 on iron balance.

40SD02 (CHF1540)

40SD02 (CHF1540) is a new entity synthesized by chemically attaching DFO to a modified starch polymer. The resulting high molecular weight chelator has a prolonged half-life. A phase I study in 10 patients with thalassemia and chronic iron overload showed that single doses of up to 600 mg/kg of the compound were safe and well-tolerated and stimulated a clinically significant amount of iron excretion.

Transfusion Transmitted Infections

Hepatitis B in Thalassemia

All thalassemics who are negative for the hepatitis B surface antigen and antibody should receive hepatitis B vaccine, 4 doses at day 0, 1 month, 2 months and 12 months intramuscularly. It also can be given intradermal in the dose of 0.1 mL, thus reducing the cost. This has been found to be effective by some workers. However, efficacy is not well proven. Medications approved by FDA for the treatment of children with HBV include IFN-alpha, lamivudine and adefovir. The recommended treatment regime for IFN-alpha is 5–10 million units/mm^2 thrice weekly by subcutaneous injection for 4–6 months. The dose for lamivudine is 3 mg/kg/day.

HIV in Thalassemia

Although sensitive and specific laboratory serologic tests became available soon after the discovery and description of HIV, a number of patients with thalassemia who received transfusions previous to HIV screening have been infected. Many more are still being infected in countries where effective protective measures for blood safety, including blood donor selection and testing, have yet to be applied. Patients with thalassemia identified with HIV infection should be managed in collaboration with an infectious diseases unit with expertise in HIV.

Hepatitis C Virus Infection in Thalassemia

Patients treated with peg-interferon alfa (PegIFN) and ribavirin (RBV) combination therapy demonstrate overall 50–55% sustained viral response (SVR) with rates as high as 80% in patients with genotypes 2 and 3. The optimal dose of PEG-IFN-alpha-2b is 60 mg/m^2/week given subcutaneously and PEG-IFN-alpha-2a at a dose of 180 mg/m^2 weekly subcutaneously. Either of two should be given in combination with ribavirin at a dose of 15 mg/kg/day twice daily. The recommended length of therapy is 48 weeks of treatment for genotypes 1 or 4 and 24 weeks duration of treatment for genotypes 2 or 3 in children.

Human Cytomegalovirus

Transfusion-associated CMV has a wide clinical spectrum. In the immunocompetent patient-host, it is usually subclinical or may appear as an infectious mononucleosis-like syndrome. The increasing use of bone marrow transplantation (BMT) as a treatment for thalassemia demands special attention to the serological status of CMV. Prevention of transmission through blood products is effectively achieved by the use of anti-CMV negative donation, but this policy may be applied only in special conditions, such as stem cell transplantation, because exclusion of CMV positive donors (50–75% of the adult population are anti-HCMV positive) will affect significantly the national pool of blood supply. As CMV is WBC-associated virus, the widespread use of leukocyte filtration, in recent years recommended for all patients with thalassemia, no matter what their condition, constitutes an effective preventative measure.

Bacterial Infections

Yersinia Enterocolitica

Yersinia species are common cause of infection in severe iron overloaded patients or in those undergoing iron chelation with DFO. Transfusion-associated transmission of *Yersinia enterocolitica* may occur from apparently healthy donors. The rate of mortality among recipients of contaminated blood is >50%. Treatment includes stopping iron chelation therapy with injection desferrioxamine immediately. IV cotrimoxazole, gentamycin, ceftriaxone, doxycycline and ciprofloxacin are the common antibiotics used in the treatment of Yersinia species.

■ MANAGEMENT OF COMPLICATIONS

Hypersplenism

Hypersplenism may occur due to inadequate transfusions, alloimmunization and rarely autoimmune hemolysis complicating thalassemia major and chronic liver disease. With the advent of hyper- and super-transfusion therapy, splenomegaly and hypersplenism have become a rarity and hence splenectomy is usually not needed in these patients. If the child has already developed splenomegaly and signs of hypersplenism and is above 5 years of age, splenectomy is indicated.

Splenectomy

Splenectomy should be considered—(1) when annual blood requirement exceeds 1.5 times the basal requirement for a patient maintaining pretransfusion Hb about 10 g/dL (transfusion requirement increases to more than 200–220 mL/kg/year of packed red cells); (2) massive spleen enlargement posing a risk of splenic rupture or when splenic enlargement is associated with left upper quadrant pain or early satiety; and (3) in the presence of leukopenia or thrombocytopenia.

All patients undergoing splenectomy should receive immunization to protect against capsulated organisms. These include pneumococcal, Hib, meningococcal vaccines, *Salmonella typhi*, which should be given at least

4 weeks before surgery. Lifelong postsplenectomy penicillin prophylaxis 125 mg twice a day for children up to 2 years and 250 mg twice a day for children 2 years and above is recommended. Chemoprophylaxis is recommended for at least 2 years while some advocate this for whole life. In the presence of early signs of infection treatment should be started immediately with broad-spectrum antibiotics without waiting for the result of laboratory tests. Post-splenectomy, there may be transient or persistent thrombocytosis. Aspirin therapy should be considered in splenectomized NTDT patients with elevated platelet counts ($\geq 500 \times 10^9$) in a dose of 50-100 mg/day. In endemic areas, prophylactic antimalarial treatment may be given to prevent malaria.

Osteopenia and Osteoporosis

Osteoporosis as defined by WHO is a "progressive systemic skeletal disease characterized by low bone mass and microarchitectural deterioration of bone tissue, with consequent increase in bone fragility and susceptibility to fracture." This can be diagnosed by dual energy X-ray absorptiometry (DEXA) scan for bone density and biochemical studies of serum calcium, inorganic phosphate, alkaline phosphatase, urinary calcium/creatinine ratio (>0.2) and urinary phosphorus/creatinine ratio (> 0.6). DEXA scan is recommended beginning by age of 10 years (**Figs. 13.1.6A and B**). Bone density T score > 1.5 SD below the mean is diagnostic of osteopenia whereas T score > 2.5 SD below the mean is termed osteoporosis.

Treatment of osteopenia and osteoporosis include diet, rich in calcium and vitamin D as well as calcium supplementation (500–1,000 mg/day and vitamin D 800–1,000 units/day); calcitonin (inhibitor of osteoclasts), IV pamidronate (15 mg/kg, every 3 months for 1 year); bisphosphonates such as Osteofos 75 mg once a week; moderate and high impact activities—walking, ballet dancing, aerobics jogging, etc.; and hormone replacement therapy for endocrine abnormalities.

Cardiac Complications

Cardiac complication such as cardiac decompensation secondary to myopathy, iron overload, and congestive cardiac failure resulting from anemia should be treated promptly. Extensive cardiac iron deposits result in chamber hypertrophy, myocardial degeneration and fibrosis leading to cardiac stiffness and reduction in cardiac contractility. Adequate chelation and symptomatic therapy can reverse the cardiac damage caused by iron overload.

Leg Ulcers

Leg ulcers are more common in thalassemia intermedia and thalassemia minor. Bed rest, regular transfusions and wound care are adequate. Local

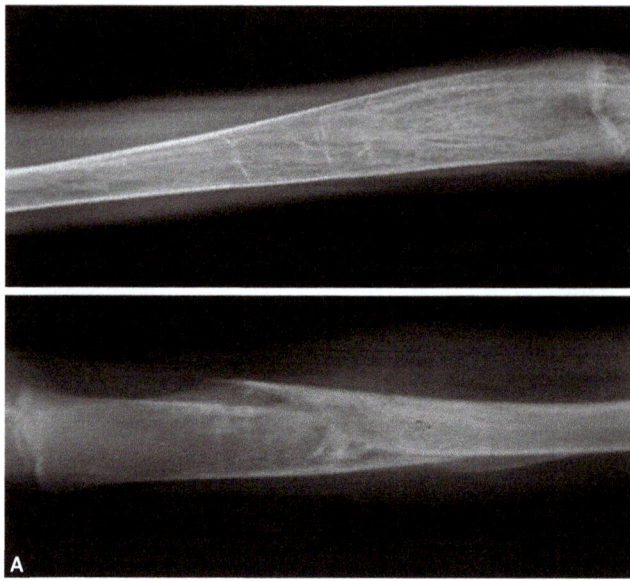

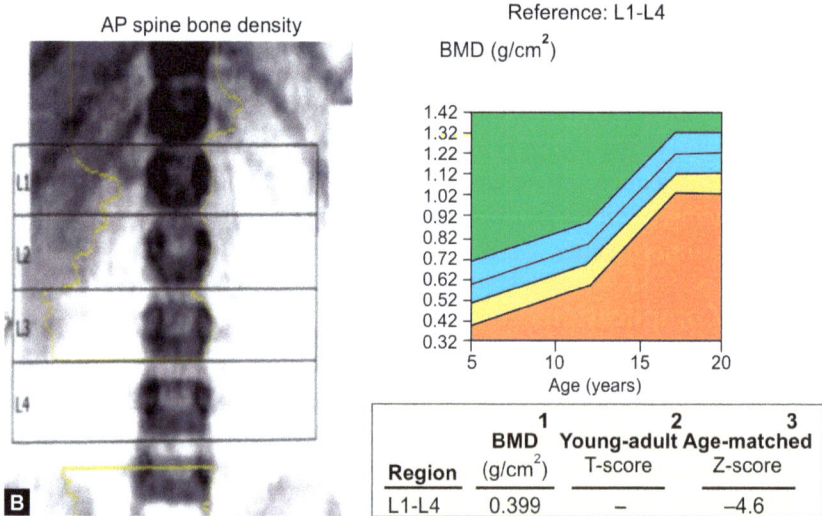

Figs. 13.1.6A and B: (A) Osteopenia and osteoporosis of the long bone; (B) Bone mineral density (BMD) study – DEXA Scan.
(AP: anteroposterior)
Source: Dr MR Lokeshwar and Dr Mamta Manglani

infiltration of growth factors such as granulocyte colony stimulating factor (G-CSF) has been found useful.

Gallstones

Gallstones are more commonly seen in children receiving irregular treatment as well as in thalassemia minor. In asymptomatic cases no active treatment is required. However, they may be removed along with splenectomy (if splenectomy is indicated).

Hepatic Dysfunction

Liver dysfunction is secondary to plasma-borne infections and iron overload. It is thus necessary to do the liver function tests and hepatitis markers particularly HBsAg and HCV antibodies every 6 months.

Endocrine Evaluation and Growth and Development

Growth retardation, hypogonadotropic hypogonadism, diabetes mellitus, hypothyroidism, hypoparathyroidism, osteopenia and osteoporosis are the common endocrine abnormalities of thalassemia. Iron deposition in the pituitary, pancreas and other endocrine organs leads to significant morbidity in transfusion dependent thalassemic patients. Patients should undergo annual endocrine screening should be initiated from the age of 9 years or earlier if indicated. The following tests should be included: thyroid functions particularly FT4 and thyroid stimulating hormone (TSH), serum calcium, magnesium, phosphorus and alkaline phosphatase, fasting and postprandial blood glucose levels and if necessary glucose tolerance test, and luteinizing hormone (LH), follicle stimulating hormone (FSH) and sex steroids in those with delayed puberty. In pediatric patients, height, weight, head circumference and growth velocity should be assessed ideally every 3 months.

Abnormal thyroid function may be reversible at an early stage through intensive chelation. In case of mild or overt hypothyroidism in addition to chelation therapy L-thyroxine is required.

Patients with thalassemia major should be regularly screened for impaired glucose tolerance test at least once every 2 years starting from 10 years of age. Management includes oral chelation therapy, dietary modifications, strict adherence to diabetic diet and weight reduction.

Growth hormone (GH) levels, serum IGF-IGFBP-3 and I are done in children with slow growth velocity after ruling out other causes of short stature. GH therapy is initiated with recombinant human GH at a dose of 0.025–0.05 mg/kg/day subcutaneous daily at night. Dose should be adjusted according to the clinical response. Adrenal function should be assessed mainly in GH deficient patients during GH therapy.

Anti-endomyseal and antitissue transglutaminase antibodies are done to rule out celiac disease. Assessment of height, weight, growth, velocity, cardiac work-up, endocrine study and bone studies evaluation are required from 10 years of age onward. This helps in early detection and better management.

CURATIVE OPTIONS

Bone Marrow Transplant or Stem Cell Transplant

Bone marrow transplantation is effective and offers the potential permanent cure if a human leukocyte antigen (HLA)-matched sibling donor is available when compared with the long-term ideal treatment. The credit of first BMT in thalassemia major goes to E Donald Thomas who performed this procedure in an 18-month-old thalassemic child in 1982 using HLA matched elder sister as donor. This child was cured of thalassemia. Dr M Chandi at Christian Medical College, Vellore, successfully did the first BMT in thalassemia in India. All over the world, transplantations have been done with a 70–80% cure rate **(Fig. 13.1.7)**.

The principles of BMT in thalassemia are:
- To destroy and prevent regeneration of defective stem cell.
- Sufficient immune suppression for good engraftment of normal marrow.

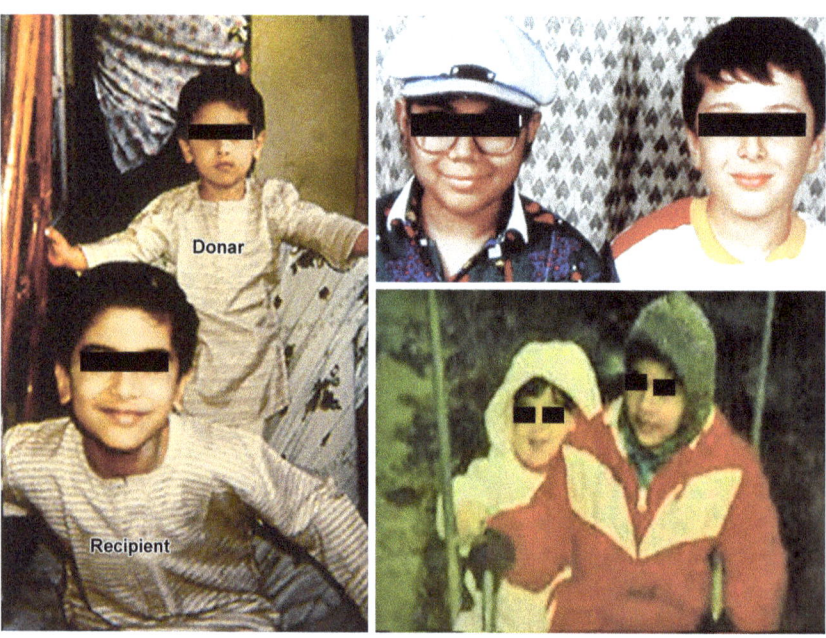

Fig. 13.1.7: Children cured by bone marrow transplant.

- To infuse stem cells with normal gene for beta-globin.
- To prevent graft versus host disease (GVHD) with high doses therapy of busulfan, cyclophosphamide, total body irradiation and other modalities.

The three most important adverse prognostic factors for survival and event-free survival are: (1) presence of hepatomegaly (liver more than 2 cm below costal margin), (2) portal fibrosis and (3) iron overload. BMT is most successful in patients who are young, properly transfused and well chelated and in good clinical shape without hepatomegaly. Ideal age of transplantation is between 2 years and 5 years. Younger the child, lesser the iron overload and other complications and hence better the results. Transplant outcomes are better with a fully HLA matched related donor. Cord blood from a matched related donor can also potentially provide good outcomes. The cost of BMT in India is around INR 1,000,000–1,500,000 and is being done at Vellore, Mumbai, Chennai, Ahmadabad, and Bengaluru, etc.

Pharmacological Methods to Increase Gamma Chain Production and Gene Manipulation

Drugs such as hydroxyurea, butyrate, 5-azacytidine and erythropoietin have been tried to induce HbF production with varying success. Hydroxyurea has been found to be useful particularly in thalassemia intermedia, double heterozygotes and sickle cell disease.

5-azacytidine

It is recommended in the dose of 2 mg/kg/day IV infusion in ringer lactate or saline solution at the rate of 6 mg/hour for 7 days. This leads to an increase in Hb from 8 to 10.8 g/dL in 2–3 weeks and an increase in fetal Hb from 1.06% to 20% on the 40th day. Side effects like nausea, vomiting, suppression of bone marrow and potential carcinogenesis have put limitations on its use in practice and unless a more effective compound with less toxicity becomes available such therapy is not recommended for thalassemia major.

Butyrates

These are found naturally increased in diabetic mothers. Their babies at birth have 100% HbF. In vitro trials found the efficacy of these drugs in increasing the HbF production. This drug is given as IV infusion slowly over 68-hours in dose of 200–400 mg/kg/day and has shown to increase HbF to 8–12% and cause a rise in Hb by 2–3 g/dL. The problem with this drug is the tedious IV route. Oral analog, sodium butyrate is useful in some patients to sustain the response after IV therapy. The side effects are few and include nausea, vomiting, electrolyte disturbances and occasional seizures. The actual efficacy of this drug is found to be lacking in many patients with sickle cell anemia and thalassemia intermedia.

Hydroxyurea

Hydroxyurea is a short-acting cytotoxic drug and is the only FDA-approved drug for the treatment of thalassemia and severe sickle cell disease. However, it is less effective in thalassemia and more likely to be useful in thalassemia intermedia. Hydroxyurea is started at dose of 5–10 mg/kg per day and slowly escalated as tolerated to 20 mg/kg per day.

Hemoglobin F induction with hydroxyurea may increase fetal hemoglobin and thus reduce transfusion requirements, decrease extramedullary erythropoietic masses, decrease leg ulcers and increase the general sense of wellbeing.

Erythropoietin

It has shown no benefit when used alone but in combination with hydroxyurea an additive effect has been found.

Metformin

Metformin is a FDA approved drug for the treatment of diabetes mellitus type 2. In a phase I study conducted in children more than 12 years with NTDT and sickle cell disease, it has been shown that metformin induces expression of HbF in primary erythroid cell cultures and is additive with hydroxyurea.

Thalidomide

Thalidomide is a drug known for its immunomodulating and antiangiogenic properties. It is known to induce γ globin gene expression and to increase the proliferation of erythroid cells. There are not enough clinical data to prove the efficacy of thalidomide. It is known to cause serious life-threatening episode of thrombosis even with a single course of the drug.

Amlodipine

Amlodipine is a calcium channel blocker broadly used in adults and children for the treatment of hypertension.

In a small phase III randomized trial conducted recently it has been shown that amlodipine at the dose of 5 mg per day (5 mg/day for patients weighing more than 30 kg or 2.5 mg/day for patients weighing 30 kg and less) has been shown to improve the myocardial iron overload without increasing the adverse effects when given in combination with standard iron chelation therapy.

There are evidences of studies done in animals, which suggest that iron enters cardiomyocytes through L-type calcium channels.

■ GENE THERAPY

In 2010, the first human gene therapy trial for β-thalassemia was published. Zynteglo is a genetically modified autologous CD34+ cell enriched population that contains hematopoietic stem cells (HSC) transduced with lentiviral vector (LVV) encoding the βA-T87Q-globin gene formerly known as *LentiGlobin BB305*. Bluebird Bio Inc. received approval for its gene therapy with Zynteglo (autologous CD34+ cells encoding βA-T87Q-globin gene) for patients ages 12 years and over with transfusion-dependent β-thalassemia who do not have the β0/β0 genotype from the European Medicines Agency (EMA) on June 3rd, 2019. It is specifically recommended for patients for whom HSC transplantation is appropriate but an HLA-matched, related HSC donor is not available. The estimated price is around $1.8 million. The EMA approval is based on the clinical data from two phase I/II trials in 22 patients out of which in 9 patients, the need for packed cell transfusion was reduced by 73% and 3 patients became transfusion independent. Global Data expects the positive interim data, two ongoing phase III trials, and a long-term follow-up study to be sufficient for Zynteglo's approval in 2020.

Outcomes were good for pediatric patients of age groups (6–13 years) in another phase I/II trial (NCT02453477) using GLOBE LVV expressing human β globin with 3 out of 4 patients obtaining elimination of transfusion requirement.

Another phase I trial (NCT01639690) using TNS9.3 LVV expressing wild type human β globin with a variant vector is under trial.

Fetal Globin Reactivation

BCL11A is being currently studied as a therapeutic target in β-thalassemia. It has been observed in phase I/II trial (NCT03432364) that disrupting the erythroid enhancer of the *BCL11A* gene, substantially increases HbF production in erythroid progeny of genome-edited CD34$^+$ hematopoietic stem/progenitor cells (HSPCs) using engineered zinc finger nucleases (ZFNs). The autologous modified HSPC drug product is named as ST-400 (BT). Some other phase I/II study uses CRISPR-Cas 9 genome editing technology.

Activin Receptor–II Ligand Traps

Sotatercept (ACE-011) and Luspatercept (ACE-536) are activin type IIA receptor fusion protein that binds to activin A and other transforming growth factor-β superfamily ligands such as BMP4, GDF11 AND GDF 15 to target late-stage erythropoiesis. They were initially produced to treat osteoporosis in postmenopausal women.

Sotatercept showed improvement in hemoglobin level and decreased transfusion burden in NTDT and TDT in phase II study with a dose of ≥0.3 mg/kg and ≥0.5 mg/kg, respectively. Doses were administered by subcutaneous injection every 3 weeks.

Luspatercept is being evaluated in phase III studies in TDT (BELIEVE, NCT02604433) and phase II in NTDT (BEYOND, NCT03342404). Luspatercept was administered subcutaneously every 3weeks at doses of 1 mg/kg in phase 3, double-blind, randomized, placebo-controlled, multicenter study (BELIEVE trial) which showed ≥ 33% reduction from baseline in RBC count transfusion burden with a reduction of at least two units from week 13 to week 24 compared to the 12-week. Luspatercept improved anemia and disease complications in patients with beta-thalassemia.

A Janus kinase (JAK2) inhibitor, ruxolitinib was assessed in 30 TDT patients with splenomegaly in a single arm open label phase II a study which showed reduction in spleen size and decrease in transfusion requirements of 5.9% from baseline administered orally at a starting dose of 10 mg twice daily.

Role of Hepcidin in Iron Overload

Hepcidin is a 25-amino acid peptide hormone and acts as an acute phase reactant. It is primarily produced in the liver in response to inflammation and increased iron stores. Hepcidin levels were reduced than expected in patients with β-thalassemia major who are highly iron overloaded because of active erythropoiesis in a study conducted by Pasricha et al. In murine model of thalassemia intermedia, it has shown to reduce iron overload. There are ongoing trials for hepcidin targeting drugs including hepcidin mimetics (LJPC-401, PTG-300), agonists of hepcidin regulator TMPRSS6 (Ionis-TMPRSS6-LRx) and ferroportin inhibitors (VIT -2763).

Role of Macrophage Manipulation Therapy

Role of macrophage manipulation therapy is still under experimental stage. Other approaches targeting iron dysregulation as mini-hepcidins, exogenous transferrin and erythroferrone inhibitors are in preclinical studies.

Wheatgrass

Wheatgrass acts as an antioxidant and detoxifier. It is also rich in many nutrients and also has amino acids. Oral intake of aqueous extract of Triticumaestivum (Wheatgrass) has shown to play a promising role in children with thalassemia receiving chronic blood transfusions in a study conducted by Mutha AS et al. and pilot study conducted by Marwaha et al. has shown to reduce transfusion requirement in TDT.

BMT in Utero

Research is underway on BMT in utero, at 14 weeks of gestation. Since the immune system is not developed at that time, there would be no rejection and mother's purified stem cells could be used, although the risk of GVHD would have to be looked into.

■ PREVENTION OF THALASSEMIA

The birth of a thalassemic child thus places considerable strain not only on affected child and family but on society at large. Therefore, there is an emphasis for shift from treatment to prevention of birth of such children in future. Not even 5–10% of thalassemic children born in India receive optimal treatment. Cost of treatment of a 4-year-old thalassemic child is around INR 100,000 annually. BMT as a curative treatment is out of reach for majority of children, which costs around INR 1,000,000–2,000,000.

Carrier Screening

The various strategies for carrier screening include the following:
- Population education
- Mass screening—screening of target population of high-risk communities
- Genetic counseling of "minor" couples and of those who test positive for thalassemia minor
- Genetic counseling
- Prenatal diagnosis of thalassemia.

Prenatal Diagnosis of Thalassemia

The incidence of misdiagnosis in prenatal testing is less than 1%. The reasons for failure include technical failure to amplify target DNA fragment, doubtful paternity, maternal contamination of samples and sample exchange.

Both preimplantation diagnosis and preconception diagnosis are available especially for couples who do not wish to undergo Medical Termination of Pregnancy (MTP) who are at a risk for transmitting a genetic disease or condition to their children. However, the procedures are technically demanding, difficult to organize and involve enormous cost. It is not an alternative to prenatal diagnosis.

■ CONCLUSION

Until last few decades thalassemia was regarded as a uniformly fatal disease and death was expected during the second decade of life before adulthood.

However, progress in the understanding and management of the disease in last three decades has improved prospects of survival such that they survive now into 3rd and 4th decades of life. This is possible provided that they receive the ideal treatment with good compliance. Thalassemia should no longer be, therefore, seen as a disease of childhood. Better management and improved survival has opened a new chapter in the management of thalassemia beyond transfusions and chelation therapy. The advent of advanced technology, with better management modalities and facilities, have metamorphosed thalassemia major from a fatal to a preventable, manageable as well as a curable disease.

■ BIBLIOGRAPHY

1. Agarwal MB. Advances in management of thalassemia. Indian J Pediatr. 2009;76:176-84.
2. Cappellini MD, Porter JB, Viprakasi V, et al. A paradigm shift on beta-thalassaemia treatment: How will we manage this old disease with new therapies? Blood Rev. 2018;32(4):300-11.
3. Casu C, Nemeth E, Rivella S. Hepcidin agonists as therapeutic tools. Blood. 2018;131(16);1790-4.
4. Casu C, Presti VL, Oikonomidou PR, et al. Short-term administration of JAK2 inhibitors reduces splenomegaly in mouse models of β-thalassemia intermedia and major. Haematologica. 2018;103(2):e46-9.
5. Dussiot M, Maciel TT, Fricot A, et al. An activin receptor IIA ligand trap corrects ineffective erythropoiesis in β-thalassemia. Nat Med. 2014;20(4):398-407.
6. Fernandes JL, Loggetto SR, Veríssimo MP, et al. A randomized trial of amlodipine in addition to standard chelation therapy in patients with thalassemia major. Blood. 2016;128(12):1555-61.
7. Khandros E, Kwiatkowski JL. Beta thalassemia monitoring and new treatment approaches. Hematol Oncol Clin N Am. 2019:33(3):339-53.
8. Lokeshwar MR. Thalassemia Syndromes. In: Parthasarathy A, Menon PSN, Nair MKC, (Eds). IAP Textbook of Pediatrics, 7th edition. New Delhi: Jaypee Brothers Medical Publishers (P) Ltd.; 2019. pp. 881-98.
9. Manglani MV, Kini PS. Management of ß-thalassemia—Consensus and controversies! Pediatr Hematol Oncol J. 2017;(2):94-7.
10. Marktel S, Cicalese MP, Giglio F, et al. Gene therapy for beta thalassemia: preliminary results from the phase1/2 Tiget-B thal trial of autologous hematopoietic stem cells genetically modified with GLOBE lentiviral vector. Blood. 2017;130(Suppl 1):355.
11. Taher AT, Karakas Z, Cassinerio E, et al. Efficacy and safety of ruxolitinib in regularly transfused patients with thalassemia: results from a phase 2a study. Blood. 2018;131(2):263-5.

13.2 NUTRITIONAL IRON DEFICIENCY ANEMIA

MR Lokeshwar, Sheikh Minhaj Ahmed

■ INTRODUCTION

Nutritional anemia is a major public health problem that affects children of all age groups especially during the periods of rapid growth where there is a demand supply mismatch. It has long-term implications if not addressed on time. It is a clinical state wherein the hemoglobin (Hb) and hematocrit (Hct) are below normal levels due to deficiency of one or more nutritional substrate required for hematopoiesis. These nutritional substrates include iron, folate, protein, vitamin B_{12}, vitamin E, ascorbic acid, and trace elements such as selenium, zinc, and copper. Supplementation of involved nutrients increases the Hb level to normal value.

It is estimated that 30% of the world population (1,200 million) suffers from nutritional anemia and of these, 90% are in the developing countries. In India, iron deficiency anemia (IDA) is the leading cause of nutritional anemia in children.

■ HISTORY OF IRON THERAPY

The nearest correlation of IDA can be made with *Pandu Roga* in Ayurveda. Father of *Pandavas* was known as Pandu as he was looking pale white. *Loha Bhasma* and *Mandura Bhasma* have been in use in Ayurveda for more than 5,000 years.

Therapeutic use of iron was known in Greek mythology—drinking wine in which sword rusted was a line of treatment. In ancient Greece, iron was thought to be imparted from the mythological figure Mars and therefore associated with "force" and "strength". It was thus primarily used therapeutically in war wounds.

In the 17th century, Sydenham used medicinal syrup of iron fillings steeped in cold wine to reduce symptoms of chlorosis or green sickness in young women. The treatment improved their headache, greenish nonicteric skin color, and consumption of stones and dirt. In the 19th century, IDA was confirmed as the cause of chlorosis based on identification of reduced iron concentration in the blood. In 1831, Blaud described iron treatment for chlorosis and developed the first modern day pill, a combination of ferrous sulfate and potassium carbonate.

■ EPIDEMIOLOGY

Iron deficiency anemia is common in children in age group 6–24 months. It affects preschool children, pregnant women, and old-aged persons. In

2010, global anemia prevalence was 32.9%. More than 2.2 billion people were affected with anemia wherein iron deficiency was the most common cause. WHO estimated that between 1993 and 2005, worldwide prevalence of anemia was 24.8% in general population—12.7% in men and 47.4% in children aged 0-5 years. Reported prevalence of anemia was 30.2% in women and 41.8% in pregnant women. Between 1995 and 2011, worldwide prevalence of anemia decreased by 4-5% in children aged 0-5 years, nonpregnant women, and pregnant women aged 15-49 years. In India, the prevalence of severe IDA was highest in Rajasthan (6.7%) followed by Uttar Pradesh (3.6%) and Madhya Pradesh (3.4%). The prevalence of anemia in rural children is higher in comparison to urban children.

■ DEFINITION

Iron deficiency anemia exists in two forms mainly as absolute and functional. When total body iron stores are normal or increased, it is termed as absolute iron deficiency. When the iron supply to the bone marrow is inadequate but the total body iron stores are normal or increased, it is called as functional iron deficiency.

WHO defines anemia as Hb of <110 g/L in children aged 0.5-4.9 years and Hb <115 g/L in those of 5-12 years of age **(Table 13.2.1)**. IDA is defined as ferritin level of <12 µg/L in children less than 5 years, and <15 µg/L in children between 5 years and 12 years without evidence of any anemia or fall in Hb below normal standard range.

Table 13.2.1: Criteria for diagnosis of anemia [Hemoglobin levels to diagnose anemia (g/dL)].

Age group	No anemia	Mild	Moderate	Severe
Children 6–59 months of age	>11	10–10.9	7–99	<7
Children 5–11 years of age	>11.5	11–11.4	8–10.9	<8
Children 12–14 years of age	>12	11–11.9	8–10.9	<8
Nonpregnant women (>15 years of age)	>12	11–11.9	8–10.9	<8
Pregnant women	>11	10–10.9	7–9.9	<7
Men	>13	11–12.9	8–10.9	<8

Source: Adapted from—World Health Organization. (2011). Haemoglobin concentrations for the diagnosis of anaemia and assessment of severity. [Online] Available from https://www.who.int/vmnis/indicators/haemoglobin/en/ [Last accessed December, 2019].

■ CAUSES

The etiology of IDA may be briefly classified as follows:
- *Decreased intake*: Prolonged breastfeeding and delayed introduction of iron-rich complementary feeds after the age of 6 months may predispose to IDA.
- *Increased requirement*:
    - During periods of growth as preterm infants, toddlers, puberty, reproductive age in females, pregnancy, and lactation.
    - Adolescence is a period of rapid growth, weight gain, and blood volume expansion. Iron requirement increases from preadolescent level of 0.7 mg to 0.9 mg iron per day to as much as 2.2 mg iron per day or more particularly in heavily menstruating girls. During this time, false concern about the body figure, food fads, and ignorance, particularly in girls, led to iron deficiency.
    - Lack of knowledge of nutritional factors further adds on to the problem.
- *Diet containing low iron or nonbioavailable dietary iron:*
    - It is estimated that in the wheat millet-based diet, iron absorption is around 2% and in rice-based diet, iron absorption is around 5–8%.
    - Cow's milk allergy also contributes to a high prevalence of anemia. Milk-induced enteropathy is the most common cause of occult gastrointestinal (GI) bleeding seen in approximately more than 50% of infants with IDA in western world.
- *Poor iron absorption*: Malnutrition, iron poor diet, malabsorption syndromes, chronic infections, chronic diarrhea, celiac disease, giardiasis, helminthiasis, sprue, hypoproteinemia, GI surgery, polyps, Meckel's diverticulum, hemorrhagic telangiectasia, peptic ulcer, and diverticulitis are other causes of bleeding diathesis and iron loss.
- Absorption of iron is enhanced by ascorbic acid, free hydrochloric acid, presence of sugars and amino acids in the diet; whereas presence of heme iron (nonvegetarian source of iron), and calcium in the form of milk, cheese depresses iron absorption. Ferrous iron is better absorbed compared to ferric iron.
- *Decreased iron stores*: This is seen in preterms and small for date neonates.
- *Increased losses*:
    - *GI bleeding*: In GI bleeding, the chronic loss of few milliliters of blood daily is enough to deplete iron stores and leads to iron deficiency. The GI bleeding may be due to diverticulitis, polyps, and repeated blood sampling.
    - *Blood losses in the menstrual cycle (menorrhagia)*: Females lose average of 40 mL blood per month in the menstrual cycle thus increasing the daily iron loss to 1.5 mg/day.

- *Intestinal parasites—hookworm infestation and giardiasis*: Infants are exposed to intestinal helminths from the time they start to crawl. Such infants may suffer from gastroenteritis and other infections further depleting their iron stores. 450 million people all over the world harbor hookworms and about 0.2 mL of blood/worm of *Ankylostoma* per day may be lost. With *Necator* infestation each worm accounts for blood loss of about 0.1–0.5 mL/day. Female subjects harboring more than 100 worms (5 mL/day blood loss) and male subjects harboring more than 250 worms (12.5 mL/day blood loss) tend to become anemic.
- *Fetomaternal hemorrhage*: This is a common cause of blood loss leading to anemia in the newborn. In about 50% of all pregnancies, there is some degree of fetomaternal hemorrhage. 8% are significant (0.5–40 mL fetal blood loss).
- *Repeated venipunctures* for investigations and hemodialysis are important iatrogenic causes of iron deficiency due to chronic blood loss.
- *Inadequate transport*: Atransferrinemia and antitransferrin receptor antibodies are the reasons for inadequate transport.
- *Genetic disorders*: Divalent metal transporter 1 deficiency anemia, Fanconi anemia, pyruvate kinase deficiency, etc. are causes of IDA. Rarely mutations in *STEP3* (*STEAP3*), *DMT1* (*SLC11A2*), and *TMPRSS6* genes may cause iron-refractory iron deficiency anemia (IRIDA). Gene sequencing may be necessary to rule out rare inherited iron-related anemias.

PATHOPHYSIOLOGY

Iron Requirements

Iron requirements per day are dependent on age, gender, weight, health, and physiological status of an individual. Thus, full-term infants with normal weight have adequate body iron store and do not suffer from iron deficiency at birth. On the contrary, preterm infants are deprived of time to build up body iron store and become susceptible to iron depletion and IDA.

According to the Institute of Medicine/Food and Nutrition Board (2001), daily iron intake is expected to be 7.8–11 mg/day at 6–12 months, 5.8–9.0 mg/day at 1–3 years, 6.1–10 mg at 4–8 years, and 8–11 mg/day at 9–13 years, corresponding to 0.9–1.3, 0.5–0.8, 0.3–0.5, and 0.2–0.3 mg/kg/day. Further, daily iron intake is maximum (7.8–11 mg) at the age between 6 months and 12 months, whereas its intake becomes minimum (5.8–9 mg) between 1 year and 3 years of age. In an adolescent child, iron requirement increases from preadolescent level of 0.7 mg to 0.9 mg iron per day to as much as 2.2 mg iron per day **(Table 13.2.2)**.

Table 13.2.2: Daily iron requirement in different age groups (mg/day).

Age	Male	Female
Birth to 6 months	0.27	0.27
7–12 months	11	11
1–3 years	7	7
4–8 years	10	10
9–13 years	8	8

Source: Institute of Medicine, Food/Nutrition Board (2001) and WHO/FAO (2004).

Iron Metabolism

Iron is an essential component of Hb in red blood cells (RBCs) and myoglobin in muscles, which is necessary for the functioning of various cellular mechanisms like enzymatic processes, DNA synthesis, and generation of mitochondrial energy. Dietary iron is available as heme and nonheme iron.

Heme iron is highly bioavailable since it is absorbed intact within the porphyrin ring. The absorption of this is not affected by food or any other factors in the gut. It is absorbed better than nonheme iron. It is the richest source of iron containing 10-18 mg of iron per 100 g. The nonvegetarian foods have Hb and myoglobin as in meat, fish, and poultry.

Nonheme iron is available in the form of ferric complexes. Nonheme iron is markedly affected by promotive and inhibitory iron-binding ligands. Foods rich in nonheme iron include cereals, pulses, legumes, bajra, nuts, dates, jaggery, and green leafy vegetables. The absorption of nonheme iron is retarded by alkaline pH, and presence of phosphates, phytates, bran, starch, tannins, calcium, antacids, other metals [Cobalt (Co) and lead (Pb)], etc. Phytates, which constitute 1-2% of many cereals, nuts and legumes, play a major role in the causation of nutritional anemia in the developing world.

Mucosal Cell Control

Iron is absorbed from the first and second parts of the duodenum, and at times jejunum. Maximum absorption of iron occurs from the duodenum. Two steps are involved in the absorption of iron—entry of iron from the intestinal lumen into the mucosal cell, and its passage from the mucosal cell into the plasma.

Appropriate iron balance in the body is achieved by mucosal cell control through transferrin and apoferritin receptors. The iron molecule that is taken into the mucosal cell across the brush border, can bind either to the apoferritin molecule or the ferroportin molecule in the mucosa. Iron status of the body at the time of the formation of the mucosal lining cells determines the amount of iron that is absorbed.

If iron in the plasma is adequate or there are increased iron stores, there is increased messenger iron in the mucosal cell. This messenger iron stimulates the production of apoferritin. Iron binds to apoferritin, which remains in the mucosal cell. There is increased transferrin saturation. Thus, whenever there is increased transferrin saturation or serum iron is normal and adequate, a larger fraction of the iron entering the mucosal cell is held back as ferritin and discarded, as the cell is desquamated, excreted, and gets denuded with the cell within 3 to 4 days.

If iron is required in the body, it is bound to the ferroportin, which is then transferred to the transferrin (produced in the liver), which carries it across the mucosa. It is then utilized in the bone marrow for Hb production, in the muscle tissue for myoglobin and in the body for various other enzymes. Any excess iron is stored in the form of ferritin in the liver.

The RBCs have a life span of approximately 120 days and are then destroyed in the spleen, liberating the free iron, which is then retransported to the bone marrow and other tissues for its reutilization. Thus, most of the iron is cycled continuously in the body, with only 1–1.5 mg/day of iron being excreted through the intestinal epithelial cells.

Since 10% of ingested iron is absorbed and the daily loss is only 1–1.5 mg, one needs to ingest about 10 mg of iron daily, except during periods of extra needs. Iron is stored in the body in the form of ferritin and hemosiderin.

In iron-deficiency state, the mucosal cell transports the iron rapidly to the circulation, where it combines with transferrin and is transported to the site of utilization and storage. Only one-tenth of the dietary iron is absorbed by the GI mucosa.

Hepcidin and its Role in Iron Metabolism

Hepatocytes produce the peptide hormone hepcidin (which is rich in cysteine rich). Hepcidin controls the release of iron from a variety of cells such as macrophages, hepatocytes, and enterocytes to plasma. It primarily controls iron absorption. The recycling of the iron from red cell lysis and release of iron from tissue iron stores is carried by interaction of hepcidin with ferroprotein, which is a cellular iron exporter. Release of ferroprotein is controlled by hepcidin.

Hepcidin expression is upregulated by high concentrations of iron in the liver and plasma, inflammation and physical activity whereas it is downregulated by iron deficiency, erythropoiesis, and hypoxia. A new hormone called erythroferrone was identified in 2014. It is produced by erythroblasts in response to erythropoietin and mediates hepcidin suppression.

Iron Transport and Storage

Transferrin helps in transport of iron from the intestines to the site of its utilization.

Transport of iron across the placenta: The transport of iron across placenta occurs against a gradient, thereby protecting fetus against iron deficiency. Babies with low iron stores may be born to mothers who are severely iron deficient during pregnancy. Most of the placental transfer of the iron occurs during the third trimester of pregnancy. Because of this, all preterm babies invariably develop anemia unless supplemented by iron and iron deficiency in the mother may cause preterm labor. About 3-4 mg of iron is passed from maternal circulation into the fetus during the last trimester of pregnancy.

Normal infants at birth have about 75 mg of iron per kg body weight, two-thirds of which is present in RBCs. Once the iron is assimilated in the body, it is not excreted. Normal body losses of iron are about 20 µg/kg/day. Most of these losses occur by shedding of cells from intestinal mucosa. Average loss of iron per day in children is 0.9 mg/day or 0.5 mg/m^2/day. Around 0.6 mg/day is lost in the GIT in the form of RBCs, bile or exfoliated mucosal cells. The rest is lost from the sweat, desquamated cells of the skin, and the urinary tract.

■ CLINICAL FEATURES

The spectrum of iron nutrition status can be divided into three stages:
1. *First stage—storage iron depletion*: Iron reserve is decreased or absent. It is characterized by reduced serum ferritin and reduced iron concentration in marrow and liver tissue. Hb, serum iron, and transferrin levels and saturation are within normal limits.
2. *Second stage—iron limited erythropoiesis (Iron deficiency without anemia)*: This refers to a milder form of iron deficiency where Hb has not fallen enough to meet the criteria of anemia. It may be transient and consists of a decrease in the transportation of iron. Hb level may still be normal or in the low normal range. Serum iron is low and total iron binding capacity (TIBC) is increased with low transferrin saturation and low serum ferritin levels.
3. *Third stage—iron deficiency anemia*: It represents the more severe form of iron deficiency. The supply of iron to erythroid cells in marrow is impaired, causing a reduction in Hb concentration, with progressive microcytic hypochromic anemia. Hb concentration has fallen with decreased serum iron, transferrin saturation, and serum ferritin levels. There is an increase in the free erythrocyte protoporphyrin (FEP), with detectable anemia, microcytosis, hypochromia on the peripheral smear with low mean corpuscular volume (MCV) and mean corpuscular hemoglobin (MCH) and high RBC distribution width (RDW).

Iron deficiency anemia is a multisystemic disease rather than pure anemia and hence the manifestations are many. Signs and symptoms are related to not only Hb level but also rate of fall of Hb and hemostatic adjustment of various systems in the body and underlying pathology. Common symptoms seen in infancy and childhood are vague such as pallor, loss of appetite, anorexia, failure to grow, recurrent infections, perspiration over the forehead, lethargy, lack of interest, and irritability. Hyperdynamic circulation may lead to palpitation, easy fatigue and shortness of breath, decreased exercise intolerance, and congestive heart failure.

If fall of Hb is gradual, the onset of symptoms may be insidious as there is cardiorespiratory adjustment. If the rate of fall of Hb is acute and rapid, child may be brought in a serious condition as in congestive failure and should be considered and treated as medical emergency.

Symptoms seen in adults like koilonychias, platynychia, angular stomatitis, bald tongue, and loss of papillae and angular cheilosis are not commonly seen in children and infants but may be seen in adolescent children. The triad of dysphasia which is much more for solids than liquids due to formation of esophageal webs at the pharyngoesophageal junction, koilonychia, and splenomegaly in a patient with IDA, known as the Plummer-Vinson or Patterson–Kelly syndrome is uncommon in infants and children. Mild splenomegaly is seen in 10–15% of patients.

Pica is a well-documented feature of anemia in children. Craving to eat substances (perverted appetite) such as eating dirt, clay (geophagia), ice (phagophagia), laundry starch (amylophagia), uncooked rice, salt, cardboard etc. are seen in almost 70–80% of patients and usually are cured by iron supplementation. Skull changes like those seen in congenital hemolytic anemia may also be seen in children with IDA present since early life. These skeletal changes do not reverse with iron therapy.

Development, Distractibility, and Cognitive Functions

Children with IDA are at high-risk of long-term impairment scores in IQ test, lack of concentration, short attention span, impaired mental, motor development, and distractibility. Teachers may complain that child is not doing well in the school. IDA in a growing child affects growth and development of brain and produces irreversible and permanent abnormalities of its function. Such deficits in cognitive functions may eventually result in school dropouts.

INVESTIGATIONS

Hemoglobin, RBC counts, and indices including reticulocyte count and peripheral smear examination are initial tests performed for the evaluation of IDA.

Hemoglobin Concentration

A fall in Hb or Hct represents anemia without any indication to its etiology. Hb estimation by cyanmethemoglobin method is considered a sensitive, rapid, and inexpensive investigation for routine practice and at field level. Hb estimation by HemoCue hemoglobin photometer has also been found to be simple and reliable, though costly.

Erythrocyte Morphology and Red Cell Indices

In a mild iron deficiency, red cell morphology and other red cell indices, e.g. MCV, MCH, and MCHC are not altered. However, in IDA, anisocytosis, microcytosis and hypochromia, presence of target cells and elongated (so-called pencil) cells is seen. Red cell indices become low, i.e. MCV <80 fl, MCH <27 pg, and MCHC <33%. MCV is more sensitive than MCH. Up to 30% cases of IDA could be misdiagnosed if only these indices are relied upon **(Flowchart 13.2.1)**.

Low Hb, low RBC count, low MCV, and high RDW suggest IDA. Low Hb, high RBC count, low MCV, and normal RDW suggest thalassemia minor or anemia of chronic infection **(Table 13.2.3)**.

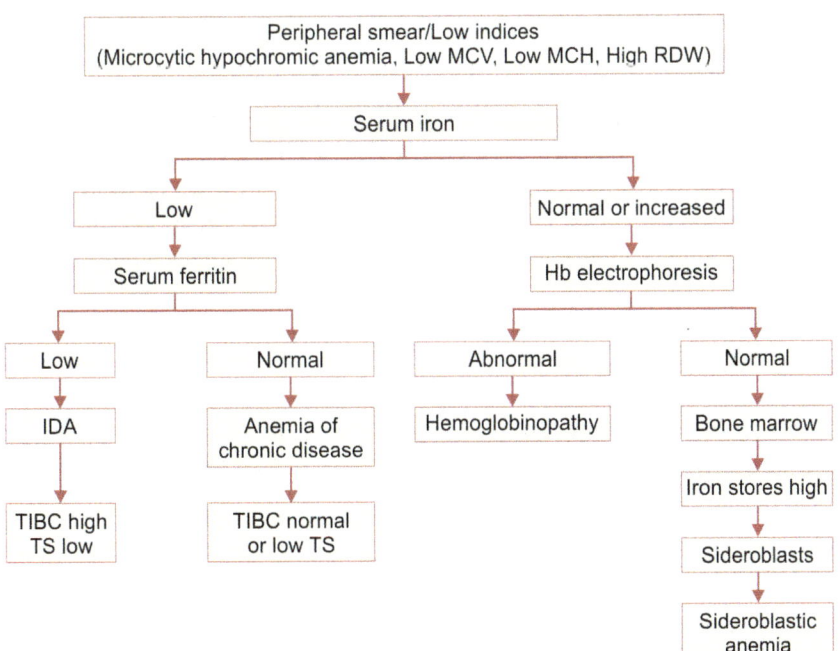

Flowchart 13.2.1: Approach to a child with microcytic hypochromic anemia.

(IDA: iron deficiency anemia; MCV: mean corpuscular volume; MCH: mean corpuscular hemoglobin; RDW: RBC distribution width; TIBC; total iron binding capacity; TS: transferrin saturation)

Table 13.2.3: Conventional test results in the progression of iron deficiency.

	Iron depletion	Iron-restricted erythropoiesis	Iron deficiency anemia
Hemoglobin (Hb) concentration	Normal	Normal	Reduced
Mean corpuscular volume (MCV)	Normal	Normal or reduced	Reduced
Reticulocyte hemoglobin content (CHr)	Normal	Reduced	Reduced
Serum iron (Fe) concentration	Normal	Reduced	Reduced
Serum ferritin concentration	Reduced	Reduced	Reduced
Total iron binding capacity (TIBC)	Normal	Increased	Increased
Soluble transferrin receptor	Normal	Increased	Increased

Red Cell Size Distribution

Electronic counters can provide red cell size distribution. The variability in red cell volume is reported as red cell distribution width (RDW). In IDA, RDW is more than 14.5%. RDW is highly sensitive (90–100%) but low in specificity (50–70%) in detecting IDA. In thalassemia trait and anemia of chronic disease, the RDW is normal.

Serum Ferritin

It is the best noninvasive test for evaluating body iron stores. It is also an acute phase reactant elevated in inflammatory disease such as ulcerative colitis and Crohn's disease. C-reactive protein (CRP) supports an inflammatory cause for elevated ferritin. Though decreased in IDA (< 12 ng/ dL), it may be increased when associated with infection and chronic disorders, e.g. chronic infection and inflammation, malignancies, and chronic liver disorders. ELISA is mostly used to assess serum ferritin level, besides the immunoradiometric assay (IRMA) and radioimmunoassay (RIA).

Serum Iron, Total Iron Binding Capacity, and Transferrin Saturation

These are useful tools in differentiating from other causes of microcytic, hypochromic anemia like thalassemia minor, anemia of chronic infection, sideroblastic anemia, and lead poisoning. Serum iron and transferrin saturation are decreased whereas TIBC is increased in IDA. The normal serum iron level varies considerably as it has a diurnal variation and peaks in the morning and decreases in the evening. Serum iron concentration may also be affected by chronic infection, malignancy, and chemotherapy. Values below 40 µg/dL (<12 µg/dL in young children) are considered diagnostic of iron deficiency (in the absence of infection or other disorders which affect iron metabolism). TIBC is the measure of transferrin circulating in the blood. In iron deficiency states, TIBC is increased (> 350 µg/dL) and transferrin saturation level is less than 16% (<14% for children).

Serum Soluble Transferrin Receptor

Serum soluble transferrin receptor is increased in anemia with increased erythropoiesis and also in IDA.

Free Erythrocyte Protoporphyrin and Protoporphyrin–Heme Ratio

The FEP value in a normal person is 15.5 ± 8.3 µg/dL of RBC. Levels more than 80 µg/dL of RBC below the age of 4 years, and more than 70 µg/dL of RBC above 4 years of age, are significant values to detect IDA. The mean protoporphyrin–heme ratio is 16.0.

Zinc Protoporphyrin

The measurement of ZPP concentration provides a reliable index of functional iron deficiency and may be used as an alternative to indices of red cell hypochromia or reticulocyte Hb content (CH_r), although it is less sensitive to acute changes in iron availability.

Hepcidin

Hepcidin is a regulator of iron metabolism. In IDA it is elevated.

Reticulocyte Count

It is usually normal. However, it may be increased, normal or decreased depending upon whether on treatment, there is recent blood loss and anemia is long-standing.

Reticulocyte Hemoglobin Content

The mean CHr and reticulocyte Hb equivalent (Ret-He) are two equivalent parameters that capture the amount of Hb available to the reticulocytes within the previous 3–4 days. The automated hematology analyzer can also report a measurement of reticulocyte-specific Hb content as mean CHr or Ret-He, depending on the type of instrument used. A decreased value (reduced < 27.5) generally reflects reduced cellular Hb content and is reliable in identifying functional iron deficiency. Furthermore, this parameter is the strongest predictor of IDA in children.

Bone Marrow Examination

Bone marrow examination is not required routinely for the diagnosis of IDA. It may be indicated in cases of IDA which are refractory to iron therapy. However, when done, it may show depletion of stainable iron in the marrow smear and erythroid hyperplasia. Bone marrow aspirates can be stained for hemosiderin by Perl's reaction and iron content is graded from 0 to 4. Although it is the most accurate technique to evaluate iron status, it is an invasive procedure and therefore impractical.

Other Supporting Tests

Routine stool and urine examination must be done to rule out associated helminthiasis, occult blood in stool, and RBC and pus cells in urine. Suspected inflammatory bowel disease can be investigated using a fecal calprotectin level. Tissue transglutaminase antibody levels help to rule out celiac disease.

Genetic Studies

Iron-refractory IDA (IRIDA) was first described by Buchanan and Sheehan in 1981 in three siblings who presented with IDA despite adequate nutritional intake of iron and had no visible evidence of GI blood loss. The siblings had no rise in Hb following oral ferrous sulfate ($FeSO_4$) therapy and responded only partially to parenteral iron treatment. In 2008, Finberg et al. classified these presentations as IRIDA and defined the key abnormalities along with mutations in *TMPRSS6* gene. The *TMPRSS6* gene is located on chromosome 22 and encodes for a transmembrane type II serine protease that suppresses hepcidin secretion by cleaving hemojuvelin, a surface coreceptor in BMP-6-SMAD signaling pathway.

Iron-refractory IDA has overlapping hematological features with classical IDA especially presence of low indices and low serum iron and transferrin saturation. Hepcidin/transferrin saturation ratio if high is a sensitive marker to identify cases of IRIDA phenotype and these cases should be subjected to *TMPRSS6* gene analysis. All 18 exons and exon–intron boundaries of *TMPRSS6* gene should be sequenced and to genetically confirm a case of IRIDA. Treatment in confirmed cases with IRIDA should be initiated with oral iron and vitamin C for 6–8 weeks as guidelines. Cases not responding or very minimally responding to above regimen should be planned for intravenous (IV) iron treatment.

Molecular genetic studies of iron deficiency involving human transferrin gene have reported human transferrin *G2775* mutation as a risk factor for iron deficiency.

Therapeutic Test

If facilities are not available for advanced tests, a simple therapeutic test done. This involves the evaluation of reticulocyte count after oral iron therapy,

Table 13.2.4: Response to iron therapy in iron deficiency anemia.

Time after iron administration	Response to iron therapy in iron deficiency anemia
12–24 hours	Replacement of iron enzymes, subjective improvement, decreased irritability, increased appetite
36–48 hours	Initial bone marrow response, erythroid hyperplasia
48–72 hours	Reticulocytosis, peaking at 5–7 days
4–30 days	Increase in Hb level

which starts increasing with 2-4 days of therapy. Hb increases by 1 g/week and reaches of normal Hb level by 3-6 months **(Table 13.2.4)**.

■ MANAGEMENT

The basic principles of management of IDA include of the following:
- Confirm the diagnosis
- Correction of anemia—iron therapy orally or parenterally, including replenishment of stores
- Treat the basic etiological factor to prevent failure of therapy and recurrence of deficiency
- Prevention of worm infestation
- Prevention and treatment of infection particularly chronic infections
- Taking care of nutrition deficient diet—diet counseling
- Treatment of bleeding—occult and persistent
- Preventive measures like iron supplementation and iron fortification.

Treatment of iron deficiency anemia depends upon the severity and associated complications. Those with very severe anemia and or in congestive heart failure, with a Hb <5 g/dL require hospitalization. Packed red cell transfusion is required for those in congestive heart failure irrespective of the level of Hb. It is preferable to give packed red blood cell (PRBC) transfusion 10-15 mL/kg. However, in children with signs of failure, PRBC as low as 2-5 mL/kg may be given at a time slowly administered over 2-4 hours to avoid volume overload and repeated 2-3 times a day. Exchange transfusion with packed cells should be considered if child is in failure. A small dose of furosemide may be administered before transfusion and may be required subsequently.

■ MEDICINAL IRON THERAPY

The aims of iron therapy are to confirm the diagnosis of IDA and to give iron in enough doses, for enough number of days to normalize the Hb levels and replenish stores, in a convenient way with least number of side effects.

It can be given either orally or parenterally. Oral iron therapy is the ideal treatment for IDA. It is safe, economical and as effective as parenteral therapy. Advantages of oral iron therapy are that it is cheap, effective, safe, convenient, and well tolerated. The desired Hb level is usually reached in 2 months and iron therapy should continue for another 2–3 months to build up iron stores. For infants and children, the recommended therapeutic dose is 3–5 mg of elemental iron per kg body weight per day. Higher doses are unnecessary and may increase side effects and reduce patient compliance. Oral iron therapy with monitoring is adequate for those without evidence of congestive heart failure. The oral iron preparations available in India are listed in **Table 13.2.5**.

Table 13.2.5: Various oral iron salts available.

Oral iron preparation	Iron compound mg/tab or 5 mL	Elemental iron mg/tab/mL	Comments	Brand name
Ferrous sulfate (hydrous)	300	60	Formulation of choice, low cost Higher GI side effects; staining of teeth Salty taste Poor acceptance	Folfer-Z (Tab)
Ferrous sulfate (dried)	200	65	Same as above	Ferrochelate–Z
Ferrous fumarate	100	33	Readily absorbed than ferrous sulfate hence less GI side effects Almost tasteless	Hemsi Vitcofol with Iron
Ferrous gluconate	259/10 mL	30	Similar efficacy and tolerability as ferrous sulfate	R B Tone
Ferrous succinate	100/tab	35	More completely absorbed, hence less GI side effects Costly	Hematrin
Ferrous bisglycinate	150/tab	30	An iron-amino acid chelate; high bioavailability Less GI intolerance than ferrous sulfate gluconate or ferrous fumarate Costly	Ferose

Contd...

Contd...

Oral iron preparation	Iron compound mg/tab or 5 mL	Elemental iron mg/ tab/mL	Comments	Brand name
Ferrous glycine sulfate	225 mg/tab	40	An iron-amino acid chelate Relatively high bioavailability	Hemfer-A
Ferrous ascorbate	100/5 mL	30	Promotes iron absorption Increased frequency of side effects	Ferronia-xt
Carbonyl iron	100/tab	98	Useful preparation for food fortification Poor oral iron absorption	Kool Z Hemogold
Sodium feredetate	231/tab	33	Effectively increase Hb profile and is tolerated well	Ferisan
Ferric ammonium citrate	150 mg/5 mL	30.75	Most commonly used ferric salt Requires reduction to ferrous form in the intestinal lumen Poor oral bioavailability Higher doses required for efficacy	Minmin Heme up
Polymaltose-iron complex (IPC)	100 mg	50 mg/mL	Ferric iron is complexed to hydrolyzed starch, making it tasteless and odorless Similar bioavailability as ferrous sulfate Promoted to cause less GI irritation, but the claim is unproven Costly Variable efficacy in different studies	Orofer, Fevorit
Colloidal iron	–	80/mL	Iron in colloidal form undergoes ready conversion to soluble form by action of gastric acid and is easily reduced to ferrous form; hence causes minimal gastric irritation	Tonoferon Ped syrup
Ferrous calcium citrate	–	25 mg	Low iron content and does not supply adequate elemental iron unless several tablets are taken which is inconvenient for the patient	Raricap-L

Supplementation of Iron Element—Oral and Parenteral

It is best absorbed when given on an empty stomach or in between the meals in divided doses. Compliance in the first month of treatment is important as maximal iron absorption occurs during this time. We recommend administering iron preparation before sleep 1-2 hours after dinner. Reduced gut motility during sleep improves absorption and reduces the side effects and has better compliance.

Dose for Preventive Supplementation

Elemental iron dosage is 2 mg/kg per day for children of all age groups. The highly bioavailable iron in breastmilk protects an infant from IDA up to 6 months. Supplementation with medicinal iron has been recommended by WHO for all children beyond 4 to 6 months of age and low birth weight babies from 2 months onward.

Therapeutic dose is given in the dose of 4-6 mg/kg/day of elemental iron till the Hb normalizes and is then continued for 3 more months to replenish stores. Compliance in the first month of treatment is important as maximal iron absorption occurs during this time. Children of 6-35 months of age should receive a daily uniform dose of iron and folic acid (IFA) supplement (20 mg elemental iron + 100 μg folic acid) in liquid form.

For women (15 years +) with severe anemia (Hb <7 g/dL), National Nutritional Anemia Control Program (NNACP) recommends two tablets of iron-folate tablet per day (each tablet containing 100 mg of elemental iron and 500 g of folic acid) for a minimum of 100 days. Prolonged duration of treatment may be required.

Combination with Other Nutrients

Addition of vitamin C (200 mg) increases the absorption of iron by about 30%. But addition of vitamin C may add to the cost significantly. Folic acid can be combined with iron at negligible extra cost. Vitamin B_{12} may need to be given to those with evidence of megaloblastic anemia. There is however no rationale in combining iron with multitude of vitamins, minerals and other hematinic in public health programs.

Daily versus Weekly Supplementation

In humans, intestinal mucosal turnover time is 5-6 days and is used as the basis for the weekly preventive supplemental regimen. The rise in Hb is nearly as effective as daily supplementation. Weekly supplementation has the advantage of being offered under supervised conditions and improves compliance. Based on a recent multicentric study in India, national consultation has now recommended that adolescent girls on attaining menarche should consume weekly dosage of one IFA tablet containing 100 mg elemental iron and 500 µg folic acid accompanied by appropriate dietary consumption. Weekly dose is considered as cost effective, with fewer side effects and better compliance.

Parenteral Iron Therapy

There is no evidence that the rate of Hb response is different in oral or parenteral therapy. Parenteral iron therapy should usually be avoided as it has severe side effects. Iron dextran complex is the most commonly used preparation. Newer preparations include iron gluconate and iron sucrose. But experience with these compounds is limited, however hence minimal side effects.

Parenteral route should be used only in specific indications:
- Severe intolerance to oral iron
- GI bleeding aggravated by oral iron therapy
- Bleeding more than the increase in Hb with oral iron, child not responding to oral iron therapy due to persistent significant bleeding like epistaxis (telangiectasia), gastrointestinal (GI) bleed, hookworm infestations, etc.
- Preoperative in urgent surgeries
- Decreased absorption as seen in various GI disorders and malabsorption syndromes such as chronic diarrhea, cystic fibrosis, Crohn's disease, surgery, etc.
- Noncompliance.

Total dose needed can be given including replenishing of stores, calculated by one of the following formula:

1. $\text{Iron (mg)} = \dfrac{\text{Weight (Kg)} \times \text{Hb deficit (g/dL)} \times 80 \times 3.4 \times 1.5}{100}$

2. Iron (mg) = Weight (Kg) × Hb deficit (g/dL) × 4

Sprinkles

A novel approach currently under study is "sprinkler" which contains microencapsulated ferrous sulfate or microencapsulated ferrous fumarate. These can be sprinkled on any complementary food at the table given by caregiver. Iron being encapsulated does not change the color and the taste of the food. It is available as Tasiron sachet and has good compliance and effective. Sprinkles have been shown to be efficacious in the treatment of anemia in many developing countries. In Sprinkles, the iron (ferrous fumarate/pyrophosphate) is encapsulated within a thin lipid layer to prevent the iron from interacting with food.

Side Effects of Iron Therapy

These include nausea, vomiting, abdominal cramps, discomfort, diarrhea, constipation, staining of tongue and teeth, and blackish discoloration of teeth, tongue, and of stools. Though most of the reaction is mild and transient, anaphylactic reactions may be life-threatening and hence one should always keep injection adrenaline, inj. hydrocortisone, and resuscitative measures handy before injecting.

Causes for not Responding to Oral Iron Therapy

- Ineffective, inadequate or improper dose
- Associated infections
- Associated occult hemorrhage
- False failure can occur due to wrong diagnosis
- Poor compliance.

■ PREVENTION

Basic approach to prevention of IDA includes dietary modification, food-based interventions, and iron supplementation.

Dietary Modification

The iron content of commonly consumed food articles is given in **Table 13.2.6**.

Individual level prevention by dietary advice and iron supplementation consists of the following steps:
- *Exclusive breastfeeding* till the age of 4 to 6 months. *Avoid bottle feeding.* An infant taking 600–650 mL of breastmilk daily ingests approximately 0.3 mg of iron/day. However, the bioavailability of this iron is quite high. As much as 0.15 mg of iron per day is absorbed which is sufficient for an exclusively breastfed baby. From 6 months of age, the iron requirement increases markedly and hence the iron from breastmilk alone is no longer sufficient.
- *Premature babies and growing babies* should be given oral iron supplemental iron after the age of 2 months.
- *Weaning foods.* Commercially prepared iron-rich weaning foods though available in developed countries, are very expensive and beyond the reach of most of the families and so not recommended. Complementary foods rich in iron and vitamin C (such as cooked vegetables and raw fruits) are not difficult to prepare at home and hence parents should be taught how to prepare mashed vegetables, citrus fruit juices, egg preparations, minced mutton etc. and motivated to introduce these to the infants in early life after 4–6 months of age. Encouraging the timely introduction of iron-containing weaning food is an important step in prevention of anemia in

Table 13.2.6: Iron content of food articles.

Food	Iron content (mg/100 g)	Articles rich in iron
Cereals	2.5–14.0	Bajra, wild barley, *kangri* ragi, rice flakes, whole wheat flour, *kodra (Harik)*
Pulses and legumes	2.7–11.0	Bengal gram, cow gram, soybean
Leafy vegetables	0.9–40.0	Amaranth, beet, greens, Bengal gram leaves, coriander, *alu* leaves, *pudina, neem*, radish top, *rajgira* leaves, turnip greens, all types of green *bhajis* (spinach, *methi*, lettuce, etc.)
Roots and tubers	0.4–13.9	
Other vegetables	0.2–22.2	Amaranth seeds, *dhaincha* seeds
Nuts and oil seeds	2.5–10.0	Garden cress, gingelly, mustard
Fruits	0.1–10.0	Dates, *karwands*, raisins
Seafood	1.0–11.5	Most Indian fish, crab
Meat	2.0–18.8	Beef
Milk	0.2–0.8	
Miscellaneous	11 mg	Jaggery
	3.3 mg	Yeast

Source: Indian Council of Medical Research. Dietary Guidelines for Indians – a Manual. National Institute of Nutrition, Indian Council of Medical Research. Hyderabad, 1998.
Mehta MN, Mehta NJ. Nutrition and Diet for Children Simplified, 1st edition. New Delhi: Jaypee Brothers Medical Publishers Pvt Ltd; 2014.

early infancy and childhood. Introduction of iron containing food after the age of 4–6 months is the most important step in prevention of anemia of infancy.

- *Older children:* Encourage taking diet containing iron such as sprouted cereals, green and leafy vegetables, nonvegetarian food like mutton, chicken, fish, egg, and liver preparations.
- Fortification of staple food with iron and introduce iron containing food in the diet. Salt and food fortification particularly with salt (1 mg of iron/g of salt) is one of the effective ways to control IDA.

Dietary modification, for older children and adult for iron supplementation can be done by:

- Increasing total consumption of habitual food so that their energy needs are fully met.
- Enhancing the bioavailability of iron ingested by promoting the intake of iron absorption enhancer including heme iron, vitamin C, meat, fish, and

other seafood and simultaneously reducing the ingestion of inhibitors of iron absorption like phytic acid, tannin, etc.
- *Heme iron* is present in meat, fish, poultry as well as in blood products (nonvegetarian food). However, it is a very small fraction of the total iron intake particularly in persons from developing poor countries.
- *Cooking of food in iron pots* may increase the iron content of a meal several fold. This is especially true for soups containing vegetables. Frying in iron pans does not increase the food's iron content.
- *Iron absorption enhancers.* In developing countries where meat intake is low, vitamin C (ascorbic acid) is the single most important enhancer of iron absorption. Adding as little as 50 mg of ascorbic acid to a meal **(Table 13.2.7)**, will double the iron absorption (an orange or lemon, or cabbage 100 g or 200 g of amaranth will provide sufficient amount of vitamin C). Germinating, malting, and fermenting also increases iron

Table 13.2.7: Approximate ascorbic acid content—fruits and vegetables.

Food	Vitamin C content (mg/100 g)
Fruits	
Guava	326
Lemon, fresh (juice)	37–50
Orange, fresh	46
Pineapple fresh	37
Mango fresh	42
Vegetables	
Cabbage (raw)	54–60
Cabbage (boiled)	15
Cauliflower (raw)	60–96
Cauliflower (boiled)	20
Potato (raw)	21
Potato (boiled)	12–18
Sweet potato (raw)	25–37
Sweet potato (boiled)	15
Spinach (boiled)	7–25
Tomato (raw)	20–26
Turnip (boiled)	17

Source: Indian Council of Medical Research. Dietary Guidelines for Indians – a Manual. National Institute of Nutrition, Indian Council of Medical Research. Hyderabad, 1998.
Mehta MN, Mehta NJ. Nutrition and Diet for Children Simplified, 1st edition. New Delhi: Jaypee Brothers Medical Publishers Pvt Ltd; 2014.

absorption by increasing the vitamin C content and lowering tannin and phytic acid. Germination increases the bioavailability by almost 2-fold.
- Nonvegetarian foods not only have a rich amount of heme iron, but they enhance the absorption of the nonheme iron contained in the rest of the meal. However, enhancing meat consumption by the poor rural people will be unrealistic.
- Avoid junk food.

Food-based Interventions

At Community Level

- Fortification of widely consumed and centrally processed staple food with iron has been successfully used in many countries. Food fortification is one of the most effective ways of prevention of iron deficiency.
- Fortification of suitable food vehicles with absorbable forms of iron is a highly desirable approach in controlling iron deficiency. Fortify a staple food that is consumed in significant quantity regularly by most people. Another approach is to fortify a widely consumed condiment—fish sauce, curry powder, salt, and sugar have all been successfully fortified with iron.
- In South America, both dried and liquid milk as well as milk products like yoghurt have been fortified with iron. In infants who receive complementary feeds, fortified infant food is an important component of control of IDA and has been successfully tried in United States and Latin America. However, this is beyond the reach of the poor parents of the developing countries.
- Ferrous fumarate, ferrous gluconate, lactate, and ferous sulfate have been extensively used for the fortification of wheat flour, bread and other bakery products, corn-soya-milk preparation (CSM), salt, sugar, fish sauce, rice, etc. The combined use of ferric orthophosphate and sodium acid sulfate or ferrous sulfate, orthophosphoric acid in the fortification of table salt has recently been reported to produce acceptable long-term bioavailability with only slight discoloration. This gives additional 10–15 mg of iron to adult per day. Iron salt EDTA (ethylene diamine tetra acetate) has been successfully used to fortify sugar or wheat flour in Guatemala (13 mg of iron/100 mg sugar).

Iron Supplementation

Supplementation with oral iron tablet or syrup is the most widely used approach to control global problem of IDA.

Advantages of supplementation of medicinal iron include that it can provide a rapid result to an ongoing problem. It can be targeted at population group at great risk and "captive audience" who can receive the supplements at school or work such as pregnant women, adolescent girls, school children, preschool children, infants, and plantation workers.

In India, prophylactic supplementation of oral tablets of iron (20 mg iron + folic acid 10 mg) once a day every year for 100 days has been recommended by National Nutritional Anemia Control Program. The age-specific interventions are based on WHO recommendations, synthesis of global evidence on IFA supplementation and the recommendations of national experts **(Table 13.2.8)**.

Other Health Measures

Helminth Control (Deworming) (Table 13.2.9)

Where hookworm infection is endemic (prevalence 20–30% or higher) and anemia is very prevalent, hookworm infection is likely to be an important cause of anemia, especially moderate-to-severe anemia. Hookworms (*Necator americanus* and *Ankylostoma duodenale*) infect approximately 1 billion of the world's population.

At the population level, endemic hookworm infection contributes to the prevalence of anemia and has the greatest effect on the prevalence of moderate and severe anemia. Hence anthelminthic therapy should be given presumptively to anyone with severe anemia, because treatment is safe and much less expensive than diagnosing hookworm infection. Anthelminthic treatment to schoolchildren without prior screening is currently recommended in the school setting and combined with IFA supplementation in antenatal care. School-based anthelminthic chemotherapy (deworming) alone may help prevent moderate-to-severe anemia in school children, but the most effective

Table 13.2.8: Iron and folic acid (IFA) supplementation program.

Age group	Intervention/Dose	Regime
6–60 months	1 mL of IFA syrup containing 20 mg of elemental iron and 100 µg of folic acid	Biweekly throughout the period 6–60 months of age and de-worming for children 12 months and above
5–10 years	Tablets of 45 mg elemental iron and 400 µg of folic acid	Weekly throughout the period 5–10 years of age and biannual de-worming

Table 13.2.9: Dosage of albendazole tablets for biannual deworming:

Age	Dose (Albendazole 400 mg tablet)
1–2 years	Half tablet
2 years upward	One tablet

strategy for anemia control is to combine anthelminthic chemotherapy with iron supplementation.

Prevention of Malaria

Plasmodium falciparum malaria causes profound anemia during and after acute infection. Detecting and treating malaria are essential for treating severe anemia where *P. falciparum* malaria is endemic. Where *P. falciparum* malaria is endemic, the use of insecticide-impregnated bed nets in communities decreases the prevalence of severe anemia in young children. Malaria prophylaxis during pregnancy may reduce the prevalence of anemia in first and second pregnancies and improve birth weight.

Infections

Certain chronic diseases, such as cancer, HIV/AIDS, rheumatoid arthritis, Crohn's disease and other chronic inflammatory diseases, can interfere with the production of RBCs, resulting in chronic anemia.

Celiac Disease

The British Society of Gastroenterology (BSG) recommends all IDA patients should be screened for celiac disease. It is implicated in 4–6% of cases.

Helicobacter pylori

H. pylori is responsible for less than 5% of cases and impairs iron absorption. It is often a missed cause of IDA. It will not respond to iron and symptoms may be masked by the side effects of iron treatment.

■ ONGOING RESEARCH

In a pilot study, vitamin D supplementation was associated with a 34% decrease in circulating concentrations of hepcidin ($p < 0.05$). A fully human anti-hepcidin antibody affected iron metabolism in both mice and non-human primates, and early phase clinical studies are beginning to be reported.

■ CONCLUSION

Nutritional anemia is a pathological condition in which Hb and Hct levels becomes abnormally low because of deficiency of one or more essential nutrients needed for Hb formation and hemopoiesis, regardless of the cause of these deficiencies. When anemia is due to nutritional deficiency, increasing the person's intake of deficient nutrients will raise the Hb and Hct.

Iron deficiency is the most common malady known to mankind since ages, though iron is available in plenty in environment. The reasons for IDA are mainly faulty dietary habits especially during growth period. Exclusive breastfeeding and proper weaning will prevent IDA in most cases. Iron supplementation in high-risk group is another alternative. IDA in early life can permanently reduce the intellectual potential. All it needs is realization of magnitude of problem of IDA and open eyes to prevent, detect, and treat IDA in time! Paradox is "Poverty in the midst of plenty".

Review of the combination of CBC, reticulocyte count, CHr or Ret-He, and peripheral smear along with serum iron, serum ferritin, and TIBC often provides evidence to support the diagnosis of IDA. However, the most convincing evidence of IDA is an increase in the Hb concentration after a therapeutic trial of medicinal iron.

Initial therapy for IDA is an oral iron medication for a minimum of 3 months, while attempting to identify and correct the underlying cause. Nevertheless, firm data regarding optimal dose, duration of therapy, and monitoring of the hematologic response are unavailable. The administration of parenteral iron to patients who fail oral iron treatment warrants further investigation and strong consideration as a potentially safe and effective option to oral iron dosing. IRIDA is a relatively recently described autosomal recessive condition that results from mutations in *TMPRSS6* gene likely being missed or underdiagnosed in our iron-deficient endemic setting due to lack of general awareness amongst physicians in establishing the diagnosing or due to lack of availability of proper genetic testing.

■ BIBLIOGRAPHY

1. Bacchetta J, Zabriskie JJ, Sea JL, et al. Suppression of iron-regulatory hepcidin by vitamin D. J Am Soc Nephrol. 2014;25(3):564-72.
2. Bhatia P, Jain R, Singh A. A structured approach to iron refractory iron deficiency anemia (IRIDA) diagnosis (SAID): The more is "SAID" about iron, the less it is. Pediatr Hematol Oncol J. 2017;2(2):48-53.
3. Gupta A. Nutritional Anemia in Preschool Children. Germany: Springer; 2017.
4. Kautz L, Jung G, Valore EV, et al. Identification of erythroferrone as an erythroid regulator of iron metabolism. Nat Genet. 2014;46(7):678-84.
5. Kotwal A. Iron deficiency anaemia among children in South East Asia: Determinants, importance, prevention and control strategies. Current Medicine Research and Practice. 2016;6(3):117-22.
6. Lokeshwar MR, Shah NK. Nutritional anemia in infancy, childhood and adolescents. In: Lokeshwar MR, Shah NK, Agarwal BR, Manglani MV, Sachdeva A (Eds). Textbook of Pediatric Hematology and Hemato-Oncology, 1st edition. New Delhi: Jaypee Brothers Medical Publishers Pvt Ltd; 2016. pp. 100-25.
7. Lopez A, Cacoub P, Macdougall IC, et al. Iron deficiency anaemia. Lancet. 2016;387(10021):907-16.
8. Mehta MN, Mehta NJ. Nutrition and Diet for Children Simplified, 1st edition. New Delhi: Jaypee Brothers Medical Publishers Pvt Ltd; 2014.

9. National Health Mission. National Iron Plus Initiative for Anaemia Control Among 6 Months Onwards Population. [Online] Available from http://www.nrhmhp.gov.in/sites/default/files/files/Iron%20plus%20initiative%20for%206%20months%20-5%20years.pdf [Last accessed December, 2019].
10. National Institute of Nutrition, Indian Council of Medical Research, Hyderabad. (1998). Dietary Guidelines for Indians – a Manual. [Online] Available from http://ninindia.org/DietaryGuidelinesforNINwebsite.pdf [Last accessed December, 2019].
11. Van Eijk LT, John AS, Schwoebel F, et al. Effect of the antihepcidin Spiegelmer lexaptepid on inflammation-induced decrease in serum iron in humans. Blood. 2014;124(17):2643-6.
12. Wong C. Iron deficiency anemia. Paediatr Child Health. 2017;27(11):527-9.
13. World Health Organization. (2011). Haemoglobin concentrations for the diagnosis of anaemia and assessment of severity. [Online] Available from https://www.who.int/vmnis/indicators/haemoglobin/en/ [Last accessed December, 2019].

CHAPTER 14

ONCOLOGY

14.1 Acute Lymphoblastic Leukemia
Anupama Borker, Narendra Chaudhary

14.1 ACUTE LYMPHOBLASTIC LEUKEMIA

Anupama Borker, Narendra Chaudhary

■ INTRODUCTION

The progress in the treatment of childhood acute lymphoblastic leukemia (ALL) is in a way the story of modern medical oncology. Starting from the 1940s when the disease was almost uniformly fatal to the current decade, the treatment of childhood leukemia has been the torchbearer of medical oncology.

It was Sidney Farber at the Children's Hospital in Boston who first experimented with treating childhood leukemia with folic acid. The hypothesis was that—if folic acid could cure pernicious anemia, it could cure leukemia. The experiment failed miserably, accelerating leukemia and hastening the death of all those children. This led Farber to think that if folic acid was food for the leukemia, could there be a drug that worked as an antifolate to stop its growth? That led to the next experiment using the antifolate aminopterin to treat children with leukemia. The miraculous results of this trial led to the first paper on the treatment of childhood ALL in the New England Journal of Medicine in 1948.[1] Since then, there has been no looking back. From temporary remissions lasting for a few months in the 1940s to 90% cure rates in the 2010s, it has been a relentless and heady journey.

As other drugs were discovered, there were attempts to combine the available drugs in various permutations and combinations to achieve the best possible results.[2] This led to the evolution of the principles of combination chemotherapy using drugs synergistically to potentiate anti-leukemia effect while keeping toxicity within acceptable limits. As the need to enroll more patients was realized, multicentric trials spanning continents were conducted and these systematic efforts began to show results in the 1970s when survival rates started rising from 10–20% to over 50%.[3,4] The introduction of high-dose methotrexate was a turning point in the progress against childhood ALL.[5]

Understanding that childhood ALL was a heterogeneous disease with differences in biological characteristics having impact on the clinical outcomes was paramount to individualizing therapy in various subtypes.[6] With the human genome project, gene expression profiling of ALL became feasible and provided insights into various new subtypes.[7] The use of minimal residual disease (MRD) monitoring and incorporating it into risk stratification and treatment planning led to improvements in outcomes for high-risk patients, while decreasing toxicity and treatment sequelae in low-risk patients.[8,9]

Relapse remains a major challenge in treating childhood ALL. Till a decade ago, bone marrow transplant was the only hope for children with early and high-risk relapse. The advent of immunotherapy and chimeric antigen receptor (CAR) therapy now offers more options for these children.

In this review, we will focus on the new risk stratification schema, some of the newer subtypes of ALL, optimal use of MRD monitoring in treatment, and current treatment options for relapsed ALL.

■ NEWER RISK STRATIFICATION

Risk-based treatment of ALL started in the 1970s when it was realized that not all children with ALL need the same intensity of treatment to get cured. The stratification though has got complex over the years. In the early trials, only two risk factors were used, viz. age and presenting white blood cell (WBC) count, and there were only two groups. Standard risk group according to the National Cancer Institute (NCI) included children in the age group of 1–10 years and with a presenting WBC count of less than 50,000/mm^3. Children less than 1 year or older than 10 years, and those with a presenting WBC count greater than 50,000/mm^3 were considered as high-risk patients. The presence of extramedullary disease in the form of central nervous system (CNS) or testicular involvement was later recognized as a risk factor. The inability of antileukemia drugs to penetrate the blood–brain barrier and the blood testicular barrier made these areas sanctuary sites for leukemic blasts.

Leukemia-related factors like the immunophenotype and cytogenetic features were then incorporated into risk stratification. T-cell ALL was recognized as a high-risk leukemia needing more intensive treatment. Certain recurrent chromosomal aberrations like hypo- and hyperdiploidy and t(9,22),[9,10] *mixed-lineage leukemia (MLL)* gene rearrangement and t(12,21)[11,12] were included as risk factors.

What emerged after all this was the fact that despite risk stratification, some patients in each risk category responded well to initial therapy and some did not. Those that did not were shown to fare poorly. Two indicators demonstrated this early response. First was the response to 1-week prephase of steroids. Patients who cleared blasts from peripheral blood with 1 week of steroid therapy were termed as good prednisone responders and those who did not were poor prednisone responders. Early prednisone responders had a much better chance of cure. The second indicator was clearance of MRD from the bone marrow at the end of induction chemotherapy.

Over the years, this MRD negativity at the end of induction has emerged as the single most important prognostic factor in determining long-term outcome.[13] Most current ALL protocols incorporate MRD at the end of induction; and some at the end of consolidation in further risk stratification of patients.

Current risk stratification systems include four risk groups—low, standard, high, and very high risk for B-ALL **(Table 14.1.1)**. Those with standard risk features but with good risk cytogenetic features are classified as low risk and are spared long-term toxicity by de-escalating treatment.[14]

Table 14.1.1: Risk stratification of acute lymphoblastic leukemia/lymphoma.

Risk group	Features	Recommended therapy	Expected outcomes

Low	All the following:
	• NCI standard risk group*
	• Low-risk cytogenetics—Trisomy 4 and 10:
	  – ETV-RUNX1
	  – Hyperdiploidy
	• Rapid response to therapy
		Conventional antimetabolite based therapy	>95%

Average	Either of the following: • NCI standard risk group and rapid response to therapy • NCI standard risk group and Lesser risk cytogenetics and slow response to therapy	Intensified antimetabolite therapy	90–95%
High	Any one of the following: • NCI high-risk group** and rapid response to therapy# • NCI standard risk group and slow response to therapy@ • CNS-positive leukemia • Testicular leukemia	Intensive multiagent therapy	88–90%
Very high	Any of the following: • MRD+ at day 29 • Induction failures • *MLL* rearrangement or iAMP21 amplification • Age < 1 year	• Consider allogeneic hematopoietic stem cell transplant in first remission • (Not recommended for infants)	<80%
Special	T-cell ALL	Intensive multiagent therapy	66–80%
	Philadelphia chromosome t(9-22)[9,11]	Intensive multiagent therapy with a BCR/ABL tyrosine kinase inhibitor	70%

(CNS: central nervous system; MRD: minimal residual disease; NCI: National Cancer Institute; MLL: mixed-lineage leukemia; iAMP21: intrachromosomal amplification of chromosome 21)
Note:
*NCI standard risk group: WBC <50,000/mm^3 *and* age 1 to <10 years.
#*Rapid response to therapy*: MRD negative at days 8 and 29.
@*Slow response to therapy*: MRD positive at day 8 and negative at day 29.
**NCI high-risk group: WBC ≥50,000/mm^3 *or* age ≥10 years.
Source: Adapted from: Hunger SP, Loh ML, Whitlock JA, et al. Children's Oncology Group's 2013 Blueprint for Research: Acute Lymphoblastic Leukemia. Pediatr Blood Cancer. 2013;60(6):957-63.

■ NEWER SUBTYPES OF ALL

Acute lymphoblastic leukemia was first classified into three subtypes (L1, L2, and L3) based on French American British (FAB) morphological criteria. The World Health Organization (WHO) in 1997 classified ALL into three types (B-cell, T-cell, and Burkitt's) based on immunophenotypic characteristics. Later in 2008, WHO revised this classification. Burkitt's leukemia was removed from ALL classification, as it was like Burkitt's lymphoma in morphology as well as management. Also, B-cell ALL was subdivided into two subtypes: (1) B-cell ALL with recurrent genetic abnormalities and (2) B-cell ALL not otherwise specified. In the 2016 update, WHO added two new provisional entities in the list of recurrent genetic abnormalities (Ph-like and iAMP21) in B-cell ALL and one new provisional entity (early T-cell precursor ALL) in T-cell ALL **(Box 14.1.1)**.[15] The underlying genetic abnormalities can be grouped as good risk or poor risk according to observed response to treatment **(Box 14.1.2)**.

Philadelphia Chromosome-like ALL

Philadelphia chromosome-like acute lymphoblastic leukemia (Ph-like ALL) is a new entity of B-cell ALL characterized by gene expression profile like Ph-positive ALL but not having typical *BCR-ABL1* translocation. This entity is seen among 10–20% of pediatric and 20–30% of adult ALL. It is associated with

---

Box 14.1.1: World Health Organization (WHO), 2016 classification of acute lymphoblastic leukemia/lymphoma.

B-lymphoblastic leukemia/lymphoma:
- B-lymphoblastic leukemia/lymphoma, NOS
- B-lymphoblastic leukemia/lymphoma with recurrent genetic abnormalities:
    - B-lymphoblastic leukemia/lymphoma with t(9;22) (q34.1;q11.2); *BCR-ABL1*
    - B-lymphoblastic leukemia/lymphoma with t(v;11q23.3); *KMT2A* rearranged
    - B-lymphoblastic leukemia/lymphoma with t(12;21) (p13.2;q22.1); *ETV6-RUNX1*
    - B-lymphoblastic leukemia/lymphoma with hyperdiploidy
    - B-lymphoblastic leukemia/lymphoma with hypodiploidy
    - B-lymphoblastic leukemia/lymphoma with t(5;14) (q31.1;q32.3); *IL3-IGH*
    - B-lymphoblastic leukemia/lymphoma with t(1;19) (q23;p13.3); *TCF3-PBX1*
    - Provisional entity: B-lymphoblastic leukemia/lymphoma, *BCR-ABL1*–like
    - Provisional entity: B-lymphoblastic leukemia/lymphoma with iAMP21

T-lymphoblastic leukemia/lymphoma:
- Provisional entity: Early T-cell precursor lymphoblastic leukemia
- Provisional entity: Natural killer (NK) cell lymphoblastic leukemia/lymphoma

(iAMP21: intrachromosomal amplification of chromosome 21; NOS: not otherwise specified)

Source: Arber DA, Orazi A, Hasserjian R, et al. The 2016 revision to the World Health Organization classification of myeloid neoplasms and acute leukemia. Blood. 2016;127(20):2391-405.

> **Box 14.1.2:** Novel genetic risk groups in acute lymphoblastic leukemia.
>
> *Good risk genetic abnormalities (GEN-GR):*
> - Good risk cytogenetic (CYTO-GR):
>   – ETV6-RUNX1
>   – High hyperploidy (51–65)
> - Good risk copy number alterations (CNA-GR):
>   – No deletions
>   – Isolated deletions of *ETV6*, *PAX5*, or *BTG1*
>   – *ETV6* deletions with single additional deletion of *BTG1*, *PAX5*, or *CDKN2A/B*
>
> *Poor-risk genetic abnormalities (GEN-PR):*
> - High-risk cytogenetics (CYTO-HR):
>   – BCR-ABL1
>   – MLL
>   – Near haploidy (<30)
>   – Low hypodiploidy (30–39)/near triploidy (60–78)
>   – iAMP21
>   – TCF3-HLF
> - Intermediate- and poor-risk copy number alterations (CNA-IR and CNA-PR):
>   – Any deletion of *IKZF1*, *PAR1*, *EBF1*, or *RB1*
>   – Other CNA profiles
>
> (iAMP21: intrachromosomal amplification of chromosome 21; MLL: mixed-lineage leukemia)
>
> *Source*: Moorman AV, Enshaei A, Schwab C, et al. A novel integrated cytogenetic and genomic classification refines risk stratification in pediatric acute lymphoblastic leukemia. Blood. 2014;124(9):1434-44.

poor prognostic factors like higher age, high WBC counts at diagnosis, poor prednisolone response, persistent MRD, and induction failure. The genetic change activates tyrosine kinase or Janus kinase (JAK)/signal transducer and activator of transcription (STAT) pathway. Hence, there is a potential role of targeted therapy to improve survival among these patients. The Children's Oncology Group (COG) and St Jude Hospital Total XVII trial will assess efficacy of type-1 JAK inhibitor ruxolitinib in children with JAK pathway alterations.[16] Recently, tyrosine kinase inhibitors (TKIs), like imatinib, were used successfully to increase remission rate and overall survival among Ph-like ALL patients. Frontline use of TKIs led to increased 3-year overall survival to 77% as against poor 5-year overall survival ranging from 22% to 27% among historical controls of Ph-like ALL. Hence, it is recommended to screen all children with intermediate and high-risk B-cell ALL except Ph+ or t(12;21)(p13.2;q22.1) *ETV6-RUNX1*-positive patients.

Intrachromosomal Amplification of Chromosome 21

First identified in 2003, intrachromosomal amplification of chromosome 21 (iAMP21) is seen on cytogenetics as dup(21) and can be detected by fluorescent in situ hybridization (FISH) for *AML1 (RUNX1)* amplification.

It is defined as three or more additional copies (total 5 or more) of *RUNX1* per cell. It is found in 2% of childhood B-cell ALL and is associated with older age at presentation (median age 9 years), and poor prognosis despite having low WBC counts.[17]

Both the British and the American cooperative groups have shown that the outcomes can be improved by treating these patients with high-risk regimens, and proceeding to transplant, if they are MRD positive at the end of induction chemotherapy.[18]

Early T-cell Precursor Acute Lymphoblastic Leukemia

Early T-cell precursor acute lymphoblastic leukemia (ETP ALL) is recently recognized as immature form of T-ALL characterized by absent CD1a and CD8 expression, weak CD5 expression, and expression of one or more myeloid antigens.[19] It is found in about 11–16% of pediatric T-ALL. Genetically, it is quite heterogeneous with more frequent occurrence of myeloid mutations like FLT3 and RAS pathway mutations.

Initial reports suggested extremely poor survival among ETP leukemia, but results of further cooperative group studies showed noninferior survival compared to non-ETP T-ALL probably due to response-based treatment protocols. A retrospective study of pediatric ETP ALL on AIEP-BFM protocol showed poor early response, but consolidation treatment was enough to overcome the effect of positive MRD.[20] Currently in Britain, ETP ALL is not treated differently from non-ETP ALL, and nelarabine-based chemotherapy and stem cell transplantation reserved only for induction failure, persistent MRD positivity after consolidation, and relapse patients. Some researchers consider acute myeloid leukemia (AML) like therapy especially in relapse setting, as CD33 expression and FLT3 mutations are frequent in ETP ALL. Development of targeted therapy using anti-CD33 therapy or FLT3 inhibitor needs further clinical evaluation for their potential role in treatment of ETP ALL.

■ TREATMENT OF ALL WITH MINIMAL RESIDUAL DISEASE MONITORING

Treatment of ALL is categorized into four components—induction, consolidation, CNS prophylaxis, and maintenance.

Induction chemotherapy lasts for 4–6 weeks, including 1 week of pre-phase steroids. Standard induction chemotherapy protocols use three or four drugs, i.e. vincristine, L-asparaginase, and steroids with or without daunorubicin. Intrathecal chemotherapy with methotrexate is an integral part of induction chemotherapy. Some intensive protocols use up to eight drugs for induction. The aim of induction chemotherapy is to achieve a three-log cell kill and decrease the leukemic cell burden to below detectable levels.

Morphologically, the bone marrow is said to be in remission when there are less than 5% blasts in the bone marrow. MRD is measured by flow cytometry or polymerase chain reaction (PCR). The sensitivity of flow cytometry to detect leukemic blasts is 1 in 10,000 cells and of PCR is 1 in 100,000 cells.

End of induction MRD has prognostic significance because it reflects not only the effect of host factors (age and tumor burden) and disease factors (immunophenotype and cytogenetic abnormalities) but also the nonmeasurable effect of cooperative genomic abnormalities, self-renewal capacity, and drug resistance of the leukemic cells and pharmacogenetics of the host.

According to a study from St Jude, the MRD on day 19 reflects the short-term response to prednisone, vincristine, daunorubicin, and asparaginase and is useful for patients with favorable presenting features for identifying candidates for treatment de-intensification. On day 46, MRD reflects response to the preceding four drugs plus cyclophosphamide, cytarabine, and mercaptopurine, which are used in phase B of induction and helps to identify patients at an increased risk of relapse and who definitely need augmented treatment.[21]

Minimal residual disease monitoring has now been integrated in risk stratification by all cooperative groups.[13] Sequential MRD monitoring at the end of induction and at the end of consolidation and augmentation of therapy can over-ride some poor prognostic factors and can tease out patients who can be cured with chemotherapy alone.

Certain high-risk groups like hypodiploidy and Ph+ ALL have conventionally been offered stem cell transplant in first remission because chemotherapy-only protocols had demonstrated poor survival in these patients. Incorporating MRD monitoring into treatment strategies has shown that among these high-risk patients, those who achieve MRD negativity at the end of induction can be treated with chemotherapy (with tyrosine kinase therapy in Ph+ and Ph-like ALL) with good survival rates.[12]

Children, who do not achieve MRD negativity at the end of induction, may become MRD negative at the end of consolidation therapy after receiving high-dose methotrexate, mercaptopurine, and cytarabine. Thus, serial monitoring of MRD can identify patients who can be cured by chemotherapy only. Those who fail to clear MRD after consolidation are clear candidates for stem cell transplantation. These patients should receive additional treatment before proceeding to transplant because MRD levels pretransplant are directly related to post-transplant relapse.[11]

Consolidation or reinduction chemotherapy uses noncross-resistant drugs to those used in induction to further bring down the leukemic cell burden. High-dose methotrexate, high-dose cytosine arabinoside, and high doses of L-asparaginase or polyethylene glycol (PEG) asparaginase form the backbone of consolidation chemotherapy.

■ CENTRAL NERVOUS SYSTEM-DIRECTED THERAPY

The concept of CNS-preventive therapy assumes that undetectable CNS leukemia is present at diagnosis. Since systemic chemotherapy may not achieve adequate drug levels across the blood–brain barrier, cranial irradiation with intrathecal chemotherapy has been in use since the 1970s as CNS-preventive therapy. This is associated with neurocognitive dysfunction, endocrine abnormalities, growth retardation, and secondary malignancies in some survivors. High-dose chemotherapy using methotrexate or cytosine arabinoside achieves good CNS penetrance and newer protocols reserve cranial irradiation for patients with CNS disease at presentation and for those who are at high risk for CNS relapse.[22]

Maintenance chemotherapy using oral mercaptopurine and methotrexate is given for 18–24 months in order to eradicate dormant leukemic cells and affect a cure.

■ TREATMENT OF RELAPSED ALL

Relapsed ALL is the fourth common malignancy in children. Akin to initial diagnosis, risk stratification of relapsed ALL helps to tailor therapy. The BFM stratification of relapsed ALL takes into consideration duration of first remission, site of relapse as marrow relapse, isolated extramedullary relapse, or combined relapse and the immunophenotype.[10] It classifies patients as S1, S2, S3, and S4. Patients in groups S1 and S2, i.e. those with late relapse and early isolated extramedullary relapse in non-T-cell ALL, have a 40–70% chance of being cured with chemotherapy alone. Patients with early relapse and T-cell relapse have only a 25–30% chance of being cured even with hematopoietic stem cell transplant (HSCT).

Newer Chemotherapeutic Agents

Clofarabine

It is a second-generation purine nucleoside analog that inhibits ribonucleotide reductase and induces apoptosis. It is approved for the treatment of children with relapsed ALL after two prior treatment regimens. As a single agent, it has shown 30% response rates. It has also been used in combination with cyclophosphamide and etoposide and with cytarabine.[23] The toxicity of combination therapy is high with severe and prolonged myelosuppression.

Nelarabine

Nelarabine, a purine nucleoside analog, is a prodrug of ara-G triphosphate (ara-GTP), which causes cytotoxicity by inhibiting DNA synthesis. A large German multicenter study proved the safety and efficacy of nelarabine as a single agent in relapse or refractory T-cell ALL serving as a bridge to transplant.[24] A COG study incorporated nelarabine into the augmented the Berlin-Frankfurt-Münster (BFM) backbone for high-risk T-cell ALL and found good efficacy but with high incidence of peripheral neuropathy and other neurotoxicity. Nelarabine used as a continuous infusion rather than short infusion may overcome its neurotoxicity.

Hematopoietic Stem Cell Transplant

Hematopoietic stem cell transplant involves high-dose chemotherapy with or without total body irradiation as the conditioning regimen followed by infusion of human leukocyte antigen (HLA) matched stem cells from the donor. It depends on two mechanisms of leukemic cell kill to achieve cures. First is direct cytotoxicity of the conditioning regimen used to eliminate all remaining leukemic cells. The second is the graft-versus-leukemia (GVL) effect wherein the donor lymphocytes launch an immune attack on the residual leukemic cells to get rid of them. A small degree of graft-versus-host disease (GVHD) is desired to ensure the GVL effect.

Only a fourth of patients with relapsed ALL who could benefit from a HSCT have a HLA-identical family donor. With the establishment of donor registries worldwide, the chance of finding a matched unrelated donor (MUD) has vastly increased and with high resolution HLA typing, the results of MUD transplants are encouraging.[25] Indian patients find it difficult to find matched donors in European and North American registries due to different racial backgrounds.

Umbilical cord blood registries offer the option of HSCT to patients lacking a matched donor. Since cord blood stem cells are immunologically naïve, some degree of mismatch gives equally good results.[26]

Haploidentical Stem Cell Transplantation

Recent progress in the field of haploidentical transplantation has made it a good option for those patients who cannot find a matched donor. Since a haploidentical donor is usually available within the family, patients can proceed to transplant without waiting for the donor search. Due to up to 50% HLA mismatch between donor and recipient, T-cell–mediated host-versus-graft response leading to graft rejection and graft-versus-host response leading to GVHD are common. The last two decades have seen extensive research and trials trying to curb GVHD and maintain donor chimerism. T-cell depletion of the graft is carried out to achieve this.[27] The major drawback was the slow immune reconstitution that led to 40% nonrelapse mortality.

Other strategies have included:
- The use of an unmanipulated graft followed by post-transplant high-dose cyclophosphamide.[28]
- Alemtuzumab providing in vivo T-cell depletion of the graft.[29]

- Granulocyte colony-stimulating factor (GCSF)-primed blood or bone marrow grafts and intensified post-transplant immunosuppression.[30]

Choosing the right haploidentical donor among available family members is also important. Data from the European Bone Marrow Transplant registry shows that transplant from mother donors compared to any other family donor is an independent prognostic factor predicting lower relapse rates, lower non-relapse mortality, and better survival.[31] The scientific rationale is that transplacental movement of maternal and fetal cells during pregnancy establishes long-term reciprocal microchimerism between mother and child. As a result, the immune system of the mother is sensitized to paternal HLA antigens. Thus, T-cell depletion removes enough T-cells to prevent GVHD but allows the transfer of sufficient number of tolerant or educated T-cells to protect the child from relapse and infections.

Immunotherapy

With the advent of immunotherapy, the options for children with relapsed ALL have increased. Unlike cytotoxic chemotherapy, which kills rapidly dividing tumor cells and normal rapidly dividing cells too, immunotherapy recruits the body's immune system to mount an immune attack specifically against tumor cells. Presently, immunotherapy options for relapsed ALL include monoclonal antibodies and chimeric antigen receptor T-cells (CAR T-cells).[32] Checkpoint inhibitors have a limited role but are being investigated.

Monoclonal Antibodies for Relapsed ALL

Monoclonal antibodies targeted to antigens commonly found on the surface of leukemic cells include the following:
- Anti-CD20—rituximab, obintumumab, and ofatumumab
- Anti-CD22—epratuzumab and inotuzumab ozogamicin (IO)
- Anti-CD19—blinatumomab.

Rituximab: It is a chimeric anti-CD20 monoclonal antibody containing a murine and a human region. Presence of CD20 has been noted in about 30-50% precursor B-cell leukemia. Rituximab binds to CD20 on the surface of leukemic blasts and causes cell lysis by three different mechanisms, viz. antibody-dependent cell-mediated cytotoxicity (ADCC), complement-mediated cytotoxicity, and apoptosis. Rituximab in combination with chemotherapy is accepted as standard of care in adults and children with B-cell lymphomas. It has produced improvement in remission rates and better MRD negativity when used in adolescents and adults with ALL in combination with chemotherapy. Its use in relapsed ALL is restricted due to the availability of better drugs.

Ofatumumab: It is a fully humanized second-generation anti-CD20 antibody with better complement-mediated cytotoxicity than rituximab.

Obintumumab: It is a glycol-engineered type II anti-CD20 antibody with more potent cytotoxicity and ADCC.

Epratuzumab: It is an unconjugated anti-CD22 antibody that gets rapidly internalized after binding to CD22. The CD22 antigen is present on the surface of leukemic blasts in more than 90% patients with ALL. Postulated mechanism of action of epratuzumab is by ADCC, CD22 phosphorylation, and inhibition of proliferation. The lack of direct cytotoxicity is the reason that epratuzumab is not used alone but in combination with chemotherapy. Several phase I and phase II studies of epratuzumab along with chemotherapy in relapsed ALL have shown response rates of 40–50%.

Inotuzumab ozogamicin: It is a humanized anti-CD22 antibody linked to a cytotoxic agent calicheamicin. Binding to CD22 leads to rapid internalization followed by fusion with intracellular lysosome that in turn degrades the linker releasing calicheamicin. Calicheamicin binds to the double-stranded nucleus causing cell death. Phase III trial of IO versus chemotherapy has shown impressive response rates of 80% versus 29% with similar rates for MRD negativity. Two phase II trials of IO with hyper-CVAD chemotherapy have shown response rates upward of 95%.

Blinatumomab (bispecific T-cell engager, BiTE): It is a bispecific monoclonal antibody with a CD19-directed CD3 T-cell engager **(Fig. 14.1.1)**. CD19 is

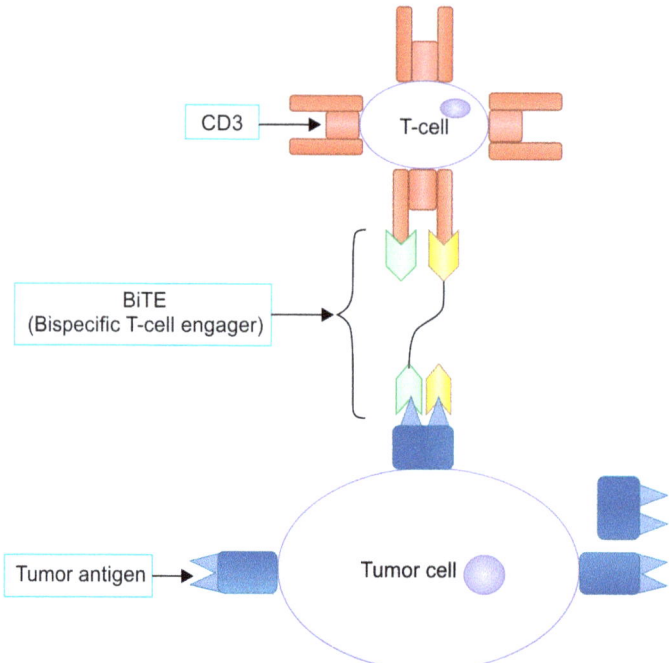

Fig. 14.1.1: Blinatumomab.

a pan B-cell marker except for plasma cells. Blinatumomab binds to both CD19 on the leukemic cell and to CD3 on T-cells thus engaging T-cells with leukemic cells leading to cell death. The direct activation of the connected T-cell leads to perforin-mediated cytotoxicity and causes the apoptosis of CD19+ leukemic cells. It also leads to marked T-cell proliferation giving rise to an army of blinatumomab-activated T-cells, which then continue the serial killing of CD19+ cells. This cytotoxicity and proliferation continue as long as there are CD19+ leukemic cells for blinatumomab to engage with. Blinatumomab activates both the CD8 cytotoxic and the CD4 helper T-cells. Since blinatumomab lacks the fragment crystallizable region of the antibody, its half-life is only 2 hours and it needs to be administered as a continuous IV infusion over 4 weeks followed by 2 weeks rest. In a phase I/phase II study of the 49 relapsed refractory children treated with blinatumomab, 39% achieved a complete remission.[33] The most severe and life-threatening toxicity of blinatumomab includes cytokine release syndrome (CRS) and neurotoxicity.

Chimeric Antigen Receptor T-cell Therapy

Chimeric antigen receptor T-cell refers to a genetically engineered T-cell that is capable of mounting an immune attack on the target cell. CAR T-cells have an extracellular domain consisting of a single chain variable fragment that can recognize a specific tumor antigen and a transmembrane domain, which is in turn linked to an intracellular domain consisting of a signaling unit (CD3 delta) and a costimulatory unit (CD28, 4-1BB) **(Fig. 14.1.2)**. These costimulatory domains enhance cytokine production, proliferation, and survivability.

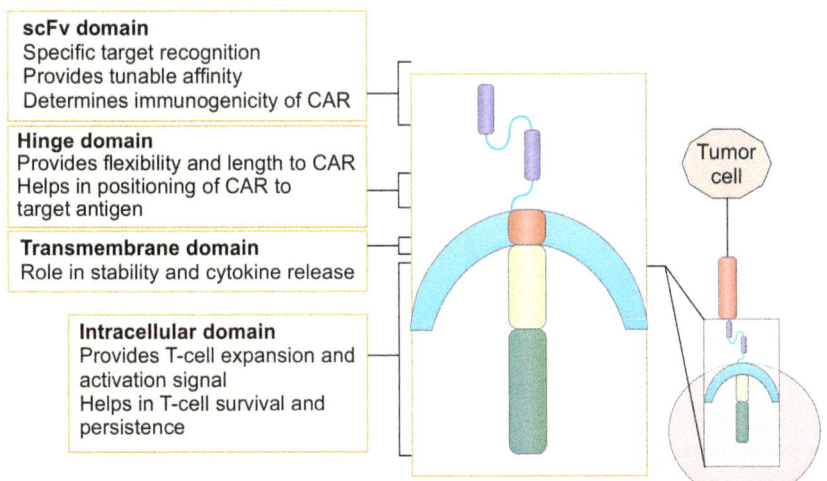

Fig. 14.1.2: Chimeric antigen receptor T-cell (CAR T-cell).
(scFv: single-chain variable fragment)

The patient's T-cells are harvested by apheresis and are then transduced with a viral vector and modified to express CARs on their surface. These modified cells are then expanded in vitro, checked for sterility, and infused back into the patient. These CAR T-cells recognize tumor cells without needing major histocompatibility complex (MHC) antigens to express them and mount an immune response to destroy them. The CAR T-cells generate memory cells that carry out surveillance and thus prevent tumor recurrence.

CD19 is a B-cell marker present on the surface of all normal B-cells except stem cells and plasma cells and on all B-cell malignancies except myeloma. There are two CD19 CAR T-cells that are approved.

Tisagenlecleucel is a CD19-directed CAR T-cell approved for the treatment of relapsed or refractory B-cell ALL in children up to 18 years of age and relapsed/refractory B-cell lymphoma in adults.[34]

Axicabtagene ciloleucel is CD19-directed CAR T-cell approved for the treatment of relapsed or refractory B-cell lymphoma in adults.

Recently, the Food and Drug Administration (FDA) has approved a CD22 CAR T-cell for achieving 70% complete remission rate in patients who had relapsed after CD19 CAR T-cell therapy.

The toxicity of CAR T-cells includes CRS, neurotoxicity, and B-cell aplasia necessitating replacement immunoglobulin therapy. CRS is a systemic inflammatory response caused by the release of inflammatory cytokines like interleukin-6 (IL-6), interferon-γ (IFN-γ), tumor necrosis factor-α (TNF-α), IL-2, and IL-10, which are released by lymphocytes and lead to a constellation of symptoms like fever, hypotension, and multiorgan dysfunction. It may range in severity from mild flu-like symptoms of fever and myalgia, to a full-fledged syndrome of vascular leak, hypotension, pulmonary edema, cardiac dysfunction, renal and hepatic failure, coagulopathy, and death. There are several grading systems developed to assess the severity of CRS. These help to guide therapy, which range from analgesics and antipyretics for mild cases to the use of corticosteroids and anti-IL6 antibody tocilizumab.

The neurotoxicity of blinatumomab varies from tremors and dizziness to seizures, strokes, mutism, and altered sensorium. The neurotoxicity is mostly reversible and does not leave behind any sequelae.

■ CONCLUSION

The developments in the last two decades have seen major advances in immunotherapy in the treatment of cancer in general and childhood leukemia in particular. The challenge of the next two decades is going to be to incorporate these advances into frontline therapy and maintain the excellent cure rates while further decreasing toxicity and long-term sequelae.

■ REFERENCES

1. Farber S, Diamond LK. Temporary remissions in acute leukemia in children produced by folic acid antagonist, 4-aminopteroyl-glutamic acid (Aminopterin). N Engl J Med. 1948;238(23):787-93.
2. Frei E 3rd, Holland JF, Schneiderman MA, et al. A comparative study of two regimens of combination chemotherapy in acute leukemia. Blood. 1958;13(12):1126-48.
3. Aur RJ, Simone J, Hustu HO, et al. Central nervous system therapy and combination chemotherapy of childhood lymphocytic leukemia. Blood. 1971;37(3):272-81.
4. Henze G, Langermann HJ, Brämswig J, et al. The BFM 76/79 acute lymphoblastic leukemia therapy study (author's translation). Klin Padiatr. 1981;193(3):145-54.
5. Evans WE, Crom WR, Abromowitch M, et al. Clinical pharmacodynamics of high-dose methotrexate in acute lymphocytic leukemia. Identification of a relation between concentration and effect. N Engl J Med. 1986;314(8):471-7.
6. Secker-Walker LM, Lawler SD, Hardisty RM. Prognostic implications of chromosomal findings in acute lymphoblastic leukaemia at diagnosis. Br Med J. 1978;2(6151):1529-30.
7. Mullighan CG, Goorha S, Radtke I, et al. Genome-wide analysis of genetic alterations in acute lymphoblastic leukaemia. Nature. 2007;446(7137):758-64.
8. Yamaji K, Okamoto T, Yokota S, et al. Minimal residual disease-based augmented therapy in childhood acute lymphoblastic leukemia: a report from the Japanese Childhood Cancer and Leukemia Study Group. Pediatr Blood Cancer. 2010;55(7):1287-95.
9. Yeoh AE, Ariffin H, Chai EL, et al. Minimal residual disease-guided treatment deintensification for children with acute lymphoblastic leukemia: results from the Malaysia-Singapore acute lymphoblastic leukemia 2003 study. J Clin Oncol. 2012;30(19):2384-92.
10. Henze G, Fengler R, Hartmann R, et al. Six-year experience with a comprehensive approach to the treatment of recurrent childhood acute lymphoblastic leukemia (ALL-REZ BFM 85). A relapse study of the BFM group. Blood. 1991;78(5):1166-72.
11. Campana D, Leung W. Clinical significance of minimal residual disease in patients with acute leukaemia undergoing haematopoietic stem cell transplantation. Br J Haematol. 2013;162(2):147-61.
12. Pui CH, Campana D, Pei D, et al. Treating childhood acute lymphoblastic leukemia without cranial irradiation. N Engl J Med. 2009;360(26):2730-41.
13. Conter V, Bartram CR, Valsecchi MG, et al. Molecular response to treatment redefines all prognostic factors in children and adolescents with B-cell precursor acute lymphoblastic leukemia: results in 3184 patients of the AIEOP-BFM ALL 2000 study. Blood. 2010;115(16):3206-14.
14. Borowitz MJ, Devidas M, Hunger SP, et al. Clinical significance of minimal residual disease in childhood acute lymphoblastic leukemia and its relationship to other prognostic factors: a Children's Oncology Group study. Blood. 2008;111(12): 5477-85.
15. Arber DA, Orazi A, Hasserjian R, et al. The 2016 revision to the World Health Organization classification of myeloid neoplasms and acute leukemia. Blood. 2016;127(20):2391-405.

16. Roberts KG. Why and how to treat Ph-like ALL? Best Pract Res Clin Haematol. 2018;31(4):351-6.
17. Harrison CJ. Blood Spotlight on iAMP21 acute lymphoblastic leukemia (ALL), a high-risk pediatric disease. Blood. 2015;125(9):1383-6.
18. Heerema NA, Carroll AJ, Devidas M, et al. Intrachromosomal amplification of chromosome 21 is associated with inferior outcomes in children with acute lymphoblastic leukemia treated in contemporary standard-risk children's oncology group studies: a report from the children's oncology group. J Clin Oncol. 2013;31(27):3397-402.
19. Coustan-Smith E, Mullighan CG, Onciu M, et al. Early T-cell precursor leukaemia: a subtype of very high-risk acute lymphoblastic leukaemia. Lancet Oncol. 2009;10(2):147-56.
20. Conter V, Valsecchi MG, Buldini B, et al. Early T-cell precursor acute lymphoblastic leukaemia in children treated in AIEOP centres with AIEOP-BFM protocols: a retrospective analysis. Lancet Haematol. 2016;3(2):e80-6.
21. Pui CH, Pei D, Raimondi SC, et al. Clinical impact of minimal residual disease in children with different subtypes of acute lymphoblastic leukaemia treated with Response-Adapted therapy. Leukemia. 2017;31(2):333-9.
22. Pui CH, Yang JJ, Hunger SP, et al. Childhood acute lymphoblastic leukemia: progress through collaboration. J Clin Oncol. 2015;33(27):2938-48.
23. Locatelli F, Testi AM, Bernardo ME, et al. Clofarabine, cyclophosphamide and etoposide as single-course re-induction therapy for children with refractory/multiple relapsed acute lymphoblastic leukaemia. Br J Haematol. 2009;147(3):371-8.
24. Gökbuget N, Basara N, Baurmann H, et al. High single-drug activity of nelarabine in relapsed T-lymphoblastic leukemia/lymphoma offers curative option with subsequent stem cell transplantation. Blood. 2011;118(13):3504-11.
25. Saarinen-Pihkala UM, Gustafsson G, Ringdén O, et al. No disadvantage in outcome of using matched unrelated donors as compared with matched sibling donors for bone marrow transplantation in children with acute lymphoblastic leukemia in second remission. J Clin Oncol. 2001;19(14):3406-14.
26. Smith AR, Baker KS, Defor TE, et al. Hematopoietic cell transplantation for children with acute lymphoblastic leukemia in second complete remission: similar outcomes in recipients of unrelated marrow and umbilical cord blood versus marrow from HLA matched sibling donors. Biol Blood Marrow Transplant. 2009;15(9):1086-93.
27. Aversa F, Tabilio A, Velardi A, et al. Treatment of high-risk acute leukemia with T-cell-depleted stem cells from related donors with one fully mismatched HLA haplotype. N Engl J Med. 1998;339(17):1186-93.
28. McCurdy SR, Kanakry JA, Showel MM, et al. Risk-stratified outcomes of nonmyeloablative HLA-haploidentical BMT with high-dose post-transplantation cyclophosphamide. Blood. 2015;125(19):3024-31.
29. Rizzieri DA, Koh LP, Long GD, et al. Partially matched, nonmyeloablative allogeneic transplantation: clinical outcomes and immune reconstitution. J Clin Oncol. 2007;25(6):690-7.

30. Di Bartolomeo P, Santarone S, De Angelis G, et al. Haploidentical, unmanipulated, G-CSF-primed bone marrow transplantation for patients with high-risk hematologic malignancies. Blood. 2013;121(5):849-57.
31. Velardi A, Ziagkos D, van Biezen A, et al. Mother donors improve outcomes after HLA haploidentical T-cell–depleted hematopoietic transplantation: a retrospective study by the Cell Therapy and Immunobiology Working Party of the EBMT. Bone Marrow Transplant. 2016;51(Suppl 1):S150.
32. Jabbour E, O'Brien S, Ravandi F, et al. Monoclonal antibodies in acute lymphoblastic leukemia. Blood. 2015;125:4010-6.
33. von Stackelberg A, Locatelli F, Zugmaier G, et al. Phase I/Phase II study of blinatumomab in pediatric patients with relapsed/refractory acute lymphoblastic leukemia. J Clin Oncol. 2016;34(36):4381-9.
34. Maude SL, Laetsch TW, Buechner J, et al. Tisagenlecleucel in children and young adults with B-cell lymphoblastic leukemia. N Engl J Med. 2018:378(5):439-48.

CHAPTER 15

ENDOCRINOLOGY

15.1 Newborn Screening for Congenital Hypothyroidism
M Vijayakumar, PSN Menon

15.1 NEWBORN SCREENING FOR CONGENITAL HYPOTHYROIDISM

M Vijayakumar, PSN Menon

■ INTRODUCTION

Thyroid hormones are essential for the smooth functioning of almost all organ systems in human body and play a crucial role in the neurologic development and physical growth of children. Congenital hypothyroidism (CH) is a common clinical condition with an incidence as high as 1 in 2000 as reported in various recent studies.[1] If not diagnosed and treated early in the neonatal period, CH causes permanent damage to the developing brain, leading to neurocognitive impairment and developmental delay.[2,3] CH is the commonest cause of preventable intellectual disability and the commonest endocrine disorder that affects children.[4] Even though the introduction of universal newborn screening (NBS) has practically eliminated late diagnosis of CH and resulting permanent neurodevelopmental impairment in most developed countries, it still remains the leading cause of preventable intellectual disability in several developing nations.[5,6] In India, barring a few isolated centers, screening for CH is not practised, leading to late diagnosis leaving thousands of children intellectually disabled. Universal newborn thyroid screening is an obligation to the society and policy planners should include NBS in national health programs.

■ THYROID DEVELOPMENT

A short discussion on thyroid development and physiology as well as CH will help to understand the principles and practice of NBS for CH. The fetal thyroid gland begins to develop as a thickening in the floor of the primitive pharynx called as median thyroid anlage in addition to a pair of lateral anlages from the fourth pharyngeal pouches at three weeks after conception. They fuse by 50 days and subsequently the thyroid gland descends to its definitive location in the anterior neck. Its connection to the pharynx (thyroglossal duct) then gets obliterated.

Thyrotropin releasing hormone (TRH) can be demonstrated in fetal hypothalamus by 8-9 weeks of gestation.[7] By ten weeks, iodine trapping followed by production of thyroid hormones ensues in the gland. Human placenta expresses the sodium–iodine symporter (NIS) throughout the gestation, which actively transports iodine from the mother to fetus.[8] Fetal thyroid gland starts secreting thyroxine (T4) by 12 weeks of gestation. Nearly 90% of the circulating triiodothyronine (T3) is derived from monodeiodination of T4 and the rest from direct glandular secretion. Type 1 deiodinase is predominantly expressed in liver, kidney and thyroid. Type 2 deiodinase is located in brain, pituitary and placenta. Type 3 deiodinase is seen in most of the fetal cells including placenta, which will convert T4 to inactive reverse T3 (rT3). There is an inverse correlation between type 2 and type 3 actions. Conversion of T4 to rT3 is more in early fetal life. Separation of placenta reduces type 3 deiodinase activity, which results in fall of rT3 and rise of T3.[7]

Thyroid hormones are essential for normal neuronal development, myelination, differentiation, dendritic and axonal proliferation and development of various neurotransmitters during intrauterine life and also in childhood.[9] There is a critical period of thyroid hormone action on brain development in intrauterine phase, and T4 is essential for postnatal brain development as well. During the first trimester, before the newborn can synthesize thyroid hormones, the fetus depends on maternal supply of T4 through placenta. This transplacental transfer continues throughout the gestation and constitutes a significant proportion of thyroid hormones present in the fetal blood. This reduces the fetal brain damage due to CH to a great extent. Defective thyroid status of the mother (hypothyroidism, iodine deficiency or thyroid stimulating hormone [TSH] receptor blocking antibodies) will result in severe damage to development of fetal nervous system compared to isolated fetal hypothyroidism. Inadequate intake of iodine by the pregnant mother results in fetal hypothyroidism and leads to irreversible brain damage (cretinism). If the mother is already on levothyroxine therapy, 30–50% increase in the dose is required during gestation due to estradiol-induced increase in serum thyroid binding globulin (TBG).[10]

■ EXTRAUTERINE THYROID ADAPTATION

During the initial hours after birth, there is a rapid increase in TSH secretion from the pituitary gland of the neonate, which in turn is stimulated by a rise in TRH from the hypothalamus. This TSH surge is believed to be an adaptation for cold exposure and stress of delivery and peaks during the first 24 hours after birth reaching up to 80 mIU/L. This surge is followed by a rise in serum T4 level, which peaks during the second day of life. TSH surge is transient, and the levels begin to decrease soon and reach almost normal levels by 4–5 days. Serum T4 levels will remain elevated for several weeks and gradually decline over 4–5 weeks of life. TSH and T4 surges are also seen in preterm babies, but with lower amplitude.[11]

■ EPIDEMIOLOGY OF CONGENITAL HYPOTHYROIDISM

Congenital hypothyroidism is considered as the commonest congenital endocrine disorder. Initially, in the prescreening era, the incidence of CH was reported as 1 in 4000 neonates. After universal screening in many industrialized countries, the incidence has almost doubled and currently 1 in 1400 to 1 in 2000 neonates are affected by CH. Another reason for this apparent increase in recent years is the lowering the screening cut-off for thyroid hormones resulting in early detection of milder cases of CH.[5]

ETIOLOGY OF CONGENITAL HYPOTHYROIDISM

A brief description of the major causes of CH will help to understand the criteria used in diagnosis of CH during NBS and the principles of early replacement therapy and follow-up monitoring.[1-4]

Thyroid Dysgenesis

Congenital hypothyroidism may result from defective development of the gland in utero (thyroid dysgenesis) or failure of the thyroid gland to produce sufficient thyroid hormones (dyshormonogenesis). Most cases (85%) of permanent primary CH are due to thyroid dysgenesis. Dysgenesis includes complete absence of the gland (agenesis, ~20%), aberrant migration (ectopic gland, ~75%) and a normally placed hypoplastic gland or thyroid hemiagenesis (~5%). Ectopic thyroid appears oval in shape due to lack of lateral lobes. Thyroid dysgenesis is a sporadic condition in most neonates, but off late a number of genetic mutations are being identified (2-5%).[12] These include several genes involved in thyroid gland formation including TSH receptor (*TSHR*) and transcription factors (*PAX8, NKX2-1, FOXE 1, NKX2-5, JAG1* and *GLIS3*) **(Table 15.1.1).**[13] It is important to note that these mutations are often associated with other congenital anomalies.

Dyshormonogenesis

Thyroid dyshormonogenesis results from genetic defects in any one of the steps involved in the biosynthesis of thyroid hormones.[14] The following steps are usually affected with varying clinical severity and associated malformations.
1. Transport of iodide across the basolateral membrane of the thyroid follicular cells (NIS).

Table 15.1.1: Some genetic syndromes associated with congenital hypothyroidism with associated clinical features.[2,12]

Genetic mutation	Associated anomalies
PAX 8	Urogenital abnormalities
NKX2-1	Interstitial lung disease, chorea
FOXE 1	Cleft palate, choanal atresia, spiky hair
NKX2 5	Congenital heart disease
JAG 1	Alagille syndrome, congenital heart disease
GLS 3	Neonatal diabetes mellitus, developmental delay, congenital glaucoma, hepatic fibrosis, polycystic disease

2. Transport of iodide from the cell into colloid lumen through pendrin (PDS: *SLC26A4*). This condition causes Pendred syndrome, which is associated with nonprogressive sensorineural deafness.[15]
3. Thyroid oxidase system consisting of two proteins DUOX1 and DUOX2. Monoallelic mutation manifests as transient CH whereas biallelic variety manifests as permanent variety.[16,17]
4. Iodide organification and iodotyrosine coupling via the thyroid peroxidase (TPO), which is encoded in the gene located on chromosome 2p25. TPO deficiency is the most common cause of dyshormonogenesis worldwide.
5. Synthesis of thyroglobulin as a result of mutations of the *TG* gene.[18]
6. Iodine recycling via iodotyrosine deiodinase; the gene is located on chromosome 6q24-25.

Most of the defects in hormonogenesis are inherited as autosomal recessive traits and occur with high incidence in consanguineous couples. A goiter will be present but may not be clinically detectable in a neonate.

Central Hypothyroidism

Central hypothyroidism is rare with earlier data showing an estimated incidence of 1 in 30,000 to 1 in 50,000. A more recent data from the Netherlands shows that the incidence may actually be higher, around 1 in 16,000. These conditions result from structural or developmental abnormalities of hypothalamus or pituitary gland and are often associated with (75%) deficiencies of other pituitary hormones. Many are due to genetic mutations in transcription factors involved in the differentiation of hypothalamus or pituitary gland (*HESX1, LHX3, LHX4, SOX3, PROP1*, and *POU1F1*).[12,19] Children with central hypothyroidism are not usually identified by clinical features of hypothyroidism because of other features of hypopituitarism such as growth failure or features of adrenocorticotropic hormone (ACTH) deficiency.

Transient Congenital Hypothyroidism

Severe iodine deficiency is an important cause of transient CH in areas where iodine deficiency is prevalent. Application of iodinated antiseptic agents (povidone iodine) to the neonates or pregnant and lactating mothers can produce transient reduction in thyroid hormone levels. Maternal therapy with antithyroid drugs and transplacental transfer of TSH blocking antibodies also cause transient hypothyroidism. Many premature babies present with low or normal TSH with low free T4 (FT4), a condition called as hypothyroxinemia of prematurity. Thyroid function will ultimately normalize as and when maturity is attained.

Recently a few genetic causes of transient CH have been described. Patients carrying one mutated allele of *DUOX2, DUOXA2, PAX8,* and *TSHR* may develop transient hypothyroidism.[19]

Table 15.1.2: Prevalence of various types of congenital hypothyroidism[20]

Thyroid dysgenesis	
• Ectopic thyroid	1:5,000
• Agenesis	1:15,000
Dyshormonogenesis	1:30,000
Central hypothyroidism	1:21,000
Thyroid hormone resistance	1:40,000

Rare Forms of Congenital Hypothyroidism

In the cell membrane, T3 is actively transported by binding to membrane protein MCT8. Defects in this protein are associated with severe psychomotor retardation associated with very high T3 levels, low rT3 and T4 with mild elevation of TSH. Resistance to thyroid hormone occurs due to mutations in the thyroid hormone receptor B *(THRB)* gene, which is characterized by increased TSH, T4 and FT4 levels.

The prevalence of various types of CH is shown in **Table 15.1.2**.

CLINICAL PRESENTATION

At birth, most cases of CH are asymptomatic and CH is suspected clinically in less than 1% of cases, underscoring the importance of NBS. The usual clinical features include macrosomia, open anterior and posterior fontanels, presence of wormian bones, large head, hypotonia, hypothermia, constipation, prolonged physiological jaundice, abdominal distension, umbilical hernia, mottled skin, macroglossia, hoarse cry and myxedematous appearance which generally manifest as the child grows older.[1-4] It is important to seek a family history of consanguinity and a history of similar condition in relatives in any infant recalled based on the results of screening test. Maternal history of congenital or acquired hypothyroidism and the treatment details should be recorded. A detailed cardiac examination and hearing assessment is a must in any infant suspected to have CH. Careful examination should be done to detect dysmorphic features.

Most cases of dyshormonogenesis develop thyroid enlargement due to trophic action of TSH, but often this is not detected in newborn period.

Central hypothyroidism manifests with symptoms of other pituitary hormone deficiencies. Symptoms due to hypothyroidism are usually mild. Major clinical findings are hypoglycemia (deficiency of ACTH or growth hormone), micropenis and cryptorchidism (deficiency of gonadotropins), and cholestasis (deficiency of ACTH). They may have associated midline malformations like cleft lip, palate, single central incisors or optic nerve hypoplasia.

NEWBORN SCREENING

Historical Aspects

Newborn screening is a preventive strategy aimed to diagnose treatable disorders early enough to provide interventions before the onset of damaging effects.[20-22] Studies conducted in 70s and early 80s showed that 20-30% of children with CH had intellectual subnormality (IQ < 70). Only 1% of children were diagnosed clinically during neonatal period. The greatest brain vulnerability due to CH is during the first few weeks of life. Thus intellectual subnormality in affected offspring can be prevented only if treatment is started before 14 days of life, which can be accomplished by NBS.

In 1934, Ivar Asbjørn Følling discovered a method for detecting phenylketonuria (PKU).[23] In 1961, Robert Guthrie, who is considered as "father of newborn screening" created the first simple inexpensive NBS for PKU by taking heel prick blood samples, on a filter paper (dried blood spot) and undertaking the necessary investigations.[24] In 1973, Jean Dussault from Quebec, Canada, developed screening method for CH using T4 and in 1975, William Morphey from Oregon, USA pioneered a mass screening program for CH which was first successfully conducted in Quebec and Pittsburg.[25,26] In 1977, Songya Pang developed screening for congenital adrenal hyperplasia.[27] By 2000 all states in USA had started regular CH screening. Radioimmunoassay (RIA) was developed as the testing method later. In 1990, David Millington developed the technique to use tandem mass spectrometry (TMS) in NBS.[28,29]

Screening for CH has been regarded as a clear success story in most developing countries. In 1968, JMG Wilson and G Jungner in their paper on "principles and practice of screening for diseases" put forward the ten principles to include a disease in the mass NBS program.[30] Important principles among these are:
- The disease should be an important health problem.
- There should be an accepted treatment for the disease.
- Facilities for diagnosis and treatment should be available.
- The cost of case finding should be economically balanced to the treatment expenditure and medical care.
- The natural history of the condition should be adequately understood.
Congenital hypothyroidism satisfies all the criteria.

In 2006, American College of Medical Genetics and Genomics (ACMG) put forward an article outlining a procedure of standardization of NBS process, which included recommendation for a uniform panel.[31,32] The guidelines divided the diseases into "primary" or "core" disorders in which NBS is a must and "secondary" disorders which are screened as a byproduct of the screening for the primary disorders. The Department of Health and Human Service, USA brought out the "recommended uniform screening panel" (RUSP), which currently includes 35 primary and 26 secondary disorders.

National Screening Programs

Now NBS is a norm in almost all developed countries. The timing of blood collection by heel prick method is between 24 and 48 hours and the samples are collected in a dried blood spot (DBS). These samples are air dried and transported to a regional laboratory where the blood spots are punched out and the screening testing are performed. Any abnormal test result is communicated to the authorized personnel in the concerned hospital. This person is responsible for contacting the family and arranging the confirmatory testing and subsequent follow-up of the confirmed cases.

A countrywide NBS program (NBS) involving all the states and union territories has not been initiated in India yet. The first pilot NBS program was conducted in Bai Jerbai Wadia Hospital, Mumbai in 1982 using cord blood TSH.[33] A longstanding NBS is ongoing at Christian Medical College Hospital, Vellore, Tamil Nadu for more than two decades.[34] State government sponsored programs are being conducted in many states like Goa and short term feasibility studies funded by various governmental agencies are being conducted in various centers.[35-37] In Kerala, the State Government is funding NBS program for four diseases including CH from 2013 onwards and is ongoing. Studies conducted in various parts of India have reported a higher prevalence of CH compared to global standards. This increased incidence is attributed to increased incidence of consanguinity, nutritional factors like iodine deficiency, and environmental as well as ethnic factors.

Timing of Sampling and Sampling Methods

The point to be considered while selecting the time of sampling is the phenomenon of TSH surge in the newborn period where TSH can be as high as 80 mIU/L. The cord blood is an ideal sample because it will be collected before the surge. Other advantages of selecting cord blood include that it is a painless procedure and that it can be collected in all neonates at any time if a written protocol is maintained in the labor room. But if thyroid screening has to be combined with screening of other metabolic illnesses, cord blood method cannot be used, since metabolic illness like PKU and galactosemia require ingestion of breastmilk for accumulation of substrates. If the sample is taken during TSH surge, especially during the first 24 hours, high false positive reports resulting in high recall rate will ensue.[38] TSH levels will come down to near normal level by 48–72 hours and hence samples taken after 48 hours are likely to show a relatively normal TSH value thus decreasing high false positive rates. Hence except in unusual situations like planning to give blood transfusions, blood collection should be delayed for at least 48 hours.

The sample is taken by heel prick and blood drops are collected in a filter paper (dried blood spot, DBS). The main advantage of using DBS is that other disorders like congenital adrenal hyperplasia (CAH) and metabolic conditions like galactosemia and PKU also can be screened. The disadvantages include pain of heel prick and the chance of unnecessary hospital stay. **Annexure 15.1.1** provides the protocol of blood sample collection for NBS in detail.

Testing the Blood Samples

Cord blood samples are sent to the in-house laboratory in a plain vacutainer for assay. The filter paper blood samples are sent to a central NBS laboratory after drying effectively. Sample collection is extremely important for getting a good result and the nursing and supporting staff should be educated about the correct technique **(Figs. 15.1.1A to H)**.

Screening Assays

There are two main screening strategies for CH:
1. Primary TSH testing
2. Primary T4 with back-up TSH testing.

The main disadvantages of primary TSH include:
1. It fails to detect central hypothyroidism where TSH levels are normal or low
2. It fails to detect a delayed rise of TSH, a condition noted in premature babies and sick neonates.

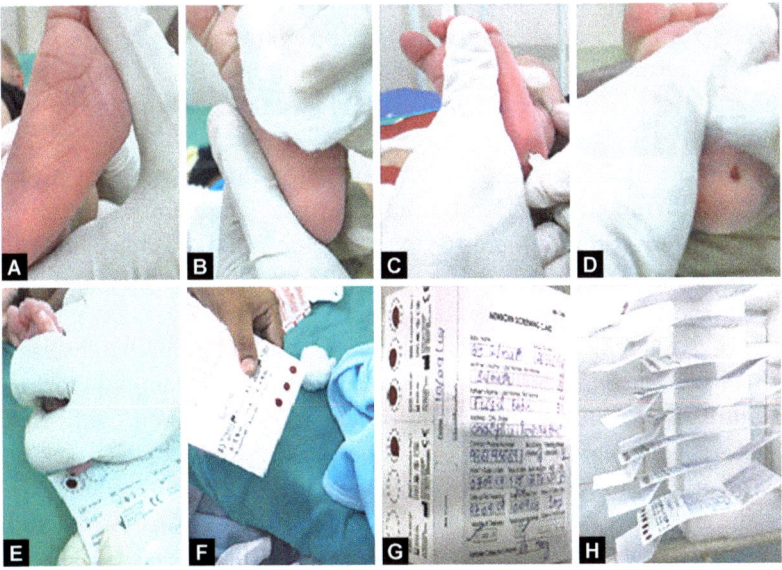

Figs. 15.1.1A to H: Steps in collection of dried blood spots from heel prick in newborns and storing.

In primary T4 method, central hypothyroidism can be detected but it misses compensatory or subclinical hypothyroidism (normal T4 with elevated TSH), which is commonly seen in ectopic thyroid.[38,39] This method also has a high false-positive rate especially in preterm, sick neonates and babies with thyroid-binding globulin deficiency. Hence a back-up TSH assay should follow this method.[40]

Primary TSH based screening is a more sensitive, specific, practical and cost-effective strategy and this method is being adopted in most countries.[22,29,40] The Netherlands, Israel and some states in USA follow primary T4 with back-up TSH assay. Some states in USA have adopted combined T4 and TSH assays, which may not be cost-effective for developing nations. Many countries have shifted from T4 to TSH-based screening protocol.

TSH is measured on DBS using either immunofluorescence or colorimetric method at a centralized laboratory where DBS samples from various centers reach. Serum samples can be analyzed by ELISA or chemiluminescence methods. The TSH measured from DBS is expressed in whole blood units. Serum units can be derived from whole blood units by multiplying the whole blood value by 2.2 (to adjust for the hematocrit). Usually the central monitoring laboratory reports TSH in serum units.

TSH Cut-off and Decision-making

The optimal time to collect a screening blood sample is between 48–72 hours of life. Various levels of cut-off are used in different studies but a value of > 20 mIU/L is usually taken as the standard.[41] All neonates with positive screening results are recalled immediately and confirmatory testing is done by measuring serum concentrations of both TSH and T4/FT4. The results should be interpreted based on gestational age and postnatal age-specific reference ranges.[11,42]

An infant in whom the TSH is elevated is diagnosed with primary hypothyroidism and in general, the higher the value, more severe is the disease and more prompt should be the treatment initiation. **Flowchart 15.1.1** provides a simplified algorithm based on the guidelines provided by the Indian Society for Pediatric and Adolescent Endocrinology (ISPAE).[38,43] If the TSH is above 80 mIU/L, the baby should be recalled immediately and the treatment should be initiated as soon as the confirmatory samples are drawn, without further waiting for the confirmatory results. When confirmatory results are available, treatment should be commenced if the serum TSH is above 20 mIU/L in the first 2 weeks of age or above 10 mIU/L after 2 weeks. If serum T4 is below 8 µg/dL (< 100 nmol/L) or FT4 less than 1.1 ng/dL (< 12 pmol/L), levothyroxine therapy is initiated (regardless of TSH levels). Caregivers of neonates with mild TSH elevation (6–20 mIU/L) and normal FT4/T4 levels are advised to bring the babies for follow-up thyroid hormone

Flowchart 15.1.1: A simplified algorithm for newborn screening for congenital hypothyroidism and subsequent follow-up and management.

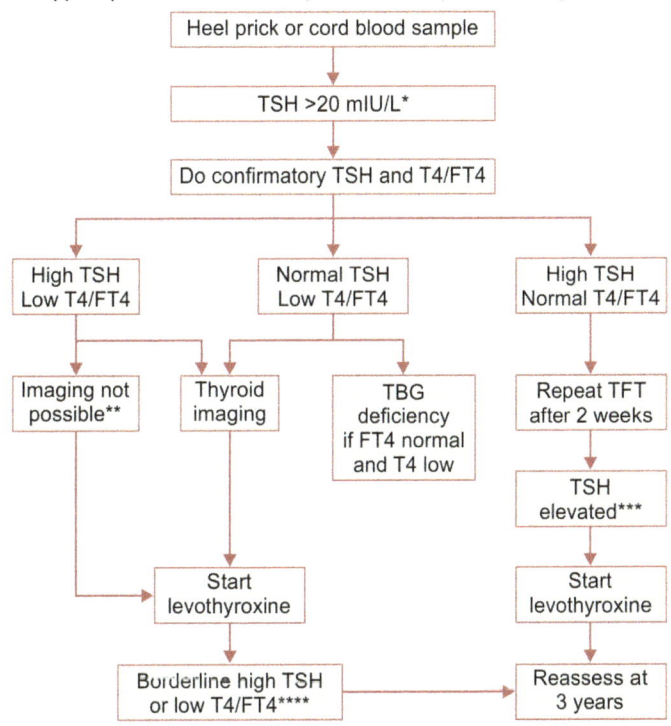

*If the TSH is above 80 mIU/L, the baby should be recalled immediately and the treatment should be initiated as soon as the confirmatory samples are drawn, without waiting for the confirmatory results.
**Delay in imaging should not prevent the neonate from getting early LT4 treatment.
***LT4 treatment is started if TSH is rising (above 20 mIU/L in neonates < 2 weeks and above 10 mIU/L in children > 2 weeks) or if FT4/T4 values are below normal.
****In this situation levothyroxine dose needs to be adjusted with further monitoring preferably after a review by a pediatric endocrinologist.
TSH: thyroid stimulating hormone; TFT: thyroid function test

tests closely (every 1-2 weeks) and treatment is started if TSH is rising (above 20 mIU/L in neonates < 2 weeks and above 10 mIU/L in children > 2 weeks) or if FT4/T4 values are below normal. Expert opinions however vary on these levels of cut-off. Since this is a contentious issue, many pediatricians prefer to continue observation. Every day of delay may result in potential loss of IQ in these children. Hence it is safer to initiate treatment in those children even with a marginal value. Many of these children have transient hypothyroidism requiring trial off therapy at a later age.[44]

TSH-based screening program may have up to 10–15% false-negative rates.[45] In some children, especially premature or very low birth weight babies (< 1500 g) elevation of TSH is often delayed as a result of immaturity of hypothalamic-pituitary-thyroid (HPT) axis, and may occur after several weeks of life. A similar picture is seen in very sick neonates due to their illness (sick euthyroid syndrome) or as a result of medications (e.g. dopamine, glucocorticoids, or iodinated compounds like povidone-iodine). In monozygotic twins who share a placental circulation, the normal baby's thyroid may compensate for the hypothyroid twin in utero; hence the initial thyroid function results may be normal. Because of these issues, repeat NBS at 2–4 weeks of postnatal age should be considered in children at risk of false-negative screening including preterm, LBW babies, very sick neonates in neonatal intensive care unit (NICU), homozygous twins, neonates on dopamine or corticosteroids, trisomy 21 and those at risk of iodine excess or iodine deficiency.

Infants with low T4 and normal TSH require some additional information before starting treatment. If the child is male and FT4 levels are normal, measurement of TBG levels is essential to rule out TBG deficiency. If serum FT4 levels are low, central hypothyroidism is a possibility. Always look for features of hypopituitarism in this setting, which include hypoglycemia, midline defects, micropenis and undescended testes. If the baby is premature, hypothyroxinemia of prematurity should be considered. This may be due to the immaturity of HPT axis, or associated nonthyroidal illness or medications, which affect thyroid hormone metabolism.

Annexure 15.1.2 provides some examples of difficult decision making during screening.

Confirmation by Investigations

Thyroid imaging, either by ultrasonography or scintigraphy is done in order to establish the diagnosis of thyroid dysgenesis.[46] In such cases treatment is ideally lifelong. Presence of a normal thyroid gland indicates the possibility of transient hypothyroidism. *But delay in imaging should not prevent the neonate from getting early treatment.* Tc-99m pertechnetate ($^{99m}TcO_4$) scans provide good anatomic details in 20–30 minutes. Feeding the baby before technetium injection and after scanning will empty the salivary gland so that any uptake in the lingual area can be confirmed as due to presence of thyroid tissue. Radioactive iodine (^{123}I) is useful in diagnosing organification disorders when combined with perchlorate test.[47]

If there is no uptake, serum thyroglobulin (TG) measurement is helpful. Serum concentration of TG indicates the presence of functional thyroid tissue. If TG is undetectable, it denotes thyroid agenesis or rarely a mutation of thyroglobulin gene. If TG is normal or high, the possibility of mutations inactivating TSH receptor or transplacental transfer of TSH receptor blocking antibodies should be considered.[48]

If the scintigraphy could not be performed before initiation of treatment, it should be considered at 3 years while performing trial off therapy. If TSH gets elevated after one month of stopping the treatment, scintigraphy can be performed to identify the etiology of hypothyroidism.

The chronicity of hypothyroidism can be estimated from radiography of knee. Absence of both femoral and tibial epiphyseal centers in a term baby denotes hypothyroidism has started in intrauterine period itself and this is a fairly reliable sign to predict greater risk of developmental subnormality in future.

Molecular genetic analysis is performed if there is a positive family history, consanguinity or if the baby is having specific symptoms like cardiac defects, choreoathetosis or hypotonia.

■ TREATMENT

Levothyroxine (LT4) is the drug of choice for CH.[1-4] Treatment should be initiated as soon as the diagnosis is confirmed and ideally within 14 days of delivery.[49] During therapy it is necessary to titrate the dose of LT4 on a regular basis as LT4 dose requirement depends on many extrinsic and intrinsic factors.[50] Both poorly controlled hypothyroidism as well as a moderate degree of undertreatment and overtreatment are associated with impaired cognitive outcomes.[51,52] The recommended dose is 10-15 µg/kg; the dose is individualized based on the severity. Infants with complete agenesis require higher dose compared to ectopic thyroid, and those with dyshormonogenesis require relatively lower doses. A scintigraphy report will aid in deciding the initial treatment dose. Many studies have observed that late initiation of treatment and insufficient doses have resulted in poor neurodevelopmental outcome.

Levothyroxine is generally available in tablet form in India, which needs to be crushed and mixed with 1-2 mL of milk or water and administered orally. LT4 liquid and injectable preparations are not available easily. In older children it should be given in empty stomach. Iron, vitamin D, calcium, soy preparations, simethicone (an ingredient of drops prescribed for infantile colic) should not be administered along with LT4 tablets. The tablets should not be diluted in excess water and kept for days. A missed dose can be given later on the same day, but repeated missing of the doses results in higher intellectual disability. The dose should be repeated if the infant vomits within an hour of ingestion. The dose of intravenous thyroxine (if available) is three-fourth of the oral dose. Addition of T3 has no benefit and it is not routinely advised.[53]

The goal of treatment is to attain a normal thyroid hormone status as quickly as possible and to maintain it consistently thereafter. Undertreatment in the initial years leads to poor neurodevelopmental and cognitive outcome. Monitoring and dose titration is based on periodic review with repeat thyroid function tests. First follow-up visit should be planned after 2 weeks of initiation of treatment, thereafter once a month for initial few months. More frequent visits are planned and dose adjustment is done if thyroid hormone tests have not normalized. The aim of the treatment is to maintain TSH at the lower range of normal age-specific range and FT4 in the upper normal range. The required dose decreases from 15 µg/day to 4 µg/day as age advances, probably due to low turnover rate of thyroxine at older age. In general, review should be planned once in every 1–2 months for first 6 months, every 2–3 months in the first year and 4–6 months till 3 years. After 3 years, and when the general condition and laboratory values are stable, less frequent visits (once in 6–12 months) are planned, as irreversible damage to the brain is less common after 3 years of age. More frequent review and monitoring of thyroid function should be done after each dose alteration.[53,54]

Poor adherence to treatment or wrong method of administration should be suspected if failure to achieve euthyroid status is happening despite repeated dose alterations. In such cases a treatment diary should be kept and should be checked regularly during each visit. Another reason for abnormal result is the time of blood collection. Ideally blood should be collected at least 4 hours after giving the tablets. If TSH concentration is normal or high in the presence of high FT4 levels, early blood collection (before 4 hours of tablet intake) should be suspected. A second reason for this abnormal test is frequent missing of the dose followed by making up by taking multiple doses before the blood test. When a child whose compliance is good and technique of LT4 administration is correct requires high doses of LT4 to keep TSH in normal range, he/she should be suspected to have thyroid hormone resistance at hypothalamic or pituitary level which may improve over time.

Trial off Therapy (Testing for Permanence)

An important concern of the family will be whether their child should take the medications lifelong and whether CH will affect his/her scholastic performance. If thyroid dysgenesis is confirmed, lifelong treatment is the only option. Many conditions, with a normal thyroid gland on imaging, are transient which include the effect of maternal antithyroid drugs or TSH receptor blocking antibodies. Children requiring less than 2 µg/kg of LT4 tablet daily have a higher chance of having transient hypothyroidism. Such children may be offered trial off therapy at 3 years. The dose should be reduced to half of the initial dose and child is followed up for a month. If thyroid functions remain normal, the tablet is stopped and the child is reviewed next month to assess thyronormalcy. Frequent follow-up with serial monitoring of thyroid function is required for a few more months (even if the child is not on medication). In a study done in USA about 40% of children labeled as having CH in the screening program were finally found to be having transient hypothyroidism and LT4 could be stopped in them.

■ PROGNOSIS

Prognosis of a child who was initiated the treatment before 2 weeks of birth is excellent.[52] Adequate treatment assures near normal neurocognitive function, school performance and normal IQ.[5] Mild defects in motor development, attention span, verbal skills, memory and IQ may occur in some patients especially who suffer severe intrauterine thyroxine depletion. Growth parameters like height, weight and bone maturation were comparable with normal children but there is a mild (one standard deviation) increase in head circumference in various studies.[55] Adoption of lowering of cut-offs has helped to identify more infants who have CH. However it is still not clear whether milder cases benefit from long-term therapy.[11]

Impact of Newborn Screening on the Neurocognitive Outcome of Children with CH

According to available studies, there is a remarkable improvement in neurodevelopmental outcome in children who were initiated LT4 therapy well in advance compared to those who were diagnosed in the prescreening era, based on clinical features. Klein et al. in their study had demonstrated that those who were diagnosed between 3 and 6 months of age in the prescreening period (based on clinical symptoms) had a mean IQ of 71 (range 35–36) and those who were diagnosed beyond 6 months of age had a lower mean IQ of 54 (range 25–50).[49] Children who were diagnosed by NBS had better results. New England Congenital Hypothyroidism Collaborative had documented a verbal IQ score of 109; a performance IQ score of 107 and a full-scale IQ score of 109 at 6 years of age in children diagnosed by screening and put on LT4 therapy sufficiently early.[56] These results were identical to their classroom controls. La Franchi S et al. in a systematic review of 51 articles found that age of initiation of treatment and severity of CH were the two most important factors affecting IQ.[57,58] Infants in whom LT4 therapy was initiated sufficiently early (12–30 days of age) had a mean IQ 15.7 points higher than those who had received the treatment late (>30 days of age). Studies have also found out that starting LT4 at a dose of 10–15 µg/kg/day had a better IQ outcome than starting at a lower dose. Most of the recent studies underscore the importance of NBS for CH and early initiation of optimum dose of LT4 for a better neurodevelopmental outcome. It is important to strengthen the surveillance system to ensure timely visits to the pediatrician and efficient control of serum thyroid hormone levels to assure a euthyroid state in children with CH.[59]

Genetics and Future Risk Stratification

Most of the cases of CH detected by NBS are sporadic. The risk of this disease in first-degree relatives is 1% and familial forms are uncommon.[60]

In dyshormonogenesis, the risk for subsequent offsprings is 25%. Girls with congenital or acquired hypothyroidism should have measurement of TSH and FT4 well in advance before pregnancy and should be monitored throughout the gestational period.[60] Requirement of LT4 increases during pregnancy.

■ SUMMARY

Congenital hypothyroidism is the commonest cause of preventable intellectual disability. Early diagnosis, prompt initiation of treatment and efficient follow-up can optimize long-term outcome and reduce the neurodevelopmental subnormality in affected children. Universal NBS is the only way to pick up CH in the newborn period, as the child is asymptomatic in his/her early days, even though NBS has its own limitations.[61] Screening for CH should be performed between 24 and 72 hours of life and abnormal screening results should be confirmed immediately by measuring serum TSH and FT4. Even if the screening results are normal, high index of clinical suspicion and repeat screening in the selected group help to pick up the cases that are likely to be missed during screening. Imaging studies are used as an adjunct in managing the newborn and assessing the prognosis and duration of treatment. Treatment with oral LT4 tablet should be initiated as early as possible, ideally within 14 days of life. Careful and regular monitoring is the key for the success of therapy. Trial off therapy is considered in a probable child with transient hypothyroidism at 3 years. Outcome in a successfully managed child is excellent barring some subtle defects in children who suffer severe intrauterine deficiency of thyroid hormone.

■ ANNEXURE 15.1.1: BLOOD SAMPLE COLLECTION FOR NEWBORN SCREENING

Timing of Heel Prick Sampling

- Ideally after 48 hours, except in special situations where it can be done after 24 hours
- Do not collect blood before 24 hours of delivery
- Repeat sampling should be done at a later date (after 1–2 weeks) in sick neonates, preterm babies and twins.

Steps for Collecting the Sample

- The following items should be kept ready before the procedure. Warm water, hot water bag, warm towels, soft cloth, alcohol, sterile gauze pad, lancet, gloves, and ball pen
- Take a written consent
- Expose baby's heel, warm the area with prewarmed towels or hot water bag for 3–5 minutes so that local blood circulation is enhanced

- Clean the area with alcohol and wipe dry with sterile gauze pad
- Keep the heel lower than the level of heart to enhance circulation
- Make a single prick on the lateral aspect of heel to a depth of 2 mm
- Discard the first drop of blood by wiping with a dry swab
- Do not squeeze
- Allow an appropriately sized blood drop to form and then carefully touch with the filter paper so that the blood is soaked through
- Blood drop should completely fill the circle and should be allowed to soak through to other side of the filter paper
- All the circles provided in the filter paper should be filled with the blood
- Avoid taking multiple blood drops over a blood drop which is already there in the filter paper (over-layering)
- Apply blood to one side of filter paper only
- Do not contaminate the circles by touching the circle before or after blood collection
- Keep the filter paper in a nonabsorbent open surface (drying rack) in horizontal position for 3-4 hours to allow the blood spot to get air-dried
- Do not keep the papers one over the other
- Do not expose to heat or direct sunlight
- Complete the information in the place provided in the filter paper
- The specimen should be transported to the regional laboratory in an envelop as soon as it is dry and no later than 24 hours.

Reasons for Invalid Blood Samples

- Removing the filter paper early, before completely filling the circle
- If the puncture site is wet
- If the puncture site is squeezed
- When the blood spot is touched with hands or other objects
- Using capillary tube or syringe for applying blood
- If sufficient time (3-4 hours) was not allotted for drying the sample
- Applying excess blood or applying blood to both sides of filter paper
- If filter paper is exposed to heat or direct sunlight
- If multiple blood drops are used in the same circle (over-layering)

■ ANNEXURE 15.1.2: CASE SCENARIOS SHOWING SPECIFIC SITUATIONS

1. Newborn screening of a premature baby revealed a TSH of 18 mIU/L. How should I proceed further?

Premature babies have an attenuated TSH surge due to immaturity of HPT axis. Concomitant illnesses like sepsis, respiratory distress and drugs like dopamine and iodinated antiseptics can further attenuate the axis. The TSH may not be as high as expected during initial few days and may rise subsequently after few weeks (delayed elevation of TSH). Hence a repeat screening is recommended after the baby has recovered from associated problems (preferably after 2–4 weeks).

2. A second screening at 25th day showed TSH 23 mIU/L and T4 6 µg/dL. Does this baby require treatment?

In this case, the T4 level is low and it may be as a result of CH per se or because of low TBG production (hypothyroxinemia of prematurity). Estimation of FT4 estimation is more appropriate in such cases. The TSH level is considered as elevated if it is above 20 mIU/L if age is <14 days and above 10 mIU/L if age is >14 days. If FT4 is also low, this child should be put on LT4 therapy. Imaging will help to assess the status of thyroid gland. Experts differ in their opinion whether to treat if FT4 is normal with a moderate elevation of TSH. A recommendation is to place the child on a lower dose of LT4 (10 µg/kg), preferably after a review by a pediatric endocrinologist, with regular follow-up. A trial for assessing permanence can be done at 3 years of age.

3. A term baby was recalled after getting a screening result of mildly elevated TSH (22 mIU/L). The confirmatory test result done on day 7 showed TSH is 1.5 mIU/L and T4 is 4 µg/dL. How will you manage this child?

In this situation also, measurement of FT4 is ideally done initially. Since T4 is low and TSH is in the lower range of normal, possibility of central hypothyroidism should be considered especially if FT4 level is also low. The child should be evaluated for features of central hypothyroidism, e.g. micropenis, midfacial defects, conjugated jaundice, hypoglycemia or polyuria.

If FT4 is normal and there are no features of central hypothyroidism, TBG measurement should be done to rule out TBG deficiency. TBG deficiency is a benign condition requiring no treatment; hence this case can be followed-up with repeat thyroid function measurements after few weeks.

If the child was sick at the time of initial sampling, with very low birth weight, or had received blood transfusion before sample collection, or is one of the monozygotic twins or sample collection was inappropriate, thyroid function tests should be repeated after 2–3 weeks of life.

If FT4 remains low after second testing, the child is asymptomatic and the possibility of central hypothyroidism has been ruled out, this child should be followed up with serial thyroid testing and developmental assessment. If FT4 is persistently low, treatment can be initiated with a lower dose of LT4 (preferably after a review by a pediatric endocrinologist) and imaging is mandatory. Assessment of permanence by performing trial off therapy should be done at 3 years.

REFERENCES

1. Desai MP. The thyroid gland. In: Desai MP, Menon PSN, Bhatia V (Eds). Pediatric Endocrine Disorders, 3rd edn. Universities Press; Hyderabad 2014. Pp. 189-94.
2. Van Villet G, Deladoëy J. Disorders of the thyroid in the newborn and infant. In: Sperling MA (Ed). Pediatric Endocrinology, 4th edn. Elsevier Saunders; Philadelphia. 2014. Pp. 186-208.
3. Salvatore D, Davies TF, Martin JS, et al. Thyroid physiology and diagnostic evaluation of patients with thyroid disorders. In: S Melmed, K S Polonsky, P Reed Larsen, H Kronenberg (Eds). Williams Textbook of Endocrinology, 13th edn. Elsevier Saunders; Philadelphia. 2016. Pp. 333-68.
4. Wassner AJ. Congenital hypothyroidism. Clin Perinatol. 2018;45(1):1-18.
5. Ford G, LaFranchi SH. Screening for congenital hypothyroidism: a worldwide view of strategies. Best Pract Res Clin Endocrinol Metab. 2014;28:175-87.
6. Therell BL Jr, Padilla CD. Newborn screening in the developing countries. Curr Opin Pediatr. 2018;30:734-9.
7. Polak M, Luton D. Fetal thyroïdology. Best Pract Res Clin Endocrinol Metab. 2014;28:161-73.
8. Dohan O, De la Vieja A, Paroder V, et al. The sodium/iodide symporter (NIS): characterization, regulation and medical significance. Endocr Rev. 2003;24:48-77.
9. de Escobar GM, Obregon MJ, Del Rey FE. Role of thyroid hormone during early brain development. Eur J Endocrinol. 2004;151:U25-U37.
10. Ghassabian A, Henrichs J, Tiemeier H. Impact of mild thyroid hormone deficiency in pregnancy on cognitive function in children: lessons from the Generation R Study. Best Pract Res Clin Endocrinol Metab. 2014;28:221-32.
11. Kaplowitz PB. Neonatal thyroid disease testing and management. Pediatr Clin N Am. 2019;66:343-52.
12. Persani L, Rurale G, de Filippis T, et al. Genetics and management of congenital hypothyroidism. Best Pract Res Clin Endocrinol Metab. 2018;32:387-96.
13. Mio C, Grani G, Durante C, Damante G. Molecular defects in thyroid dysgenesis. Clin Genet. 2019 Aug 21. Doi: 10.1111/cge.13627.
14. Fu J, Dumitrescu AM. Inherited defects in thyroid hormone cell-membrane transport and metabolism. Best Pract Res Clin Endocrinol Metab. 2014;28:189-201.
15. Wemeau JL, Kopp P. Pendred syndrome. Best Pract Res Clin Endocrinol Metab. 2017;31:213-24.
16. Sasivari Z, Szinnai G, Seebauer B, et al. Double variants in TSHR and DUOX2 in patient with hypothyroidism: case report. J Pediatr Endocrinol Metab.2019; sep 21. Doi: 10.1515/jpem-209-0051.
17. Peters C, Nicholas AK, Schoenmakers E, et al. DUOX2/DUOXA2 mutations frequently cause congenital hypothyroidism that evades detection on newborn screening in the United Kingdom. Thyroid. 2019;29:790-801.
18. Heo S, Jang JH, Yu J. Congenital hypothyroidism due to thyroglobulin deficiency: a case report with a novel mutation in TG gene. Ann Pediatr Endocrinol Metab. 2019;24:199-202.

19. Polak M, Refeloff S, Szimmai G, et al. Disorders of thyroid gland. In: Sarafoglou K (Ed). Pediatric Endocrinology and Inborn Errors of Metabolism. 2nd edn. McGraw Hill Educations. New York. 2017. pp. 481-509.
20. Rose SR, Brown RS, Foley T, et al. Update on newborn screening and therapy for congenital hypothyroidism. Pediatrics. 2006;117:2290-303.
21. Deladoey J, Ruel J, Giguere Y, et al. Is the incidence of congenital hypothyroidism really increasing? A 20-year retrospective population-based study in Quebec. J Clin Endocrinol Metab. 2011;96:2422-9.
22. Leger J, Olivieri A, Donaldson, et al. ESPE-PES-SLEP-JSPE-APEG-APES-ISPAE; Congenital Hypothyroidism consensus Conference Group. European Society for Paediatric Endocrinology consensus guidelines on screening, diagnosis, and management of congenital hypothyroidism. J Clin Endocrinol Metab. 2014;99:363-84.
23. Brosco JP, Paul DB. The political history of PKU: Reflections on 50 years of newborn screening. Pediatrics. 2013;132(6):987-9.
24. Guthrie R. Screening for inborn errors of metabolism in the newborn infant- a multiple test program. Birth Defects Original Article, Series IV 1962. pp. 92-8).
25. Dussault JH. The anecdotal history of screening for congenital hypothyroidism. J Clin Endocrinol Metab. 1999;84:4332-4.
26. American College of Medical Genetics Newborn Screening Expert Group. Newborn Screening: Towards a Uniform Screening Panel and System. Genetic Med. 2006; 8(5)Suppl:S12–S252.
27. Pang S. Newborn screening for congenital adrenal hyperplasia. Pediatr Ann. 2003;32:516-23.
28. Fisher DA, Dussault JH, Foley TP Jr, et al. Screening for congenital hypothyroidism: results of screening one million North American infants. J Pediatr. 1984;21:695-700.
29. Fabie NAV, Pappas KB, Feldman GL. The current state of newborn screening in the United States. Pediatr Clin N Am. 2019;66(2):369–86.
30. Wilson JMG, Jungner G. Principles and practice of screening for disease. Geneva: WHO; 1968. Available from: http://www.who.int/bulletin/volumes/86/4/07-050112BP.pdf.
31. Watson MS, Mann MY, Lloyd-Puryear MA, Ronaldo P, Howell RR and American College of Medical Genetics Newborn Screening Expert Group. Newborn screening: Toward a uniform screening panel and system-Executive Summary. Pediatrics. 2006;117(5 Pt 2):S296-307.101097/01.gim.0000223891.82390.ad.
32. Sweetman L, Millington DS, Therrell BL, et al. Naming and counting disorders (conditions) included in new born screening panels. Pediatrics. 2006;117(5 Pt2):S308–14.
33. Colaco MP, Desai MP, Ajgaonkar AR, et al. Neonatal screening for hypothyroidism. Indian Pediatr. 1984;21:695-700.
34. Mathai S. Newborn screening for congenital hypothyroidism—experience from India. Abstract presented at 8th Asia Pacific Regional Meeting of the International Society for Neonatal Screening. New Delhi. September 2013.
35. Desai MP, Upadhye P, Colaco MP. Neonatal screening for congenital hypothyroidism using the filter paper thyroxine technique. Indian J Med Res. 1994:100:36–42.

36. Kaur G, Srivastav J, Jain S, et al. Preliminary report on neonatal screening for congenital hypothyroidism, congenital adrenal hyperplasia and glucose-6-phosphate dehydrogenase deficiency: a Chandigarh experience. Indian J Pediatr. 2010;77:969-73.
37. Gopalakrishnan V, Joshi K, Phadke SR, et al. Newborn screening for congenital hypothyroidism, galactosemia and biotinidase deficiency in Uttar Pradesh, India. Indian Pediatr. 2014;51:701-5.
38. Desai MP, Sharma R, Riaz I, et al. New born screening guidelines for congenital hypothyroidism in India: recommendation of the Indian Society for Paediatric and Adolescent Endocrinology (ISPAE)-Part 1: Screening and confirmation of diagnosis. Indian J Pediatr. 2018;85(6):40-7.
39. Delange F. Neonatal screening for congenital hypothyroidism: results and perspectives. Horm Res. 1997;48:51-61.
40. Walfish PG. Evaluation of three thyroid-function screening tests for detecting neonatal hypothyroidism. Lancet. 1976;1:1208-10.
41. Verma P, Kapoor S, Kalivani M, et al. An optimal capillary screen cut-off on thyroid stimulating hormone for diagnosing congenital hypothyroidism: data from a pilot newborn screening program in Delhi. Indian Pediatr. 2019;56:281-6.
42. Esfandiari NH, Papaleontiou M. Biochemical testing in thyroid disorders. Endocrinol Metab Clin N Am. 2017;46:631-48.
43. Sudhanshu S, Riaz I, Sharma R, et al. New born screening guidelines for congenital hypothyroidism in India: Recommendation of the Indian Society for Paediatric and Adolescent Endocrinology (ISPAE)-Part 2: Imaging, treatment and follow up. Indian J Pediatr. 2018;85(6):448-53.
44. Itonaga T, Higuchi S, Shimura K, et al. Levothyroxine dosage as predictor of permanent and transient congenital hypothyroidism: a multicenter retrospective study in Japan. Horm Res Paediatr. 2019;92:45-51.
45. Koulouri O, Moran C, Halsall D, et al. Pitfalls in the measurement and interpretation of thyroid function tests. Best Pract Res Clin Endocrinol Metab. 2013;27:745-62.
46. Livett T, LaFranchi S. Imaging in congenital hypothyroidism. Curr Opin Pediatr. 2019;31:555-61.
47. Vliet GV, Deladoëy J. Interpreting minor variations in thyroid function or echo structure: treating patients, not numbers or images. Pediatr Clin N Am. 2015;62:929-42.
48. Clerc J. Imaging the thyroid in children. Best Pract Res Clin Endocrinol Metab. 2014;28:203-20.
49. Klein AH, Meltzer S, Kenny FM. Improved prognosis in congenital hypothyroidism treated before age three months. J Pediatr. 1972;81:912-5.
50. Hindmarsh PC. Optimization of thyroxine dose in congenital hypothyroidism. Arch Dis Child. 2002;86:73-5.
51. Bongers-Schokking JJ, de Muinck Keizer-Schrama SM. Influence of timing and dose of thyroid hormone replacement on mental, psychomotor, and behavioral development in children with congenital hypothyroidism. J Pediatr. 2005;147:768-74.
52. Bongers-Schokking JJ, Resing WC, de Rijke YB, et al. Cognitive development in congenital hypothyroidism: is overtreatment a greater threat than undertreatment? J Clin Endocrinol Metab. 2013;98:499-506.

53. Cherella CE, Wassner AJ. Congenital hypothyroidism: insights into pathogenesis and treatment. Int J Pediatr Endocrinol. (2017) 2017:11 .DOI 10.1186/s13633-017-0051-0.
54. Taylor PN, Lazarus JH. Hypothyroidism in pregnancy. Endocrinol Metab Clin N Am. 2019;48:547–56.
55. Pimentel J, Chambers M, Shahid M, et al. Comorbidities of thyroid disease in children. Adv Pediatr. 2016;63(1):211-26.
56. New England Congenital Hypothyroidism Collaborative. Neonatal hypothyroidism screening: status of patients at 6 years of age. J Pediatr. 1985;107:915–9.
57. LaFranchi S, Austin J. How should we be treating children with congenital hypothyroidism? J Pediatr Endocrinol Metab. 2007;20:559–78.
58. LaFranchi SH, Hanna CE, Krainz PL, et al. Screening for congenital hypothyroidism with specimen collection at two time periods: results of the Northwest Regional Screening Program. Pediatrics. 1985;76:734–40.
59. Menon PSN. Prevention of neurocognitive impairment in children through newborn screening for congenital hypothyroidism. India Pediatr. 2018;55:113-4.
60. Persani L, Rurale G, de Filippis T, et al. Genetics and management of congenital hypothyroidism. Best Pract Res Clin Endocrinol Metab. 2018;32:387-96.
61. Therrell BL Jr. Newborn screening for congenital hypothyroidism in India: let's just do it! Indian Pediatr. 2019;56:275-6.

CHAPTER 16

GENETICS

16.1 Down Syndrome: Rising Up
Shubha R Phadke

16.1 DOWN SYNDROME: RISING UP

Shubha R Phadke

■ INTRODUCTION

Down syndrome (DS) has a long history and it may not be wrong to state that the specialty of medical genetics began with the disorder named as DS. It is the most common cause of intellectual disability. The characteristic phenotype makes the clinical diagnosis easy. The British clinician, Langdon Down, described it as a Mongolian idiocy in 1862 and the disorder got the name, DS. With development of karyotyping techniques in 1956, Lejeune identified trisomy of chromosome 21 as the cause of DS.[1]

A lot of developments in genetics and technology got reflected in the understanding of trisomy 21. It led to improved investigations for not only the diagnosis, but also population-based screening for trisomy 21. The developments in diagnosis and management of trisomy 21 parallel the genetic approach to other chromosomal and monogenic disorders, especially those with intellectual disability.

Not only there were developments in genetic technologies over last few decades, the societal change in the perspective toward and facilities for children with special needs changed the scenario for the families with DS children. Now, individuals with DS or other neurodevelopmental disabilities have opportunities to get incorporated in the society and contribute to it by living a fruitful and happy life **(Fig. 16.1.1)**. The words like "mental retardation" and "intellectual disability" are getting replaced by special children or individuals

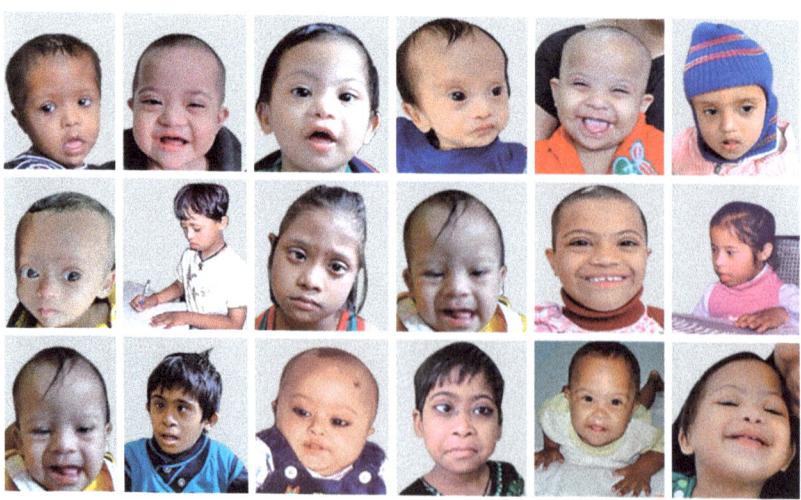

Fig. 16.1.1: Facial features of children of various ages with trisomy 21.

Table 16.1.1: Possibility of giving birth to a child with Down syndrome with increasing maternal age.

Age of the mother (in years)	Possibility of a child with Down syndrome
20	1:1,925
25	1:1,205
30	1:885
35	1:365
40	1:110
45	1:32

with special needs and abilities. This is a major step in opening the arms of society to take these "special individuals" in its folds. This chapter in the 21st century plans to present the positive aspects of children with DS along with clinical features, diagnostic tests, genetic counseling issues, and population-based prevention.

■ EPIDEMIOLOGY

The birth prevalence of DS is reported to be 1 in 700 worldwide[2] and 1 in 1,200 in India.[3] The difference is likely to be due to the average age of women at childbirth as the possibility of birth of a child with trisomy 21 increases as the mother's age increases **(Table 16.1.1)**. In India, most of the children with trisomy 21 are born to young mothers. As DS is the most common genetic disorder, all pediatricians and neonatologists need to be well-conversant with diagnosis, management, and genetic counseling for this disorder.

■ ETIOLOGY

Extra copy of chromosome 21 is the etiology of DS. In around 95% of cases, the extra chromosome 21 is free **(Fig. 16.1.2)** and the total number of chromosomes is 47 (47, XX, +21 or 47, XY, +21). In about 4% cases of DS, the extra chromosome 21 is attached to another chromosome **(Figs. 16.1.3A to C)**, usually some acrocentric chromosome (21, 22, or 14). In such cases with translocation, karyotyping of the parents is necessary for giving risk of recurrence in the next child as some cases might have received the translocated chromosome from one of the parents who is a balanced carrier of the translocation. Remaining 1% cases are mosaic with trisomy 21 in some cells and some cells with normal cell line with 46 chromosomes.

Percentage of normal cell line is not the only factor to predict the outcome regarding cognitive function and presence of mosaicism does not always predict better intelligence quotient (IQ). Though the definite clinical

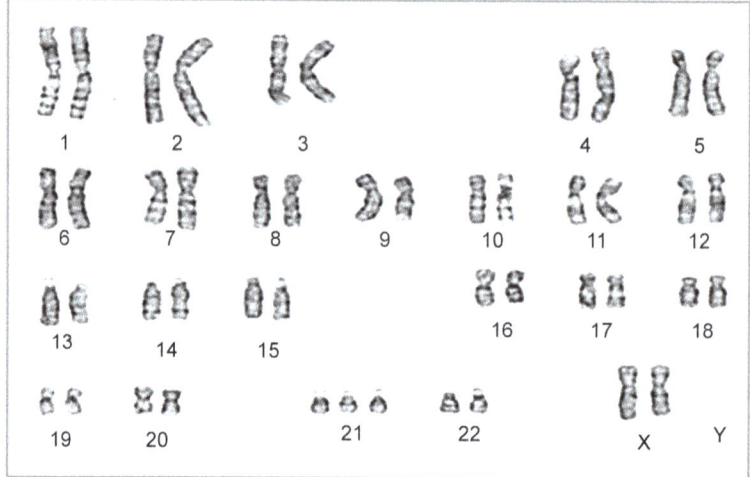

Fig. 16.1.2: 47, XX, +21. Karyotype of a girl with Down syndrome with free trisomy 21.

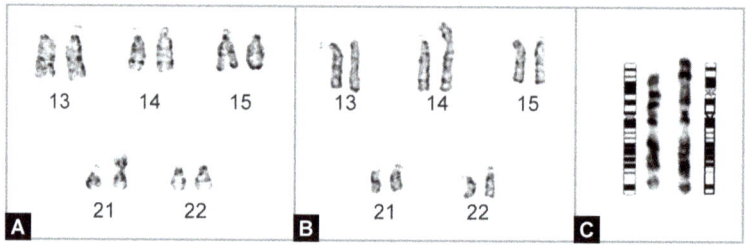

Figs. 16.1.3A to C: Partial karyotypes showing translocation of chromosome 21 to other chromosome. (A) Translocation between chromosome 21 and chromosome 21; (B) Translocation between chromosome 14 and chromosome 21; and (C) Chromosome 21 is attached to chromosome 11.

diagnosis is possible in most of the children with DS, karyotyping is essential as the risk of recurrence in the siblings and other relatives will depend on the chromosomal abnormality. Chromosomal analysis of parents of a child with free trisomy 21 (47, +21) is not indicated. Rarely, the child with DS is not alive and, in such situation, karyotyping of parents can provide useful information for genetic counseling.

■ PATHOGENESIS

Presence of extra copy of chromosome 21 (trisomy instead of normal disomy) leads to presence of three copies of genes on chromosome 21 and attempts have been made to find out the critical region of chromosome 21 for the features of DS. Study of genotype-phenotype correlation in cases with partial trisomy of a small part of chromosome 21 suggested region from 21q21 to 21q22.3 to be the critical region for manifestations of DS. However, study of these cases suggested that it was not possible to attribute all features to one critical region on chromosome 21. There are at least 300 genes on chromosome 21 and studies have shown that 22% of them are expressed 1.5 times of the normal and may be responsible for the features of DS. Contribution of genes important for specific features has been discussed.[2] Premature aging and decreased function of the immune system may be caused by the overexpression of superoxide dismutase 1 (*SOD1*) gene (OMIM 147450). Neuropathological changes of Alzheimer disease are seen in all individuals with DS more than 40 years old. Association of amyloid beta A4 precursor protein (*APP*) gene on chromosome 21 with Alzheimer disease is being investigated. Better understanding of effects of various genes may be useful in planning novel therapeutic strategies.

■ AUTOIMMUNE DISORDERS IN CHILDREN WITH DOWN SYNDROME

Increased risk of autoimmune disorders and leukemia in children with DS is well-known. Celiac disease has a prevalence of 4.5–7%, autoimmune thyroiditis is diagnosed in 5–54% of DS subjects, and type 1 diabetes (T1D) is present in 1% of these individuals. Increased risk of infections and autoimmune diseases suggests abnormalities of immune function in DS, though the exact mechanisms of pathogenesis are not understood. Though organ-specific autoimmune diseases are common in DS patients, systemic autoimmune diseases like systemic lupus erythematosus are not more common than the general population. Natural T regulatory cells play an important role in autoimmunity by suppressing the autoreactive T cells that escape the thymic negative selection in circulation. It has been shown that in DS patients, the circulating T regulatory cells are increased in number compared to the healthy control, whereas their function is impaired.[4]

Other factor thought to be implicated in autoimmune disorders in DS is autoimmune regulator (AIRE) protein, a transcription factor located on chromosome 21 that plays a crucial role in autoimmunity by regulating promiscuous gene expression.[5] *AIRE* gene is located on chromosome 21 and is a transcription factor for many genes that encode for peripheral tissue-restricted antigens. The role of this gene was evaluated because the spectrum of autoimmune diseases in DS subjects is similar to that seen in the rare autosomal recessive disease namely autoimmune polyendocrinopathy-candidiasis-ectodermal dystrophy syndrome, also called autoimmune polyendocrine syndrome type 1 which is caused by mutations in *AIRE* gene. In spite of being located on chromosome 21, the gene expression is reduced to half of the normal in thymuses of DS individuals rather than being increased to 1.5 times. It was confirmed that all three copies of the gene were expressing but significantly fewer AIRE-positive cells were found in the thymic medulla of DS patients compared with those in the control group. This suggests that reduced AIRE expression may be playing a role in change in immune tolerance in DS.

LEUKEMIA IN CHILDREN WITH DOWN SYNDROME

Children with DS have a significantly increased risk of childhood leukemia. Acute megakaryoblastic leukemia (AMKL) and DS-acute lymphoblastic leukemia (DS-ALL) are 500 times and 20 times, respectively, more common in DS than normal children. A preleukemia, called transient myeloproliferative disorder (TMD), characterized by a GATA-binding protein 1 (*GATA1*) mutation, affects up to 30% of newborns with DS. Though spontaneous regression is common, life-threatening issues and progression to AMKL or myelodysplastic syndrome (MDS) are seen in one-fourth of the cases. Other than *GATA1* gene, genetic variations and epigenetic changes in other genes are implicated in the progression to leukemia which is a multistage process. DS-ALL is a high-risk leukemia and mutations in the Janus kinase-signal transducer and activator of transcription (JAK-STAT) pathway are frequently observed. JAK inhibitors may improve outcome for this type of leukemia. Key candidate genes in leukemogenesis on chromosome 21 include *ERG, ETS2, RUNX1, GABPA, BACH1,* and *DYRK1A*. Mateos et al.[6] have provided an extensive review of leukemia and MDS in DS.

CLINICAL FEATURES

The clinical features of patients with DS are shown in **Box 16.1.1**. Intellectual disability is the most serious manifestation. The clinical diagnosis is possible based on the characteristic facial phenotype due to the combination of variations of eyes, nose, and ears (**see Fig. 16.1.1**). The IQ of children with the disease is usually between 40 and 60 but may be higher in many, like variability of cognitive function among normal children. Most of the affected children walk, talk in simple language and can be trained in self-care and a vocation that requires simple and repetitive tasks.

Major malformations associated with trisomy 21 are cardiac malformations especially atrioventricular canal defects, duodenal atresia, tracheoesophageal fistula, congenital cataract, and Hirschsprung disease. Other important problems are epilepsy, hypothyroidism, deafness, atlantoaxial instability, and increased risk of leukemia. Other than hypothyroidism, the risk for other autoimmune disorders like celiac disease, alopecia areata, and vitiligo is increased. When serious malformations are present and are untreated, death may occur during infancy but otherwise life expectancy is not markedly reduced. In adults with DS, there is increased prevalence of dementia and neuropathological changes like those seen in Alzheimer disease.

Small teeth, missing teeth, and increased risk of periodontal disease need special mention. Large tongue and small jaw are other contributory factors to the dental problems which can be looked for and prevented by training and supervising dental care.

> **Box 16.1.1:** Clinical features of patients with trisomy 21.
>
> - Brachycephaly
> - Flattened facial features
> - Flat occiput
> - Epicanthic folds
> - Oblique palpebral fissures
> - Hypertelorism
> - Brushfield spots
> - Dysplastic ears
> - Low-set ears
> - Small nose
> - Depressed nasal bridge
> - Excess skin at the nape of the neck
> - Short and broad neck
> - Open mouth
> - Protruding tongue
> - Furrowed tongue
> - Narrow and high-arched palate
> - Dental abnormalities
> - Broad hand and short fingers
> - Short fifth middle phalanx
> - Clinodactyly of the fifth finger
> - Short limbs
> - Transverse palmar crease
> - Increased gap between the first and second toes
> - Hyperextensibility of the joints
> - Rough skin on the dorsum of the hands
> - Hypotonia
> - Intellectual disability
> - Congenital heart disease
> - Duodenal atresia
> - Hirschsprung disease

◼ NEONATAL PRESENTATION

Down syndrome is usually detected at neonatal stage. It is sometimes a surprise to the obstetrician, pediatrician, and the family who is expecting a normal healthy child. Most of the babies with trisomy 21 do not have any obvious external anomalies and the parents and family members do not have any clue to the existence of a major chromosomal abnormality in the baby. To break the news that the child has a serious birth defect which is associated with subnormal intelligence is a challenging task for the clinician and hence, it must be handled carefully by the senior obstetrician or pediatrician.[7] The diagnosis should be declared as early as possible to the family. This is important not only for the family but also for the neonate who needs to be evaluated for serious internal malformations, which may require urgent attention. Preferably, both the parents should be present and if appropriate elder or other family members may be involved in the session. There is no correct way to provide the news of existence of a problem with long-term implications, but an attempt may be made to reduce the emotional trauma to the family. Positive but realistic information about outcome and ways to help the baby by providing supportive care need to be provided. Rare complications should not be mentioned in the beginning. The diagnosis should be confirmed by chromosomal analysis in each case, though usually clinical diagnosis is correct. In some neonates, especially premature babies, the phenotype may be subtle, and the clinician may like to wait for the report before disclosing the diagnosis.

In current era of population-based screening for DS, rarely a child with DS may be born to a family who had low risk of trisomy 21 on biochemical screening done on maternal blood during first or second trimester. Counseling such a family is a difficult task and needs a lot of empathy, understanding of principle of screening test, and their detection rates.

■ ANTENATAL PRESENTATION

Detection of duodenal atresia or cardiac malformation or other ultrasonographic markers like increased nuchal translucency during prenatal ultrasonography may suggest the possibility of DS in the fetus. 30% of prenatally detected fetuses with duodenal atresia have trisomy 21 **(Figs. 16.1.4A to E)**. Amniocentesis and chromosomal analysis by rapid test namely—fluorescence in situ hybridization (FISH) or quantitative fluorescent polymerase chain reaction (QF-PCR) for common trisomies (chromosomes 21, 13, and 18)—are indicated to plan the further management. A pediatrician may be required to be a part of counseling team.

Prenatal diagnosis of trisomy 21 is also done by fetal chromosomal analysis done by chorionic villus sampling or amniocentesis done due to detection of increased risk of trisomy 21 by biochemical screening [first trimester double marker test or second trimester quadruple test or noninvasive prenatal screening (NIPS) on free fetal DNA (ffDNA) in maternal plasma] or identification of ultrasonographic markers for trisomy 21 like increased nuchal thickening and absent nasal bone. Mother's plasma contains ffDNA shade from broken down trophoblastic cells of placenta. New technology of next generation sequencing (NGS) can identify the chromosomal aneuploidies in fetus by testing ffDNA and the test is known as NIPS. NIPS can detect almost all fetuses with trisomy 21, but rarely false-positive and false-negative results are reported. Thus, this costly test which is a technological marvel continues to remain a screening test with high sensitivity. If NIPS shows high risk of trisomy 21, it is essential to do confirmation on fetal sample collected by invasive method like amniocentesis before taking irreversible decision like termination of pregnancy. In such situations, most of the families may

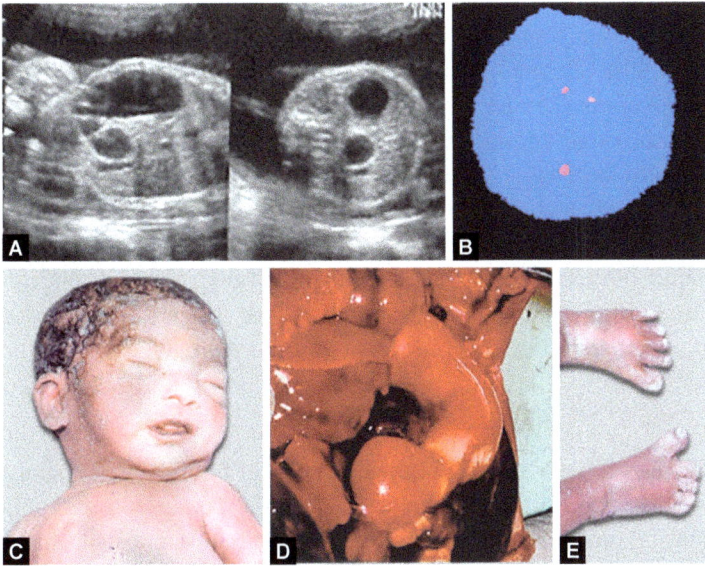

Figs. 16.1.4A to E: Prenatally detected duodenal atresia in a fetus with Down syndrome. (A) Double bubble appearance on antenatal USG; (B) Interphase FISH showing three signals for chromosome 21 probes; (C) Subtle facial phenotype of Down syndrome; (D) Distended duodenal bulb; and (E) Increased gap between first and second toes. (FISH: fluorescence in situ hybridization; USG: ultrasonography)

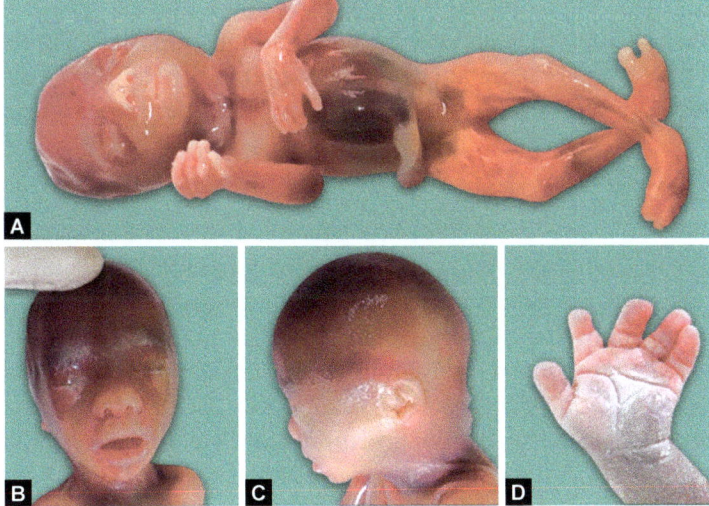

Figs. 16.1.5A to D: Fetus with trisomy 21.

opt for termination of pregnancy within the legal limits allowed by medical termination of pregnancy act. Pediatrician may be involved to examine the fetus after termination.[8] It should be noted that most of the fetuses with trisomy 21 do not have external malformations and characteristic facial phenotype is not obvious till later part of pregnancy **(Figs. 16.1.5A to D)**.

STILLBIRTHS

More than 50% of conceptuses with trisomy 21 are lost before birth. Most of them are spontaneously aborted and chromosomal analysis of products of conception may identify trisomy 21. Chromosomal abnormalities are seen in 5% of stillbirths. Though the chromosomal analysis of products of conception from each spontaneous abortion is not indicated, fetal autopsy and chromosomal analysis of stillborn baby is essential to provide genetic counseling. Pediatrician can play an important role in explaining the importance of fetal autopsy for providing risk of recurrence and also in examining fetuses for dysmorphic features and helping in diagnosis.

INFANCY AND CHILDHOOD

Many families are not told about the diagnosis of DS during neonatal period or infancy. The parents note developmental delay in the later part of infancy or childhood and then the child may be given the diagnosis of DS. Indian experience showed that parents of only 27% of children with DS were communicated about the diagnosis during infancy and most of them were not aware about the association of intellectual disability and lack of curative treatment for that.[9] At whatever age, a child with DS is seen by a sensitive pediatrician who must assess the knowledge of the family about the condition and attitude toward the disorder and their child with DS. Based on the assessment, appropriate counseling and accurate but positive information should be provided. Acceptance of the disorder in the child is the first and most important step toward the direction of evaluation and starting therapies.

INVESTIGATIONS

As mentioned above, every child with clinically diagnosed or suspected DS should be evaluated by karyotyping. Karyotype, in addition to confirming the diagnosis, gives the specific chromosomal abnormality, which is essential for genetic counseling. Rarely, extra chromosome may be attached to a chromosome other than G or D group of chromosomes (*see* **Fig. 16.1.3C**). Karyotype report is available usually within 2-3 weeks. In babies with serious malformation and the need to confirm the diagnosis at the earliest, molecular techniques like FISH (which can be done on interphase nuclei) or QF-PCR can be done. The reporting time for these tests is 3-4 days. The other advantage of QF-PCR is that it does not need live cells and hence sample [1-2 mL of blood in ethylenediaminetetraacetic acid (EDTA) vial or a small part of umbilical cord] from stillborn baby or dead neonate can be collected and stored for long time and the test done as per the family's convenience.

It is important to remember that the phenotypes of other disorders like Zellweger syndrome, other chromosomal abnormalities like duplication of part of q arm of chromosome 10 or p arm of chromosome 9 are similar to DS and need to be suspected if trisomy 21 is not detected.

Investigations to look for associated anomalies and disorders are discussed in the management section.

■ MANAGEMENT

Management of DS has multiple components including lifelong surveillance for complications, surgical management of malformations, supportive therapies, special education, employment opportunities, and efforts to incorporate them in the society in fruitful and fulfilling ways. Pediatricians should not only give the diagnosis, but has to become the central pillar to coordinate various modalities of evaluation and treatment. The surgical management of major malformations, occupational and physical therapies, and timely diagnosis of associated illnesses like hypothyroidism, celiac disease, and anemia has improved life expectancy of individuals with DS and hence, parents, pediatricians, and society have to make the best efforts to help the special individuals with one extra chromosome to lead happy, healthy, and useful life. Guidelines for health supervision of children with DS are available[10] and the pediatricians must take up the responsibility of management of these children. This is especially important, as there are hardly any special clinics for DS in India though the need for such special clinics at medical college level is strongly felt. Pediatricians also have responsibility to transfer the adolescent to adult care facilities and ensure that the transition is smooth. Providing emotional support and maintain positivity are very important to develop correct attitude in the parents who play a major role in deciding outcome of the child **(Box 16.1.2)**.

Box 16.1.2: Achievements of son shared by proud parents of a young man (Fig. 16.1.6) with Down syndrome.

- Special Olympics Bharat National Games (December 2005) in New Delhi—Gold medal in softball throw
- Special Olympics Asia-Pacific Regional Games (December 2013) at Newcastle, Australia—Silver medal in Aquatics
- Young Achiever's Award by Lucknow Management Association (LMA) in December 2014 in recognition of his exemplary bold and indomitable spirit—the first intellectually disabled person to receive such an award
- UP State Award for "Outstanding Role Model" in mental disability by "Viklang Jan Vikas Vibhag" of the Uttar Pradesh Government in 2014
- First District Yogasana Championship (September 2015) in Lucknow—second position among normally abled
- National Basketball Championship organized by SOB at Chennai in August 2016—fourth position
- Qualified Senior Secondary School Examination (12th class) of the National Institute of Open Schooling (NIOS) in April 2019
- National Floor Hockey Championship in November 2018—Gold medal for UP team

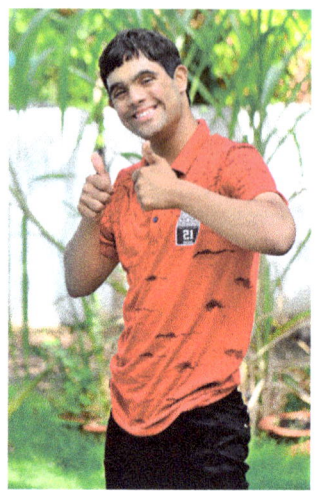

Fig. 16.1.6: Achiever who makes his parents feel proud of him.

TREATMENT OF MALFORMATIONS

Cardiac anomalies are present in 40–50% of children with DS and need urgent attention after birth. Immediately after birth, evaluation for life-threatening anomalies like tracheoesophageal anomalies, cardiac anomalies, gastrointestinal anomalies including anal atresia, etc. need to be looked for. If clinically stable, cardiac evaluation by echocardiogram and electrocardiogram can be done within first week to first month after birth. Even if there are no clinical findings suggestive of cardiac anomaly, each child should be evaluated by echocardiography. Surgical interventions are curative for the cardiac anomalies, gastrointestinal tract anomalies, and craniovertebral junction anomalies. They have a good outcome on the functioning of the organ. However, the family should be informed that the developmental delay and intellectual disability associated with DS does not have curative treatment. Surgical treatment of cardiac and other system anomalies is lifesaving and is very important to avoid sufferings of the child in later life. These include cleft lip, gastrointestinal malformations, and Hirschsprung disease.

NEURODEVELOPMENTAL PROBLEMS

During neonatal period and early infancy, it is difficult to understand the severity of intellectual disability in the figures of IQ. The realistic description about the outcome in simple understandable form is essential. Most of the children with DS learn to walk, talk, take care of self, and express and feel love and emotions. These children are mostly pleasant with happy demeanor, trainable, and can work and live under partially supervised setups. Better upbringing and training have shown that grown-up individuals with DS do very well in special Olympics, hospitality industry and make their parents feel proud of them (*see* **Fig. 16.1.6 and Box 16.1.2**). Evidence suggests that by late teenage years and early adulthood individuals with DS achieve an adequate level of autonomy in daily personal care and improve their independence skills outside the home.[11]

Evaluation for deafness during neonatal period and then at regular intervals is essential as untreated deafness will affect the development of speech as well as other fields. Hearing evaluation should be yearly as the children with DS are at increased risk of otitis media which may affect hearing. Same is true for congenital and later onset hypothyroidism and presymptomatic diagnosis and treatment are essential for good outcome. **Table 16.1.2** shows the simplified protocol for evaluation.[10] Frequent evaluation for behavioral problems, sleep apnea, swallowing study, etc. can be done as the need arises.

Table 16.1.2: Evaluation essential for a child with Down syndrome since birth.

Evaluation	Age	Remark
Evaluation for tracheoesophageal fistula, duodenal atresia, anal atresia, and cardiac anomaly	Day 1	Need urgent management
Karyotype and explaining the diagnosis	Birth to 1 month	As early as possible
Electrocardiogram (ECG) and echocardiography	Birth to 1 month	Immediate if clinical symptoms suggest the need
Eye examination for cataract	Birth to 1 month	–
Hearing evaluation	Birth to 1 month	After 6 months and then every 2 years
Congenital hypothyroidism	Days 3–7 along with other tests done for newborn screening	6 monthly in first year and then yearly
Ophthalmological evaluation for squint, refractive errors, etc.	6 months and then every 2 years	
Clinical evaluation for dentition, anemia, symptoms of celiac disease*, behavioral problems, gait abnormality, muscle weakness, upper motor neuron signs, and neck pain	Yearly	If signs and symptoms indicate, imaging for atlantoaxial dislocation needs to be done
Behavioral assessment, speech problems	Yearly	Evaluation and management by specialist may be needed

*Symptoms of celiac disease like constipation, nausea, diarrhea, and behavioral problems are seen in many, but biopsy proved celiac disease is seen in 1–6% of children.[12]

SURVEILLANCE FOR COMPLICATIONS

Table 16.1.2 shows the timeline for surveillance. Feeding difficulties, gastroesophageal reflux, and hypotonia may need special attention during infancy. Rare associations like atlantoaxial dislocation and risk of leukemia need not be mentioned to the parents. As evaluation by plain radiograph for atlantoaxial joint is not reliable, careful evaluation by history and examination should be done to look for spinal cord compression during every follow-up visit. Detailed neuroimaging may be needed, if there are any signs or symptoms or the child has to take part in contact sports and special Olympics. Dentition may be delayed, and parents can be assured for the concern. Risk of leukemia is 1%, but transient MDS is found in 10% of newborns. It usually resolves by 3 months, but can be fatal or preleukemic. Evaluation for hematological malignancies and *GATA1* mutations is not advised for all neonates and children with DS. Hypothyroidism is reported in 4–10% of cases. There is increased prevalence of other autoimmune disorders like alopecia areata and vitiligo. Hirschsprung disease is a known association and needs to be picked based on symptoms. Behavioral problems, speech problems, bowel habits, and dribbling of saliva may need guidance by a pediatric psychologist or a developmental pediatrician. As the child grows, anticipatory guidance about puberty, vocational education, and employment needs to be initiated.

SUPPORTIVE THERAPY

For special issues, each child may need management. Hypotonia is very common during infancy and developmental delay is universal. Social milestones are usually not markedly delayed and often the parents refuse to accept the delay during infancy as the child keeps on gaining milestones and delay may not be appreciable to the laypersons, especially those in stages of denial. Parents should be encouraged to enroll the child in early intervention program. It is useful to the child and also gives a meaning to the life to parents who wish from their heart to do contribute to the development of the child. The gain of milestones during physiotherapy gives positivity to the parents. Normal vaccination, admission to preschool with normal children, and encouragement to parents to treat the child like a normal child help to change the attitude of the family to the child. Supportive therapy includes assessment of the emotional status of parents and intrafamilial relationships. The continued involvement of the pediatrician comfortable with DS goes long way in family's acceptance and emotional adjustments. Discussions about the differently abled child and what to tell the family and friends should be initiated and the siblings and grandparents should be involved in that.

■ EDUCATION AND OCCUPATION

Like normal population, there is a great variability in the cognitive function of the children with trisomy 21. Presence of mosaicism does not mean that the IQ will be better. Continued follow-up of development and IQ estimation during childhood give some idea about the functional outcome during adulthood. Availability of special educators, opportunity to mix with other children, and changing attitude of parents and society in this era are reducing the gap between the lives of individual with DS and those without them. The right to education is fundamental as per our constitution and employment of teachers for students with special needs will go a long way in providing opportunities to children with DS and other neurodevelopmental disorders and appreciating their contribution to the society. Such school atmosphere is also good for the emotional growth and development of sense of responsibility for future citizens of the country. Schooling with normal children prepares the children with DS to integrate in the society as adults.

■ EXPERIMENTAL THERAPIES

Available options of occupational therapy, behavioral therapy, and special education are not curative. Though they bypass some components and train using available strengths, the disability cannot be completely eliminated. Trials using megavitamin therapy, piracetam, cholinesterase inhibitors, stem cell therapy, etc. have not provided evidence of their efficacy on improving cognitive function.[13] The counseling sessions should initiate the topic and scientifically correct and up-to-date information will satisfy the parents.

■ GENETIC COUNSELING

Counseling begins as soon as a neonate is seen with the face suggestive of DS. Extreme sensitivity, good communication, and positive and careful use of words are the requisite for the pediatrician to break the news. Emotional care of the parents is as essential as the parents who were expecting a perfectly normal baby and are seeing one. The laypersons cannot appreciate the facial phenotype and do not feel that anything is unusual about the child, if there are no structural malformations. For a pediatrician to be able to give positive but realistic scenario, he or she has to be aware of the improved facilities for training and the satisfactory outcome of the children with intellectual disabilities including DS. All parents go through the various stages of coping and acceptance, but many parents never forget the day and the way the diagnosis of DS was disclosed to them. Diagnosis of DS is easy, but disclosing it to the parents is difficult. Pediatrician needs to provide follow-up for medical care and helps in organization of supportive care facilities including connecting to the DS care facilities, medical genetics center, and parents' support group. The continued involvement of the pediatrician is an important aspect of the management. For a newborn or infant with DS after preliminary counseling, ordering chromosomal analysis and evaluation for associated treatable malformations and illnesses need immediate attention. Special mention needs for the babies with major malformation or serious life-threatening neonatal illness. A photograph and urgent chromosomal analysis are essential. If the neonate dies, the accurate diagnosis will be useful for genetic counseling regarding the risk of recurrence. If there is no access to karyotyping facilities, 1 or 2 mL of blood in EDTA vial stored at 4°C can be used later for confirming the diagnosis by QF-PCR.

The next part of genetic counseling is providing information regarding risk of recurrence during next pregnancy. It should be a part of initial counseling session even if the family may not think of next pregnancy now. The risk of recurrence is given in **Table 16.1.3**. It should be noted that the risk of recurrence in siblings in most of the cases is only 1%, but indicates the need of prenatal diagnosis. If one of the parents is a carrier of a balanced translocation, the risk of recurrence increases and depends on the carrier parent. Balanced translocation between both copies of chromosome 21 is a rare situation and will need other reproductive options like gamete donation to prevent a child with trisomy 21.

Table 16.1.3: Down syndrome due to translocation: Types, relative prevalence, and risk of Down syndrome in the offspring of the carriers of translocation.

Chromosomes involved in the translocation	Relative frequency among the cases with Down syndrome due to translocation	Prevalence of de novo* translocation	Prevalence of inherited translocation	Risk of Down syndrome in the offspring of a translocation carrier	
				Carrier mother	Carrier father
Dq21q [t(14;21) or others]	54.2%	55%	45%	10–15%	1–5%
21qGq t(21;21) t(21;22)	40.9%	96%	4%	– 100% 5–10%	– 100% 1–5%
21 with chromosomes other than G and D groups	4.9%	Few	Most	10–15%	1–5%

*The risk of recurrence of Down syndrome in the siblings of a case with *de novo* translocation or mosaic trisomy 21 is 1%.

Note: D—D group of chromosomes, i.e. 13, 14, or 15; G—Group of chromosomes, i.e. 21 or 22.

PRENATAL DIAGNOSIS AND POPULATION-BASED SCREENING

Prenatal diagnosis and population-based screening are the domains of the obstetricians and clinical geneticists. But being a part of genetic counseling and population-based screening being offered to all pregnant women, pediatricians can help in providing information required for the family to make informed decision. Prenatal diagnosis with the objective of terminating the pregnancy if the fetus has trisomy 21 and proactive management to help a child with DS may appear superficially contradictory to each other unless one appreciates different perspectives of the two entirely different situations. Every family wants a healthy normal child and option of prenatal diagnosis and termination of pregnancy, if the fetus has a serious disorder, is acceptable to most of the families and is legally possible before 20 weeks of gestation in India. The families who love their child and are taking the best care of the child with DS may opt for prenatal diagnosis and they need not feel guilty about it.

The other important scientific aspect about DS is an important part of history of medical genetics and that is population-based screening. Association of advanced maternal age with increased risk of a child with trisomy 21 was identified and prenatal screening based on maternal age using cutoff of 35 years was introduced in 1980s. This could detect 30% of fetuses with trisomy. Later, various biochemical markers were identified and currently first trimester double marker [free beta human chorionic gonadotropin (hCG) and pregnancy-associated plasma protein A (PAPP-A)] in maternal blood combined with ultrasonography for nuchal thickening (ultrasonographically measured subcutaneous thickness behind the neck of the fetus) or second trimester quadruple test identifies about 90% of fetuses with trisomy 21. The cut-off used for screen positivity is 1 in 250 and the false-positive rates are 5%. Quadruple test includes testing for alpha-fetoprotein (AFP), a protein made by the fetus, hCG, a hormone made by the placenta, estriol, a hormone made by the placenta and the baby's liver, and inhibin A, another hormone made by the placenta. This test using four biochemical markers done around 16 weeks of gestation is the cost-effective method and it includes AFP, which screens for neural tube defects which is five times more common than trisomy 21.

NONINVASIVE PRENATAL SCREENING

The latest development is detection of fetal aneuploidy by studying cell-free fetal DNA (cffDNA) in maternal plasma. This test has detection rate of 99% and minimizes the need of invasive testing for fetal karyotyping. Though the sensitivity of testing on cffDNA is very high, occasionally false-positive and false-negative results are reported. Hence, the test continues to be a screening test. At present, very high cost of test on cffDNA does not justify its use for population-based screening and its use needs to be limited to the high-risk pregnancies or the families wish to avoid for invasive testing.

The availability of various screening tests of different costs and with various detection rates makes choice of test difficult. Guidelines for screening test for DS in Indian setup are needed to make the protocol-based testing and this is discussed in Indian Journal of Medical Genetics.[14] An uptake of screening test, invasive test, and termination of fetus with trisomy 21 are personal decisions for the family and depend on many factors like the previous obstetric history, family history, and personal views and values. Therefore, appropriate pretest and posttest counseling in nondirective fashion is essential for the success of population-based screening program for trisomy 21. Equally important is to stress cost-effectiveness of such a program and needs to remember that many other genetic disorders of severe nature and disability need attention. Medical fraternity in India and all over world is trying to increase the detection rates for DS by screening methods at all costs; may be with the objective of eradicating the disorder. One has to ponder about it and there will be many people and doctor who do not feel it justified. Also, need to remind everyone that prevention of DS is an option and not a compulsion.

Taking a three-generation pedigree is the most important screening test to prevent birth of children with many other disabilities and disorders with poor outcome.

With facilities for management of medical issues in children with DS and opportunities to integrate in the society, individuals with DS are contributing to the society by leading happy and meaningful life **(Fig. 16.1.7)**. A small study on the coping strategies of parents of children with DS from India showed that

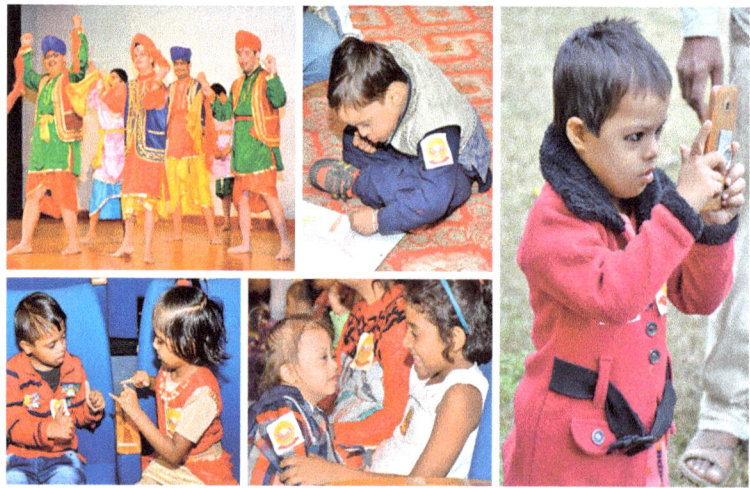

Fig. 16.1.7: Star performers, photographer, and the audience on a special children's day: Dreams come true.

both mother and father have good acceptance for the situation and have used refocus on planning.[15] It is the time that pediatricians feel positive about the outcome of children with DS and take care of the different issues proactively. There is great variability in IQ and capabilities of so-called "normal" people and the artificially created boundaries between "normal" and those with intellectual disability need to be wiped out. Efforts to integrate everyone in the society are needed. Pediatricians caring children with DS will play a major role by organizing the comprehensive care of these children with beautiful faces and minds, thus changing the views of society toward DS.

■ PEEPING INTO THE FUTURE

Shutting the function of genes on the extra copy of chromosome 21 can be the curative treatment of DS. Though far from clinical application, a study has provided proof of this concept in cell lines of trisomy 21.[16] Jiang et al. inserted a single gene, X-inactive specific transcript (*XIST*) (the X-inactivation gene), in chromosome 21 of a pluripotent stem cells derived from DS patient. *XIST* gene is normally present on X chromosome and is responsible for silencing of genes from one X chromosome in females. The XIST noncoding RNA coated chromosome 21 and triggered stable heterochromatin modifications, chromosome-wide transcriptional silencing, and DNA methylation to form a "chromosome 21 Barr body". The cells with one "lyonized" chromosome 21 showed that the expression of the genes on chromosome 21 (which are expressed 1.5 times in patients with trisomy 21) returned to normal level. When these stem cells were transformed to neurons, the rate of proliferation of the neurons was normal as compared to slow growing neurons with all three copies of chromosome 21 functioning. Successful trisomy silencing *in vitro* also surmounts the major first step toward potential development of "chromosome therapy".

■ CONCLUSION

Down syndrome being the commonest cause of intellectual disability, the pediatricians need to be conversant with the management of the children with DS and their families. In addition to scientific aspects of diagnosis and management an extra allowance of empathy, communication skills and positivity is needed in pediatricians taking care of children with DS. The involvement of pediatrician starts from the day of birth and sometimes on prenatal diagnosis of DS. There is a need of special clinics for DS children and adults at medical college and tertiary care hospitals to provide comprehensive care for DS. Pediatricians can be the in-charge coordinating supportive care facilities and providing regular surveillance as per protocol. As the facilities and approach of the society, government and schools towards individuals with different abilities and special needs are getting incorporated in the society and leading healthy, happy and fruitful lives. Pediatricians need to play a proactive role for children with DS. Everyone working with DS realises that the attempts to help the children with DS and their families brings peace to the mind and soul.

■ REFERENCES

1. Lejeune J, Gautier M, Turpin R. Study of somatic chromosomes from 9 mongoloid children. C R Hebd Seances Acad Sci. 1959;248(11):1721-2.
2. Mégarbané A, Ravel A, Mircher C, et al. The 50th anniversary of the discovery of trisomy 21: the past, present, and future of research and treatment of Down syndrome. Genet Med. 2009;11(9):611-6.
3. Verma IC, Anand NK, Kabra M, et al. Study of Malformations and Down Syndrome in India (SOMDI): Delhi Region. Indian J Hum Genet. 1998;4(2):84-7.
4. Pellegrini FP, Marinoni M, Frangione V, et al. Down syndrome, autoimmunity and T regulatory cells. Clin Exp Immunol. 2012;169(3):238-43.
5. Giménez-Barcons M, Casteràs A, Armengol Mdel P, et al. Autoimmune predisposition in Down syndrome may result from a partial central tolerance failure due to insufficient intrathymic expression of AIRE and peripheral antigens. J Immunol. 2014;193(8):3872-9.
6. Mateos MK, Barbaric D, Byatt SA, et al. Down syndrome and leukemia: insights into leukemogenesis and translational targets. Transl Pediatr. 2015;4(2):76-92.
7. Gupta R, Phadke S. Newborn with Down Syndrome: Care and Counseling. Genet Clin. 2011;4(2):7-9.
8. Radhakrishnan P, Nayak SS, Shukla A, et al. Facial profile and additional features in fetuses with trisomy 21. Clin Dysmorphol. 2018;27(4):126-9.
9. Girisha KM, Sharda SV, Phadke SR. Issues in counseling for Down syndrome. Indian Pediatr. 2007;44(2):131-3.
10. Bull MJ. Health supervision for children with Down syndrome. Pediatrics. 2011;128(2):393-406.
11. Rofail D, Froggatt D, de la Torre R, et al. Health-Related Quality of Life in Individuals with Down Syndrome: Results from a Non-Interventional Longitudinal Multi-National Study. Adv Ther. 2017;34(8):2058-69.
12. Bhat AS, Chaturvedi MK, Saini S, et al. Prevalence of celiac disease in Indian children with Down syndrome and its clinical and laboratory predictors. Indian J Pediatr. 2013;80(2):114-7.
13. Hart SJ, Visootsak J, Tamburri P, et al. Pharmacological interventions to improve cognition and adaptive functioning in Down syndrome: Strides to date. Am J Med Genet A. 2017;173(11):3029-41.
14. Phadke SR, Puri RD, Ranganath P. Prenatal screening for genetic disorders: suggested guidelines for the Indian Scenario. Indian J Med Res. 2017;146(6):689-99.
15. Gupta N, Sapra S, Kabra M. Coping strategies of parents of Down syndrome children in India. Indian J Pediatr. 2013;80(7):534-5.
16. Jiang J, Jing Y, Cost GJ, et al. Translating dosage compensation to trisomy 21. Nature. 2013;500(7462):296-300.

CHAPTER 17

ADOLESCENT MEDICINE

17.1 Suicide in Adolescents: Causes and Prevention
Swati Bhave, Anuradha Sovani

17.1 SUICIDE IN ADOLESCENTS: CAUSES AND PREVENTION

Swati Bhave, Anuradha Sovani

■ INTRODUCTION

Mental disorders account for a large proportion of the disease burden in young people in all societies. Most mental disorders begin during youth (12–24 years of age), although they are often first detected later in life. Poor mental health is strongly related to other health and development concerns in young people, notably lower educational achievements, substance abuse, violence, and poor reproductive and sexual health.[1]

Suicide occurs throughout the life span and is the second leading cause of global deaths between the ages of 15 years and 29 years. Suicide and suicidal patients represent a significant public health problem.[2] The rising incidence of depression in young people and lack of coping skills have contributed to the increasing number of suicides in the very young people.[3] Multiple dimensions whether biological, dynamic, or psychological affect suicide. Adolescents who are identified and treated for suicidal behavior continue to be at risk. They require a therapeutic alliance, and frequently our ability to bind psychosocial interventions and judicious hospitalization in addition to drug treatment.[4] A study in Denmark presents an interesting case in point, wherein concerted attempts have shown a decline in suicide rates.[5]

The occurrence of suicidal behavior can be divided into behaviors that are successful in ending life—*completed suicide*—and those that for one reason or another fail at ending life—*suicide attempts or parasuicides*. Suicides are always underreported and underdiagnosed as the cause of death or disability mainly because of the social and legal consequences.

In USA, the leading methods of suicide for the 15–19-year age group in 2013 were suffocation (43%), discharge of firearms (42%), poisoning (6%), and falling (3%).[6] The prominent methods that were most commonly used to commit suicide in India during 2015 included "hanging" (45.6%), consuming "poison" (27.9%), "self-immolation" (7.2%), and "drowning" (5.4%).[7,8] In another estimate from India, the leading cause of suicide in both men and women above the age of 15 years was poisoning, mostly from agricultural pesticides (chiefly organophosphates) resulting in about 92,000 deaths nationally.[9]

■ INDIAN SCENARIO

In the Indian culture, the family unit has both a positive and a negative impact on suicide. The family serves as a protective factor that provides a strong support for the individual, but alternately creates an inseparable individual when seeking mental health care, which often complicates the situation. Indian culture and mentality do not embrace the need of mental health professionals and care as openly as in the Western culture of today. There is a stigma attached and mental illness is perceived as shameful and hence going to quacks is preferred.

The allopathic medicines are perceived as very toxic and herbal remedies are preferred. Religion is integral to the Indian culture and hence mental illness is often portrayed as due to past or present sins, perceived as evil and a curse from black magic, etc., and most people seek help from *tantriks* or from religious leaders, and attend religious establishments prior to obtaining a mental health evaluation.

Causes of Suicides in India

Suicide risks were higher in educated versus illiterate adults. About half of the suicides were from poisoning, much of which was pesticide. At ages 15–29 years, suicide accounted for nearly as many deaths as traffic accidents in men and maternal deaths in women.[1]

About 3% of deaths at ages 15 years and older (2,684/95,335) were due to suicide. This corresponds to about 187,000 suicide deaths in India in 2010 at these ages (115,000 men and 72,000 women; age-standardized rates per 100,000 at ages 15 years and older of 26.3 for men and 17.5 for women). A 15-year-old in India had an approximate cumulative risk of 1.3% of dying before age 80 years by suicide; men had higher risk (1.7%) than women (1.0%), with especially high risks in South India (3.5% among men and 1.8% among women).[9]

"Family problems (other than marriage-related issues)" (34.0%) and "illness" (17.2%) have together accounted for 51.1% of total suicides in the country during the year 2015. The main causes for suicides below 18 years have been "family problems" (2,139), "failure in examination" (1,360), and "illness" (904).[7]

The number of suicides in the country during the decade (2005–2015) had recorded an increase of 17.3% (133,623 in 2015 from 113,914 in 2005). The increase in number of suicides was reported each year till 2011; thereafter, a declining trend has been noticed till 2014 and it again increased by 1.5% in 2015.[7]

During the year 2015, the share of "drowning" (from 5.6% in 2014 to 5.4% in 2015) and "coming under running vehicle/train" (from 2.6% in 2014 to 2.5% in 2015) as mode adopted by suicide victims has decreased while shares of "fire/self-immolation" (from 6.9% in 2014 to 7.2% in 2015), "hanging" (from 41.8% in 2014 to 45.6% in 2015), "by poison" (from 26.0% in 2014 to 27.9% in 2015), "by jumping from building or other sites of moving trains/vehicles" (from 1.1%

in 2014 to 1.8% in 2015), and "by touching an electric wire" (from 0.6% in 2014 to 0.7% in 2015) have increased during 2015 over 2014.[7]

The overall male:female ratio of suicide victims for the year 2015 was 68:32. However, the proportion of boys:girls suicide victims (below 18 years of age) was 47:53. The overall male:female ratio of suicide victims for the year 2015 was 68.5:31.5, showing a marginal increase of male and marginal decrease of female ratio as compared to the year 2014 (67.7:32.3).[7]

For suicide deaths at ages 15 years and older, 40% of male suicides and 56% of female suicides occurred at ages 15–29 years.[9]

LEGAL ASPECTS

Earlier, as per the law in India, attempted suicide was treated as a criminal offense and was considered punishable under IPC (Indian Penal Code) Section 309. Attempted suicide was decriminalized with the passage of the Mental Healthcare Bill. The Rajya Sabha passed the Bill on August 8, 2016, and the Lok Sabha on March 27, 2017.[10] Suicide attempters are recognized by the law as being under severe stress. In clinical practice, however, all patients at the risk of suicide are considered medicolegal cases; at the same time, healthcare practitioners must not stigmatize these patients or discriminate against them. They need to be handled with sensitivity and empathy.

VARIOUS THEORIES AND HYPOTHESIS OF ADOLESCENT SUICIDES

Dynamic Hypothesis

Researchers have made attempts to understand patients and their difficulties. One of the most important finding is of cognitive rigidity, with inability to revise expectations of the self, leading to hopelessness and suicidality.

Neurobiology

Neurobiology of suicide has been studied using peripheral tissues, such as platelets, lymphocytes, and cerebral spinal fluid obtained from suicidal patients or from the postmortem brains of suicide victims. They show an abnormality of serotoninergic mechanism, such as increased serotonin receptor subtypes and decreased serotonin metabolites, such as 5-hydroxyindoleacetic acid. These studies also suggest abnormalities of receptor-linked signaling mechanisms, such as phosphoinositide and adenylyl cyclase signaling mechanisms. Other biological systems that appear to be dysregulated in suicide are the hypothalamic-pituitary-adrenal (HPA) axis, and abnormalities of neurotropins and neurotropin receptors. More recently, several studies also indicate abnormalities of neuroimmune functions in suicide.[11]

■ IMPULSIVE SUICIDES IN CHILDREN AND ADOLESCENTS

Due to the high preponderance of the hypothalamic limbic system in the adolescent and poor control of the developing prefrontal cortex, adolescents are prone to impulsive high-risk behavior. Sudden impulsive suicides due to inability to cope with academic failures, romantic rejections, denial of screen gadgets, not getting permission to go for trips or picnics, and removal of mobile phones or screen gadgets as a punishment have all resulted in suicides by both children and adolescents as seen in newspaper reports. The main way to prevent such suicides is by increasing the coping skills of young people by World Health Organization (WHO) life skill education program for all teens and improving parenting skills through awareness and education. Suicide prevention awareness is very important in community and in educational institutes. Making everyone aware of suicide helplines is also very vital for suicide prevention.[12,13]

■ RISK FACTORS FOR SUICIDE IN ADOLESCENTS

There have been many studies to identify risk factors in adolescent suicide. However, it should be also kept in mind that not all adolescents with high risk factors will commit suicide and many suicides may not have documented risk factors.

Suicide affects young people from all races and socioeconomic groups, although some groups have higher rates than others. History taking is very important to elicit these factors because early intervention in adolescents with risk factors does reduce the incidence of suicide.[14] All the risk factors either singly or with their interplay increase the suicidal behavior.[15]

Risk factors and protective factors for suicide are summarized in **Table 17.1.1**.

Different Sexual Orientation

These adolescents have more than twice the rate of suicidal ideation.[16]

Male:Female Ratios

Global data and Indian data show that the percentage of completed suicides is higher in males, while attempted suicides may be higher in females.[17] Suicide is much more common in adolescent and young adult males than females (the ratio grows from 3:1 in the rare prepubertal suicides to approximately 5.5:1 in 15–24-year olds), but many of the risk factors are the same for both sexes. Suicide attempts are more common in girls than boys (approximately 1.6:1). Panic attacks are a risk factor for ideation or attempt in females, while aggressiveness increases the risk of suicidal ideation or attempt in males.[18]

Table 17.1.1: Suicide—risk and protective factors.

Risk factors for suicide	Protective factors for suicide
• A combination of individual, relationship, community, and societal factors contribute to the risk of suicide • Risk factors are those characteristics associated with suicide—they might not be direct causes	• Protective factors buffer individuals from suicidal thoughts and behavior. • To date, protective factors have not been studied as extensively or rigorously as risk factors • Identifying and understanding protective factors are, however, equally important as researching risk factors
• Family history of suicide • Family history of child maltreatment • Previous suicide attempt(s) • History of mental disorders, particularly clinical depression • History of alcohol and substance abuse • Feelings of hopelessness • Impulsive or aggressive tendencies • Cultural and religious beliefs (e.g. belief that suicide is noble resolution of a personal dilemma) • Local epidemics of suicide • Isolation—a feeling of being cut off from other people • Barriers to accessing mental health treatment • Loss (relational, social, work, or financial) • Physical illness • Easy access to lethal methods • Unwillingness to seek help because of the stigma attached to mental health and substance abuse disorders or to suicidal thoughts	• Effective clinical care for mental, physical, and substance abuse disorders • Easy access to a variety of clinical interventions and support for help seeking • Family and community support (connectedness) • Support from ongoing medical and mental healthcare relationships • Skills in problem-solving, conflict resolution, and nonviolent ways of handling disputes • Cultural and religious beliefs that discourage suicide and support instincts for self-preservation

Source: Centers for Disease Control and Prevention. Risk and protective factors. [online] Available from: https://www.cdc.gov/violenceprevention/suicide/riskprotectivefactors.html. [Last accessed December, 2019].

Past Attempts

These are one of the strongest predictors of suicidal behavior and suicide completion.[19] After an attempt, the risk of suicide remains high for more than a decade and the risk factors may change over a period of time.[20]

Adoption

History of adoption is also seen as a risk factor in some. The odds for reported suicide attempt are elevated in individuals who are adopted relative to those who are not adopted. The relationship between adoption status and suicide attempt is partially mediated by factors known to be associated with suicidal behavior. Continued study of the risk of suicide attempt in adopted offspring may inform the larger investigation of suicidality in all adolescents and young adults. The odds of a reported suicide attempt were ~4 times greater in adoptees compared with nonadoptees (odds ratio: 4.23). After adjustment for factors associated with suicidal behavior, the odds of reporting a suicide attempt were reduced but remained significantly elevated (odds ratio: 3.70).[21]

Guns and Firearms at Home

There are various reports on the impact of accessibility to gun arms kept at home—some showing impact and others not showing significant correlation.[22-24] In their nationally representative survey of US adults in households with children and/or teenagers, the authors found that gun prevalence and storage status did not differ by the presence of youth in the home with high-risk conditions. Firearms were present in ~42% of all households, and ownership prevalence did not differ between homes with or without youth at risk for self-harm.[25]

Bullying: Both Cyberbullying and Real Life

This is a high-risk factor for suicide attempts. Childhood bullying can have a long-term risk of suicide in adolescence.[26] In a long-term study, factors such as age, gender, history of abuse, history of bullying, type and time of bullying, and diagnoses were documented. While controlling for age, gender, grade, psychiatric diagnosis, and abuse, a history of bullying was the most significant predictor of suicidal ideation. Nearly 77% of the adolescents had experienced bullying, while 68.9% had suicide ideation at presentation. Individuals in this study who reported cyberbullying were 11.5 times more likely to have suicidal ideation documented on presentation, while individuals reporting verbal bullying were 8.4 times more likely.[27]

Impact of Media Exposure

Media exposure of suicide can have a major impact on young people and can result in imitation and cluster suicides.[28] A prospective study found increased suicidality with exposure to the suicide of a schoolmate.[15,29,30] Professional associations and the Government need to issue guidelines to press about the reporting on suicide by young persons. More than 50 research studies worldwide have found that certain types of news coverage can increase the likelihood of suicide in vulnerable individuals. The magnitude of the increase is related to the amount, duration, and prominence of coverage. Very detailed and graphic reporting of suicides, especially on the front page in newspapers, can increase clustering. Risk of additional suicides increases when the story explicitly describes the suicide method and uses dramatic/graphic headlines or images, and repeated/extensive coverage sensationalizes or glamorizes a death. Covering suicide carefully, even briefly, can change public misperceptions and correct myths, which can encourage those who are vulnerable or at risk to seek help. The National Institute of Mental Health (NIMH) suggests best practices for media and online reporting of deaths by suicide.[31]

Psychiatric Disorders and Substance Abuse

Such adolescents are at a high risk for suicidality.[32] Anxiety disorders, especially of severe variety and agitation, may be an important risk factor of acute suicide attempt. Substances of all variety are associated with risk of suicide. Psychosis in both mood disorder and schizophrenia can increase the risk. Adolescents with borderline traits have a high prevalence of suicidal ideations, impulsivity, and self-injurious behavior. These patients are at a risk for unexpected unintentional and accidental deaths. Substance can be used to control anxiety and agitation produced before attempting suicide. Substance can be used as a form of slow poisoning to kill oneself; here, most of the adolescents have comorbid depressive disorder. Mental illness and substance abuse in family members are also risk factors.[33,34] Sleep disturbances preceding suicide can also be a risk factor.[35]

Internet Use

Self-reported daily use of video games and internet exceeding 5 hours was strongly associated with higher levels of depression and suicidality (ideation and attempts) in adolescents.[36] Suicide-related searches were found to be associated with completed suicides among young adults.[37] Learning of another's suicide online may be another risk factor for youth.[38] Suicide attempts by susceptible individuals discussed on chat rooms and various forums appear to have been encouraged by such conversations.[39]

Websites and Games that Guide and Force Teens into Suicide

Prosuicide websites and online suicide pacts facilitate suicidal behavior, with adolescents and young adults at particular risk.[40] Browsing through websites that advocate suicide or describe methods in detail is a high risk for suicide attempts and suicide.[41,42]

Websites and games like "Blue Whale" are designed to systematically make adolescents progressively harm themselves and ultimately force them into suicide. The Blue Whale challenge is an online game. The game is named so because sometimes whales beach themselves intentionally and die. In this game, an online administrator assigns tasks to its participants. The participants are given a period of 50 days to complete each task. The players are expected to take photos of them undertaking the challenge and upload them as proofs for the curator's approval. The last challenge is to commit suicide. Players of this game cannot stop playing because they are blackmailed and cyberbullied into completing the game. This deadly game has spread all over the globe, and in India, there have been reports of children harming themselves and, in a few cases, even committing suicides, which are allegedly linked to Blue Whale Challenge. More than six children across India in the age group of 12–19 years have taken their lives allegedly playing this game within a span of 2 weeks.

Blue Whale is not a freely downloadable game, application, or software. Children cannot access it on their smartphones through app stores or on social media platforms such as Facebook. It is shared among secretive groups on social media networks. The creators seek out their players/victims and send them an invitation to join.[43,44]

■ DELIBERATE SELF-HARM

This involves intentional self-poisoning or self-injury, irrespective of the apparent purpose of the act. Deliberate self-harm in adolescents is associated with histories of broken home, family history of psychiatric disorder, and child abuse. An unsupported social environment for lesbian, gay, bisexual, and transgender adolescents, for example, increases the risk of suicide attempts.[16]

Various forms of deliberate self-harm are self-cutting; drug overdose, most commonly anxiolytics, analgesics, and multivitamin drugs; jumping from heights; or jumping in front of a running vehicle. Large proportion of deliberate self-harm is carried out impulsively in a way that invites discovery and may not be dangerous.

The distinction between suicide and deliberate self-harm is not absolute. There is an important overlap. Some people who had no intention of dying succumb to the effects of an overdose. Others who intend to die are revived. Moreover, many patients were ambivalent at the time, uncertain whether they wished to die or live.

Nonsuicidal Self-injury and Suicide Risk

The most common method of deliberate self-injury is laceration, usually of forearm or wrists. Superficial self-lacerations, which are not dangerous to life, are more common among young adolescents. They generally have severe personality problems characterized by low self-esteem, impulsive or aggressive behavior, unstable mood, difficulty in interpersonal relationships, and tendency to abuse alcohol and drugs. Usually, increased irritability and tension precede self-laceration and are then relived by it. Self-cutting in adolescents may not include a suicide wish and is practiced as it releases endorphins and relieves the distress in some emotionally disturbed adolescents. However, some studies do show that there is an increased risk of suicidal attempts and suicidal ideation. Pathologic internet use correlates with suicidal ideation and nonsuicidal self-injury (NSSI).[45-48]

■ PROTECTIVE FACTORS FOR PREVENTION OF SUICIDE

These include religious involvement and connection between the adolescent and parents, school, and peers.[49] Community and parental awareness along with awareness in teachers and peers is also a supportive factor. Good parent–adolescent bonding and a stable family are very important.[50,51]

■ PREVENTION OF SUICIDE

Identification and Prevention of Depression and Treatment of Severe Depression

Since the main aim of this chapter is prevention of suicide, we are not giving in-depth discussion on screening, management, and diagnosis of depression. But it is extremely important to know that depression is strongly associated with high risk of suicide, especially when it occurs as comorbidity in other mental illnesses.[52] Though many child and adolescent suicides are impulsive on-the-spot reactions to negative events in their life and their inability to cope, many adolescent suicides are also planned and are due to chronic depression. Hence, identification of red flag signs of depression and timely intervention to prevent it from becoming a chronic and/or severe depression are the need of the hour.[53]

It must be also remembered that adolescent depression may be missed as they can put a mask of happiness and pretend that they are very happy. In fact, parents are often surprised when we show them screening results that show depression. A complete physical examination and necessary tests should also be done to rule out medical conditions such as anemia, hypothyroidism, and neurological problems that can mimic depression.[54,55]

Antidepressant Medication Prescription and Increased Danger of Suicide in Adolescents

Serotonin receptors in the brain increase their activity in persons with major depression and suicidality, which explains why medications that desensitize or downregulate these receptors (such as the selective serotonin reuptake inhibitors or SSRIs) have been found effective in treating depression. Hence, it is important to give medications in severe depression in adolescents.[56]

However, adolescents, who are prescribed antidepressant medications, need to be carefully monitored. The United States Food and Drug

Administration (FDA) has required manufacturers to include a "black box" warning label on antidepressants that alerts healthcare providers and consumers to an increased risk of suicidal thinking and behavior in children and adolescents being treated with these medications.[57] This warning has prompted further discussion of the relative risks and benefits of use of antidepressants in children and adolescents. The Society for Adolescent Medicine (SAM) has issued a position statement to urge a balanced approach to the treatment of depression in adolescents, a serious and prevalent problem for this age group.[28]

Interventions for Prevention of Suicide

Intervention in public health or mental health domains is typically divided into the following:
- "Universal intervention" where one targets the population as a whole with the premise that all would be equally at risk.[58]
- "Selective intervention" where only certain subgroups are targeted and administered the intervention.
- "Indicated intervention" where the persons who are given the intervention are already showing signs of being affected by the problem at hand.[59]

Universal Intervention

Offering universal prevention, i.e. conducting school mental health programs or college-based interventions with suicide prevention as the central theme, works on the premise that adolescents have greater difficulty in expressing their internal stress.[60] They may not be as verbal and expressive about it as adults and may feel more stigmatized to reveal their emotional issues. Their depression or other emotional concerns may thus manifest as somatic symptoms, irritable mood, and poor academic performance.

Selective Intervention

The mental health professionals in touch with adolescents while conducting group sessions and in school or college workshops may do well to ask the question:

"Sometimes when young people are faced with stress or multiple problems, they wish that it would all end by putting an end to their life. Has it ever happened with you?"

- If the answer is "no," one can use positive reinforcement and try to ensure that things stay that way. The adolescent's coping can be strengthened, and they can be praised and encouraged to continue to face the challenges they have encountered in life.

- You can announce that if the answer is "yes," they can meet you or contact you after the session. One can check for a suicide plan and continue to manage the case. One can use tools for screening for suicidal thoughts.

Screening

In adolescent clinical practice, use of the home, education/employment, eating, activities, drugs and alcohol, suicide and depression, sexuality and safety (HEEADSSS) tool is very useful in identifying symptoms of depression.[61] Those adolescents who show signs and symptoms of depression are to be screened and assessed by various tools such as patient health questionnaires 2 (PHQ 2), PHQ 9, and Beck's Depression Inventory.[62-64]

Questionnaires for Assessing Suicide Behaviors

Suicide Behaviors Questionnaire Substance Abuse and Mental Health Services Administration, 2001

This screening tool assesses suicide-related thoughts and behaviors.[65]

ASK Q—Ask Suicide Screening Questions

The Ask Suicide-Screening Questions (ASQ) toolkit is a free resource for medical settings (emergency department, inpatient medical/surgical units, and outpatient clinics/primary care) that can help nurses or physicians successfully identify youth at risk for suicide.[66] The ASQ is a set of four screening questions that takes 20 seconds to administer. In an NIMH study, a "yes" response to one or more of the four questions identified 97% of youth (aged 10–21 years) at a risk for suicide. By enabling early identification and assessment of young patients at a high risk for suicide, the ASQ toolkit can play a key role in suicide prevention.

Columbia-Suicide Severity Rating Scale, 2008

The Columbia-Suicide Severity Rating Scale (C-SSRS) is a questionnaire used for suicide assessment.[67] It is available in 114 country-specific languages. Mental health training is not required to administer the C-SSRS. Various professionals can administer this scale, including physicians, nurses, psychologists, social workers, peer counselors, coordinators, research assistants, high school students, teachers, and clergy.

■ MANAGEMENT OF SUICIDAL BEHAVIOR

All adolescent stakeholders need to be conversant with identifying and managing suicidal behavior.[68-70]

Factors Facilitating Teen Suicide

- *Predisposition*: Mostly some mental health problem (e.g. depression)
- *Trigger*: Something happened that made adolescents feel unhappy, afraid, or angry, e.g. conflicts in relationship, exam failure, and disciplinary crisis.
- *Facilitator*: Under the influence of alcohol/drugs, ready plan (copycat suicide), and lack of religious inhibition.
- *Opportunity*: Access to the means of suicide, availability of the circumstances as planned.

How to Identify the High-Risk Adolescents

- There have been suicides in the family.
- The young person has attempted suicide previously.
- There are other comorbid psychiatric disorders (e.g. mood disorders such as depression, substance abuse, and internet addiction), impulsivity, and aggression.
- They have access to lethal means (e.g. firearms).
- They have experienced negative events (e.g. disciplinary crises and physical or sexual abuse) among others.

How to Ask?

It is not easy to ask patients about their suicidal ideas.[69] It is helpful to lead into the topic gradually. A sequence of useful questions is:
- Do you feel unhappy and helpless?
- Do you feel desperate?
- Do you feel unable to face each day?
- Do you feel life is a burden?
- Do you feel life is not worth living?
- Do you feel like committing suicide?

When to Ask?

It is important to ask these questions:
- After a rapport has been established.
- When the patient feels comfortable about expressing his or her feelings.
- When the patient is in the process of expressing negative feelings.

Further Questions

The process does not end with confirmation of the presence of suicidal ideas. It continues with further questions aimed at assessing the frequency and severity of the idea and the possibility of suicide. It is crucial for questions

not to be demanding or coercive, but to be asked in a warm way showing the physician's empathy with the patient. Such questions might include:
- Have you made any plans for ending your life?
- How are you planning to do it?
- Do you have in your possession pills/guns/other means?
- Have you considered when to do it?

If a patient has planned a method and is in possession of the means (e.g. pills) or if the proposed means are easily accessible, the suicide risk is higher.

Caution

Misleading or false improvement—when an agitated patient suddenly appears calm, he or she may have made the decision to commit suicide and hence feel calm after making the decision.

Denial—patients who have very serious intentions of killing themselves may deliberately deny such ideas.

How to Refer?

After deciding to refer a patient, the pediatrician should:
- Take the time to explain to the patient the reason for the referral
- Allay anxiety about stigma and about psychotropic medication
- Make clear that pharmacological and psychological therapies are effective
- Emphasize that referral does not mean "abandonment"
- Arrange an appointment with the psychiatrist
- Allocate a time for the patient after his or her appointment with the psychiatrist
- Ensure that the relationship with the patient continues.

Enlisting Support

The physician should assess the available support systems; identify a relative, friend, acquaintance, or other person who would be supportive to the patient; and solicit that person's help.

Steps in the Treatment of Suicidal Attempt

1. Management of associated mental illness
2. Following a proper discharge and follow-up protocol.

Acute Management of Suicidal Behavior

All the teens with suicidality should be referred to the psychiatrist.

Hospitalization

Indications for immediate hospitalization are as follows:
- Recurrent thoughts of suicide
- High level of intent to die in the immediate future (the next few hours or days)
- Agitation or panic
- Existence of a plan to use a violent and immediate method
- All who express a persistent wish to die or who have a clearly abnormal mental state.

Regardless of the apparent mildness of the patient's suicidal behavior, the clinician must obtain information from a third party.

How to Hospitalize the Patient?

- Do not leave the patient alone.
- Arrange for hospitalization.
- Arrange for transfer to the hospital by ambulance or the police.
- Inform the concerned authorities and family.

Inpatient treatment should continue until their mental state or level of suicidality has stabilized.

Contracting

Entering into a *"no suicide" contract* is a useful technique in suicide prevention.[69] Other people close to the patient can be included in negotiating the contract. The negotiation of the contract can promote discussion of various relevant issues. In the majority of instances, patients respect the promises they give to a physician. Contracting is appropriate only when patients have control over their actions. The value of "no-suicide contracts," in which the child or adolescent agrees not to engage in self-harming behavior and to tell an adult if he or she is having suicidal urges, is not known. The child or adolescent might not be in a mental state to accept or understand the contract and both family and clinician should know not to relax their vigilance just because a contract has been signed.

The clinician who has treated the suicidal child or adolescent during the days following an attempt should be available to the patient and family (e.g. receive and make phone calls outside of therapeutic hours) or have adequate coverage if away, by a physician having experience managing suicidal crises, and have support available for himself or herself.

Once a therapeutic alliance is established and the adolescent attends the first treatment sessions, he or she is more likely to continue treatment.

Psychotherapy

This is very important for treatment of mental disorders associated with suicidal behavior:
- Cognitive behavioral therapy (CBT)
- Interpersonal psychotherapy for adolescents (IPT-A)
- Dialectical behavioral therapy (DBT)
- Psychodynamic therapy
- Family therapy.

Psychopharmacology

- Lithium greatly reduces the rate of both suicides and suicide attempts in adults with bipolar disorder. Discontinuing lithium treatment in bipolar patients is associated with an increase in suicide morbidity and mortality.
- Selective serotonin reuptake inhibitors reduce suicidal ideation and suicide attempts. They are safe in children and adolescents. There have been some reports that SSRIs may have a disinhibiting effect (especially in patients with SSRI-induced akathisia) and increase suicidal ideation in a small number of adults not previously suicidal. However, it would be prudent to carefully monitor children and adolescents on SSRIs to ensure that new suicidal ideation or akathisia (movement disorder that makes it hard to stay still) is noted.
- Tricyclic antidepressants should not be prescribed for the suicidal child or adolescent as a first-line of treatment. They are potentially lethal, because of the small difference between therapeutic and toxic levels of the drug, and have not been proven effective in children or adolescents.
- Other medications that may increase disinhibition or impulsivity, such as the benzodiazepines and phenobarbital, should be prescribed with caution.
- Any and all medications prescribed to the suicidal child or adolescent must be carefully monitored by a third party, and any change of behavior or side effects must be reported.

Discharge and Follow-up

It is important to ensure that the adolescent will have adequate supervision and support over the next few days. A responsible adult should agree to "sanitize" the environment by securing or disposing of potentially lethal medications and firearms. The clinician should warn the adolescent (and the parents) about the dangerous disinhibiting effects of alcohol and other drugs.

Teens require support for longer than 2 or 3 months and the focus of the support should be providing hope, encouraging independence, and helping the patient to learn different ways of coping with life stressors.

GUIDELINES FOR SUICIDE PREVENTION

Many professional organizations have published guidelines on this subject.

The American Academy of Pediatrics (AAP) Guidelines

These are intended to assist pediatricians, in collaboration with other child and adolescent health care professionals, in the identification and management of the adolescent at risk for suicide.[70] Suicide risk can only be reduced, not eliminated, and risk factors provide no more than guidance. Nonetheless, care for suicidal adolescents may be improved with the pediatricians' knowledge, skill, and comfort with the topic, as well as ready access to appropriate community resources and mental health professionals.

The American Psychiatric Association (APA), 2003 Practice Guideline for the Treatment of Patients with Suicidal Behaviors

This practice guideline consists of three parts: Assessment, Treatment and Risk Management Recommendations, Background Information and Review of Available Evidence, and Future Research Needs.[71] A quick reference guide is also available.

The American Academy of Child and Adolescent Psychiatry (AACAP), 2001 Practice Parameter for the Assessment and Treatment of Children and Adolescents with Suicidal Behavior

These guidelines review what is known about the epidemiology, causes, management, and prevention of suicide and attempted suicide in young people. Detailed guidelines are provided concerning the assessment and emergency management of the children and adolescents who present with suicidal behavior. The guidelines also present suggestions on how clinicians can interface with the community.

Self-harm Guidance by National Institute for Health and Care Excellence, 2015

This resource by National Institute for Health and Care Excellence (NICE), which gives national guidance and advice to improve health and social care, provides guidance, guidelines, and advice for self-harm as well as useful pathways to care.

Indian Academy of Pediatrics

The Indian Academy of Pediatrics recently had a consultative meeting on August 16, 2019, to come out with guidelines for suicide prevention, which will soon be published.

Other Useful Websites

Self-Harm and Suicidal Behaviors Guidelines—Headspace from Australia

This list of authoritative guidelines provides evidence-based information about the practical treatment of self-harm and suicidal behaviors.

World Suicide Prevention Day

The World Suicide Prevention Day (WSPD) is an awareness day observed on September 10, every year, in order to provide worldwide commitment and action to prevent suicides, with various activities around the world since 2003. The International Association for Suicide Prevention (IASP) collaborates with the WHO and the World Federation for Mental Health (WFMH) to host WSPD.

SUMMARY

- Suicide is an unfortunate permanent solution to a temporary and in most cases a solvable problem.
- Mental illnesses are a major cause of adolescent suicides. All efforts must be made to increase awareness, establish screening, and early intervention to manage mental illnesses.
- The second cause is lack of resilience and copings skills—inability to control impulsive behavior, lack of resilience, not able to accept rejections, or failures.
- The third is lack of connectedness to parents, community, school, and peers. If we can establish connectedness through school and community programs, this will be a protective shield to prevent suicides.
- Increasing awareness about causes of suicide, warning signs, helplines, etc., in schools and colleges, and community will reduce the rising incidence of adolescent suicides.

REFERENCES

1. Patel V, Fisher AJ, Hetrick S, et al. Mental Health of young people a global public health challenge. Lancet. 2007;369(9569):1302-13.
2. World Health Organization. Suicide data. [online] Available from: https://www.who.int/mental_health/prevention/suicide/suicideprevent/en/. [Last accessed December, 2019].
3. Wagner KD, Brent DA. Depressive disorders and suicide in children and adolescents. In: Sadock BJ, Sadock VA, Ruiz P, (Eds). Kaplan and Sadock's Comprehensive Textbook of Psychiatry, 9th edition, Volume 2. Philadelphia: Lippincott Williams & Wilkins; 2009; p. 3652.

4. Shastri PC, Shastri JP. Adolescent suicide and suicide prevention. In: Bhave SY, Menon PSN, Parthasarathy A (Eds). Bhave's Text Book of Adolescent Medicine, 1st edition. New Delhi: Jaypee Brothers Medical Publishers; 2006.
5. Nordentoft M. Prevention of suicide and attempted suicide in Denmark. Epidemiological studies of suicide and intervention studies in selected risk groups. Dan Med Bull. 2007;54(4):306-69.
6. Levine DA; Committee on Adolescence. Office-based care for lesbian, gay, bisexual, transgender, and questioning youth. Pediatrics. 2013;132(1):e297-313.
7. National Crime Records Bureau. Ministry of Home Affairs. (2015). Accidental deaths and suicides in India. [online] Available from: http://ncrb.gov.in/StatPublications/ADSI/ADSI2015/adsi-2015-full-report.pdf. [Last accessed December, 2019].
8. Samuel D, Sher L. Suicidal behavior in Indian adolescents. Int J Adolesc Med Health. 2013;25(3):207-12.
9. Patel V, Ramasundarahettige C, Vijayakumar L, et al.; Million Death Study Collaborators. Suicide mortality in India: a nationally representative survey. Lancet. 2012;379(9834):2343-51.
10. Rao GP, Math SB, Raju MS, et al. Mental Health Care Bill, 2016: A boon or bane? Indian J Psychiatry. 2016;58(3):244-9.
11. Pandey GN. Biological basis of suicide and suicidal behavior. Bipolar Disord. 2013;15(5):524-41.
12. The Better India. (2017). 13 helplines that hear and help people struggling with depression and suicidal thoughts. [online] Available from: https://www.thebetterindia.com/94553/suicide-helplines-india/. [Last accessed December, 2019].
13. LBB. (2019). 5 suicide prevention helplines in india you need to know about. https://lbb.in/delhi/suicide-helplines-india/. [Last accessed December, 2019].
14. American Academy of Child and Adolescent Psychiatry. Practice parameter for the assessment and treatment of children and adolescents with suicidal behavior. J Am Acad Child Adolesc Psychiatry. 2001;40(7 Suppl):24S-51S.
15. Gould MS, Kleinman MH, Lake AM, et al. Newspaper coverage of suicide and initiation of suicide clusters in teenagers in the USA, 1988-96: a retrospective, population-based, case-control study. Lancet Psychiatry. 2014;1(1):34-43.
16. Hatzenbuehler ML. The social environment and suicide attempts in lesbian, gay, and bisexual youth. Pediatrics. 2011;127(5):896-903.
17. Our World in Data. (2017). Male-to-female ratio of suicide rates. [online] Available from: https://ourworldindata.org/grapher/male-female-ratio-of-suicide-rates. [Last accessed December, 2019].
18. Practice guideline for the assessment and treatment of patients with suicidal survivors. Am J Psychiatry. 2003;160(11 Suppl):1-60.
19. Bostwick JM, Pabbati C, Geske JR, et al. Suicide attempt as a risk factor for completed suicide: even more lethal than we knew. Am J Psychiatry. 2016;173(11):1094-100.
20. Centers for Disease Control and Prevention. Risk and protective factors. [online] Available from: https://www.cdc.gov/violenceprevention/suicide/riskprotectivefactors.html. [Last accessed December, 2019].

21. Keyes MA, Malone SM, Sharma A, et al. Risk of suicide attempt in adopted and nonadopted offspring. Pediatrics. 2013;132(4):639-46.
22. Brent DA, Perper JA, Allman CJ, et al. The presence and accessibility of firearms in the homes of adolescent suicides. A case-control study. JAMA. 1991;266(21): 2989-95.
23. American Academy of Pediatrics; Committee on Injury and Poison Prevention. Firearm injuries affecting the paediatric population. Pediatrics. 1992; 89(4 pt 2):788-90.
24. Grossman DC, Mueller BA, Riedy C, et al. Gun storage practices and risk of youth suicide and unintentional firearm injuries. JAMA. 2005;293(6):707-14.
25. Scott J, Azrael D, Miller M. Firearm storage in homes with children with self-harm risk factors. Pediatrics. 2018;141(3):pii: e20172600.
26. Brunstein Klomek A, Sourander A, Gould M. The association of suicide and bullying in childhood to young adulthood: a review of cross-sectional and longitudinal research findings. Can J Psychiatry. 2010;55(5):282-8.
27. Alavi N, Reshetukha T, Prost E, et al. Relationship between bullying and suicidal behaviour in youth presenting to the emergency department. J Can Acad Child Adolesc Psychiatry. 2017;26(2):70-7.
28. Gould MS, Greenberg T, Velting DM, et al. Youth suicide risk and preventive interventions: a review of the past 10 years. J Am Acad Child Adolesc Psychiatry. 2003;42(4):386-405.
29. Swanson SA, Colman I. Association between exposure to suicide and suicidality outcomes in youth. CMAJ. 2013;185(10):870-7.
30. Haw C, Hawton K, Niedzwiedz C, et al. Suicide clusters: a review of risk factors and mechanisms. Suicide Life Threat Behav. 2013;43(1):97-108.
31. National Institute of Mental Health. Recommendations for reporting on suicide. [online] Available from: www.nimh.nih.gov/health/topics/suicide-prevention/recommendations-for-reporting-on-suicide.shtml. [Last accessed December, 2019].
32. Kelleher I, Corcoran P, Keeley H, et al. Psychotic symptoms and population risk for suicide attempt: a prospective cohort study. JAMA Psychiatry. 2013;70(9): 940-8.
33. Asarnow JR, Porta G, Spirito A, et al. Suicide attempts and nonsuicidal self-injury in the treatment of resistant depression in adolescents: findings from the TORDIA trial. J Am Acad Child Adolesc Psychiatry. 2011;50(8):772-81.
34. VanWicklin JE. Adolescent depression: a systematic overview. J Psychol Christianity. 1990:9:5-14.
35. Goldstein TR, Bridge JA, Brent DA. Sleep disturbance preceding completed suicide in adolescents. J Consult Clin Psychol. 2008;76(1):84-91.
36. Messias E, Castro J, Saini A, et al. Sadness, suicide, and their association with video game and internet overuse among teens: results from the youth risk behavior survey 2007 and 2009. Suicide Life Threat Behav. 2011;41(3):307-15.
37. Katsumata Y, Matsumoto T, Kitani M, et al. Electronic media use and suicidal ideation in Japanese adolescents. Psychiatry Clin Neurosci. 2008;62(6):744-6.
38. Dunlop SM, More E, Romer D. Where do youth learn about suicides on the Internet, and what influence does this have on suicidal ideation? J Child Psychol Psychiatry. 2011;52(10):1073-80.

39. Becker K, Schmidt MH. Internet chat rooms and suicide. J Am Acad Child Adolesc Psychiatry. 2004;43(3):246-7.
40. Westerlund M, Hadlaczky G, Wasserman D. The representation of suicide on the Internet: implications for clinicians. J Med Internet Res. 2012;14(5):e122.
41. Becker K, Mayer M, Nagenborg M, et al. Parasuicide online: Can suicide websites trigger suicidal behaviour in predisposed adolescents? Nord J Psychiatry. 2004;58(2):111-4.
42. Hagihara A, Miyazaki S, Abe T. Internet suicide searches and the incidence of suicide in young people in Japan. Eur Arch Psychiatry Clin Neurosci. 2012;262(1):39-46.
43. UNICEF. What is the blue whale challenge and why should parents be concerned about this game? [online] Available from: http://www.unicef.in/STAYSAFEONLINE/Story-What-is-the-Blue-Whale-Challenge-and-why-should-parents-be-concerned-about-this-game-.html. [Last accessed December, 2019].
44. Express. (2017). Blue Whale Game - Suicide Challenge EXPLAINED, how many have died, has it come to the UK? [online] Available from: https://www.express.co.uk/life-style/science-technology/806384/Blue-Whale-Game-Suicide-Challenge-UK. [Last accessed December, 2019].
45. Wilkinson P. Nonsuicidal self-injury: a clear marker for suicide risk. J Am Acad Child Adolesc Psychiatry. 2011;50(8):741-3.
46. Durkee T, Hadlaczky G, Westerlund M, et al. Internet pathways in suicidality: a review of the evidence. Int J Environ Res Public Health. 2011;8(10):3938-52.
47. American Academy of Child and Adolescent Psychiatry. [online] Available from: www.aacap.org. [Last accessed December, 2019].
48. Walsh E, Eggert LL. Suicide risk and protective factors among youth experiencing school difficulties. Int J Ment Health Nurs. 2007;16(5):349-59.
49. Flouri E, Buchanan A. The protective role of parental involvement in adolescent suicide. Crisis. 2002;23(1):17-22.
50. American Psychiatric Association. Diagnostic and Statistical Manual of Mental Disorders (DSM-5). [online] Available from: https://www.psychiatry.org/psychiatrists/practice/dsm. [Last accessed December, 2019].
51. Nelson FL. Evaluation of a youth suicide prevention school program. Adolescence. 1987;22(88):813-25.
52. Cook MN, Peterson J, Sheldon C. Adolescent depression: an update and guide to clinical decision making. Psychiatry (Edgmont). 2009;6(9):17-31.
53. Son SE, Kirchner JT. Depression in children and adolescents. Am Fam Physician. 2000;62(10):2297-308.
54. HHS.gov. U.S. Department of Health and Human Services. What biological factors increase risk for suicide? [online] Available form: https://www.hhs.gov/answers/mental-health-and-substance-abuse/what-biological-factors-increase-risk-of-suicide/index.html. [Last accessed December, 2019].
55. FDA Public Health Advisory. (2004). Suicidality in children and adolescents being treated with antidepressant medications. [online] Available from: http://www.fda.gov/cder/drug/antidepressants/SSRIPHA200410.html. [Last accessed December, 2019].
56. Lock J, Walker LR, Rickert VI, et al. Suicidality in adolescents being treated with antidepressant medications and the black box label: Position paper of the Society for Adolescent Medicine. J Adolesc Health. 2005;36(1):92-3.

57. Centers for Disease Control and Prevention (2017). Preventing suicide: a technical package of policies, programs, and practices. [online] Available from: https://www.cdc.gov/violenceprevention/pdf/suicideTechnicalPackage.pdf. [Last accessed December, 2019].
58. Kalafat J, Elias MJ. An evaluation of a school-based suicide awareness intervention. Suicide Life Threat Behav. 1994;24(3);224-33.
59. Cohen E; Contemporary Pediatrics (1988). Getting into adolescent heads. [online] Available from: https://www.contemporarypediatrics.com/pediatrics/getting-adolescent-heads. [Last accessed December, 2019].
60. National HIV Curriculum. Patient Health Questionnaire-2 (PHQ-2). [online] Available from: https://www.hiv.uw.edu/page/mental-health-screening/phq-2. [Last accessed December, 2019].
61. Kroenke K, Spitzer RL, Williams JB. The PHQ-9: validity of a brief depression severity measure. J Gen Intern Med. 2001;16(9):606-13.
62. American Psychological Association. Beck Depression Inventory (BDI). Construct: Depressive symptoms. [online] Available from: https://www.apa.org/pi/about/publications/caregivers/practice-settings/assessment/tools/beck-depression. [Last accessed December, 2019].
63. Substance Abuse and Mental Health Services Administration. (2001). Suicide Behaviors Questionnaire (SBQ-R). [online] Available from: https://www.integration.samhsa.gov/images/res/SBQ.pdf. [Last accessed December, 2019].
64. National Institute of Mental Health. Ask Suicide-Screening Questions (ASQ) Toolkit. [online] Available from: https://www.nimh.nih.gov/research/research-conducted-at-nimh/asq-toolkit-materials/index.shtml. [Last accessed December, 2019].
65. General, Healthcare. The Columbia-Suicide Severity Rating Scale (C-SSRS)... Substance Abuse and Mental Health Service Administration. SAMHSA. 3. https://www.jointcommission.org › assets › Suicide_Prevention_Resources. [Last accessed December, 2019].
66. Zametkin AJ, Alter MR, Yemini T. Suicide in teenagers: assessment, management, and prevention. JAMA. 2001;286:3120-5.
67. Mental and Behavioural Disorders Department of Mental Health. World Health Organization (2000). Preventing Suicide: A Resource for General Physicians. [online] Available from: https://www.who.int/mental_health/media/en/56.pdf. [Last accessed December, 2019].
68. Shain B; Committee on Adolescence. Guidelines from the American Academy of Pediatrics. Suicide and Suicide Attempts in Adolescents. Pediatrics. 2016;138(1):pii: e20161420.
69. National Institute for Health and Care Excellence. (2013). Self-Harm. [online] Available at https://www.nice.org.uk/guidance/qs34/resources/selfharm-pdf-2098606243525. [Last accessed December, 2019].
70. Headspace for health professionals. [online] Available from: https://headspace.org.au/health-professionals/headspace-for-health-professionals/#guidelines. [Last accessed December, 2019].
71. International Association for Suicide Prevention. (2010). World Suicide Prevention Day - 10th September, 2010 - Activities. [online] Available from: https://www.iasp.info/wspd/pdf/2010_wspd_activities.pdf. [Last accessed December, 2019].

CHAPTER 18

INTENSIVE CARE

18.1 Acute Respiratory Distress Syndrome
Santosh T Soans, K Siddhanth Shetty

18.1 ACUTE RESPIRATORY DISTRESS SYNDROME

Santosh T Soans, K Siddhanth Shetty

■ INTRODUCTION

Recognition of acute respiratory distress syndrome (ARDS) since the first description in 1967 by Ash Baugh et al. in adults to the current day scenario has evolved to include children with more definitive guidelines and clear management strategies.[1]

Acute respiratory distress syndrome is considered as one of the most challenging clinical syndromes to manage for a clinician due to its heterogeneous etiology. Though they represent a small percentage of admissions in the pediatric intensive care unit (PICU), morbidity and mortality are still high in children.[1,2]

Acute respiratory distress syndrome is primarily caused by damage to alveolar epithelial-endothelial permeability barrier, thus resulting in pathobiological changes leading to the clinical hallmarks of ARDS, which include hypoxemia, increasing radiographic opacities, increased ventilation-perfusion mismatch, decreased functional residual capacity (FRC), increased physiologic dead space, and decreased lung compliance, which is now better termed in children as "pediatric acute respiratory distress syndrome (PARDS)".[1]

Mechanical ventilation (MV) is the cornerstone in the treatment of PARDS. There is great scope and need for further studies in treatment strategies for better outcomes in PARDS. These include (but are not limited to) ventilator modes, i.e. nonconventional ventilation including airway pressure release ventilation (APRV), high-frequency ventilation (HFV), and neutrally adjusted ventilation assist (NAVA), as well as ancillary strategies in fluid management, neuromuscular blocking agents (NMB), surfactant, steroids, and prevention of ventilator-induced lung injury (VILI).[1]

The use of newer modalities such as extracorporeal life support (ECLS) for refractory ARDS continues to increase, both in the adult and children. Despite decades of use, the optimal timing for cannulation remains uncertain and continues to be controversial.[1] The Pediatric Acute Lung Injury Consensus Conference (PALICC) reported a mortality rate for PARDS of 40% when the oxygenation index (OI) exceeds 16. Therefore, the key to optimal outcomes for severe PARDS is balancing risk and benefit to cannulate for ECLS for the right patient at the right time.[2]

■ DEFINITION

American–European Consensus Conference (AECC) definition in 1994 for acute lung injury (ALI) and ARDS was "acute onset of severe hypoxia, ratio of

the partial pressure of arterial oxygen (PaO_2) to the fraction of inspired oxygen (FiO_2) or P/F ratio < 300 for ALI and <200 for ARDS with bilateral opacities on chest radiograph in the absence of clinical evidence of left ventricular failure".[1] Then came the Berlin definition in 2012, which included several changes such as:
- P/F ratio-based severity grading—mild (200–300), moderate (100–200), and severe (<100)
- Use of positive end-expiratory pressure (PEEP) ≥ 5 cmH_2O with minimal settings
- Removal of pulmonary capillary wedge pressure.[2]

The second consensus conference held in 2015 by the PALICC group has given the current definition for PARDS, i.e. hypoxia in the presence of

Table 18.1.1: Pediatric acute respiratory syndrome (PARDS)—definition.

Age	Exclude patients with perinatal-related lung disease			
Timing	Within 7 days of known clinical insult			
Origin of edema	Respiratory failure not fully explained by cardiac failure or fluid overload			
Chest imaging	Chest imaging findings of new infiltrates consistent with acute pulmonary parenchymal disease			
Oxygenation	Noninvasive mechanical ventilation	Invasive mechanical ventilation		
	PARDS (no severity stratification)	Mild	Moderate	Severe
	Full face mask bi-level ventilation or CPAP ≥ H_2O P/F ratio ≤ 300 S/F ratio ≤ 264	4 ≤ OI ≤ 8 5 ≤ OS ≤ 7.5	8 ≤ OI ≤ 16 7.5 ≤ OSI ≤ 12.3	OI ≥ 16 OSI ≥ 12.3

Special populations:

Cyanotic heart disease	Standard criteria with an acute deterioration in oxygenation not explained by underlying cardiac disease
Chronic lung disease	Standard criteria with chest imaging consistent with new infiltrate and acute deterioration in oxygenation from baseline
Left ventricular dysfunction	Standard criteria with chest imaging changes and acute deterioration in oxygenation not fully explained by left ventricular dysfunction

(CPAP: continuous positive airway pressure)
Note:
OI = Oxygenation index = (FiO_2 × mean airway pressure × 100)/PaO_2
OSI = Oxygen saturation index = (FiO_2 × mean airway pressure × 100)/SpO_2
Wean FiO_2 to maintain SpO_2 ≤ 97% to calculate OSI or SF ratio (SpO_2/FiO_2 ratio)
Source: Pediatric Acute Lung Injury Consensus Conference Group. Pediatric acute respiratory distress syndrome: consensus recommendations from the Pediatric Acute Lung Injury Consensus Conference. Pediatr Crit Care Med. 2015;16(5):428-39.

Table 18.1.2: At-risk criteria for pediatric acute respiratory distress syndrome (PARDS).

Age: Exclude patients with perinatal-related lung disease	*Oxygenation*
Timing: Within 7 days of known clinical insult	Nasal mask CPAP or BiPAP $FiO_2 \geq 40\%$ to attain SpO_2 88–97%
Origin of edema: Respiratory failure not fully explained by cardiac failure or fluid overload	Oxygen via mask, nasal cannula, or high flow SpO_2 88–97% with oxygen supplementation at minimum flow:
Chest imaging: Chest imaging findings of new infiltrate(s) consistent with acute pulmonary parenchymal disease	• <1 year: 2 L/min • 1–5 years: 4 L/min • 5–10 years: 6 L/min • >10 years: 8 L/min Invasive mechanical ventilation
	Invasive mechanical ventilation Oxygen supplementation to maintain $SpO_2 \geq 88\%$ but OI < 4 or OSI < 5

(BiPAP: bi-level positive airway pressure; CPAP: continuous positive airway pressure; FiO_2: fraction of inspired oxygen; SpO_2: peripheral capillary oxygen saturation; OI: oxygenation index; OSI: oxygen saturation index)

Note: If PaO_2 is not available, wean FiO_2 to maintain $SpO_2 \leq 97\%$ to calculate OSI
Given lack of available data, for patients on an oxygen blender, flow for at-risk calculation = FiO_2 × flow rate (L/min) (e.g. 6 L/min flow at 0.35 FiO_2 = 2.1 L/min)

Source: Pediatric Acute Lung Injury Consensus Conference Group. Pediatric acute respiratory distress syndrome: consensus recommendations from the Pediatric Acute Lung Injury Consensus Conference. Pediatr Crit Care Med. 2015;16(5):428-39.

a new lung infiltrate occurring within 7 days of a known insult and severity of hypoxia being defined by oxygenation index (OI) [mean airway pressure (MAP × FiO_2/PaO_2] in positive pressure ventilation with PEEP ≥ 5 cmH_2O.

It also allows the use of pulse oximetry saturation to calculate peripheral capillary oxygen saturation (SpO_2)/FiO_2 (S/F) ratio when PaO_2 is not available. There is no age limit for PARDS, but the guidelines exclude perinatal-related lung diseases **(Table 18.1.1)**.[2] Those at risk for PARDS have also been defined **(Table 18.1.2)**.[2]

■ EPIDEMIOLOGY, RISK STRATIFICATION, AND MORTALITY

Pediatric acute respiratory distress syndrome accounts for 1–10% of PICU admissions with mortality rates as high as 60–70% with a declining trend in the last three decades due to better clinical guidelines and management strategies.[3]

The Pediatric Acute Respiratory Distress Syndrome Incidence and Epidemiology (PARDIE) study was the first to differentiate mortality risk by PARDS severity grading as defined by PALICC guidelines, showing a significant rise in mortality with increasing disease severity: 10–15% for mild or moderate PARDS versus 33% for severe PARDS.[4]

Also measuring OI at 6–12 hours and 24 hours after onset of PARDS was found to be more accurate in stratifying the degree of lung injury than prognostication at onset of disease.[5] The PARDIE study corroborated this finding, revealing that PARDS severity level at 6 hours was more predictive of mortality.[4]

There is high variability in mortality data in PARDS because of the heterogeneous etiology and comorbid conditions at the time of presentation. Although PARDS is defined and graded based on OI and oxygen saturation index (OSI), a large retrospective study reveals that neurologic failure and multiorgan dysfunction syndrome (MODS) were the primary causes of early and late deaths rather than refractory hypoxemia.[6]

In pediatric population, mortality rate ranges from 35% to 46% with mild-to-severe ARDS, which is quite lower than adult populations.[6] As mortality is still significant in the pediatric population, we need early identification, risk stratification, protocolled management, and further research for better outcome.

ETIOLOGY

Pediatric acute respiratory distress syndrome can occur due to direct or indirect injury to the lungs. The most common underlying condition for PARDS is viral respiratory infection. Also, it is associated with many different underlying clinical conditions including sepsis, trauma, burns, acute pancreatitis, aspiration, toxic inhalation, transfusion, and cardiopulmonary bypass surgery **(Table 18.1.3)**.[2,7]

Table 18.1.3: Causes of acute respiratory distress syndrome (ARDS).

Direct lung injury (Alveolar-epithelial)	Indirect lung injury (Alveolar-capillary)
• Pneumonia • Aspiration • Inhalation injury • Drowning • Pulmonary contusion	• Sepsis/Systemic inflammatory response syndrome • Major trauma • Pancreatitis • Severe burns • Massive transfusion or TRALI • Shock • Cardiopulmonary bypass • Head injury • Drug overdose

(TRALI: transfusion-related acute lung injury)

PATHOBIOLOGY

Alveolar Epithelial Injury and Dysfunction

There are two types of alveolar cells: type 1 and type 2 cells, which make up 90% and 10% of the alveolar surface area, respectively. Type 1 cells are large, flat, and thin cells and are the main site of gas exchange. Type 2 cells are responsible for surfactant production and ion transport; they also proliferate and differentiate to type I cells after injury and are also responsible for the removal of excess alveolar fluid through sodium-dependent intracellular transport **(Figs. 18.1.1A and B)**.[7,8]

The alveolar epithelium capillary structure has a large surface area for gas exchange and comprises the alveolar epithelium, capillary endothelium, and a thin layer of liquid coating the alveolar epithelium, which is required for gas exchange, protection against pathogens, dispersion of surfactant, and maintenance of aqueous and gas compartments.

Disruption of alveolar epithelium capillary structure leads to the accumulation of protein-rich fluid, proinflammatory mediators like interleukins (IL-1 and IL-8), tumor necrosis factor-α (TNF-α), and leukotriene B4, which lead to neutrophil recruitment into the alveoli resulting in surfactant degradation,[7,8] decreased FRC, increased dead space, reduced lung compliance, and impaired gas exchange leading to atelectasis and hypoxia **(Figs. 18.1.1A and B)**.[8]

Lung Endothelial Injury

Injury to the pulmonary endothelium is more commonly seen due to indirect lung injury than direct lung injury.[7] It causes activation of coagulation and inflammatory cascade leading to the release of endothelial-specific proteins such as von Willebrand (VW) factor, angiotensin-converting enzyme, and thrombomodulin, which are known to cause endothelial damage. Elevation of these proteins is also associated with MODS and higher mortality in children.[7,8] Disruption of endothelial barrier leads to sepsis in bacterial pneumonia by creating open interface between alveolar and circulating compartment.[9]

Inflammatory Dysfunction

Many human studies have demonstrated evidence of inflammatory dysfunction in ARDS and their relationship with outcome.[7,8,10] A multicenter study of inflammatory pathways in PARDS identified a strong relationship between mortality and elevated plasma levels of both proinflammatory IL-6, IL-8, IL-18, MIP-1b, TNF-α and anti-inflammatory cytokines IL-1RA, IL-10, and TNF-R2.[10] These cytokines were also noted to be associated with ARDS illness severity.[10,11]

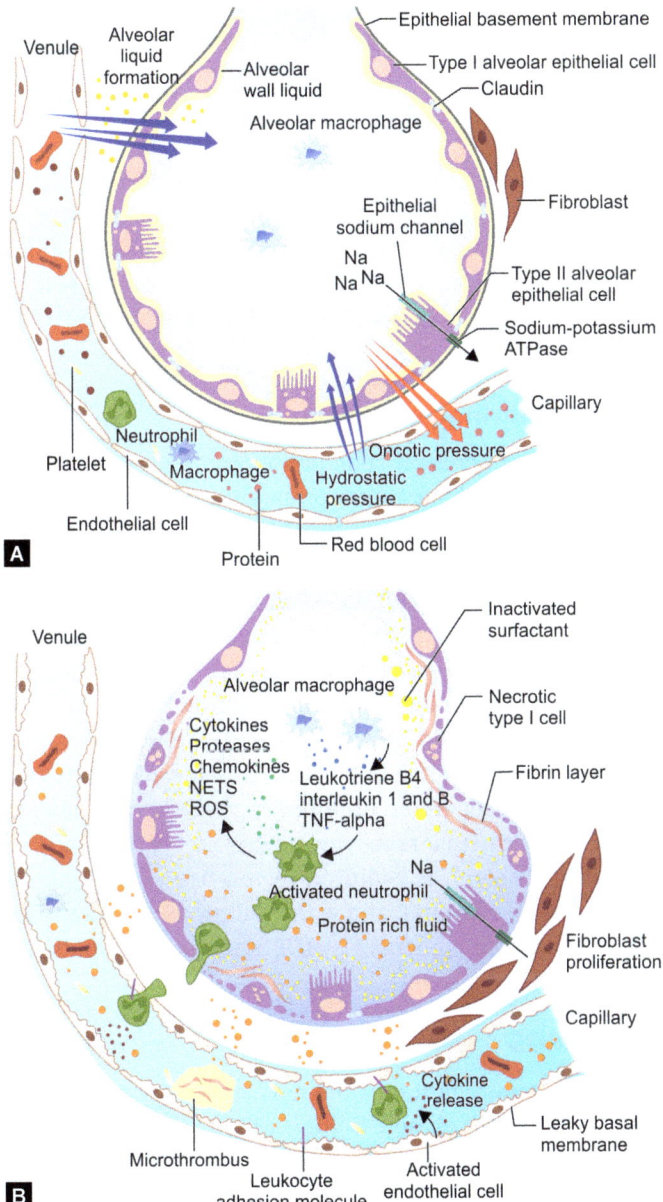

Figs. 18.1.1A and B: Schematic representation of alveolus in healthy children and in acute respiratory distress syndrome (ARDS).
(NETs: neutrophil extracellular traps; ROS: reactive oxygen species; TNF: tumor necrosis factor)
Source: Sapru A, Flori H, Quasney MW, et al.; Pediatric Acute Lung Injury Consensus Conference Group. Pathobiology of acute respiratory distress syndrome. Pediatr Crit Care Med. 2015;16(5 Suppl 1):S6-22.

Macrophages in the alveolar interstitium are primarily responsible for recruiting neutrophils and circulatory macrophages to the alveoli; these in turn cause endothelial injury by interacting with the vessel wall and platelets.[7]

Surfactant Dysfunction

Type 2 alveolar cells produce surfactant, which reduces the surface tension in air–water level. There are four important surfactants proteins—A, B, C, and D, of which B and C are mainly responsible for reducing surface tension; A and D play an important role in innate and adaptive immune responses.[8] Decrease or dysfunction in surfactant leads to low FRC and compliance leading to atelectasis and hypoxia.[7,8]

Thrombosis and Fibrinolysis Dysfunction

The imbalance caused between coagulation and fibrinolysis due to host response to infection and injury leads to microthrombosis and pulmonary vascular injury, which occur early in ARDS.[7] The pulmonary capillary endothelium provides the surface that integrates inflammatory pathways of the innate immune system with the coagulation cascade; the immediate response of endothelial cells to stimuli results in shifting from their normal antithrombotic and anti-inflammatory phenotype to an "activated" state of endothelial "dysfunction," characterized by prothrombotic and proadhesive properties, i.e. expression of adhesion molecules, tissue factor, and VWF factor, plasminogen activator inhibitor-1.[7,8,10] This alters the barrier function of alveolar capillaries, regulates pulmonary vascular permeability, and influences pulmonary vascular reactivity.[7]

Hence, further research is required in the use of therapies such as heparinoids, antiplatelet agents, and activated protein C as anticoagulant and profibrinolytic in the treatment of PARDS among select groups of patients with specific biomarkers or genetic profiles.[7,8,10]

Resolution of ARDS

Acute respiratory distress syndrome does not cause any long-lasting residual change in the lung such as change in lung structure or functions, as it can fully resolve. However, re-establishing the balance of proinflammatory and anti-inflammatory responses is key to prevent lung fibrosis. Repair of the epithelium occurs in a complex process, which consists of epithelial cell spreading, migration, proliferation, and differentiation. Scar tissue is formed during healing to preserve alveolar integrity and prevent further alveolar edema. The scar tissue is then removed by matrix metalloproteinases.[7]

It is also thought that multipotent mesenchymal stem cells may have a role in repair of lung alveoli. There is an ongoing phase 2 clinical trial to test the role of mesenchymal stem cells in ARDS in adults.[7,8]

In brief, ARDS occurs in three phases:
1. *Exudative phase*: This is characterized by tachypnea, hypoxemia, decreased lung compliance, and hypercarbia.
2. *Fibroproliferative phase*: There is chronic inflammation with scarring of the alveolar capillary unit causing an increase in the alveolar dead space and refractory pulmonary hypertension.
3. *Recovery phase*: There is restoration of the alveolar epithelial barrier, increased lung compliance, improvement in oxygenation, and eventual return to premorbid lung function (*see* **Fig. 18.1.1B**).[12]

■ MANAGEMENT

Targeted Therapy

Since ARDS is a clinical syndrome of impaired gas exchange, support of oxygenation and ventilation (i.e. noninvasive ventilation and invasive MV) are key in the management, although MV may worsen or even initiate lung injury/inflammation and has, thus, been identified as a risk factor for poor patient outcomes.[1,8]

The development of VILI has led to the concept of "lung-protective ventilation" strategies. Such an approach is based on two principles. The first is to avoid overdistension (i.e. volutrauma) and the other is to avoid or minimize the cyclic opening and closing of alveoli (i.e. atelectrauma).[13]

Recent advances in understanding VILI have thrown light into newer subtle form of lung injury such as ergotrauma (airway-driving pressure) and biotrauma that can induce or aggravate lung injury within the ambit of lung-protective ventilation.

Statistical analysis of clinical trials showed that driving pressure (Dp), as compared to tidal volume (VT) and PEEP, was best related to mortality. Dp is the difference between plateau pressure (Ppl) and PEEP. Static compliance (ability of lungs to stretch and expand) of the respiratory system (C_{RS}) is the quotient between VT and Dp. Therefore, Dp represents VT corrected for the patients C_{RS}. Thus using Dp as safety limit is a way of decreasing cyclic or dynamic strain, the lung parenchyma is subjected to during each ventilator cycle by adjusting VT and PEEP during MV accordingly to keep the Dp below 15 cmH$_2$O.[14]

> *Driving pressure (Dp) = Plateau pressure (Ppl) − PEEP*
> *Static compliance of respiratory system (C_{RS}) = VT ÷ (Ppl − PEEP) = VT ÷ Dp*
> *Dp = VT ÷ C_{RS}*

Biotrauma is the release of inflammatory mediators by various ventilator strategies that cause or worsen lung and other organ injury by cross-reactivity. Bronchoalveolar lavage (BAL) fluid and plasma concentrations of various proinflammatory cytokines as described in pathobiology were studied and it was observed that patients receiving lung-protective ventilation had comparatively lesser concentrations to traditional volumes and PEEP.[15]

In the following discussion, the authors review current and recent advances in management, citing relevant adult and pediatric studies along with the recently published PALICC recommendations.

■ OXYGENATION AND GAS EXCHANGE

High-flow Nasal Cannula and Noninvasive Ventilation

The use of noninvasive positive-pressure ventilation (NPPV) has increased over the last three decades and is an attractive strategy for children with impending respiratory failure. Noninvasive delivery of ventilation via mask or other interface can reduce atelectasis, and also ease out fatigued respiratory muscles while keeping the child's natural airway and airway clearance mechanisms intact. NPPV avoids some of the complications, which are associated with invasive therapies, as well as the need for sedation or muscle relaxation to facilitate these therapies.[8,16]

The indications for NPPV include the following:
- Select populations (immunodeficiency to avoid infective complication of MV)
- Mild-to-moderate ARDS
- Early in disease for at risk patients
- Postextubation respiratory support in severe ARDS.[16]

Patients Ventilator Interface

The outcomes of NPPV are attributed to a good patient ventilator interface. Appropriate fitting masks will improve tolerance of this therapy. Usually, facial or oronasal masks are advised, as they provide superior support over nasal and helmet interfaces in PARDS due to reduced air leaks and increased patient-ventilator synchrony.[16]

Heated humidifier is strongly recommended for NPPV in children. Children using NPPV should be closely monitored for potential problems, such as skin breakdown, conjunctivitis, and gastric distention.[16]

Modes of Noninvasive Ventilation

Pressure support ventilation with PEEP is strongly recommended, as it improves oxygenation and decreases muscle fatigue in patients with PARDS. In case of patient-ventilator asynchrony, HFNC or continuous positive airway pressure (CPAP) may be used. Physiologic and clinical experience suggests the use of bi-level positive airway pressure, which is superior to CPAP.[16]

Identification of NPPV Failure

Severe hypoxemia on NPPV indicates failure (gas exchange alterations within the 1st hour). Factors that indicate worsening are:
- Increased respiratory rate
- Increased oxygen requirement
- Decrease in PaO_2/FiO_2 ratio, an increased $PaCO_2$
- Altered level of consciousness.

Any worsening change in the above parameters warrants intubation and ventilation.

Sedation should be used with caution in children receiving NPPV for PARDS. Although sedation can sometimes facilitate tolerance of this therapy, it can also depress the respiratory efforts and level of consciousness leading to difficulty in assessment of NPPV failure.[17]

Invasive Ventilation

The mainstay of invasive ventilation is to balance adequate gas exchange and oxygenation with prevention of VILI.[8,15] In a landmark study on lung-protective ventilation, the ARDS Network found a decrease in mortality with lower tidal volume ventilation (6 mL/kg of predicted body weight) when compared with conventional ventilation volumes at that time (12 mL/kg of predicted body weight).[18]

There is no strong evidence for most of the recommendations described in this section because of limited studies in the pediatric population and most studies are largely based on the experience in the adult population for patients with ARDS with consensus-based modifications for children.[2,8,17,19]

Intubation

Physiological Difficult Airway

In a critically ill child, airway management involves identification of any untoward complications due to underlying physiological derangements, which might potentially lead to cardiovascular collapse during airway management.

Hypoxemia, hypotension, metabolic acidosis, and right ventricular (RV) failure are clinically important physiological parameters, which are deranged in critically ill child and hence anticipated as difficult airway during intubation.

Hypoxemia: Preoxygenation in children having ARDS is important, as they are primarily hypoxic during intubation. The goal in preoxygenation should be—(1) maximum hemoglobin saturation and (2) maximal PaO_2. Current methods of preoxygenation include the use of nonrebreathing mask and NPPV, although there is a risk of derecruitment while removing mask for tube placement. HFNC for preoxygenation has shown to have benefits in terms of tolerance, oxygenation, and ease of tube placement.

Hypotension: Hypotension is a major risk factor for adverse events including cardiopulmonary arrest related to airway management in ARDS. Common causes of hypotension/shock are sepsis, capillary leak, volume depletion, positive pressure ventilation-induced hypotension, and vasodilatory effects of sedation. Management with fluid resuscitation for volume responders, vasoconstrictors such as phenylephrine for sedation-induced transient drop, and inotropes for septic shock is suggested prior to intubation.

Severe acidosis: Respiratory acidosis is usually corrected easily by interventions that increase the alveolar ventilation such as bag–valve mask ventilation, NPPV, or MV. When acidemia develops from metabolic acidosis, maintenance of acid–base homeostasis depends on a compensatory respiratory alkalosis from alveolar hyperventilation. In the event that patients with severe acidemia require intubation, even a brief apneic period can lead to a precipitous drop in pH given the loss of the already inadequate respiratory compensation leading to hemodynamic deterioration after intubation. Management includes maintaining spontaneous respiration while intubating, short trial of NPPV, postintubation choosing a ventilator mode that allows the patient to set and maintain their own minute ventilation in order to best maintain their respiratory compensation such as pressure-controlled mode and helps to avoid sudden cardiovascular collapse.

Right ventricular failure: In severe PARDS, RV failure occurs because the intrathoracic pressure is transmitted to the alveolar capillary bed, leading to collapse of these small vessels and increases the pulmonary vascular resistance against which the RV must pump leading to RV dilation, retrograde flow, decreased coronary perfusion, and ultimately systemic hypotension and cardiovascular collapse. Management includes bedside echo for RV function, use of low-dose norepinephrine, preoxygenation, and inhaled nitric oxide (iNO) via nasal cannula, if available.[20]

Selection of Endotracheal Tube

Cuffed endotracheal (ET) tube is preferred to uncuffed. The advantages include that it avoids leak, prevents aspiration, and controls overventilation. The disadvantages are mucosal injury and tracheal stenosis. Maintaining cuff pressure between 20 cmH_2O and 25 cmH_2O allowing 20% leak helps to alleviate these problems.[2,17]

Modes of Ventilation

The recent consensus conference was unable to recommend, if any mode of ventilation was superior to the other, due to the limited data available in the pediatric population.[2]

Tidal Volume

There is strong recommendation by consensus conference for the use of predicted body weight (PBW) in determining the VT.[2] Two recent studies have shown increased mortality with increased VT, although the study did not show any change in ventilator-free days or mortality in children older than 1 year.[21]

The current recommendation for an invasively ventilated child states that the delivered VT should be in or below the range of physiologic VT for age/body weight (i.e. 5-8 mL/kg predicted body weight) according to lung pathology and respiratory system compliance.[2,8,19,21] Patient-specific tidal volumes are to be used according to disease severity. Tidal volumes should be 3-6 mL/kg for PBW for patients with poor respiratory system compliance and closer to the physiologic range (5-8 mL/kg ideal body weight) for patients with better preserved respiratory system compliance.[2,8,9,22]

Peak Pressures and Plateau Pressure

Limiting the plateau pressure to 28 cmH_2O and allowing a slightly higher plateau pressure of 29-30 cmH_2O in poor chest wall compliance (chest wall edema/deformity, abdominal compartment syndrome) is recommended in clinical practice to reduce VILI,[2] as high-peak pressures have been associated with increased mortality.[21,22]

Positive End-expiratory Pressure

Positive end-expiratory pressure titration is done for better oxygenation, lung recruitment, and to avoid collapse of alveoli at the end of expiration thus preventing atelectrauma, also known as open lung concept.

Optimization of PEEP

- Mild-to-moderate PARDS 7-8 cmH_2O
- Severe PARDS 10-15 cmH_2O, although higher PEEP has been tried.
- However, the target plateau pressure should be kept in mind while titrating PEEP
- Recruitment maneuvers:
  - Slow incremental and decremental PEEP in an attempt to improve severe oxygenation failure.[2,8,15,17]
  - *PEEP titration method*: Incremental PEEP titration—increase PEEP by 2 cmH_2O every 5 minutes, check for response (i.e. saturation, P_{peak}, P_{plat}, hemodynamics, and dynamic compliance), and titration is done till the above parameters are either improving or have been stable during the recruitment maneuver (optimal PEEP). Stop the maneuver, if any of the above parameters worsens. Decremental PEEP titration is another method that has been tried (i.e. starting with higher

PEEP and gradually decreasing by 2 cm) with targets as described previously.[2,8,17,19,23]
- Recruitment also depends on the type of lung disease (e.g. diffuse alveolar disease vs pneumonia-like alveolar consolidations), time course (e.g. early vs. late PARDS), and mechanics of the respiratory system (e.g. pulmonary compliance). In general, patients with predominantly increased lung elastance (i.e. decreased lung compliance) show less positive response to recruitment maneuvers than patients with increased chest wall elastance (i.e. decreased chest wall compliance).[17]

Gas Exchange Goals

The key to gas exchange is to balance between risk and benefit of ventilatory support in PARDS.

Permissive Hypoxia

For mild PARDS with PEEP $\leq$ 10 cmH$_2$O, the SpO$_2$ goal should generally be 92–97%. For those with more severe PARDS with PEEP $\geq$ 10 cmH$_2$O, the recommended SpO$_2$ of 88–92% should be considered after PEEP has been optimized.[2] FiO$_2$ should be reduced to best tolerated minimum level to avoid biotrauma.[24,25]

The short- and long-term end-organ effect of these strategies has not been well described. Hence, clinicians should be cautious while applying this strategy and keep a close watch for tissue/organ oxygenation (when SpO$_2$ is < 92%), monitor cerebral oxygenation and oxygen delivery, lactate, and central venous saturation while balancing VILI and hypoxemia/oxygen toxicity.[2,24,25]

Permissive Hypercapnia

This is a strategy primarily aimed at minimizing VILI in patients with moderate-to-severe PARDS. A pH range of 7.15–7.30 with PCO$_2$ of up to 80 mmHg is tolerated while using lung-protective ventilation (low VT and optimal PEEP). Contraindications to this include pulmonary hypertension, intracranial hypertension, congenital heart lesions, and cardiac dysfunction with hemodynamic instability.[2,8,17,19]

■ NONCONVENTIONAL VENTILATION

Different forms of nonconventional ventilation are used in children with PARDS, particularly in those with severe disease/refractory hypoxia of which high-frequency oscillatory ventilation (HFOV) and APRV will be discussed here.

High-frequency Ventilation

High-frequency ventilation is defined by high-respiratory rate (>120 bpm for adults and >150 bpm for infants and children) and delivered tidal volume that is less than anatomic dead space ventilation.[17,19] The various modes of HFV are HFOV, high-frequency jet ventilation (HFJV), high-frequency percussive ventilation (HFPV), and tracheal gas insufflation.[26] In this section, we will discuss about HFOV.

High-frequency Oscillatory Ventilation

High-frequency oscillatory ventilation provides lung-protective ventilation strategy by preventing atelectrauma and maintaining airway recruitment via a constantly applied airway pressure and preventing volutrauma by avoiding alveolar overdistension via the delivery of tidal volume less than anatomic dead space. Mean airway pressure is decreased minimizing barotrauma and better gas exchange is achieved due to gas molecules consistently agitated inside the airway due to the oscillatory mechanism.[26-28]

Recruitment in HFOV is done by increasing or decreasing the mean airway pressure (P_{aw}) in a stepwise manner while monitoring CO_2 and O_2. HFOV can also be used in air leak and secretion-induced lung collapse. Allow peritubal air leak in HFOV, provided P_{aw} could be maintained. Drawbacks include less effective exhalation, increased need for sedation.[27,28]

The OSCAR trial showed significant change in 30-day mortality between HFOV and control group,[25] although in the OSCILLATE study, interestingly an increased mortality was seen with HFOV as compared with the lung-protective conventional ventilation group. Also, larger subset of HFOV subjects required inotropic support as compared with the conventional ventilation group.[28]

Indications: PALICC guidelines suggest HFOV as an alternative ventilatory mode for those patients with moderate-to-severe PARDS in whom plateau airway pressures exceed 28 cmH_2O in the absence of clinical evidence of reduced chest-wall compliance.[2,27,28]

Airway Pressure Release Ventilation

Airway pressure release ventilation allows for spontaneous breathing, it is a pressure-limited, time-triggered, and time-cycled mode that maintains an elevated baseline pressure (*P*-high) with deflations or "releases" of gas to a lower pressure setting (*P*-low). The adult study has shown the possibility of using lower inspiratory plateau pressures for a given tidal volume when compared with volume ventilation as well as decreased sedation requirements.[29]

Alternative modes of unconventional ventilation such as APRV and HFJV or HFOV have some theoretical advantages for patients with moderate-to-severe ARDS, but there is no pediatric data available showing any superiority when compared to conventional modes of ventilation in children with PARDS.[17] Physiological and theoretical basis of using HFOV and APRV in PARDS sounds right but lack of strong evidence has discouraged clinicians from using these alternative modes.

■ PULMONARY ANCILLARY STRATEGIES

Exogenous Surfactant

Surfactant deficiency occurs due to direct lung injury in PARDS. Since the pathological changes in ARDS are similar to those seen in neonatal RDS, the rationale in the use of exogenous surfactant replacement therapy in PARDS was studied.[30]

A lot of interest was generated for the pediatric population as well, although they have shown no benefit in outcomes, further studies on dosing, time, and delivery approaches have to be undertaken.[31] However, currently, there is no recommendation that surfactant therapy be used as routine therapy for those with PARDS.[2,31]

Inhaled Nitric Oxide

Nitric oxide increases the cyclic guanosine monophosphate (cGMP), which relaxes the smooth muscles and thereby causes pulmonary vasodilation. This shunts the blood to the well-ventilated areas of the lungs from the poorly ventilated areas and reduces dead space ventilation and ventilation/perfusion mismatch.

Inhaled nitric oxide in the range of 5–40 ppm has been used with clinical improvement in PaO_2 allowing space for FiO_2 reduction in severe PARDS. Randomized control trials (RCTs) have demonstrated an oxygenation benefit with iNO in PARDS.[32]

Routine use of iNO is not recommended unless pulmonary hypertension or severe right ventricular dysfunction is documented or in severe cases of PARDS as a rescue bridge to ECLS.[2,17,19,23,31]

Prone Positioning

Prone positioning helps in improving oxygenation in ARDS by recruiting lower lobe atelectasis, decreasing ventilation perfusion (V/Q) mismatch, decreasing dead space ventilation, and maintaining open lung units thereby helping to improve P/F ratio and OI.[33] Two landmark studies done in adult and pediatric populations showed conflicting results on prone ventilation strategies.[32,24] In our practice, we follow 16 hours prone plus 8 hours supine using log roll technique and giving daily routine care during supine position.[34] PALICC recommends that it should be considered an option in cases of severe PARDS.[31]

Tracheal Suctioning

Maintaining airway patency is vital for any ventilated patient. There is a strong recommendation for maintaining a clear airway; however, clinicians must be cautious while suctioning, as there is a possibility of decruitment post-suctioning. There are no guidelines favoring the use of close (in-line) over open suction methods. Routine instillation of saline for suction is not recommended. It can be used to remove thick secretions.[31]

Extracorporeal Life Support

Extracorporeal membrane oxygenation (ECMO), also known as heart lung machine, is a modified cardiopulmonary bypass machine **(Fig. 18.1.2)**. In the next step of management of moderate-to-severe PARDS, ECMO has emerged as a lifesaving therapy. ECMO allows the injured lungs to rest and recover and helps to limit the volutrauma, barotrauma, and oxygen toxicity associated with MV.[35-38] The international Extracorporeal Life Support Organization (ELSO) registry contains data on nearly 98,000 patients supported with ECMO as of January, 2018 (www.ELSO.org). Over the last decade, there has been an exponential growth of ECMO utilization in children with severe respiratory failure.[37,39,40]

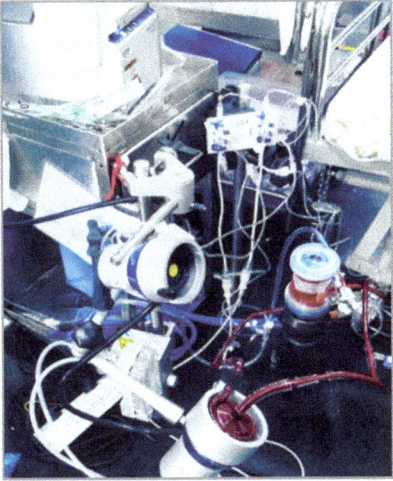

Fig. 18.1.2: Extracorporeal membrane oxygenation (ECMO) on flow in pediatric intensive care unit (PICU).

The ECMO initiation is of two modes:
1. *Venovenous (VV) ECMO:* It can replace the gas exchange functions of the native lung during the period ECMO support. Blood is both withdrawn and returned to the patient's venous circulation. It requires adequate pumping of the native heart.
2. *Venoarterial (VA) ECMO:* It can provide both respiratory gas exchange as well as circulatory support during the period of ECMO support. Blood is withdrawn from the venous circulation and returned to the arterial circulation of the patient.[30,36,37,39]

The PALICC guidelines suggest that ECMO should be considered in severe PARDS when toxic support is needed to maintain gas exchange.[36] However, ECMO should only be considered after demonstrating deteriorating trends and if the disease process is likely reversible or if lung transplant is considered.[38] Serial evaluation for ECMO eligibility should be done rather than a single point assessment.

Indications (Table 18.1.4)

- Severe respiratory failure as evidenced by sustained PaO_2/FiO_2 ratios <60–80 or OI > 40

Table 18.1.4: Indications and contraindications for extracorporeal membrane oxygenation (ECMO).

Indications	Relative contraindications	Contraindications
• PaO_2-FiO_2 ratio: <60–80 • Oxygen Index >40 • Mean airway pressure >20–25 on conventional ventilation or >30 on HFOV • Evidence of iatrogenic barotrauma • Acute unremitting hypercapnic or hypoxic respiratory failure • Air leak syndrome • Mediastinal masses • Pulmonary embolism • Cardiac failure • Cardiac arrest	• Duration of pre-ECLS mechanical ventilation >14 d • Recent neurosurgical procedures or intracranial hemorrhage (<7 d) • Pre-existing chronic illness with poor long-term prognosis • Allogeneic bone marrow transplant recipients • Solid organ tumors	• Lethal chromosomal abnormalities (Trisomy 13 or 18) • Severe neurologic compromise (intracranial hemorrhage with mass effect) • Incurable malignancy

(ECLS: extracorporeal life support; HFOV: high-frequency oscillatory ventilation; PaO_2-FiO_2: partial pressure of oxygen dissolved in blood-fractional inspired oxygen)
Source: Graeme M, Steve C, Giles P. (2015). Indications for paediatric respiratory extracorporeal life support. International Summary, Ann Arbor, March 2015. [online] Available from https://www.elso.org/Portals/0/Files/ELSO%20guidelines%20paeds%20resp_May2015.pdf. [Last accessed December, 2019].

- Poor response to conventional MV ± other forms of rescue therapy, e.g. HFOV, iNO, and prone positioning
- Elevated mean airway pressure >20–25 cm on conventional ventilation, >30 cm on HFOV
- Evidence of iatrogenic barotrauma
- Extracorporeal CO_2 removal is recommended in those with extreme hypercarbia (pH < 7.1) with mild-to-moderate hypoxemia.
- *Rate of deterioration and how quickly ECLS can be initiated:* Clinicians working in centers without the capacity to facilitate rapid ECLS (<30–45 minutes) should refer earlier, particularly if there is rapid deterioration.[40]

Contraindications

- Chromosomal abnormalities (e.g. Trisomy 13 or 18)
- Severe neurological compromise (e.g. intracranial hemorrhage with mass effect)
- Allogeneic bone marrow transplant recipients with pulmonary infiltrates
- Brain death
- Developing or poor neurological outcome
- Incurable malignancy
- Duration of pre-ECLS MV >14 days (relative).[40]

Steroids

Administration of steroids was guided by the idea that inflammation plays a key role in PARDS. The current estimation of steroid use is about 20–60% in PARDS. This is confounded by many factors (i.e. shock, pre-extubation, and hypercytokinemia) in which steroids have been used.[2,8] Use of steroids has not shown any benefit in PARDS. PALICC recommends against corticosteroids as routine therapy in PARDS pending further studies in specific populations.[2,35]

■ NONPULMONARY STRATEGIES

Sedation and Neuromuscular Blockade

The use of minimal yet effective sedation is recommended in children for better oxygenation/gas exchange by preventing ventilator-patient asynchrony. Sedation given must also be periodically assessed for duration, time, amount, and type of sedation given. Pain and sedation scales should be used; monitoring for intermediate withdrawal syndrome (IWS) should be done periodically. Complications of oversedation such as feed intolerance and autonomic disturbances should be watched for. Sedation should be weaned appropriately and should be switched over to oral sedation as early as possible.[35]

Neuromuscular blockade (NMB) should be considered only if sedation alone is not adequate for effective ventilation. If NMBs are used, then periodic NMB holiday should be considered every alternative day, especially in full chemical paralysis. The adequacy of NMB should be monitored by effective ventilation, clinical movements, and "train of four" response (a clinical tool to assess neuromuscular block in the anesthetized patient by stimulating the ulnar nerve with supramaximal twitch stimuli and studying the twitch amplitude). The usage of NMB agents has also been associated with critical illness polyneuropathy and myopathy (CIPNM). Curare-based NMB agents (cisatracurium) that are not dependent on renal clearance should preferentially be used when renal dysfunction is present or likely to develop.[35]

Nutrition

Early enteral feeding has shown to have better mortality outcomes in PARDS. Enteral feeding is preferred to parenteral nutrition and should be started as soon as feed tolerance is established. During illness, the body's need/demands are increased, which lead to acute malnutrition increasing the morbidity and mortality. Adequate delivery of nutrition meets the metabolic demands, improves immune function, clear toxic metabolites, and maintains intestinal epithelium integrity.[35]

Fluid Management

The goal of fluid administration in critically ill patients with PARDS is to maintain intravascular volume and ensure adequate end-organ perfusion while minimizing extravascular lung water and pulmonary edema.[36] However, reducing fluid administration to decrease pulmonary edema can lead to decreased intravascular pressures, making fluid management a challenge. Current practice is to administer fluid when it is required and once hemodynamically stable, the child is diuresed using diuretics.

Current consensus suggests that—biphasic fluid needs after initial fluid resuscitation and goal-directed fluid management based on individual patients should be used in order to maintain adequate intravascular volume while aiming to prevent a positive fluid balance.[2,33,35]

Blood transfusion is not recommended in children who are clinically stable and have an adequate oxygen delivery, except for those with cyanotic heart diseases, bleeding, or severe hypoxemia. Packed cells are transfused to maintain a target hemoglobin of >7 g/dL.[35]

■ IMAGING

X-ray (Figs. 18.1.3A to D)

It helps in etiological diagnosis, PEEP titration (recruitment), and detection of complications such as effusion, air leaks, etc. It is easily available bedside, major drawbacks being interobserver variability and radiation exposure.

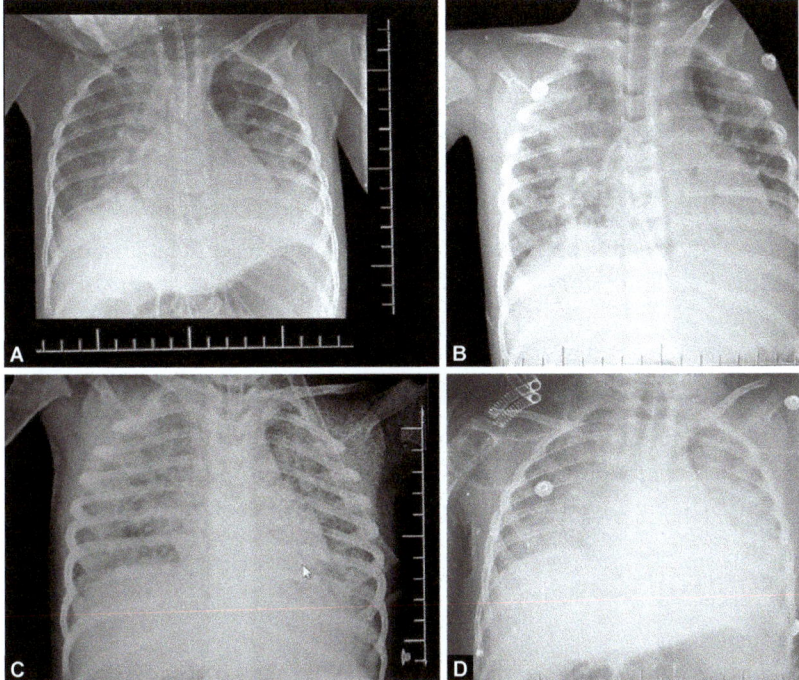

Figs. 18.1.3A to D: Child with severe acute respiratory distress syndrome (ARDS), showing various stages—(A) patchy infiltrates, (B) alveolar and reticular opacification, (C) interstitial infiltrates, and (D) complete white out lungs.

Computed Tomography Scan (Fig. 18.1.4)

It helps in etiological diagnosis and PEEP adjustment (homogeneity and recruitability). It has higher sensitivity compared to X-ray, drawbacks being radiation exposure and risk of transport.

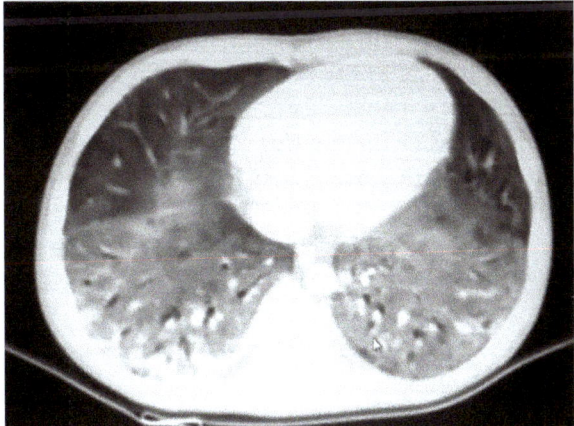

Fig. 18.1.4: Computed tomographic scan showing ground–glass appearance and air bronchogram.

Ultrasound

It helps in etiological diagnosis, PEEP adjustment (homogeneity and recruitability), and differentiates new comorbidity, heart and lung interaction, and evaluation of diaphragm function.

Positron Emission Tomography Scan

It shows regional lung perfusion, pulmonary vascular permeability, metabolic activity of inflammatory lung cells, without radiation exposure, drawback being long duration of procedure and risk of transport.

Electric Impedance Tomography

It detects regional lung perfusion, pulmonary vascular permeability, and metabolic activity of inflammatory lung cells without radiation exposure, drawbacks being long duration of procedure and risk of transport.

■ MONITORING

This includes:
- *Lung compliance monitoring* in PARDS for severity assessment using parameters such as pressure and tidal volume on the ventilator, dynamic compliance, and plateau pressure measurement.
- *Esophageal manometry* measuring transpulmonary pressure helps in PEEP adjustment and prevention of ventilator-induced lung injury. Equipment used is esophageal balloon pressure monitor or ventilator with special function.
- *Oxygenation and ventilation parameters and severity scores* P/F (S/F ratio) and OI (OSI) for severity assessment, diagnosis and prognosis assessment at a given point.
- *Lung injury score* for severity assessment using chest X-ray, arterial blood gas (ABG) compliance, PEEP, S/F or P/F ratio divided by number of components used. It is a noninvasive score used bedside.
- Ventilation index [$PaCO_2$ (in mm Hg) × peak airway pressure (in cm H_2O) × respiratory rate (breaths/min)/1,000] has been shown to have prognostic value in PARDS.
- *Continuous arterial gas monitoring* for ventilator settings and adjustment.
- *Continuous CO_2 monitoring* using capnography or transcutaneous monitors.
- *Electrical activity of diaphragm* to see the respiratory drive, synchronization, and function of diaphragm.[41]

WEANING

Weaning is a strategy in assessing patient tolerance toward extubation, wherein the amount of ventilator support is gradually decreased while continuously looking at various parameters such as improvement in the severity of PARDS, adequate gas exchange, adequate respiratory drive, and hemodynamic stability. These are the key indicators of improvement before children with ARDS can proceed to the ventilator weaning strategies.

- Weaning PEEP Q4H by 1 cmH$_2$O while maintaining SpO$_2$ ≥ 95
- Once PEEP is 5 ≤ H$_2$O start weaning FiO$_2$
- Changing to pressure support (PS) ventilation and adjustment made while keeping exhaled VT between 5 mL/kg to 7 mL/kg is key goal in weaning, wean PS every 2 cmH$_2$O and reassess in 30 minutes.
- If exhaled VT is ≤ 5 mL/kg, go back on previous PS, if more than 5 mL/kg, keep weaning to PS between 5 cmH$_2$O and 10 cmH$_2$O and review every Q4H.
- Respiratory rate (RR) while weaning should be age appropriate, any increase or decrease should be monitored and evaluated for anxiety, sedation, and withdrawal features.
- Extubation can be planned once patient is on PS for 2 hours and exhaled tidal volumes are 5 mL/kg and SpO$_2$ ≥ 92% on PEEP ≤ 5 and FiO$_2$ ≤ 0.50.[42]

OUTCOMES

Pediatric Acute Lung Injury Consensus Conference has provided the pediatric community with a consistent definition for infants, children, and adolescents. PARDS, which is a common diagnosis in critically ill children admitted in PICU, has seen a declining trend over the past few decades due to better clinical guidelines but still forms a significant proportion of all children admitted to the PICU. ALI/ARDS results in significant morbidity and mortality with prolonged stay in PICU impacting economic and social status of the family and the quality of life of the affected child.

Current data on long-term outcomes for PARDS survivors remains quite limited. Future studies on pulmonary, neurocognitive, and neuromuscular morbidities are needed in survivors of PARDS.[2,43]

REFERENCES

1. Orloff KE, Turner DA, Rehder KJ. The current state of pediatric acute respiratory distress syndrome. Pediatr Allergy Immunol Pulmonol. 2019;32(2):35-44.
2. Pediatric Acute Lung Injury Consensus Conference Group. Pediatric acute respiratory distress syndrome: consensus recommendations from the Pediatric

Acute Lung Injury Consensus Conference. Pediatr Crit Care Med. 2015;16(5): 428-39.
3. Gupta S, Sankar J, Lodha R, et al. Comparison of prevalence and outcomes of pediatric acute respiratory distress syndrome using Pediatric Acute Lung Injury Consensus Conference criteria and Berlin definition. Front Pediatr. 2018;6:93.
4. Khemani RG, Smith L, Lopez-Fernandez YM, et al. Pediatric acute respiratory distress syndrome incidence and epidemiology (PARDIE): an international, observational study. Lancet Respir Med. 2019;7(2):115-28.
5. Yehya N, Thomas NJ, Khemani RG. Risk stratification using oxygenation in the first 24 hours of pediatric acute respiratory distress syndrome. Crit Care Med. 2018;46(4):619-24.
6. Yehya N, Keim G, Thomas NJ. Subtypes of pediatric acute respiratory distress syndrome have different predictors of mortality. Intensive Care Med. 2018;44(8):1230-9.
7. Sapru A, Flori H, Quasney MW, et al.; Pediatric Acute Lung Injury Consensus Conference Group. Pathobiology of acute respiratory distress syndrome. Pediatr Crit Care Med. 2015;16(5 Suppl 1):S6-22.
8. Heidemann SM, Nair A, Bulut Y, et al. Pathophysiology and management of acute respiratory distress syndrome in children. Pediatr Clin N Am. 2017;64(5):1017-37.
9. Ware LB, Matthay MA. The acute respiratory distress syndrome. N Engl J Med. 2000;342(18):1334-49.
10. Xiang M, Fan J. Pattern recognition receptor-dependent mechanisms of acute lung injury. Mol Med. 2010;16(1-2):69-82.
11. Parsons PE, Matthay MA, Ware LB, et al.; National Heart, Lung, Blood Institute Acute Respiratory Distress Syndrome Clinical Trials Network. Elevated plasma levels of soluble TNF receptors are associated with morbidity and mortality in patients with acute lung injury. Am J Physiol Lung Cell Mol Physiol. 2005;288(3):L426-31.
12. Sharp C, Millar AB, Medford AR. Advances in understanding of the pathogenesis of Acute respiratory distress syndrome. Respiration. 2015;89(5):420-34.
13. Dreyfuss D, Saumon G. Ventilator-induced lung injury: Lessons from experimental studies. Am J Respir Crit Care Med. 1998;157(1):294-323.
14. Amato MB, Meade MO, Slutsky AS, et al. Driving pressure and survival in acute respiratory distress syndrome. N Engl Med. 2015;372(8):747-55.
15. Curley GF, Laffey JG, Zhang H, et al. Biotrauma and ventilator-induced lung injury: Clinical implications. Chest. 2016;150(5):1109-17.
16. Essouri S, Carroll C; Pediatric Acute Lung Injury Consensus Conference Group. Noninvasive support and ventilation for pediatric acute respiratory distress syndrome: Proceedings from the Pediatric Acute Lung Injury Consensus Conference. Pediatr Crit Care Med. 2015;16(5 Suppl 1):S102-10.
17. Rimensberger PC, Cheifetz IM; Pediatric Acute Lung Injury Consensus Conference Group. Ventilatory support in children with pediatric acute respiratory distress syndrome: proceedings from the Pediatric Acute Lung Injury Consensus Conference. Pediatr Crit Care Med. 2015;16(5 Suppl 1):S52-60.
18. Acute Respiratory Distress Syndrome Network, Brower RG, Matthay MA, et al. Ventilation with lower tidal volumes as compared with traditional tidal volumes for acute lung injury and the acute respiratory distress syndrome. N Engl J Med. 2000;342(18):1301-8.

19. Cheifetz IM. Pediatric ARDS. Respir Care. 2017;62(6):718-31.
20. Mosier JM, Joshi R, Hypes C, et al. The physiologically difficult airway. West J Emerg Med. 2015;16(7):1109-17.
21. Erickson S, Schibler A, Numa A, et al. Acute lung injury in pediatric intensive care in Australia and New Zealand: a prospective, multicenter, observational study. Pediatr Crit Care Med. 2007;8(4):317-23.
22. Khemani RG, Conti D, Alonzo TA, et al. Effect of tidal volume in children with acute hypoxemic respiratory failure. Intensive Care Med. 2009;35(8):1428-37.
23. Grasso S, Mascia L, Del Turco M, et al. Effects of recruiting maneuvers in patients with acute respiratory distress syndrome ventilated with protective ventilatory strategy. Anesthesiology. 2002;96(4):795-802.
24. Curley MA, Hibberd PL, Fineman LD, et al. Effect of prone positioning on clinical outcomes in children with acute lung injury: a randomized controlled trial. JAMA. 2005;294(2):229-37.
25. Abdelsalam M, Cheifetz IM. Goal-directed therapy for severely hypoxic patients with acute respiratory distress syndrome: permissive hypoxemia. Respir Care. 2010;55(11):1483-90.
26. Imai Y, Slutsky AS. High-frequency oscillatory ventilation and ventilator-induced lung injury. Crit Care Med. 2005;33(3 Suppl):S129-34.
27. Young D, Lamb SE, Shah S, et al. High-frequency oscillation for acute respiratory distress syndrome. N Engl J Med. 2013;368(9):806-13.
28. Ferguson ND, Cook DJ, Guyatt GH, et al. High-frequency oscillation in early acute respiratory distress syndrome. N Engl J Med. 2013;368(9):795-805.
29. Frawley PM, Habashi NM. Airway pressure release ventilation: Theory and practice. AACN Clin Issues. 2001;12(2):234-46.
30. Willson DF, Thomas NJ, Markovitz BP, et al. Effect of exogenous surfactant (calfactant) in pediatric acute lung injury: a randomized controlled trial. JAMA. 2005;293(4):470-6.
31. Tamburro RF, Kneyber MC; Pediatric Acute Lung Injury Consensus Conference Group. Pulmonary specific ancillary treatment for pediatric acute respiratory distress syndrome: Proceedings from the Pediatric Acute Lung Injury Consensus Conference. Pediatr Crit Care Med. 2015;16(5 Suppl 1):S61-72.
32. Ibrahim TS, El-Mohamady HS. Inhaled nitric oxide and prone position: how far they can improve oxygenation in pediatric patients with acute respiratory distress syndrome? J Med Sci. 2007;7(3):390-5.
33. Soo Hoo GW. In prone ventilation, one good turn deserves another. N Engl J Med. 2013;368(23):2227-8.
34. Guerin C, Reignier J, Richard JC, et al.; PROSEVA Study Group. Prone positioning in severe acute respiratory distress syndrome. N Engl J Med. 2013;368(23):2159-68.
35. Valentine SL, Nadkarni VM, Curley MA; Pediatric Acute Lung Injury Consensus Conference Group. Nonpulmonary treatments for pediatric acute respiratory distress syndrome: Proceedings from the Pediatric Acute Lung Injury Consensus Conference. Pediatr Crit Care Med. 2015;16(5 Suppl 1):S73-85.
36. Dalton HJ, Macrae DJ; Pediatric Acute Lung Injury Consensus Conference Group. Extracorporeal support in children with pediatric acute respiratory distress syndrome: Proceedings from the Pediatric Acute Lung Injury Consensus Conference. Pediatr Crit Care Med. 2015;16(5 Suppl 1):S111-7.

37. Bartlett RH, Gazzaniga AB, Jefferies MR, et al. Extracorporeal membrane oxygenation (ECMO) cardiopulmonary support in infancy. Trans Am Soc Artif Intern Organs. 1976;22:80-93.
38. Lewandowski K. Extracorporeal membrane oxygenation for severe acute respiratory failure. Crit Care. 2000;4(3):156-68.
39. Combes A, Hajage D, Capellier G, et al. Extracorporeal membrane oxygenation for severe acute respiratory distress syndrome. N Engl J Med. 2018;378(21): 1965-75.
40. Graeme M, Steve C, Giles P. (2015). Indications for pediatric respiratory extracorporeal life support. International Summary, Ann Arbor, March 2015. [online] Available from https://www.elso.org/Portals/0/Files/ELSO%20guidelines%20paeds%20resp_May2015.pdf. [Last accessed December, 2019].
41. Kawaguchi A, Jouvet P. Imaging and Monitoring in pediatric acute respiratory distress syndrome. In: Shein SL, Rotta AT (Eds). Pediatric acute respiratory distress syndrome: A Clinical Guide. Cham, Switzerland.Springer; 2020. pp. 33-46. [online] Available from https://doi.org/10.1007/978-3-030-21840-9. [Last accessed December, 2019].
42. Randolph A. Ventilator weaning and extubation strategies for children with PARDS. In: Shein SL, Rotta AT (Eds). Pediatric acute respiratory distress syndrome: A Clinical Guide. Cham, Switzerland: Springer; 2020. pp. 101-115. [online] Available from https://doi.org/10.1007/978-3-030-21840-9. [Last accessed December, 2019].
43. Quasney MW, Lopez-Fernandez YM, Santschi M, et al.; Pediatric Acute Liver Injury Consensus Conference Group. The Outcomes of children with pediatric acute respiratory distress syndrome: Proceedings from the Pediatric Acute Lung Injury Consensus Conference. Pediatr Crit Care Med. 2015;16(5 Suppl 1): S118-31.

CHAPTER 19

EMERGENCIES AND POISONING

19.1 Rodenticide Poisoning
P Ramachandran

19.1 RODENTICIDE POISONING

P Ramachandran

■ INTRODUCTION

The management of rodents is a great concern all over the world. Rats are ubiquitous and opportunistic animals; some such as the brown rats (*Rattus norvegicus*) and the black rats (*Rattus rattus*) are present in all continents, except Antarctica.[1] Whenever not controlled, rodents destroy grain stock in huge amounts. In India, analysis of the damage caused by rodents to the agricultural products and food grains in farms, households and storage facilities show that the damage ranges from 2% to 15% throughout the country and sometimes there is severe damage of even up to 100% loss of the field crop. According to a conservative estimate about 5–6% of the total food grains being produced are lost annually at the preharvest stage due to rodents.[2]

In USA, the estimated cost induced by rodents' damage is about 19 billion dollars.[3]

Rodenticides or rat poisons are a variety of chemical substances grouped under pesticides and are developed specifically for killing rats, which constitute a significant menace to agricultural products and human beings.[4] They are among the most toxic substances regularly found in homes. Widespread use of rodenticides of increasing potency in and around households has led to an increase of the exposure risks and the intoxication risks for non-target species such as pets, wildlife, and human beings, especially children. Pesticide poisoning including rodenticides, whether due to self, accidental, occupational, or for homicidal purpose, is a global public health problem, and self-poisoning accounts for one-third of the world's suicide rate. In fact, in some parts of developing countries, pesticide poisoning causes more deaths than infections.[5] Each year, around 300,000 deaths occur worldwide due to pesticides. Deaths are mostly associated with metal phosphides and yellow phosphorus. Most rodenticides produce their toxic effect in humans by ingestion of a large single dose. This occurs accidentally in children and intentionally in adolescents.

Though many substances are used as rodenticides, their availability and market regulations differ in countries. Besides, there are also some unapproved preparations still available in the market.

Rodenticides are a heterogeneous group of compounds that exhibit markedly different toxicities to humans and rodents. The varieties of rodenticides used over the years are legion with heavy metals like arsenic being used before mid-twentieth century and oral anticoagulants after that.

■ COMMONLY USED RODENTICIDES IN INDIA

The commonly used rodenticides in India are listed below:
- Anticoagulants such as warfarin, coumatetralyl (Racumin), and second-generation single dose superwarfarins such as brodifacoum, chlorophacinone, difenacoum, diphacinone, and bromadiolone (Rodenticide preparations)
- Aluminum phosphide and zinc phosphide (Ratnil)
- Yellow phosphorus (Ratol)
- Barium carbonate.

Highly toxic rodenticides are those substances with a single dose LD_{50} of less than 50 mg/kg body weight (LD_{50} or lethal dose$_{50}$ is the amount of poison that causes death in 50% of patients following exposure) **(Table 19.1.1)**. In India, zinc phosphide, aluminum phosphide, yellow phosphorus, superwarfarins, and barium carbonate are the most common rodenticides implicated in poisoning.

Poison baiting of rodents with zinc phosphide and burrow fumigation with aluminum phosphide is common in agricultural fields. Coumatetralyl (Racumin) and bromadiolone are used for the control of both agricultural and commensal rodent pests in India. Coumatetralyl, though of first generation, has high efficacy against the widely occurring "lesser bandicoot rats" approaching that of the second-generation anticoagulant rodenticides (ARs).[2]

In a hospital-based study from Karnataka, out of 97 adults with rodenticide poisoning, 43 (44.3%) had consumed yellow phosphorus, 28 (28.8%) zinc phosphide, 5 (5.1%) aluminum phosphide, and 21 (21.6%) superwarfarin (0.005% bromadiolone).[6] In another study of 56 adults with rodenticide poisoning over 1 year again from Karnataka, the most common poisoning agent was zinc phosphide (18 cases, 32.14%) followed by aluminum phosphide (12 cases, 21.4%), yellow phosphorus (8 cases, 14.2%), and bromadiolone (2 cases, 3.6%). An unknown compound, which was not specified on the packet, was implicated in 16 cases (28.57%) with 25% mortality.[7] A similar situation is seen in most places wherein a significant proportion of cases there is no information available on the nature of poison and the clinician will have to suspect the type of toxin based on the symptoms **(Table 19.1.2)**. Whenever

Table 19.1.1: Grades of toxicity of rodenticides.

High toxicity	Moderate toxicity	Low toxicity
Zinc phosphide, aluminum phosphide, yellow phosphorus (single dose fast-acting agents), barium carbonate	Cholecalciferol	Warfarin, superwarfarins like bromadiolone (single dose agents)

Table 19.1.2: Clinical syndromes in rodenticide poisonings.

Toxidrome	Suspected rodenticide
Cardiac arrhythmias, refractory shock, or cardiac arrest	*Early*: Zinc or aluminum phosphide, yellow phosphorus or barium carbonate *Late*: Arsenic, thallium, or fluoroacetamide
Severe liver failure: Early/late	Yellow/white phosphorus
Muscle rigidity, opisthotonus, trismus, and facial grimacing (risus sardonicus)	Strychnine
Bruising or bleeding	Anticoagulants (warfarin, superwarfarin compounds)

possible, the rodenticide package should be inspected for the brand name, the full chemical name of the product, and any other relevant warning labels. Failure in the examinations or inability to cope up with the high expectation from parents and teachers has increased the incidence of poisoning among students.[7]

METAL PHOSPHIDES

In a study based on the telephone calls to the National Poisons Information Centre (NPIC), AIIMS, New Delhi over 13 years (1999–2012), a total of 4,929 calls of pesticide poisoning were reported with 59.38% calls pertaining to household pesticides and 40.61% calls related to agricultural pesticides. Among the household pesticides, the highest number of calls were due to pyrethroids (26.23%) followed by rodenticides (17.06%); and among agricultural pesticides, the organophosphates (9.79%) ranked first followed by aluminum phosphide (9.65%).[8]

Aluminum and zinc phosphides are highly effective rodenticides and are used widely to protect grain in stores and during its transportation.[9] It is readily available in Asian markets such as India.[10]

ALUMINUM PHOSPHIDE

Aluminum phosphide (AlP) is a solid fumigant and is available in the form of tablets, pellets, granules, or as dust. Commercially, it is available as dark gray tablets of 3 g each, consisting of AlP (56%) and carbamate (44%), by the names Celphos, Alphos, and others.[11] AlP poisoning is common in all parts of the world, but is found more commonly in developing countries like India and is often implicated in accidental and suicidal poisonings in India. Many lives have been lost in the last three decades, especially among the young rural population of northern India due to AlP poisoning. It is not just limited to the agricultural society and the incidence is increasing in the urban families also.[12]

In an autopsy study of unnatural deaths in Northwest India, AlP was found to be the most common suicidal poison, causing 68.4% of total deaths due to poisoning between 1992 and 2002.[13] In countries such as UK, AlP is available, but supply is restricted under the Pesticides Act to qualified users. In European countries also, suicides by AlP ingestion are rare.

Acute poisoning with these compounds may be direct due to direct ingestion of the salts or indirectly from accidental inhalation of phosphine generated during their approved use. On contact with the moisture (H_2O) in the atmosphere or with the hydrochloric acid (HCl) in stomach, AlP releases toxic phosphine gas as shown below:

$$AlP + 3H_2O = Al(OH)_3 + PH_3 \text{ (Phosphine)}$$
$$AlP + 3HCl = AlCl_3 + PH_3 \text{ (Phosphine)}$$

The residues, aluminum hydroxide [$Al(OH)_3$] or aluminum chloride ($AlCl_3$), are nontoxic. For effective action, these preparations must be fresh, otherwise they gradually lose their potency over time due to release of phosphine gas on exposure to atmosphere and become nontoxic residues. In its pure form, phosphine gas is colorless and odorless. It is inflammable and may spontaneously ignite in air at ambient temperature at concentrations above the threshold limit range of 1.9% (v/v). Each 3 g AlP tablet can release 1 g of phosphine (PH_3) gas. The lethal dose of AlP is around 0.5 g. Those who survived had either taken a very small amount, or an expired tablet or phosphine gas evaporated because the tablet had been exposed to air. Ingestion of fresh phosphide rodenticide in the original packaging is most potent.[10] Inhalation of PH_3 at a concentration of 300 ppm is also dangerous. At 400–600 ppm, it is lethal within an hour.

Mechanism of Toxicity

Toxicity occurs in children due to ingestion of these formulations accidentally or in adolescents due to suicide attempt. Inhalation of phosphine gas is a less common mode of toxicity.

Both forms of poisoning are mediated by phosphine. On ingestion, phosphine gas is released from stomach and gets rapidly absorbed affecting the heart, lungs, kidneys, and liver. Serious cardiac arrhythmias, intractable shock, acidosis, and pulmonary edema may result. Phosphine also has a local corrosive action on intestinal mucosa. The mechanism of toxicity on various tissues includes failure of cellular respiration due to the effect on mitochondria, inhibition of cytochrome C oxidase, formation of highly reactive hydroxyl radicals, lipid peroxidation, increased activity of superoxide dismutase, and reduction of catalase and glutathione **(Flowchart 19.1.1)**. The major lethal consequence of phosphide ingestion, profound circulatory collapse, is secondary to factors including direct effects on cardiac myocytes,

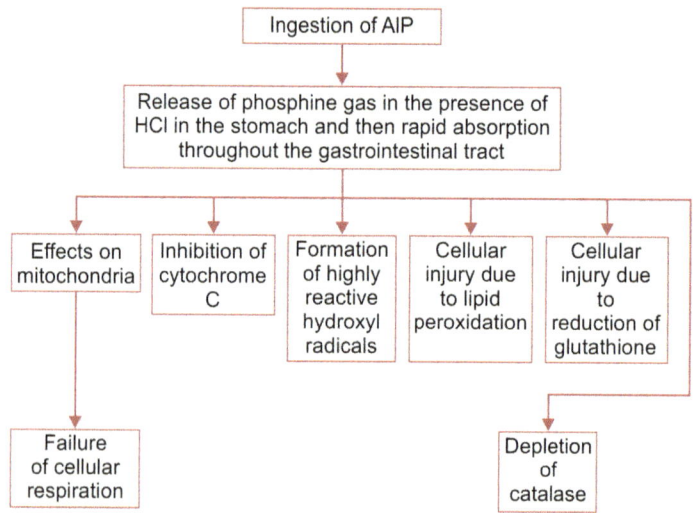

Flowchart 19.1.1: The mechanisms of aluminum phosphide (AlP) toxicity.[10]

fluid loss, and adrenal gland damage.[9] Indicators of oxidative stress (reduced glutathione and malonyldialdehyde) reach peak levels within 48 h of exposure and normalize by 5th day.[14,15] Both hypo- and hypermagnesemia can occur due to unknown reasons.[16]

Clinical Features

The clinical features are nonspecific and depend on the amount, route, and duration after exposure. After ingestion, toxic features usually develop within few minutes. In mild poisoning, nausea, repeated vomiting, diarrhea, headache, abdominal discomfort, garlic breath, and tachycardia are common features. These patients usually show recovery. On the other hand, in moderate-to-severe ingestion, the signs and symptoms of gastrointestinal (GI), cardiovascular (CVS), respiratory, and central nervous systems (CNS) appear initially, and later on, features of hepatic and renal failure and disseminated intravascular coagulation (DIC) may occur.[9,11] Endoscopy may reveal corrosive lesions of esophagus and stomach, severe gastric erosions, duodenal erosions, and esophageal strictures or fistula.

On inhalation of phosphine gas, the child may have difficulty in breathing followed by other features such as nausea, vomiting, diarrhea, dizziness, headache, ataxia, paresthesia, tremors, muscle weakness, diplopia, and jaundice. In severe inhalation toxicity, the patient may develop various organ involvements like severe toxicity following oral ingestion.

Cardiovascular system involvement is significant in AlP poisoning characterized by profound and refractory hypotension, congestive heart failure, electrocardiographic (ECG) abnormalities, myocarditis, subendocardial infarction, or pericarditis. ECG abnormalities include rhythm disturbances, ST-T changes, and conduction defects. In a study of AlP poisoning, life-threatening ventricular tachycardia was recorded in 40% cases and ventricular fibrillation (VF) in 23.3% cases. Supraventricular tachycardia and atrial flutter/fibrillation occurred in 46.7% and 20% patients, respectively. ST-T changes simulating myocardial ischemia were also present in all patients (S-T depression in 90%, S-T elevation in 10%). One-third of the patients developed variable degrees of heart block.[17] Hypotension was seen in 76-100% of severe cases.[18] Refractory shock occurs due to myocardial damage, peripheral vasodilatation, and fluid loss.

Respiratory complications occur in the form of pulmonary edema and acute respiratory distress syndrome (ARDS) leading on to respiratory failure. Metabolic acidosis is seen due to blockage of oxidative phosphorylation and poor tissue perfusion.

A study done in North India of AlP poisoning with 33 patients (18-48 years; mean age 22 years) revealed that maximum number of patients presented clinically with cardiovascular instability, either in the form of hypotension or arrhythmias (58%), 15% with respiratory distress alone, and 18% of the patients had combined symptoms related to respiratory, CVS, or CNS. Rest of the patients got admitted with other symptoms such as GI bleed or altered sensorium.[12]

Other uncommon complications are adrenal insufficiency, pancreatitis, hypo- or hyperglycemia, methemoglobinemia, microangiopathic hemolytic anemia, and DIC. Late esophageal complications like stricture are seen in some patients. Dysphagia was observed in 38.87% of survivors after a mean interval of 38.6 days. Esophageal strictures were seen in 32.2% of the survivors. Two patients reported a tracheoesophageal fistula.[19]

Aluminum phosphide poisoning has a high mortality (30-100%) and survival is unlikely, if more than 1.5 g is ingested.[20] In a study of 56 adults with rodenticide poisoning from Karnataka, the mortality rate was high with AlP (5 cases out of 12, 41.6%).[7] Most of the deaths occurred within the first 24 hours after ingestion mainly due to arrhythmia and after 24 hours due to refractory shock, acidosis, and ARDS.[21]

There are interesting reports about spontaneous ignition and burns that occurred after oral poisoning with AlP. Phosphine gas is inflammable, depending on temperature and pressure.[22]

Diagnosis

The diagnosis of AlP usually depends on the clinical suspicion or history (self-report or by attendants). In case of doubt, diagnosis can be made easily by a silver nitrate-impregnated paper test on gastric content or on breath.

For the silver nitrate test on gastric aspirate, diluted gastric content is heated up in a flask to 50°C for 15–20 minutes, keeping silver nitrate paper on the mouth of the flask. If phosphine is present, the paper will turn black due to silver phosphate. Gas chromatography with nitrogen–phosphorous detector is the most specific and sensitive test and it can be used for analysis of airtight samples (viscera and gastric content) collected during autopsy.[23]

Management

There is no antidote to phosphine or metal phosphide poisoning and many patients die, despite intensive care.[9]

Initial Stabilization

Airway, breathing, and circulation are assessed and stabilized by the standard cardiopulmonary assessment using Indian Academy of Pediatrics Advanced Life Support (IAP-ALS) guidelines.[24]

Continuous monitoring of vitals is required, and the necessary supportive care is provided. The healthcare provider must take personal protective measures, including facemask and rubber gloves during decontamination. "Spontaneous ignition" is a rare but possible finding in cases of AlP poisoning.[22]

Initial investigation should include ECG, chest X-ray, blood glucose, arterial blood gas, and electrolytes including magnesium, routine hemogram, liver function tests, and renal function tests. Repeated or continuous ECG and echocardiography can reveal cardiac dysfunction early.[25]

Decontamination

Gastrointestinal decontamination may be useful within 1–2 hours. GI decontamination should be attempted only after ensuring airway protection. Potassium permanganate (1:10,000) is used for gastric lavage through a nasogastric tube, as it oxidizes phosphine to nontoxic phosphate. This can be followed by 1 g/kg of activated charcoal (50–100 g in adolescents) to reduce absorption, if the patient arrives within 1 h after ingestion of a large amount. In vitro experimental findings suggest that fat and oil, mainly vegetable oils and liquid paraffin, inhibit phosphine release from the ingested AlP. The possible role of coconut oil in managing acute AlP poisoning is favorably concluded in a case report even 6-hour postingestion.[26]

In another study of AlP poisoning, institution of intensive care support along with gastric lavage using a combination of coconut oil with soda bicarbonate brought about a survival of 42%. The mechanism by which coconut oil reduces the toxicity of phosphides is unknown but most probably it forms a protective layer around the gastric mucosa, thereby preventing the absorption of phosphine gas. Secondly, it helps in diluting the HCl and inhibiting the breakdown of phosphide from the pellet of AlP. Soda bicarbonate neutralizes the HCl thereby diminishing the catalytic reaction of phosphide with HCl and inhibiting the release of phosphine.[12]

Cardiovascular Support

Cardiac failure and refractory shock are important contributory factors for mortality in AlP poisoning. All patients of severe AlP poisoning require continuous invasive hemodynamic monitoring and early resuscitation with fluid and vasoactive agents. Fluid therapy could be guided by central venous pressure (CVP) and invasive arterial pressure monitoring in a pediatric intensive care unit (PICU). For refractory hypotension, norepinephrine or vasopressin could be used. In view of the reversible nature of myocardial involvement, maximal cardiac support should be available including facilities for cardioversion, cardiac pacemaker, and intra-aortic balloon pump for mechanical support.[27,28]

In a study of 30 patients with AlP poisoning, IV amiodarone/xylocard could revert dangerous ventricular arrhythmias to sinus rhythm in four cases.[17] Trimetazidine, an anti-ischemic drug belonging to the group of partial fatty acid oxidation inhibitors, was found to be effective in stopping ventricular ectopic beats and preserving oxidative metabolism.[29]

Organ Support

In view of multiple organ involvement, early identification of respiratory failure and renal failure and ventilatory support and renal replacement therapy respectively should be instituted.

In the presence of metabolic acidosis, intravenous sodium bicarbonate for the "aggressive correction of acidosis" protocol resulted in significant improvement in patient outcome from 30% to 55%.[30] Optimal management of hypo- or hyperglycemia and hypokalemia and steroid use for adrenal insufficiency are other adjuncts. Cyanosis not responding to oxygen therapy may be a sign of methemoglobinemia that requires therapy with intravenous methylene blue (1% solution) in the dose of 2 mg/kg of body weight over 5 minutes.[31]

A systematic management of AlP poisoning **(Flowchart 19.1.2)** is likely to give the best possible results in this life-threatening poisoning.[25]

Prognosis

The mortality in adults who have ingested 500 mg of AlP or above is between 30% and 100%. The higher the blood phosphine, the higher is the mortality. Patients having blood phosphine levels equal to or less than 1.067 ± 0.16 mg survived, and this dose seems to be the lethal threshold of phosphine toxicity.[14]

Flowchart 19.1.2: Management of aluminum phosphide/phosphine poisoning.[25]

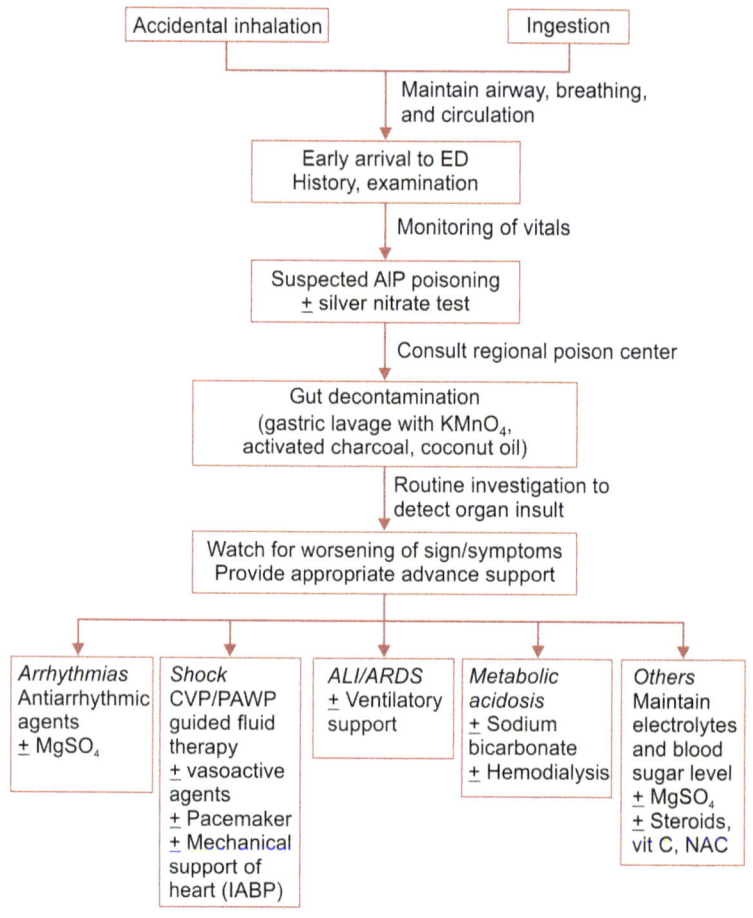

(ED: emergency department; CVP: central venous pressure; PAWP: pulmonary artery wedge pressure; IABP: intra-aortic balloon pump; ECLS: extracorporeal life support; ALI/ARDS: acute lung injury/acute respiratory distress syndrome; NAC: N-acetylcysteine)

■ ZINC PHOSPHIDE

The other metal phosphide rodenticide associated with significant mortality in our country is zinc phosphide. It is a dark gray crystalline powder with an odor like rotten fish or garlic. It is available as pellets. Inhalation or ingestion can be fatal. It is added to rodent baits in a concentration of 0.75–2.0%. Its mode of action is like AlP. It reacts with hydrochloric acid in the stomach releasing the highly toxic phosphine gas, a very potent respiratory poison.

Death occurs within 24 hours due to cardiorespiratory failure. Fatal dose is 2–10 mg/kg.[32]

Clinical Features

Symptoms following poisoning are like AlP but of slower onset because of the slow release of phosphine. Initial GI symptoms are followed by severe CVS effects such as ventricular tachycardia, VF, hypotension, and CNS manifestations such as agitation, convulsions, and coma. Death occurs due to VF.

In a hospital-based study on rodenticide poisoning, mortality in patients with ingestion of zinc phosphide was 35.7% and patients who lost for follow-up were 7.1%.[6] In another study, it was 16.6%.[7]

Treatment

As there is no specific antidote, treatment is supportive as in AlP poisoning. Zinc phosphide is radiopaque and, when positive, abdominal radiographs can help to confirm the diagnosis and support specific management.[33]

■ WHITE OR YELLOW ELEMENTAL PHOSPHORUS

Phosphorus exists in two forms—red and yellow (white). Red phosphorus is nonvolatile, insoluble, and unabsorbable and, therefore, nontoxic when ingested. Yellow phosphorus (also referred to as white phosphorus), on the other hand, is a severe local and systemic toxin causing damage to gastrointestinal, hepatic, cardiovascular, and renal systems.[7] Pastes containing phosphorus are applied on bread and used as bait for rodents.

Mechanism of Action

It is a corrosive agent and damages all tissues it comes in contact with, including skin and the gut lining. If the patient survives, a relatively symptom-free period of a few hours or days may follow. The third stage of toxicity then ensues with systemic signs indicating severe injury to the liver, myocardium, and brain. This is due to phosphine gas formed in and absorbed from the gut. Toxic dose is 15 mg; fatal dose is 50 mg. The mechanisms by which ingested (white) phosphorus causes tissue damage are direct tissue toxicity caused by an exothermic reaction, local production of phosphoric acid leading to tissue corrosion, and formation of phosphorus pentoxide, which reacts, with organic molecules. Phosphorus binds to calcium and can cause life-threatening hypocalcemia.

Clinical Features

Severe gastric irritation results, followed by cardiovascular failure. In some cases, CNS signs such as lethargy and irritability are the earliest symptoms. It can be fatal within 24 hours. In a hospital-based study of 97 adults with rodenticide poisoning from Karnataka, 44% were due to yellow phosphorus with high mortality of 27.9%. Around 23.2% of yellow phosphorus poisoning was lost to follow-up (discharged against medical advice). Initially, they developed acute liver failure and later progressed to multisystem organ failure.[7] Liver necrosis may occur later also.

Patient with yellow phosphorous ingestion may pass through three stages:[34]

1. *First stage*:
    - Occurs in the first 24 hours
    - Asymptomatic or gastrointestinal symptoms like nausea, vomiting, and diarrhea
    - Perioral and mucosal burns
    - The feces or vomitus may exhibit phosphorescence, sometimes labeled as the "smoking stool syndrome"
    - Mortality in this stage is due to cardiovascular collapse and ventricular dysrhythmias.
    - Absence of any laboratory abnormalities.
2. *Second stage*:
    - Occurs between 24 hours and 72 hours after ingestion
    - Asymptomatic period and patient may be discharged prematurely
    - Mild elevation of liver enzymes and bilirubin
    - Hematological abnormalities.
3. *Third stage (advanced)*:
    - Occurs after 72 hours up to weeks
    - Resolution of symptoms, or
    - Death.

In third stage, patient may present with:
- Gastrointestinal manifestations:
    - Acute hepatic failure—most dreaded complication
- Renal toxicity:
    - Acute tubular necrosis
    - Acute renal failure
- Central nervous system toxicity:
    - Confusion
    - Psychosis
    - Hallucinations
    - Coma
- Cardiac toxicity:
    - Arrhythmias
    - Cardiogenic shock.

Individual patients may or may not display all phases of toxicity. Overlap of toxic findings between phase I and phase III or absence of a latent period is common.

Treatment

If dry and exposed to air, white phosphorus poses a risk of burns and fire. All clothing should be removed and soaked with water to prevent spontaneous ignition. Elemental phosphorus on the patient's skin should be copiously irrigated with water or saline. Wounds should be covered with saline-soaked gauze to prevent drying. If burned area is infected, it is covered with an antimicrobial cream. Health workers should be careful not to get the dry phosphorus on their body or clothes.

Supportive Management

Control of airway and convulsions must be done, prior to considering careful GI decontamination. There is no need to attempt gastric decontamination, if the patient has already vomited.

N-acetylcysteine (NAC) has significant role in acute liver injury. This is probably attributed to the antioxidant property and hepatoprotective nature of NAC. Patients who presented early and started with NAC had good prognosis.[6]

Yellow phosphorus consumption is associated with the late manifestation of liver cell injury and multiorgan dysfunction syndrome (MODS); hence, the patient should be observed for 1 week without early discharge.[7]

■ BARIUM CARBONATE

Barium carbonate, the soluble salt of barium, was used as a rodenticide, though currently its usage is very limited. It is highly toxic and a dose of as little as 200 mg can produce toxicity. It inhibits the potassium efflux channels without interfering with potassium influx pumps resulting in severe hypokalemia. This causes serious cardiac arrhythmias and muscle paralysis.

Clinical Manifestations of Toxicity

Following GI symptoms of nausea and vomiting, there is profound muscle weakness followed by paralysis. Hypertension may be seen. Life-threatening ventricular arrhythmias follow. In suspected poisoning, immediate serum electrolyte assessment must be done and severe hypokalemia should be corrected as a priority.

Management

Airway and breathing require immediate attention as the child may develop ventilatory failure due to profound muscle weakness. Administration of oral magnesium sulfate helps in converting the toxic ionic barium to insoluble barium sulfate.

Correction of hypokalemia with large infusions of IV potassium with close monitoring is the main treatment.[35] If still not corrected, renal replacement therapy may be required. Survival depends on aggressive electrolyte correction and respiratory support.

■ ANTICOAGULANT RODENTICIDES

Anticoagulant rodenticides are one of the most common methods employed in rodent control. ARs have been used since the 1940s to control rodent populations. Warfarin was the first molecule used. The process of controlling rodent population poses challenges when the rodenticide compounds used are also toxic to humans and domestic animals. The ideal rodenticide should be highly toxic to rodents in small amounts but relatively nontoxic in small quantities to nontarget species. The anticoagulant rodenticides best fit these criteria.

The current anticoagulant rodenticide molecules belong to the family of vitamin K antagonists (VKAs). The effect of VKA was observed in the "sweet clover" poisoning of bovines resulting in a hemorrhagic disease and death of the animal. Clover, used as fodder, contains coumarin, which is a precursor of dicoumarol, a VKA. If clover fodders are not stored under proper conditions, fermentation occurs with change of clover coumarin to dicoumarol rendering the clover fodder toxic. Dicoumarol was synthesized by Paul and Stahmann in 1941, bringing into use VKA as an anticoagulant medication. These were also employed as rodenticides. Following this, other VKA molecules including warfarin and molecules more potent than dicoumarol were synthesized. After their use for more than a decade, rodents started developing resistance to ARs. To overcome this, the first generation of ARs has been supplemented by second-generation ARs, which are long-acting and are named "superwarfarins".[4]

Second-generation anticoagulants have been used successfully for rodent control in different pest situations and have been proved effective in numerous field studies against agricultural and commensal rodent pests. These molecules are more potent (nearly 100 times) than the first-generation due to their longer half-life with longer tissue-persistence and better efficacy. First-generation molecules have tissue persistence of a few days, while the second-generation molecules have tissue persistence of a few weeks. In various parts of the world, the long-acting superwarfarins have become the most common rodenticide poisoning encountered in humans **(Table 19.1.3)**.[36]

According to US National Poison Data System, over the 5-year period (2011–2015), the cumulated number of exposures is 44,095 for long-acting superwarfarin type and 1,029 for warfarin-type drugs. Children less than 5 years were involved maximally (88%). In cases associated with significant complications, severe bleedings are observed in less than 10% of cases, with fatal bleedings occurring in only eight patients among the 44,095 exposed.[4,37]

Table 19.1.3: Anticoagulant rodenticides.[32]

Anticoagulant class	Generic name	Commercial product
Coumarin	• Warfarin • Coumatetralyl	• D-Con Mouse Prufe • Fumarin • Hot shot Rat • Mouse killer Racumin
4-hydroxycoumarin (Superwarfarin)	• Brodifacoum • Bromadiolone • Difenacoum	• Havoc • Talon • Super-Caid Endox • Commercial preparation
Indandione (Superwarfarin)	• Chlorophacinone • Diphacinone • Pindone	• Caid • Drat • Rozol

Evolution of Anticoagulant Rodenticides

The first methods used to control rodent populations aimed to kill them immediately. They were based on physical traps or rapid killer molecules like strychnine. However, the neophobic behavior of rodents and their social organization make these methods ineffective because the rapidity of symptoms or death after bait eating by the fellow rats induces bait aversion in the remaining rodent population. That is how a slower onset of action by anticoagulants is advantageous as the rodents do not link their symptoms and death to bait eating and consequently do not shy away from bait.[38]

Mechanism of Action

Both short- and long-acting anticoagulants inhibit the activity of vitamin K 2,3-epoxide reductase, an enzyme involved in the synthesis of the active form of vitamin K leading to decrease in the concentration of active vitamin K-dependent clotting factors II, VII, IX, and X. This results in an increase of clotting times and then, with time, to death by hemorrhages. Some of these also damage the capillaries and increase their permeability thereby increasing the risk of hemorrhage.

Onset of anticoagulant effect is seen in 15–20 hours after ingestion. VKAs are mainly stored in liver. Their liver storage and their elimination are key factors, which determine a part of their efficiency and their persistence. The half-life of warfarin is 35 hours, brodifacoum 56 days (7 weeks), and chlorophacinone 6–11 days. Hence, large symptomatic ingestions with superwarfarins require weeks to months of medical care.

Clinical Features

Bleeding following accidental ingestion of anticoagulant rodenticides is unlikely in children, though prothrombin time (PT) may be mildly prolonged. Minor to life-threatening bleeding may occur following acute intentional ingestion of large amounts. The presence of petechiae under a blood pressure cuff may alert the physician to such coagulopathy.

The following complications have been reported:
- Spontaneous intra-abdominal hemorrhage
- Hematuria
- Hematemesis
- Spontaneous hemoperitoneum
- Extremity pain associated with compartment syndrome
- Intracerebral hemorrhage
- Death.

Suicidal large ingestions by adolescents can lead to profound and prolonged anticoagulation with serious or life-threatening hemorrhage, including GI, genitourinary, and intracranial bleeding commencing at 24–48 hours after exposure. The most common bleeding after exposure is frank hematuria with abdominal or flank pain.[39] With significant bleeding, hemorrhagic shock may occur. With intracranial bleeding, signs of increased intracranial pressure are seen.

After ingestion of second-generation agents (superwarfarins), coagulopathy may be present for many months and recurrent bleeding is possible.

Investigations

The diagnosis of anticoagulant rodenticide intoxication has to be considered for any patient with prolonged PT (increased INR) and prolonged activated partial prothrombin time (APTT). The vitamin K-dependent factor II, VII, X, and IX coagulant activities are decreased, while factor V coagulant activity and the fibrinogen levels are normal. Coagulation studies are expected to be normal immediately after exposure to anticoagulants. These patients may require serial testing for 2 days to confirm or rule out toxicity.

Management

One dose of activated charcoal can be given, if the patient is brought within 1–2 hours. For small, unintentional ingestions of an anticoagulant rodenticide, repeat PT measurements 24- and 48-hour postingestion to ensure no coagulation disturbances. Intentional exposure to AR for suicidal or other reasons may require substantial treatment with vitamin K for a protracted period of time, particularly in the face of exposure to one of the superwarfarins.

Such patients and those with bleeding should be managed in consultation with a hematologist.

If there is no coagulopathy: No treatment is required and counseling for prevention of further exposure is all that is needed.

Coagulopathy without active hemorrhage in superwarfarin poisoning:
- *If international normalized ratio (INR) < 4*: No active treatment, but periodic monitoring with advice to prevent trauma is all that is required.
- *If INR > 4*: Institution of oral vitamin K therapy is suggested.

Vitamin K1 (phytomenadione, which is the active form of vitamin K) is administered for bleeding or significant increase in PT/INR. Vitamin K3 (menadione) is not effective. Oral vitamin K1 is safest with onset of action within 6-12 hours and can be given 3-4 times/day. Oral vitamin K1 can be administered as follows—adults and children over 12 years: 15-25 mg; children under 12 years: 5-10 mg.

Coagulopathy with bleeding:
- *Minor bleed*: Oral vitamin K1 may be required for prolonged duration in superwarfarin poisoning in consultation with a hematologist.[40]
- *Major bleed (life-threatening gastrointestinal, genitourinary, or intracranial hemorrhage)*: In addition to vitamin K, prothrombin complex concentrate (25-50 IU/kg) and either recombinant factor VIIa (20 µg/kg) or fresh frozen plasma (15-20 mL/kg) may be needed to rapidly reverse anticoagulation.[41]

Vitamin K can be given by intravenous (IV) route in a dose of 0.3 mg/kg with a maximum of 10 mg per dose. The onset of action of IV K1 is rapid in 1-2 hours, but there is a risk of anaphylactic reactions; hence, it should be used only in severe cases. Other adverse reactions are flushing, hypotension, cyanosis, dizziness, diaphoresis, dyspnea, cardiac, and/or respiratory arrest. Oral K1 50-100 mg may be needed for weeks to months following initial IV therapy for ingestion of large quantities of superwarfarin compounds. Such patients will need consultation with a hematologist for management.

In contrast to other rodenticides, anticoagulant rodenticides have an effective antidote, the vitamin K. Consequently, anticoagulant poisoning is rarely fatal once recognized and treated promptly.

■ OTHER RODENTICIDES

Currently, the metal phosphides, white/yellow phosphorus, and anticoagulant rodenticides are the ones, which are implicated in rodent poisoning in Indian studies. Still, a substantial proportion is due to unknown poisons resulting from Lax market regulations and absent labeling over the packets of pesticides/rodenticides. A summary of rodenticides including ones currently not much used, mode of action, clinical signs and symptoms of poisoning, and the available treatment is given **(Table 19.1.4)**.[42]

Table 19.1.4: Rodenticides: Action, estimated fatal dose, signs, symptoms, and antidote.

Name	Mechanism of action	Estimated fetal dose	Signs and symptoms	Antidote
Highly toxic signal work: "Danger" (LD < 50 mg/kg) in rats				
Aluminum phosphide, Zinc phosphide (powder, rotten fish or phosphorus odor) normally used as 1% concentration	Releases phosphine on contact with water or acid in stomach	2–10 mg/kg	Rotten fish odor, GI and CVS toxicity ALI Coma, seizures Renal toxicity	Dilute with $NaHCO_3$ Coconut oil
Elemental phosphorus (yellow, waxy paste)	Local irritation Burns on contact GI/liver/renal damage	1 mg/kg	Skin/GI burns "Smoking" luminescent, vomiting, and stools Jaundice CVS symptoms Coma, seizures Cardiac arrest	Supportive care
Thallium (white crystals)	Combines with mitochondrial SH groups, interferes with oxidative phosphorylation	14 mg/kg	Abdominal pain Diarrhea Painful neuropathy Coma, seizures	AC Prussian blue
Sodium monofluoroacetate (SMFA) (white crystals)	Interferes with Krebs cycle	3.7 mg/kg	Seizures, coma, VT, VF	Experimental
Arsenic (Powder)	Combines with SH group and interferes with enzymatic reactions	1.4 mg/kg	GIT symptoms CVS (VT, Torsades de pointes) Altered sensorium Garlic odor (Death 1–24 hours)	Succimer, Dimercaprol Hemodialysis, if AKI
Barium (lump)	Hypokalemia, NM blockade	20–30 mg/kg	Paralysis GIT symptoms Dysrhythmia CVS and respiratory failure	Orogastric lavage with Na_2SO_4, K replacement

Contd...

Contd...

Name	Mechanism of action	Estimated fetal dose	Signs and symptoms	Antidote
Sodium fluoro-acetamide	Interferes with Krebs cycle	13–14 mg/kg	Seizures Coma VT, VF	Experimental
Moderate toxicity "Warning"				
Cholecalciferol (D3) pellets	Hypercalcemia		Lethargy weakness Polyuria, renal injury Hypercalcemia	Fluids, Furosemide, Prednisolone, Calcitonin Hemodialysis
Low toxicity "Caution"				
Anticoagulant Long-acting hydroxy-coumarin 4-hydroxycou-marin (grain-based bait)	Interferes with clotting factors II, VII, IX, and X		Increased INR Bleeding to death	Vitamin K1 FFP Activated FVII Prothrombin complex concentrate
Indanedione: Diphacinone Chlorophaci-none	Interferes with clotting factors II, VII, IX, and X		Increased INR Bleeding to death Chronic Ingestion/CVS and CNS	Vitamin K1 FFP Activated FVII Prothrombin complex concentrate

(AKI: acute kidney injury; ALI: acute lung injury; CNS: central nervous system; CVS: cardiovascular system; FFP: fresh frozen plasma; GIT: gastrointestinal tract; VF: ventricular fibrillation; VT: ventricular tachycardia; INR: international normalized ratio)
Note: Danger, Warning, and *Caution* are the signals on the package of rodenticides in other countries.
Source: Modified from—Flomenbaum NE. Pesticide: An overview of rodenticides and pesticides. In: Nelson LS, Lewin NA, Howland MA, Hoffman RS, Goldfrank LR, Flomenbaum NE (Eds). Goldfrank's Toxicologic Emergencies, 9th edition. New York: McGraw Hill Medical; 2011. pp. 1423-33.

■ CONCLUSION

Strict implementation of nationwide pesticide regulation including restriction of availability of rodenticides, usage of alternative rodenticides less toxic to humans, increasing the awareness among the public and healthcare workers about the proper use, and improved medical management in consultation with regional or national poison control centers could reduce the mortality due to rodenticide poisons especially those due to metal phosphides and phosphorus, as there is no specific antidote available presently for them.[12,25] Older children and adolescents with suicidal poisoning will require psychiatric counseling after the treatment of poisoning. Prevention of further episodes of accidental poisoning is important in young children.

REFERENCES

1. Buckle AP, Smith RH. Rodent Pests and Their Control, 2nd edition. Boston, MA: CAB; 2015. pp. 42.
2. Parshad VR. Rodent control in India. Integrated Pest Manag Rev. 1999;4(2):97-126.
3. Pimentel D, Lach L, Zuniga R, et al. Environmental and economic costs of nonindigenous species in the United States. BioScience. 2000;50(1):53-65.
4. Lefebvre S, Fourel I, Queffélec S, et al. (2017). Poisoning by Anticoagulant Rodenticides in Humans and Animals: Causes and Consequences. [online] Available from https://www.intechopen.com/books/poisoning-from-specific-toxic-agents-to-novel-rapid-and-simplified-techniques-for-analysis/poisoning-by-anticoagulant-rodenticides-in-humans-and-animals-causes-and-consequences. [Last accessed December, 2019].
5. Eddleston M, Karalliedde L, Buckley N, et al. Pesticide poisoning in the developing world—a minimum pesticides list. Lancet. 2002;360(9340):1163-7.
6. Nalabothu M, Monigari N, Acharya R. Clinical profile and outcomes of rodenticide poisoning in tertiary care hospital. Int J Sci Res Pub. 2015;8(5):1-12.
7. Suneetha DK, Inbanathan J, Kannoth S, et al. Profile of rat killer poisoning cases in a tertiary care hospital at Mysore. Int J Sci Stud. 2016;3(12):264-7.
8. Peshin S, Srivastava A, Halder N, et al. Pesticide poisoning trend analysis of 13 years: A retrospective study based on telephone calls at the National Poisons Information Centre, All India Institute of Medical Sciences, New Delhi. J Forensic Legal Med. 2014;22:57-61.
9. Proudfoot AT. Aluminium and zinc phosphide poisoning. Clin Toxicol (Phila). 2009;47(2):89-100.
10. Mehrpour O, Jafarzadeh M, Abdollahi M. A systematic review of aluminium phosphide poisoning. Arh Hig Rada Toksikol. 2012;63(1):61-73.
11. Goel A, Aggarwal P. Pesticide poisoning. Natl Med J India. 2007;20(4):182-91.
12. Bajwa SJS, Bajwa SK, Kaur J, et al. Management of celphos poisoning with a novel intervention: A ray of hope in the darkest of clouds. Anesth Essays Res. 2010;4(1):20-4.
13. Singh D, Dewan I, Pandey AN, et al. Spectrum of unnatural fatalities in the Chandigarh zone of north-west India: a 25 year autopsy study from a tertiary care hospital. J Clin Forensic Med. 2003;10(3):145-52.
14. Chugh SN, Chugh K, Arora V, et al. Blood catalase levels in acute aluminium phosphide poisoning. J Assoc Physicians India. 1997;45:379-80.
15. Hsu CH, Chi BC, Liu MY, et al. Phosphine-induced oxidative damage in rats: Role of glutathione. Toxicology. 2002;179(1-2):1-8.
16. Siwach SB, Singh P, Ahlawat S, et al. A study of serum and tissue magnesium content in patients of aluminium phosphide poisoning and critical evaluation of high dose MgSO4 therapy in reducing mortality. J Assoc Physicians India. 1994;42(2):107-10.
17. Siwach SB, Singh H, Jagdish, et al. Cardiac arrhythmias in aluminium phosphide poisoning studied by on continuous holter and cardioscopic monitoring. J Assoc Physicians India. 1998;46(7):598-601.
18. Singh RB, Rastogi SS, Singh DS. Cardiovascular manifestations of aluminium phosphide intoxication. J Assoc Physicians India. 1989;37(9):590-2.

19. Jain RK, Gouda NB, Sharma VK, et al. Esophageal complications following aluminium phosphide ingestion: an emerging issue among survivors of poisoning. Dysphagia. 2011;25(4):271-6.
20. Gupta S, Ahlawat SK. Aluminum phosphide poisoning-a review. J Toxicol Clin Toxicol. 1995;33(1):19-24.
21. Wahab A, Zaheer MS, Wahab S, et al. Acute aluminium phosphide poisoning: An update. Hong Kong J Emerg Med. 2008;15(3):152-5.
22. Shadnia S, Soltaninejad K. Spontaneous ignition due to intentional acute aluminum phosphide poisoning. J Emerg Med. 2011;40(2):179-81.
23. Musshoff F. A gas chromatographic analysis of phosphine in biological material in a case of suicide. Forensic Sci Int. 2008;177(2-3):e35-8.
24. Jayashree M, Kulgod V, Sharma A; IAP ALS Group. Recognition of a sick child: A structured approach. IAP ALS Handbook, 1st edition. New Delhi, India: IAP National Publishing House; 2018. pp. 10-27.
25. Gurjar M, Baronia AK, Azim A, et al. Managing aluminum phosphide poisonings. J Emerg Trauma Shock. 2011;4(3):378-84.
26. Shadnia S, Rahimi M, Pajoumand A, et al. Successful treatment of acute aluminium phosphide poisoning: Possible benefit of coconut oil. Hum Exp Toxicol. 2005;24(4):215-8.
27. Siddaiah L, Adhyapak S, Jaydev S, et al. Intra-aortic balloon pump in toxic myocarditis due to aluminium phosphide poisoning. J Med Toxicol. 2009;5(2):80-3.
28. Chacko J, Shivaprasad C. Fatal aluminium phosphide poisoning due to myocardial depression refractory to high dose inotropic support and intra-aortic balloon counterpulsation. Indian J Crit Care Med. 2008;12(1):37-8.
29. Duenas A, Perez-Castrillon JL, Cobos MA, et al. Treatment of the cardiovascular manifestations of phosphine poisoning with trimetazidine, a new anti-ischemic drug. Am J Emerg Med. 1999;17(2):219-20.
30. Jaiswal S, Verma RK, Tewari N. Aluminium phosphide poisoning: Effect of correction of severe metabolic acidosis on patient outcome. Indian J Crit Care Med. 2009;13(1):21-4.
31. Soltaninejad K, Nelson LS, Khodakarim N, et al. Unusual complication of aluminum phosphide poisoning: Development of hemolysis and methemoglobinemia and its successful treatment. Indian J Crit Care Med. 2011;15(2):117-9.
32. Thangavelu S, Ramachandran P, Mahender E. Rodenticide poisoning. Handbook on Poisoning in children, IJPP Series-6. Chennai, India: Alamu Printing Press; 2013. pp. 145-52.
33. Hassanian-Moghaddam H, Shahnazi M, Zamani N, et al. Abdominal imaging in zinc phosphide poisoning. Emerg Radiol. 2014;21(3):329-31.
34. González-Andrade F, López-Pulles R. White phosphorus poisoning by oral ingestion of firecrackers or little devils: current experience in Ecuador. Clin Toxicol (Phila). 2011;49(1):29-33.
35. Payen C, Dellinger A, Pulce C, et al. Intoxication by large amounts of barium nitrate overcome by early massive K supplementation and oral administration of magnesium sulphate. Hum Exp Toxicol. 2011;30(1):34-7.
36. Lung D, Tarabar A. (2015). Rodenticide Toxicity: Background, Etiology, Epidemiology. Medscape Updated: Dec 29, 2015. [online] Available from https://

emedicine.medscape.com/article/818130-overview#showall. [Last accessed December, 2019].

37. Mowry JB, Spyker DA, Brooks DE, et al. 2015 Annual Report of the American Association of Poison Control Centers' National Poison Data System (NPDS): 33rd Annual Report. Clin Toxicol (Phila). 2016;54(10):924-1109.
38. Parshad VR, Kochar JK. Potential of three rodenticides to induce conditioned aversion to their baits in the Indian mole rat, Bandicota bengalensis. Appl Anim Behav Sci. 1995;45(3):267-76.
39. Watt BE, Proudfoot AT, Bradberry SM, et al. Anticoagulant rodenticides. Toxicol Rev. 2005;24(4):259-69.
40. Bruno GR, Howland MA, McMeeking A, et al. Long-acting anticoagulant overdose: brodifacoum kinetics and optimal vitamin K dosing. Ann Emerg Med. 2000;36(3):262-7.
41. Zupancić-Salek S, Kovacević-Metelko J, Radman I. Successful reversal of anticoagulant effect of superwarfarin poisoning with recombinant activated factor VII. Blood Coagul Fibrinolysis. 2005;16(4):239-44.
42. Flomenbaum NE. Pesticide: An overview of rodenticides and pesticides. In: Nelson LS, Lewin NA, Howland MA, Hoffman RS, Goldfrank LR, Flomenbaum NE (Eds). Goldfrank's Toxicologic Emergencies, 9th edition. New York: McGraw Hill Medical; 2011. pp. 1423-33.

Index

Page numbers followed by *b* refer to box, *f* refer to figure, *fc* refer to flowchart, and *t* refer to table.

A

Abacavir 145, 148
Abdominal compartment syndrome 491
Absolute lymphocyte count 85
Absolute neutrophil count 85
Acellular pertussis, effectiveness of 65
Acid-fast bacilli 91, 190
Acidosis 509
  metabolic 489
  severe 490
Acquired immunodeficiency syndrome 261
  diagnosis 143
  management 143
Activated partial prothrombin time 520
Acute encephalitis syndrome 186
  global watchlist of 196
Acute encephalopathy 185
  causes of 187*t*
Acute heart failure 200
  diagnosis of 207*fc*
  management of 207*fc*
Acute lung injury, transfusion related 483
Acute lymphoblastic leukemia 398, 402*b*, 405, 442
  classification of 401*b*
  risk stratification of 400*t*
Acute respiratory distress syndrome 156, 480, 485*f*, 486, 511, 514
  causes of 483*t*
  resolution of 486
Adenoid measurement 135*f*
Adenoidectomy 140
Adenosine
  deaminase level, elevated 105
  monophosphate 220
Adenotonsillar hypertrophy 128, 135, 137
  treatment of 139
Adenotonsillectomy 125, 133, 138, 140
  long-term impacts of 140
  rates of 130
Adenovirus 191, 309
Adhesion molecules, expression of 486
Adolescent suicides, hypothesis of 460
Adrenomedullin 202
Advanced cardiac life support 207
Advisory Committee on Immunization Practices 122
Aedes aegypti 159
Aedes albopictus 159
  mosquito 159
Agammaglobulinemia 79, 260
Air bronchogram 499*f*
Airway pressure release ventilation 480, 493
Alagille syndrome 418
Alanine aminotransferase 206, 269, 273, 278, 279
Albinism 84
Alcohol abuse 273
Aldosterone antagonists 210
Alkaline phosphatase 46, 206
Allergic diseases
  incidence of 242
  prevalence of 242
Allergic disorders, diagnosis of 242
Allergy 241
  latex 244
  skin testing 244
    contraindications of 244
Allogeneic bone marrow transplant recipients 497
Alopecia 84
  areata 442
Alpha-fetoprotein 453
Alpha-thalassemia
  intermedia 344
  syndromes, classification of 344*t*
Aluminum 508
  chloride 509
  hydroxide 509
  phosphide 507, 508, 522
    management of 514*fc*
    toxicity, mechanisms of 510*fc*
Alveolar epithelium 484
  capillary structure, disruption of 484
Alveoli, closing of 487
Alzheimer disease 442
American Academy of Child and Adolescent Psychiatry 473
American Academy of Pediatrics 21, 122, 138
  guidelines 473
American Association for Study of Liver Diseases 276
American College of Medical Genetics and Genomics 421
American Psychiatric Association 473
American-European Consensus Conference 480
Amikacin 98, 311
Aminoglycosides 94, 95
  second-line 107

Aminosalicylic acid 257
Amlodipine 366
Amoxicillin 310, 333
Ampicillin 333
Amrinone 211
Analgesics 465
Anemia
  diagnosis of 372*t*
  microcytic hypochromic 379*fc*
Angiogenesis 43
Angiotensin converting enzyme 202, 484
  inhibitor 208, 209, 213
Angiotensin receptor
  antagonist 213
  blocker 213
Anhidrotic ectodermal dysplasia 78
Ankylostoma duodenale 392
Annual influenza
  epidemics 113
  vaccination 123
  vaccine, use of 163
Anti-asthma drugs 230*t*
Antibiotic 94, 309
  allergies, multiple 130
  intravenous 311*t*
  oral 310*t*
  therapy 121
Antibody
  based tests 119
  deficiencies, predominantly 79
  dependent cell-mediated cytotoxicity 407
  detection assays 117
  enzyme-labeled 243
  expressing B memory cells 127
  mediated rejection 292
  monoclonal 158, 165, 407
Anticoagulant rodenticides 507, 518, 519*t*, 521
  evolution of 519
Antidepressant medication 466
Antiepileptic drugs 181, 183
  multiple 175
Antigen detection tests 117, 118
Anti-hantavirus immunoglobulin G 158
Anti-human immunodeficiency virus agents, second class of 145
Anti-inflammatory medicines 128
Antileukemia drugs 399
Antineutrophil cytoplasmic antibody 253
Antioxidant 209
Antiretroviral drug 145, 146
  short course of 150
Antiretroviral therapy 145, 148, 153
Anti-saccharomyces cerevisiae 253
Antitubercular drugs 94
Antitubercular therapy 109, 261
Antiviral medicines 165

Aorta, coarctation of 201, 202
Aortic arch, interrupted 201
Aortic stenosis 201, 202
Apnea
  hypopnea index 136
  obstructive 131
Apneic spells, life-threatening 44
Apoptosis 407
Appetite, loss of 204
Arrhythmia 205
  serious cardiac 509
Arsenic 522
Arterial blood gas 500
  analysis 206
Arterial gas monitoring, continuous 500
Arterial oxygen, partial pressure of 481
Artery thrombosis, hepatic 291, 295
Arthritis
  pyogenic sterile 82
  rheumatoid 45
Ascites 204
Ascorbic acid content, approximate 390*t*
Asepsis 307
Asian Pacific Association for Study of Liver 276
Aspartate aminotransferase 206
Aspiration 483
Asthma 133, 220, 224, 229
  allergic 244
  control
    assessment of 232*t*
    questionnaire 231
  eosinophilic 224
  global initiative for 221, 228
  management of 222
  predictive index, modified 234, 235*t*
  severe uncontrolled 244
Atkins diet, modified 182, 183
Atresia
  choanae 332
  duodenal 442, 445*f*
Atrial natriuretic peptide 203
Atrioventricular canal defects 442
Attention deficit hyperactivity disorder 133
Autoimmune
  lymphoproliferative syndrome 76, 80
  polyendocrinopathy with candidiasis and ectodermal dystrophy syndrome 80, 441
Autoinflammatory disorders 81
Automated microscopy techniques 94
Automated smart microscopy 94
Autosomal recessive disease 441
Axonal proliferation 417
Aysplasia, bronchopulmonary 18
Azacytidine 365
Azathioprine 255, 295

B

Bacillus calmette-guérin 58, 60, 81, 84, 102
   reaction, disseminated 81
Bacteria 308
Bacteriuria, asymptomatic 306
Baloxavir
   marboxil 121
   single dose 121
Barium 522
   carbonate 507, 517
Basophil histamine release test 247
B-cell receptor 73
Beclomethasone 226-228
   dipropionate 228
Bedaquiline 95
Behavioral therapy, dialectical 472
Bell's muscle 326f
Beta-blockers 209, 210, 212
Beta-lactamase-producing microorganisms 128
Beta-receptor antagonists 208
Beta-thalassemia
   classification of 344t
   intermedia 344
   pathophysiology of 342fc
   prevalence of 341t
Bile canalicular transporter defects 4
Bile ducts, extrahepatic 4
Bi-level positive airway pressure 482
   use of 488
Biliary stenosis 292
Bilirubin
   damage 4
   encephalopathy 9
     acute 5
     signs of 7f
   induced neurologic dysfunction score 5, 6t
   metabolism 2, 3fc
   neurotoxicity 4, 5
   overproduction 4
   transcutaneous 5, 11
   values 4
Biochemical hypovitaminosis D, prevalence of 51
Biometric liver
   spectrometry 350
   susceptometry 350
Biopsy 106
Bio-Rad variant machine 349f
Birth weight
   low 11
   normal 40
   very low 12
Bladder
   bowel function, evaluation of 328
   diverticula 332

   dysfunction 328
     non-neurogenic 324
   neurogenic 318, 328
   outlet obstruction 328
   ultrasonography of 329
Blinatumomab 407, 408, 408f
Blood
   brain natriuretic peptide 131
   disorders 114
   fractional inspired oxygen 496
   investigations 205, 206t
   pressure 321, 336
   samples testing 423
   transfusion 160
   urea nitrogen 206
Body mass index 289
Bone
   and joints, tuberculosis of 106
   marrow
     examination 350, 382
     transplant 364, 364f
   mineral density 362f
     reduced 227
   remodelling, state of 41
Boomerang sign 193f
Borrelia burgdorferi 194
Bovine milk allergy 261
Bovine rotavirus vaccine 67
Bowel dysfunction 328
Bradyarrhythmias 205
Bradycardia 190, 210
Bradykinin 202
Brain oxygen optimization 28
Breastfeeds, cessation of 144
Breathing
   during sleep, abnormal 132
   oral 132
Breathlessness 115, 220
British Thoracic Society 222
Brodifacoum 507
Bromadiolone 507
Bronchial asthma
   diagnosis of 220
   management of 220
Bronchial provocation tests 225
Bronchoalveolar lavage 92, 104, 108, 115, 116, 234, 487
Bronchodilator 92, 220, 226
Bronchoscopy 92
Bronchospasm 210
Bruton tyrosine kinase 76
B-type natriuretic peptide 203, 206, 207
Budesonide 226-228
Burkitt's leukemia 401
Burns, mucosal 516
Butyrates 365

C

Calcineurin inhibitors 295
Calcitriol 41
Calcium 44t
  causes nutritional rickets 38
  channel defects 78
  deficiency 38
  metabolism, normal 38
  sensitizer 211
  serum 363
Calculate peripheral capillary oxygen
    saturation 482
Calicheamicin 408
Canadian Thoracic Society 222
Candidiasis, mucocutaneous 84
Capillary endothelium 484
Capnography 500
Capreomycin 98
Captopril 209
Carbapenems 312
Carbon dioxide monitoring, continuous 500
Carcinoma, hepatocellular 264, 269, 272, 287
Cardiac catheterization 206
Cardiac dysfunction 410, 492
Cardiac failure, congestive 200
Cardiac index 206
Cardiac resynchronization therapy 213, 214
Cardiomyocyte 43
  injury 201
Cardiomyopathy 44, 208, 216
  dilated 208
  precipitating factors of 201t
Cardiopulmonary bypass
  machine, modified 495
  surgery 483
Cardiovascular support 513
Cardiovascular system 523
  pathophysiology 131
Cartridge-based nucleic acid amplification
    methods 96
    test 104, 107
Carvedilol 209, 210
Catalase 509
Cataract, congenital 442
Cefixime 310
Ceftriaxone 311, 360
Celiac disease 373, 393, 442
Cellscope 94
Cellular rejection, acute 292
Cellular responsiveness, modulation of 43
Cellulose acetate electrophoresis 348f
Central nervous system 81, 399, 400, 510, 523
  directed therapy 405
  features of 92
  infection 179, 185
  pathophysiology 131
  toxicity 516
  tuberculosis 106

Central venous pressure 513, 514
Cephalexin 310, 333
Cephalhematoma 5
Cephalosporin 310, 320
Cerebellum 4
Cerebral malaria 185
Cerebrospinal fluid 91, 187, 190, 190t, 195
Cervical
  adenitis syndrome 130
  adenopathy, tuberculous 91
CHARGE syndrome 332
Chediak-Higashi syndrome 85
Chelation therapy 355
Chemiluminescent assays 47
Chemoprophylaxis 103, 123
  antiviral 124
Chemotherapeutic agents, newer 405
Chest
  pain 204
  tightness 220
  wall elastance 492
  X-ray 91, 104, 205, 207
Chikungunya 158, 189
  epidemics 165
Childhood
  adenotonsillectomy trial 137
  asthma control test 231
  epilepsy 172
  syndromes 170
Chimeric antigen receptor 398
  T-cell 407, 409
  therapy 409
Chlorophacinone 507
Cholecalciferol pellets 523
Cholestasis, progressive familial intrahepatic 290
Chondrocyte differentiation 38
Choreoathetosis 427
Choreo-athetotic movements 189
Chromatography, microcolumn 347
Chromosome
  therapy 455
  translocation of 440f
Chronic granulomatous disease 74, 80, 83, 260
Chronic hepatitis 45
  B 273, 274, 277, 278fc, 279fc
    prevalence of 264
    reactivation of 270, 277
    treatment of 279t
    virus infection 273t
Ciprofloxacin 310, 360
Cirrhosis 264, 277
Cisatracurium 498
Clean catch urine sample 306
Clobazam 178
Clofarabine 405
Clofazimine 95

Clostridium difficile 84, 259
Clover coumarin 518
Coagulopathy 410, 521
Co-amoxiclav 310, 311
Cobalt 375
Cognitive behavioral therapy 472
Cohen's cross-trigonal reimplantation 334
Colitis 80
    acute severe 259
    eosinophilic 261
Coloboma 332
Colon, multiple internal fistulae of 252*f*
Colony forming units 307, 329
Columbia-suicide severity rating scale 468
Coma 516
Compact fluorescent lamp 10, 11
Complete blood count 108, 206, 345, 353
Computed tomography 190, 260, 315
    contrast-enhanced 91, 106
    scan 499, 499*f*
Confusion 516
Congenital hypothyroidism 416, 418*t*, 420, 425*fc*
    epidemiology of 417
    etiology of 418
    types of 420*t*
Congestion 200
Conjunctivitis 488
    allergic 244
Consciousness
    altered level of 489
    level of 120, 489
Constipation 420
Continuous antibiotic prophylaxis 332
    role of 332
Continuous positive airway pressure 18, 24, 481, 482, 488
Conventional antiepileptic drug, choice of 183*b*
Coombs' test 7
    direct 7
Core antigen 265
Corn-soya-milk preparation 391
Coronavirus 157
Corpus callosotomy 184
Corticosteroids 295
    intranasal 139
    prenatal 17
    therapy 237
Cotrimoxazole 152, 310
    prophylaxis 152
Cough 220
    moist 233
    nocturnal 220
Coumatetralyl 507
C-reactive protein 108, 190, 207, 253, 380
Crigler-Najjar syndrome 297

Crimean-congo hemorrhagic fever 160, 196
    virus 160, 161
Crohn's disease 46, 106, 250, 251*t*, 254, 256, 387
    infantile 252*f*
    management of 258*fc*
Cryptosporidium 84
Cyclic guanosine monophosphate 202, 494
Cycloserine 95
Cysteinyl leukotrienes, overproduction of 134
Cystic fibrosis 80, 387
Cystitis 315, 315*f*
    hemorrhagic 309
Cystourethrogram 318
Cystourethrography 331
Cytarabine 404
Cytogenetics, high-risk 402
Cytokine
    anti-inflammatory 484
    dysregulation 114
    proinflammatory 211
    release syndrome 409
Cytomegalovirus 143, 259, 293, 352, 354
Cytosine arabinoside, high-dose 404
Cytotoxic T lymphocyte 79
    associated antigen 76
Cytotoxicity, complement-mediated 407

D

Daycare transfusion center 354
Daytime sleepiness, excessive 132
Dead space ventilation 494
Deafness 442
Deferasirox 356
Deferiprone 356
    side effects of 356
Deferitin 358
Dehydrocholesterol 41
Dendritic cells 43
Dengue 189
Deoxyribonucleic acid 77, 97, 266
    double-stranded 155
Depression, treatment of severe 466
Dermatological infection 261
Desferrioxamine 355
    chelatable iron 357
Desferrithiocin 358
Device therapy 213
Dextrocardia 233
Dextromer 333
Diabetes mellitus 45, 114, 115, 441
    neonatal 418
Diaphragm
    electrical activity of 500
    function of 500
Diarrhea, chronic 143, 373
Diastolic ventricular relaxation 211
Dietary modification 388

Difenacoum 507
Diffusion-weighted imaging 192
Dihydroxyvitamin D 41
Dimercaptosuccinic acid 314, 316, 328
Di-palmitoyl-phosphatidyl-choline 19
Diphacinone 507
Diphtheria, tetanus, and pertussis 64
    vaccines 59, 64
Direct nuclear cystogram 330
Disability-adjusted life year 2
Disseminated intravascular coagulation 186, 510
Diuresis 213
Dizziness 204, 210
Dobrava-Belgrade virus 158
Dobutamine 211
Dolutegravir 147, 148
Domino liver transplantation 289
Donation after cardiac death 288
Donor selection criteria 288, 289*t*
Doose syndrome 179
Dopamine 211, 426
Double bubble appearance 445*f*
Down syndrome 438, 439*t*, 440*f*, 441, 442, 445*f*, 447*b*, 449*t*, 452*t*
Doxycycline 360
Dravet syndrome 178
Dried blood spot 422
    collection of 423*f*
Driving pressure 487
Drug
    allergy 244
    drug interaction 148
    overdose 483
Dual energy X-ray absorptiometry 351, 361
Duodenal erosions 510
Dyshormonogenesis 418, 420, 427, 430
Dyskeratosis 78
Dysplasias, immuno-osseous 78
Dyspnea 204
Dysrhythmias 215
Dystrophic nails 84

E

Ebola
    viral disease 164
    virus 161, 196
Echocardiogram 207
Echocardiography 205
Eczema, severe 244
Edema 204, 205
    pulmonary 204, 205, 410, 498, 509
Efavirenz 146, 148, 151
Electrocardiogram 205, 207, 358
Electrochemiluminescence assay 40
Electroencephalogram 171, 181, 188, 194
Electrolyte, serum 206

Elevated mean airway pressure 497
Empiric antitubercular therapy 105
Emtricitabine 145, 147, 148
Enalapril 209
Encephalitides, emerging 194
Encephalitis 185
    acute disseminated 192
    autoimmune limbic 192
Encephalomyelitis, acute disseminated 189, 193*f*
Encephalopathy 185
    acute febrile 185, 195
    early infantile epileptic 175, 179*f*
    early myoclonic 175
    epileptic 175, 180*t*
    myoclonic epileptic 176*f*
    sepsis-associated 196
    with status epilepticus in sleep 176
Endobronchial ultrasound-guided transbronchial needle aspiration 91
Endometrial tissue 96
Endothelial dysfunction, state of 486
Endotracheal tube, selection of 490
End-tidal carbon monoxide 7
Enfurvirtide 146
Enoximone 211
Enterocolitis, necrotizing 16
Enteroviruses 162, 309
Enuresis, secondary 133
Envelope antigen 265
Enzyme 203
    immunoassay methods 119
    linked immunosorbent assay 47, 101, 144, 160
    replacement 87
Eosinophil 224
    cationic protein 247
Epicutaneous test 244
Epidermodysplasia verruciformis 81
Epilepsia partialis continua 182
Epilepsy
    benign 171
    childhood absence 174
    drug resistant 182
    early-onset childhood 172
    focal 171
    generalized 171
    juvenile
        absence 174
        myoclonic 174
    mesial temporal lobe 179
    progressive myoclonic 179*f*
    refractory 179
    seizures, juvenile myoclonic 175*f*
    self-limited focal 171
    severe myoclonic 178

syndrome 170, 171
    febrile infection-related 196
    severe 175, 176t, 180t
    type 170
Epileptic syndromes, age-wise 179f
Episode, acute 235
Epratuzumab 407
Epstein-Barr virus 80, 189, 293
Erythrocyte
    morphology 379
    sedimentation rate 108, 207
        high 253
Erythroderma 84
Erythroferrone inhibitors 368
Erythropoietin 366
Escherichia coli 259, 309
Esophageal manometry 500
Esophagus 510
Estimated glomerular filtration rate 321
Ethambutol 95
Ethylenediaminetetraacetic acid vial 446
Etravirine 146
European Association for Study of Liver 276
European Medicines Agency 367
European Society for Paediatric Gastroenterology, Hepatology and Nutrition 277
Exchange transfusion 10, 12
Exercise 220
Exhaled breath
    condensate 224, 225
    temperature 224
Exhaled nitric oxide, fraction of 223, 224, 246
Extended-spectrum beta-lactamase organisms 309
Extracorporeal life support 480, 495, 496, 514
Extracorporeal membrane oxygenation 207, 215, 494f, 495, 496t
Extrapulmonary disease 96, 99
Extrapulmonary tuberculosis 104, 105
    manifestations of 90
Extraskeletal systemic disorders 38
Extrauterine thyroid adaptation 417
Extravascular lung water 498
Extubation 501
Eyewear, protective 116

F

Failure to thrive 233
Familial hemophagocytic lymphohistiocytosis syndromes 79
Fat, autologous 333
Fatigue 204
Feed pattern 204
Ferritin, serum 349, 380
Ferrous sulphate, oral 382
Fetal globin reactivation 367

Fever
    familial mediterranean 82
    hemorrhagic 158
Fibrinolysis dysfunction 486
Fine-needle aspiration cytology 91
Fistula 510
    perianal 252f
    tracheoesophageal 442
Fixation off phenomenon 173
Flavivirus 159, 160
Flow cytometry 404
Fluid
    attenuated inversion recovery 192
    biochemistry of 91
    cytology of 91
    management 498
    supplementation 9
Fluorescein diacetate 93
Fluorescence microscopy, advantages of 93
Fluorescent *in situ* hybridization 402, 444, 445
Fluoroquinolone 98
Fluticasone 226
    furoate 227
    propionate 227, 228
Focal segmental glomerulosclerosis 328
Folate metabolism 78
Follicle stimulating hormone 363
Follow-up diagnostic test 93
Food
    allergy 45
        oral food challenge for 246
    and drug administration 213, 410
    articles, iron content of 389t
    items, vitamin D content of 43t
    protein allergy, multiple 261
Forced expiratory
    flow 221, 222
    volume 221, 222
Forced inspiratory vital capacity 222
Forced oscillation technique 222
Forced vital capacity 221, 222
Formoterol 226, 228
Frank-Starling mechanism 202
Free erythrocyte protoporphyrin 377, 381
Free fetal deoxyribonucleic acid 444
Fresh frozen plasma 523
Frontotemporal hyperintensity 191f

G

Gallop rhythm 205
Gallstones 363
Gamma chain production 365
Gamma-glutamyl transpeptidase 292
Gas exchange 488
    goals 492
Gastric
    aspirate 92, 104

distention 488
erosions, severe 510
Gastroenterology 249
Gastroesophageal reflux disease 233
Gastrointestinal bleeding 373, 387
Gastrointestinal tract 250, 354, 250, 523
Gata-binding protein 1 442
Gene
   inheritance of 343
   manipulation 365
   therapy 367
Genetic 437
   counseling 451
   disorders 374
   generalized epilepsies 173, 173t, 174
   studies 382
Genital hypoplasia 332
Gentamicin 311, 360
Gianotti-Crosti syndrome 269
Giardiasis 374
Glasgow coma scale 190
Global Consensus Recommendations 44, 47, 49, 50
Global Health Security Agenda 164
Global influenza surveillance and response system 163
Globus pallidus 4
Glomerular filtration rate 320
Glucocorticoid 426
   receptors 226
Glucose-6-phosphate dehydrogenase deficiency 80
Glutathione 509
Glycemic index treatment, low 183
Glycogen storage disease 284
Glycoproteins 163
Graft-versus-host disease 365, 406
Granulocyte colony stimulating factor 270, 363, 407
Granuloma 92, 182
Greenstick fractures 48
Ground glass appearance 499f
Growth 140
   failure 133
   hormone 363
   hormone secretion decreases 131
   plate, poor mineralization of 38
Guanylyl cyclase A 202
Guillain-Barré syndrome 160

H

H1N1 encephalitis 193f
Haemophilus influenzae 64, 128
Hand foot mouth disease 162
Hantaan virus 158
Hantavirus 158
   pulmonary syndrome 158
   zoonotic reservoirs for 158

Haploidentical stem cell transplantation 406
Head injury 483
Heart
   block 210
   disease 332
      congenital 200, 201t, 202t, 418
      cyanotic 481
   failure 200
      advanced 200
      causes of congestive 202t
      chronic 200
      end-stage 200
      pathophysiology of chronic 203fc
      signs of 204t
      symptoms of 204t
      treatment of 207
   lesions, congenital 492
   transplantation 214, 216
Heated humidified high-flow nasal cannula 26
Heel prick sampling, timing of 430
Helicobacter pylori 393
   infection 253
Helminth control 392
Helminthiasis 373
Hemagglutination inhibition test 118, 119
Hemagglutinin 163
Hematemesis 520
Hematocrit 371
Hematology 339
Hematopoietic stem cell 367
   transplant 87, 260, 405, 406
Hematuria 520
Hemispherectomy 184
Hemodynamics 491
Hemoglobin 7, 371
   concentration 378
   E beta-thalassemia 344
   fetal 341, 344, 352
   H disease 344
   pattern of 349f
   quantitation of 347
   saturation, maximum 489
Hemoperitoneum, spontaneous 520
Hemoptysis 115
Hemorrhage
   conjunctival 158
   fetomaternal 374
   intracerebral 520
   intracranial 497
   retinal 158
Henipaviral diseases 164
Henipavirus 157
   genus, paramyxovirus virus of 157
Hepatic dysfunction 363
Hepatitis
   acute viral 269

envelope antigen and antibody 267
severe acute 276
Hepatitis B 64, 359
  acute 274, 276
  core
    antigen 265
    immunoglobulin M 267*f*
  immunoglobulin, combination of 281
  spectrum of 264
  surface antigen 264, 265, 266, 354
  vaccine 59, 64
  viral infection 267*f*
  virus 265*f*, 268, 278, 279
    envelope antigen 267*f*, 273, 279, 279*fc*
    infection 264, 268*f*, 269*fc*, 275
    surface antigen 267*f*, 273, 353
    treatment of 278*fc*
Hepatitis C
  virus 353, 354
  infection 359
Hepatitis core
  antibody 267
  antigen 267
Hepatocytes 376
Hepatology 263
Hepatomegaly 204, 205
Hepatopulmonary syndrome 285
Hepatorenal syndrome 285
Hepatosplenomegaly 5, 261
Hepcidin 381
Heritable disorder 324
Herpes simplex
  encephalitis 81, 191, 191*f*, 194
  virus 81, 195
    encephalitis 188
Higher tuberculin unit, use of 102
High-performance liquid chromatography 47, 347
Hirschsprung disease 442
Homogeneity 499
Hookworm infestation 374
Hormone
  adrenocorticotropic 175, 181, 183, 419
  luteinizing 363
Human chorionic gonadotropin 453
Human cytomegalovirus 359
Human immunodeficiency virus 90, 99, 102, 143-145, 151, 153, 155, 187, 273, 352-354, 359
  antigen 144
  diagnosis of 143, 144
  disease, global 143
  infection 143, 151
    advanced 101
    serological diagnosis of 144
  management 143, 145
  perinatal transmission of 150
  treatment of 145

Human leukocyte antigen 351, 364, 406
Human metapneumoviruses 157
Human monovalent live vaccine 66
Human organ transplant Act 283
Human papilloma virus 64, 81
Human rabies immunoglobulin 70
Hyaluronic acid 333
Hydrocephalus 92, 191
Hydrochloric acid 509
Hydrochlorothiazide 210, 211
Hydronephrosis
  antenatal 324
  postnatal 336
  prenatal 336
Hydroxybenzyl-ethylenediamine-diacetic acid 357, 358
Hydroxycoumarin 523
Hydroxyindoleacetic acid 460
Hydroxylase production 41
Hydroxyurea 366
Hyperbilirubinemia 4, 7*b*, 13*t*
  neonatal 2
  nonconjugated 8
  physiologic 4
  risk factors for 3*t*
Hypercalcemia 48
Hypercapnia, permissive 28, 492
Hypercarbia, permissive 28
Hypercytokinemia 497
Hyperdiploidy 399
Hypergammaglobulinemia 261
Hyperglycemia 210, 513
Hyperimmunoglobulin syndrome 78
Hyperkalemia 210
Hypermagnesemia 510
Hyperplasia, congenital adrenal 423
Hypersplenism 360
Hypertension 132, 304, 327
  intracranial 492
  pulmonary 492, 494
Hypertonic aerosol 220
Hypochloremia 210
Hypoglycemia 420, 432
Hypokalemia 513
Hyponatremia 210
Hypopituitarism 426
Hypoplastic left heart syndrome 201, 202, 216
Hypopneas 131
Hypoproteinemia 373
Hypotension 200, 205, 209, 210, 410, 489, 490, 513, 515
  causes of 490
Hypothalamic-pituitary-adrenal axis 140, 460
Hypothalamic-pituitary-thyroid 425
Hypothermia 420
Hypothesis, dynamic 460
Hypothyroidism 442
  central 419

subclinical 424
transient congenital 419
Hypothyroxinemia 426, 432
Hypotonia 420, 427
Hypoxemia 489
  refractory 483
Hypoxia
  acute onset of severe 480
  permissive 492
Hypsarrhythmia 177*f*

I

Iatrogenic barotrauma, evidence of 497
Icterus neonatorum 2
Idiopathic thrombocytopenic purpura 143
Immune
  dysregulation 80
    diseases of 79
  reactive phase 270, 271
  system
    cells 43
    overview of 73
  tolerant phase 270, 271
Immunity 57
  adaptive 73, 86
  cell-mediated 86
  cellular 74
  humoral 74
  innate 73, 80, 85
Immunization 57
  active 280
  schedule 58
Immunofluorescence assays 119
Immunoglobulin 46, 127
  A 76
  E 76, 220, 230
  G 230
    use of 101
  intravenous 12, 182
  M 76, 101, 158
  therapy, replacement 87
Immunology 241
Immunoradiometric assay 380
Immunosuppression 293, 296
Immunotherapy 407
Imperforate anus 332
Implantable cardioverter defibrillator 213
In vitro screening tests 243, 244
  advantages of 245
Indian Academy of Pediatrics 58, 59, 104, 473
  Advanced Life Support 512
  Advisory Committee on Immunization Practices 122
  Immunization Timetable 62*t*
Indian Council of Medical Research 50, 99, 164
Indian Society for Pediatric and Adolescent Endocrinology 424

Indirect hyperbilirubinemia, exchange transfusion of 11*t*
Inducible nitric oxide synthase 246
Infections
  acute viral 112
  bacterial 360
  chronic 373
  hospital-associated 121
  perinatal 2
  prevention of 86
  respiratory 45
  sinopulmonary 261
  treatment of 87
Inferior vena cava 289
Inflammation, allergic 128
Inflammatory bowel disease 45, 250, 252*t*, 254t-256*t*
  early-onset 259
Inflammatory disease 251*t*
Inflammatory mediators, role of 128
Infliximab 256
Influenza 191
  activity, level of 117
  B viruses 122
  complicated 115t
  diagnosis of 112
  infection, control of 122
  management of 112
  tests 118
  treatment of 112
  vaccination 122
  vaccine 59, 68
    dosage of 123*t*
  virus 112, 113, 163
    epidemiology of 122
    infections 113
    neuraminidase 121
    strain of 113
Inhaled corticosteroid 225, 226, 227*t*, 228*t*, 230
  formulations 227
Inhibit reverse transcriptase enzyme 145
Injury
  alveolar epithelial 484
  inhalation 483
  renal 328
  reperfusion 290
Inotuzumab ozogamicin 407, 408
Insect bite venom allergy 244
Inspired oxygen, fraction of 19, 481, 482
Insulin resistance, homeostatic model assessment of 45
Integrase strand transfer inhibitors 145, 147
Intensive care unit 207
Interferon regulatory factor 7 76
Interferon-gamma 74
  release assays 102
Interleukin 226, 410

Intermediate withdrawal syndrome 497
International Association for Suicide
    Prevention 474
International Collaborative Infantile Spasms
    Study 176
International Committee on Taxonomy of
    Viruses 155
International Extracorporeal Life Support
    Organization 495
International Grading System 326
    of Vesicoureteral Reflux 327*f*
International League Against Epilepsy 170
    Framework of Epilepsy classification 171*f*
    seizure types 170
International normalized ratio 521, 523
Intestinal parasites 374
Intra-aortic balloon pump 514
Intrachromosomal amplification of
    chromosome 400-402
Intracranial infections 190*t*
Intracranial pressure 190
Intradermal route 65
Intradermal skin tests 245
Intranasal steroid 139
    safety and effectiveness of 140
Intraocular pressure, low 158
Intravascular pressures 498
Intravenous drug 264
Intravesical ureter 325*f*
    demonstration of 325*f*
Intubation 489
Invasive methods 107
Iron
    absorption
        enhancers 390
        poor 373
    and folic acid 386
        supplementation program 392*t*
    chelation, adverse effects of 357*t*
    deficiency anemia 371, 377, 379, 383*t*
        high incidence of 349
        nutritional 371
    deficiency, progression of 380*t*
    element, supplementation of 386
    metabolism 375
    overload, role of hepcidin in 368
    refractory iron deficiency anemia 374, 382
    requirements 374
    salts, oral 384*t*
    serum 348, 380
    studies 348
    supplementation 391
    therapy 383*t*
        history of 371
        parenteral 387
        side effects of 388
    transport and storage 376
Ischemia 205, 290

Isolation 120
Isoniazid 95
    dose of 153
    prevention therapy 153
Ivabradine 212

J

Janus kinase 402
    signal transducer and activator of
        transcription 442
Japanese encephalitis 64, 185, 191, 192*f*, 195
Jaundice 2, 6*b*, 6*f*
    conjugated 432
    early detection of 4
    management of 13*t*
Jet ventilation, high-frequency 493

K

Kanamycin 98
Karyotyping 439
Kerley lines 205
Kernicterus 2, 9
Ketogenic diet 178, 182
Kidney
    abnormal 335
    disease, chronic 115
    injury, acute 523
    ultrasonography of 329
Kikuchi disease 105
Klebsiella 309
Koilonychias 378
Kramer's criteria 5

L

Lactate dehydrogenase 206
Lamivudine 145, 147, 148
Landau Kleffner syndrome 176
L-asparaginase 403, 404
Lassa fever 164
Late allograft dysfunction 293
Latent infection
    chemoprophylaxis of 102
    detection of 91, 101
Latent tuberculosis 46
    infection, diagnosis of 102
Lead 375
Left ventricular
    assist device 215
    dysfunction 481
    ejection fraction 207
    fractional shortening 207
Leg ulcers 361
Leigh's disease 193
Lemierre syndrome 130
Lennox-Gastaut syndrome 177, 178*f*
Lentiviral vector 367
Leptospirosis 189
Lethargy 5

Leukemia 406, 442
    acute megakaryoblastic 442
    acute myeloid 403
    lymphoblastic 401
    mixed-lineage 399, 400, 402
Leukemic blasts 399
Leukocyte adhesion deficiency 74
Leukoencephalopathy, progressive multifocal 147
Leukotriene 139, 226, 484
    receptor antagonists 227
Levosalbutamol 226
Levothyroxine 427
    therapy 424
Light-emitting diode 9-11
    microscopy 93
Line probe assay 98, 107
Linear serpiginous ulcers 252f
Linezolid 94, 95
Lipid peroxidation 509
Lipoarabinomannan 101
Lipopolysaccharide-responsive beige-like anchor 76
Liposaccharides encounter
    macrophage 43
    monocyte 43
Liquid chromatography-tandem mass spectrometry 47
Lisinopril 209
Liver
    cell injury 517
    disease 281
        chronic 272
        decompensated 272
        end-stage 268f, 269
    failure
        acute 269, 270, 287
        acute-on-chronic 269, 274
    function test 190, 206, 291
    iron concentration 350
    transplantation 284b, 287, 287b, 288, 295, 296
    evolution of 282
Living donor liver transplant 283, 287
Loha bhasma 371
Long-acting beta-2 agonists 226, 228
Loop diuretics 210
Lopinavir 148
Low-dose norepinephrine, use of 490
Lucinactant 20
Lumbar puncture 188
Lung
    attack, acute 235
    collapse, secretion-induced 493
    compliance 480, 492
        monitoring 500
    disease, chronic 18, 481
    endothelial injury 484
    function 487
        tests 221
    injury 18
        acute 480, 514, 523
        direct 483
        indirect 483
        score 500
        ventilator-induced 480
        protective conventional ventilation group 493
    volumes, dynamic 221
Lymph node 104
    tuberculosis 105
Lymphadenitis, mycobacterial 105
Lymphohistiocytosis, hemophagocytic 79
Lymphoma 400t
    acute lymphoblastic 401b

M

Macrophage 43, 73
    manipulation therapy, role of 368
Magnesium sulfate 16
    therapy 16
Magnetic resonance cholangiopancreatography 292
Magnetic resonance imaging 90, 92, 158, 191, 207, 350
    cardiac 205
Major histocompatibility complex 76, 410
Malabsorption syndromes 373
Malaria, prevention of 393
Malformations, arteriovenous 184
Mallampati score 134, 134f
Malperfusion 200
Mandura bhasma 371
Maple syrup urine disease 284, 286
Marburg virus disease 164, 196
Matrix metalloproteinases 486
Mean airway pressure 481, 493
Mean cell
    hemoglobin 347
        concentration 347
    volume 347
Mean corpuscular
    hemoglobin 377, 379
    volume 377, 379
Mean platelet volume 85
Measles
    containing vaccine 59
    mumps, and rubella 59, 64, 68
    vaccines 68
Mechanical ventilation 26, 480
Meckel's diverticulum 373
Mediastinal adenopathy 91
Medical therapy 208
Medicinal iron therapy 383
Medium-chain triglyceride 288
Megacystis-megaureter association 332

Melanin, intraepidermal retention of 159
Membranes, preterm premature rupture
    of 16
Mendelian susceptibility 81
Meningitis 191
    tuberculous 106, 191
Meningococcal vaccine 64
Meningococcemia 189
Meningococcus infection 73
Meningoencephalitis 159
    tuberculous 185
Mental
    disorders 458
    status 115
Mercaptopurine 404
Meropenem 312
Mesenchymal stem cells, role of 486
Messenger ribonucleic acid 128
Metabolic disorders 286
Metabolic syndrome 45, 134
Metal phosphides 508
Metformin 366
Methemoglobinemia 513
Methotrexate 404
    high-dose 404
Methylmalonic academia 284
Metolazone 210, 211
Metoprolol 210
Microbial infection 128
Microneutralization assay 119
Micropenis 426, 432
Microscopy, field of 93
Microthrombosis 486
Micturating cystourethrogram 314, 328, 330*f*
Middle east respiratory syndrome
        coronavirus 157, 197
Midfacial defects 432
Mid-stream urine sample 306
Milrinone 211
Minimal residual disease 398, 400
    monitoring 403
Moisture 509
Molecular genetics 342
Molecular methods 95, 97, 103
    newer 99
Mometasone 226
    furoate 140
Monocytes 73
    via cathelicidin 43
Mononuclear cells 38
Monosegment liver transplantation 289
Monotherapy
    effective 150
    initiation of 146
Montelukast
    role of 139
    therapy 139

Mother-to-child transmission 150, 274
    prevention of 150
Motility, defects of 80
Mouth breathing 132
Mucopolysaccharidoses 136
Mucosal cell control 375
Multi-allergen immunoglobulin E antibody
        screening assays 243
Multicystic dysplastic kidneys 332
Multifocal discrete lesions 158
Multiorgan dysfunction 410
    syndrome 483, 517
Muzaffarpur encephalopathy 195
Mycobacteria 73
Mycobacterial disease 81
Mycobacterial growth indicator tube 94, 107
Mycobacterium
    avium complex 147
    tuberculosis 43, 95, 97, 186, 194
        genomes 101
        identification of 95
Mycophenolate, antimetabolites 295
Myelination 417
Myelitis, acute flaccid 162
Myelodysplasia 78
Myelodysplastic syndrome 442
Myelosuppression 405
Myocarditis 511
Myopathy 498
Myopia, transient 158

N

N-acetylcysteine 514, 517
Naked-eye single tube red cell osmotic
        fragility test 347
Nasal
    cannula, high-flow 488
    high-flow therapy 25
    intermittent positive pressure ventilation
        25
    swab 115, 116
Nasopharyngeal aspirates 115
Nasopharyngeal swab 115, 116
National AIDS control organization 144
National Cancer Institute 399, 400
National Centre for Disease Control 164
National Immunization Program 58
National Immunization Schedule 58, 60*t*
National Institute for Health and Care
        Excellence 183, 222, 473
National Institute of Mental Health 464
National Institute of Standards and
        Technology 48
National Institute of Virology 164
National Nutrition Survey, comprehensive 40
National Nutritional Anemia Control Program
        386
National Poisons Information Centre 508

National representative population,
    population-based health survey
    of 39
National Screening Programs 422
Natriuresis 209, 213
Natriuretic peptides 202, 203, 206
Natural killer cells 73
Near infrared spectroscopy 29
Necessitates invasive methods 108
Necrotic mediastinal nodes 91
Neisseria 73
    meningitis 82
Neonatal intensive care unit 16, 426
Neonatal jaundice
    diagnosis of 8*fc*
    management of 8*fc*
Neonatal oxygenation prospective
    meta-analysis 28
Neonatology 1
Nephrology 303
Neprilysin 203, 213
    inhibitor 213
Neurally adjusted ventilator assist 25, 27
Neuraminidase 163
Neurologic failure 483
Neuromuscular blocking agents 480
    usage of 498
Neurotoxicity 4, 409
Neutrally adjusted ventilation assist 480
Neutropenia
    congenital 80
    severe congenital 74
Neutrophil 43, 74
    extracellular traps 485
    function tests 85
Nevirapine 146, 148
    prophylaxis 152*t*
New viral infections 155
New York Heart Association 205*t*
Newborn screening 416, 421
Nipah virus 157, 193
    encephalitis 194
Nitric oxide 246
    inhaled 490, 494
Nitroblue tetrazolium reduction test 85
Nitrofurantoin 320
Nocturnal pulse oximetry 136
Nodules, endobronchial 91
Noninvasive methods, newer 350
Noninvasive positive-pressure ventilation
    short trial of 490
    use of 488
Noninvasive prenatal screening 444, 453
Noninvasive ventilation 24, 487, 488
    modes of 488
Non-nucleoside reverse transcriptase
    inhibitors 145
Nonsteroidal anti-inflammatory drugs 159

Nonsuicidal self-injury 465, 466
Nontuberculous mycobacteria 93
Norepinephrine 513
Nosocomial infections 165
Nosocomial transmission 157
Nuclear
    cystogram 330
    factor-kappa-B essential modifier 76
    scan 331*f*
Nucleic acid amplification
    assays 117
    test 117
        packed cell transfusion 354
Nucleic acid test 144
Nucleoside analogs 276
    reverse transcriptase inhibitors 145
Nucleotide analog 270
    reverse transcriptase inhibitors 145
Nutrition 37, 498
Nutritional rickets 49*t*
    diagnosis of 46
    management of 50
    overall incidence of 38
    prevention of 50
    treatment of 48
Nyctereutes procyonoides 156

O

Obesity 137, 233
Obstructive sleep
    apnea 130, 139, 141
        syndrome 131
    disordered breathing 130, 133, 134, 139
        spectrum of 131
    hypopneas 130
Ofatumumab 407
Ofloxacin 310
Oligohydramnios 321
Olprinone 211
Opportunistic infections 152
    diagnosis of 145
    treatment of 145
Optic nerves 4
Oral polio vaccine 60, 84
    bivalent 59
    efficacy of 65
Organ dysfunctions, periodic tests for 351
Organophosphates 508
Oropharyngeal aspirates 115
Oropharyngeal swab 115
Orthomyxoviridae 163
Orthopnea 204
Oscillatory ventilation, high-frequency 27,
        492, 493, 496
Oseltamivir 121, 163
    therapy, initiation of 121
Osteoid mineralization, abnormal 38

Index

Osteopenia 361, 362*f*
Osteoporosis 361, 362*f*
Otitis media 84, 133
    recurrent 133
Oversedation, complications of 497
Oxidative burst 85
Oxygen
    consumption, nonradiometric detection of 94
    dissolved, partial pressure of 496
    saturation 120, 208
        index 481-483
    target after stabilization 28
    therapy 120, 121
Oxygenation 488
    and ventilation parameters and severity scores 500
    index 480-482

P

Packed cell volume 7
Packed red blood cell 383
Paguma larvata 156
Pain, abdominal 204
Pallor 5
Palpitation 204
Panayiotopoulos syndrome 172
Pancreas, beta cells of 38
Pandu roga 371
Paper electrophoresis 348*f*
Papilledema 189
Para-aminosalicylic acid 95
Paradigm shift 130
Paradise criteria 129
Parainfluenza 191
Parasuicides 458
Parathyroid hormone 351
    secretion of 41
Parenchyma 315
Parenteral nutrition, total 284
Parent-to-child transmission
    prevention of 150
    recent protocol of prevention of 153
Partial thromboplastin time 206
Patchy restless sleep 131
Patent ductus arteriosus 24, 202
Paucibacillary disease 97
Peak pressures 491
Pedal edema 204
Pediatric Acute Lung Injury Consensus Conference 480, 501
    conference guidelines 482, 496
    recommends against corticosteroids 497
Pediatric acute respiratory distress syndrome 480, 481*t*, 482, 482*t*
    management of 495
    moderate-to-severe 495
    severity of 501
    survivors of 501
    treatment of 480
Pediatric
    Acute Liver Failure 285
    advanced life support 207
    allergic diseases 242
    cardiac transplant 216
    Crohn's disease activity index 253, 258
    Endocrine Society 50
    epilepsy syndrome, common 171
    heart failure 204
    intensive care unit 480, 495*f*, 513
    liver transplantation 282
    obstructive sleep apnea, initial cases of 126
    pulmonary tuberculosis, treatment of 105
    sleep questionnaire 136, 137
    tuberculosis 103, 106
        diagnosis of 90
    ulcerative colitis 257
        activity index 253
Pelvis, renal 329
Pelviureteric junction obstruction 331
Percussive ventilation, high-frequency 493
Pericardial fluid, analysis of 106
Periodic lateralized epileptiform discharges 194
Peripheral blood mononuclear cells 144
Peripheral capillary oxygen saturation 482
Peritonitis, spontaneous bacterial 285
Phagocyte immunodeficiency disorders 87
Phagocytic cell defects 86
Phagocytosis 85
Phagosomes, mycobacterial 43
Pharmacokinetic booster 146
Pharyngitis 130
Pharyngotonsillitis, episodes of 129
Phenobarbitone 12
Phenotypic susceptibility testing 95
Phenylketonuria 421
Phosphine 509
    gas 510
    poisoning, management of 514*fc*
Phosphodiesterase 211
Phosphorus 46
    elemental 522
    white elemental 515
    yellow 507
        elemental 515
Phototherapy 9, 10, 11*t*, 13
    devices 9*t*
    supportive care during 10*t*
Ping pong spread 130
Plasma protein A, pregnancy-associated 453
Plasminogen activator inhibitor 486
Plasmodium falciparum malaria 393
Plateau pressure 487, 491
Platynychia 378

Plethora 5
Pleural effusion 105, 204, 205
Pneumococcal conjugate vaccine 60, 64
Pneumocystis
　carinii 86
　　infection 292
　jirovecii 77, 143
　　prevention of 152
Pneumonia 113, 483
　extensive 120
　severe 120
Polio vaccine 59, 65, 66
　injectable 59, 64
Polyarteritis nodosa 269
Polyethylene glycol 404
Polymerase chain reaction 95, 97, 144, 194, 195, 274, 404
　systems, multiplex 117
　test, timing of 144
Polymorphonuclear leukocytes 190
Polyneuropathy 498
Polysomnography 136
Polytetrafluoroethylene 333
Polyuria 432
Portable digital fluorescent microscope 94
Portal vein thrombosis 291
Positive end-expiratory pressure 491
　use of 481
Positive pressure ventilation 22
Positron emission tomography 90
　scan 92, 500
Post-adenotonsillectomy 139
Postexposure prophylaxis 69, 275
Postextubation respiratory support 488
Post-liver transplant 281
Post-transplant lymphoproliferative disorder 293
Povidone-iodine 426
Pregnancy, medical termination of 369
Preoxygenation 490
　current methods of 489
Pressure support mode 27
Pressurized metered dose inhalers 228, 229
Preterm labor 304
Prick-to-prick test 244
Primary immunodeficiency disorders 73
　treatment of 86
Prohormone 38
Prophylaxis 318, 320
Propionic academia 284
Protease inhibitors 146
Protein
　interacting protein 77
　rich fluid, accumulation of 484
　surface 19
Proteinuria 328

Prothrombin
　complex concentrate 521
　time 520
Prune-Belly syndrome 332
Pseudomonas aeruginosa 81
Psoriasis 45
Psychiatric disorders 464
Psychodynamic therapy 472
Psychopharmacology 472
Psychosis 516
Psychotherapy 472
Public health interventions 165
Pulmonary artery 202
　wedge pressure 514
Pulmonary capillary wedge pressure, removal of 481
Pulmonary tuberculosis 104
　diagnosis of 104*fc*, 105, 106
Pulmonary vein stenosis 201
Puumala virus 158
Pyelograms 314
Pyoderma gangrenosum, acne syndrome 82
Pyrazinamidase enzyme
　absence of 95
　presence of 95
Pyrexia of unknown origin 92
Pyridoxal isonicotinoyl hydrazone 358
Pyrosequencing data 100

Q

Quadrivalent
　formulation 163
　vaccines 123
Quantitative fluorescent polymerase chain reaction 444
Quantitative insulin-sensitivity check index 45
Quinolones 94, 310
　newer-generation 107
　susceptibility testing of 95

R

Rabies
　human monoclonal antibody 70
　vaccine 59, 69
Raccoon dogs 156
Radio-allergosorbent test 243
Radioimmunoassay 47, 380, 421
Radiology 90, 91
Radiotracer 331
Ramipril 209
Randomized control trial 16, 45, 494
Rapamycin
　inhibitors sirolimus, mammalian target of 295
　mammalian target of 295
Rapid influenza diagnostic tests 117, 118

Rapid molecular assays 117, 118
Rattus norvegicus 506
Rattus rattus 506
Reactive oxygen species 485
Red blood
    cell 2, 342, 375
        distribution width 377, 379
        distribution width 347, 380
        indices 379
        lysis 376
        size distribution 380
Reflux 334
    bilateral high-grade 330*f*
    grade, lower 327
    high-grade 335
    intrarenal 326
    nephropathy 328, 330
    nonresolving persistent high-grade 333
Regurgitation, pulmonary 202
Renal disease, end-stage 327
Renal dysplasia 320
Renal failure 410
    acute 516
Renal function tests 190, 206
Renal syndrome 158
Renin-angiotensin-aldosterone system 202, 203
Respiratory
    burst, defects of 80
    disease, chronic 114
    distress 120, 205
        syndrome 16
    failure
        acute 120
        severe 495, 496
    infections, acute lower 68
    rate 120, 489, 501
    syncytial virus 191
    syndrome coronavirus 155
    system, static compliance of 487
    tract infection, lower 113, 115, 120
    virus 143
        encephalitis 191
Restless patchy sleep 132
Reticulocyte
    count 7, 347, 381
    hemoglobin content 381
Retinoid X receptor 43
Reverse transcriptase polymerase chain
        reaction 117, 158
    assay, real time 117
Revised National Tuberculosis Control
        Program 93, 104
Reye's encephalopathy 193
Rhinitis, allergic 233, 244
Rhythm 205
Ribavirin 359
    role of 158

Ribonucleic acid
    double-stranded 155
    single-stranded 155
Rickets, prevention of 50
Rickettsia rickettsii 194
Rifampicin 95, 97, 109
    resistance 96, 99
        diagnosis of 96
        false-positive cases of 108
        tuberculosis cases, annual incidence of 90
Rift valley fever 164, 197
Ritonavir 148
Rituximab 407
Rodenticides 506, 521, 522*t*, 523
    antidote 522*t*
    poisoning 506, 508*f*
    signs 522*t*
    symptoms 522*t*
Ross classification of heart failure, modified 205*t*
Rotavirus 64
    gastroenteritis events 66
    vaccine 59, 66, 67
        monovalent 59

S

Sacubitril 213
Salbutamol 226
Saline
    hypertonic 92
    routine instillation of 495
Salmonella typhi 67, 360
Schwartz formula 321, 322
Sclerosis, multiple 45
Seasonal influenza
    A virus 118
    B virus 118
    epidemics 113
    viruses, types of 112
Seasonal viruses 113
Second-generation line probe assay 98, 107
Sedation and neuromuscular blockade 497
Seizure
    hypocalcemic 44
    triad of 176*f*
    type 170
Seoul virus 158
Serum soluble transferrin receptor 381
Servo-controlled oxygen delivery 28
Severe acute respiratory distress syndrome 499*f*
Severe acute respiratory syndrome 197
    coronavirus 155
Shock
    causes of 490
    intractable 509
Short-acting beta-2 agonists 226

Shwachman-Diamond syndrome 80
Silicone 333
Sin Nombre virus 158
Sinapultide 20
Single-chain variable fragment 409
Single-photon emission computed
    tomography 331
Sinusitis 84
Skin tests 245
Sleep
    apnea study, assessment of 133
    clinical record 137
    disordered breathing 126, 135, 137, 138
Smoking stool syndrome 516
Society for Adolescent Medicine 467
Sodium
    fluoroacetamide 523
    hypochlorite microscopy 93
    iodine symporter 416
    monofluoroacetate 522
    potassium adenosine triphosphatase 211
Spirometry 221-223
Spironolactone 210
Splenectomy 360
Splenium, hyperintensity of 193*f*
Spondylitis, ankylosing 252
Sprinkles 387
Staphylococcus aureus 73, 81
Stem cell
    multipotent mesenchymal 486
    transplant 364
Stenosis, pulmonary 201, 202
Steroid 497
    therapy 140
Stillbirths 446
Stimuli 220
Stomach 510
Stomatitis, angular 378
Streptococcus pneumoniae 79, 81
Stridor 44
Stroke, arterial ischemic 192*f*
Substance abuse 458, 464
Sudden cardiac death 204
Suicidal attempt, treatment of 470
Suicidal behaviour
    acute management of 470
    guidelines 474
    management of 468
Suicide 458, 462*t*
    attempts 458
    causes of 458, 459
    impulsive 461
    prevention of 458, 466, 467, 473
    risk 465
        factors for 461
Sulfamethoxazole 333
Sunlight exposure, role of 50

Superconducting quantum interference
    device 350
Superoxide dismutase 509
Supportive therapy 120, 450
Suprapubic aspirate 307
Surgery, cardiac 204
Sympathetic nervous system 201, 203
Sympathomimetic amines 211
Synchondrosis, sphenobasioccipital 135*f*
Syncope 204
Systemic inflammatory response syndrome
    483
Systemic lupus erythematosus 45, 76, 82
Systemic vascular resistance 206

T

Tachycardia 200
    ventricular 523
Tacrolimus 295
    monotherapy 298
Tandem mass spectrometry 421
T-cell
    defects, regulatory 80
    precursor acute lymphoblastic leukemia,
        early 403
    receptor 73
Teflon 333
Telangiectasia, hemorrhagic 373
Tenofovir 148, 151
    alafenamide 145
    disoproxil fumerate 145
Terizidone susceptibility testing 95
Thalamic basal ganglia 192*f*
Thalassemia 340, 346*f*, 351*t*, 352, 359
    intermedia 345
    major 343*f*, 345
        inheritance of 343*f*
        management of 351, 352*t*
    minor 347, 349*f*
    nontransfusion dependent 343, 345, 346*f*,
        357
    prenatal diagnosis of 369
    prevention of 369
    syndromes 340, 345
    transfusion dependent 343, 345, 346*f*
Thalidomide 366
Thallium 522
Thiazides 210
Throat
    infections, recurrent 129
    swab 115, 116
Thrombocytopenia 261
    congenital 77
    syndrome 164, 197
Thrombomodulin 484
Thrombophlebitis 130
Thrombosis 486
Thymic defects 77

Thyroglobulin 426
Thyroid
  binding globulin 417
  development 416
  dysgenesis 418
  dyshormonogenesis 418
  follicular cells 418
  function tests 206
  hormone 418
    receptor 420*b*
  peroxidase 419
  stimulating hormone 351, 363, 417, 418
Thyrotropin releasing hormone 416
Tidal volume 491
Tisagenlecleucel 410
T-lymphocytes 43
Tonic-clonic seizures
  generalized 174, 175, 183
  myoclonic 174
Tonsillar hypertrophy 134*f*
Tonsillar infections, recurrent 128, 141
Tonsillectomy 125, 141
Tonsillitis, recurrent 128
Tonsillopharyngitis
  favorable natural history of 129
  natural history of recurrent 129
Tonsils 127
Topiramate 178
Total anomalous pulmonary venous
    connection 202
Total iron binding capacity 349, 377, 379, 380
Total serum bilirubin 5, 7*b*, 11, 13
Toxic shock syndrome 114
Toxicity
  cardiac 516
  clinical manifestations of 517
  mechanism of 509
  renal 516
Tracheal aspirates 115, 116
Tracheal suctioning 495
Transcutaneous ventricular assist device 215
Transferrin saturation 348, 379, 380
Transfusion
  therapy 352, 353*t*
    initiation of 353
    management of complications of 354
  transmitted infections 359
Transient drop, sedation-induced 490
Transient myeloproliferative disorder 442
Traumatic brain injury, severe 28
Trial off therapy 428
Tricuspid regurgitation 202
Triiodothyronine 416
Trimethoprim 320, 333
Trisomy 21 440*f*, 443*b*, 445*f*
Trivalent oral polio vaccine 65
Tuberculin skin test 101
Tuberculomas 92

Tuberculosis 58, 90, 143, 153, 195, 260*t*
  abdominal 106
  diagnosis of 90, 91, 95, 96, 99, 101, 108
  disease, diagnosis of 91
  drug resistant 100, 107, 107*fc*
  histopathological feature of 90
  meningitis 189
    diagnosis of 92
  pericardial 106
  polymerase chain reaction 190, 260
  risk of developing 153
Tubular necrosis, acute 516
Tumor necrosis factor 81, 410, 484, 485
Typhoid
  conjugate vaccine 64, 67
  vaccine 59, 67
Tyrosine kinase 402
  inhibitors 402

U

Ulcerative colitis 250, 251*t*, 252*f*, 254, 256, 257
  management of 257*fc*
Ulcers, superficial 252*f*
Ultrasonography 90, 91, 445
Ultrasound 314, 500
Ultraviolet B rays 50
Umbilical cord clamping 17
United States Agency for International
    Development 144
Upper airway resistance syndrome 131
Upper gastrointestinal
  endoscopy 253
  tract 254
Upper respiratory tract infections 83
Ureter
  intramural 325
  submucosal 325
  ultrasonography of 329
Ureteral hiatus 326*f*
Ureterovesical junction 324, 325
  normal 325*f*
  refluxing 325*f*
Urethral valves, posterior 318
Urinary tract
  dysfunction, lower 333
  infection 304, 310*t*, 311*t*, 324, 334
    documentation of 329
    radiological tests for 314*t*
  symptoms, lower 328
Urine
  output 115
  protein 321
  specimen 329

V

Vaccine 165
  composition 163
  preventable diseases 153

production purposes 117
strains 123
Valproate 178
Valsartan 213
Varicella
  encephalopathy 189
  zoster virus 195
Vascular injury, pulmonary 486
Vasculitis 189
Vasodilation, pulmonary 494
Vasopressin 513
Vedolizumab 256
Vein, internal jugular 130
Venoarterial extracorporeal membrane oxygenation 496
Ventilation
  high-frequency 480, 493
  index 500
  invasive 489
  modes of 490
  nonconventional 480, 492
  perfusion 494
  volume-targeted 26
Ventricular
  assist device 207, 215
  fibrillation 511, 523
  septal defect 202
Vesicoureteral reflux 318, 319, 324, 326, 328, 331, 332, 336
  grades of 327*f*
  natural history of 327
  management of 334, 335
Vigabatrin 175
Vincristine 403
Violence 458
Viral replication, inhibition of 121
Viral upper respiratory infections 128
Virion, release of 163
Virus
  emergence, different stages of 155
  isolation 117, 118
  neutralization tests 119
  nucleoprotein 119
  transmission of 265
Vital fluorescent staining 93
Vitamin
  B12, defects of 78
  C, role of 356
  D 44*t*
    assay 47
    content, low 43
    deficiency of 38, 39, 40*t*, 41*t*, 44, 50
    extraskeletal role of 52
    intramuscular injection of 48
    metabolism 42*f*
    physiology of 41
  receptor 38, 42
  response element 42, 43
  role of 38
  serves 38
  status 38, 39, 47*t*
  supplementation, beneficial effect of 45
  treatment doses of 49*t*
  D2 binding protein 42
  K 521
    antagonists 518
Volatile organic compounds 224, 225
Volutrauma 487
Vomiting 5, 204

W

Waldeyer's sheath 326*f*
Weaning 501
West syndrome 175
  triad of 177*f*
West-Nile virus disease 189
Wheeze 220
  recurrent 133
White blood cell 345, 399
Whole-cell pertussis vaccine 64
Wiskott-Aldrich syndrome 77, 85, 260
World Federation for Mental Health 474
World Health Organization 64, 93, 147, 148*t*, 401*b*, 461
World Suicide Prevention Day 474
Wormian bones 420

X

X-linked agammaglobulinemia 74
Xpert *Mycobacterium tuberculosis* 99

Y

Yersinia enterocolitica 360

Z

Zanamivir 163
Zellweger syndrome 446
Zidovudine 145, 147, 148
Ziehl-Neelsen
  microscopy, future of 94
  staining 93
Zika
  disease 164
  infection, treatment of 160
  virus 159
Zinc
  finger nucleases 367
  phosphide 507, 508, 514, 522
  protoporphyrin 381
Zoonotic diseases, incidence of 155
Zoster encephalitis 191, 192*f*

EU GSPR Authorised Reprsentative
Logos Europe, 9 rue Nicolas Poussin
1700, La Rochelle, France
Phone: +33 (0) 6 67 93 73 78
E-mail: contact@logoseurope.eu

www.ingramcontent.com/pod-product-compliance
Ingram Content Group UK Ltd.
Pitfield, Milton Keynes, MK11 3LW, UK
UKHW050427150426
5217IPUK00019B/1276